Applied Pharmacology for Veterinary Technicians

Fifth Edition

Boyce P. Wanamaker, DVM, MS
Director (Retired)
Veterinary Technology Program
Columbia State Community College
Columbia, Tennessee

Kathy Lockett Massey, LVMT
Veterinary Technology Department
Columbia State Community College
Columbia, Tennessee

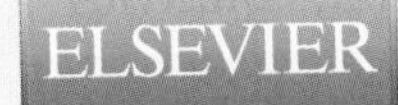

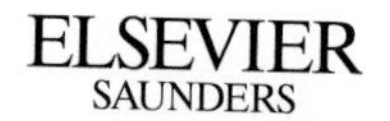

3251 Riverport Lane
St. Louis, Missouri 63043

APPLIED PHARMACOLOGY FOR VETERINARY TECHNICIANS, FIFTH EDITION ISBN: 978-0-323-18662-9

Notices

Knowledge and best practice in this field are constantly changing. As new research and experience broaden our understanding, changes in research methods, professional practices, or medical treatment may become necessary.

Practitioners and researchers must always rely on their own experience and knowledge in evaluating and using any information, methods, compounds, or experiments described herein. In using such information or methods they should be mindful of their own safety and the safety of others, including parties for whom they have a professional responsibility.

With respect to any drug or pharmaceutical products identified, readers are advised to check the most current information provided (i) on procedures featured or (ii) by the manufacturer of each product to be administered, to verify the recommended dose or formula, the method and duration of administration, and contraindications. It is the responsibility of practitioners, relying on their own experience and knowledge of their patients, to make diagnoses, to determine dosages and the best treatment for each individual patient, and to take all appropriate safety precautions.

To the fullest extent of the law, neither the Publisher nor the authors, contributors, or editors, assume any liability for any injury and/or damage to persons or property as a matter of products liability, negligence or otherwise, or from any use or operation of any methods, products, instructions, or ideas contained in the material herein.

ISBN: 978-0-323-18662-9

Library of Congress Cataloging-in-Publication Data
Wanamaker, Boyce P., author.
Applied pharmacology for veterinary technicians/Boyce P. Wanamaker, Kathy Lockett Massey. – Fifth edition.
p. ; cm.
Includes bibliographical references and index.
ISBN 978-0-323-18662-9 (pbk. : alk. paper)
I. Massey, Kathy Lockett, author. II. Title.
[DNLM: 1. Drug Therapy–veterinary. 2. Animal Technicians. 3. Pharmacology. 4. Veterinary Medicine.
SF 915]
SF915
636.08951—dc23

2014001951

Vice President and Publisher: Linda Duncan
Content Strategy Director: Penny Rudolph
Content Manager: Shelly Stringer
Publishing Services Manager: Catherine Jackson
Senior Project Manager: Mary Pohlman
Design Direction: Amy Buxton

Printed in Canada.
Last digit is the print number: 9 8 7 6 5 4

This edition is dedicated to
that sense of awe, wonder, and mystery
for nature and the animal kingdom
that inspires us to pursue careers in veterinary medicine
and to recognize the interdependency
of all living things.

B.W.

Thanks to God for the loving miracle of my parents,
Harry and Bettie Lockett, who chose me to share their lives with.

To my children, Eric and Darla, you are the light of my life.
Try to give back to the world more than you take.

To Dr. Wanamaker for his patience.

To Dr. Frankie Locklar for teaching me about tolerance and other life lessons.

To all the technicians and students I've worked with, don't ever forget that we are not just helping animals, but people too. If an animal can make a person laugh, our job may have a twofold purpose.

Perhaps mirth is the epitome of human health.

K.M.

Preface

Applied Pharmacology for Veterinary Technicians, Fifth Edition, is designed for both the graduate technician and the student. As a teaching and reference book, its purpose is to help veterinary technicians become familiar with the many veterinary pharmacologic agents and their uses, adverse side effects, and dosage forms. We believe it is very important for the technician to understand the uses of pharmacologic agents and to have the ability to provide client education under the supervision of the attending veterinarian. One of the key features of this book is that its format provides quick and easy access to important chapter content. Each chapter is introduced with learning objectives, a chapter outline, and key terms. "Technician's Notes" throughout the text provide helpful hints and important points technicians should be aware of to avoid errors and increase efficiency.

NEW TO THIS EDITION

New features have been added to the fifth edition to aid the student and technician in the study and application of pharmacology. All of the drug information throughout the book has been updated and new drugs that have entered the market since the publication of the fourth edition have been included to keep you current with the newest pharmacologic agents and their uses, adverse side effects, and dosage forms. Scientific advances in the area of stem cell treatment have been added to the chapter on immunologic drugs. Coverage of fluid therapy has been expanded to prepare veterinary technicians for the role they play in fluid, electrolyte, and therapeutic nutritional therapy, which can be critically important to the outcome of a case. The fifth edition is now in color, bringing important concepts to life.

EVOLVE SITE

The Evolve student resources offer the following features to reinforce textbook content and help students master key concepts:

- **Drug Administration Videos:** Twelve narrated video clips demonstrate drug administration techniques (oral, injectable, inhaled) and IV preparation for dogs and cats
- **Drug Calculators with Related Exercises:** Six drug calculators with accompanying word problems help students perform accurate drug calculations
- **Drug Label Image Collection:** Over 135 photos of drug labels, divided by chapters and organized alphabetically, help students become familiar with drug information and packaging encountered in practice
- **Animations:** Animations of pharmacologic processes, such as passive diffusion and receptor interaction, help students visualize and understand key concepts
- **Dosage Calculation Exercises:** Exercises reinforce calculations skills and provide valuable practice in the areas of:
  - Drug Calculation Methods
  - Oral and Enteral Medication Administration
  - Intravenous Infusion
  - Critical Care Calculations
- **Answers to Review Questions:** Answers to the chapter review questions allow students to gauge comprehension of key topics

Our intent in writing this book has been to combine the comprehensiveness of a veterinary pharmacology textbook with the coverage of pharmacologic fundamentals needed by veterinary technicians. No longer will veterinary technician educators have to draw from two sources for this type of coverage. The scope and organization of the information in this book will make it a useful reference for the practicing technician as well.

Boyce P. Wanamaker, DVM, MS
Kathy Lockett Massey, LVMT

Acknowledgments

I would like to acknowledge the editors and staff at Elsevier including Mary Pohlman and Shelly Stringer for their support and assistance in making this edition possible.

I would also like to recognize veterinary technicians and veterinary technology students everywhere whose desire for knowledge and dedication to quality animal care have made animal nursing a true profession.

I would like to thank Columbia State Community College for the opportunities it has provided me.

I would like to acknowledge the following people who have influenced my professional career in a positive way: Charles Byles, DVM; Charles Chamberlain, PhD; Karon Jennings, DVM; Mary Kirby, LVMT; Walter Martin, DVM; Kathy Massey, LVMT; G.M. Merriman, DVM; Christy Pettes, MD; H.B. Smith, DVM; Duane Tallman, DVM; and Dale Thomas, MS.

Boyce P. Wanamaker

I would like to thank: Boyce Wanamaker, DVM, Columbia State Community College, Columbia, Tennesse; Mary Kirby, LVMT, Columbia State Community College, Columbia, Tennessee; Bill Henson, DVM, Henson Animal Clinic, Corinth, Mississippi; Jim Jackson, DVM, Jackson Animal Clinic, Corinth, Mississippi; Forrest Cutlip, DVM, Milan Animal Hospital, Milan, Tennessee; C.F. Locklar, Jr., DVM, Maury County Veterinary Hospital, Columbia, Tennessee; Steve Grubbs, DVM, PhD, Princeton, New Jersey; Robert Myers, DVM, Maury County Veterinary Hospital, Columbia, Tennessee; Christi Cartwright, LVMT, Maury County Veterinary Hospital, Columbia, Tennessee.

Kathy Lockett Massey

Contents

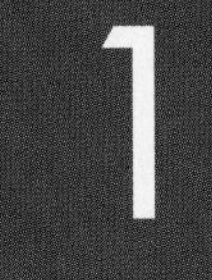

CHAPTER 1

General Pharmacology

OUTLINE

Introduction
Drug Sources
Inactive Ingredients
Pharmacotherapeutics
Pharmacokinetics
- Routes of Administration
- Drug Absorption
- Drug Distribution
- Biotransformation
- Drug Excretion

Pharmacodynamics
Drug Interactions
Drug Names
Drug Labels
Development and Approval of New Drugs
- Regulatory Agencies
- Steps in the Development of a New Drug

Federal Laws Related to Drug Development and Use
- The Animal Medicinal Drug Use Clarification Act
- Compounding of Veterinary Drugs
- The Veterinary Feed Directive
- The Minor Use and Minor Species Animal Health Act

Dispensing Versus Prescribing Drugs
Marketing of Drugs
Disposal of Unwanted Drugs

LEARNING OBJECTIVES

After studying this chapter, you should be able to

1. Define terms related to general pharmacology.
2. List common sources of drugs used in veterinary medicine.
3. Outline the basic principles of pharmacotherapeutics.
4. Define the difference between prescription and over-the-counter drugs.
5. Describe the events that occur after a drug is administered to a patient.
6. List and describe the routes used for administration of drugs.
7. Define *biotransformation,* and list common chemical reactions involved in this process.
8. List the routes of drug excretion.

KEY TERMS

Adverse drug event
Adverse drug reaction
Agonist
Antagonist
Compounding
Drug
Efficacy
Extralabel use
Half-life
Manufacturing
Metabolism (biotransformation)
Parenteral
Partition coefficient
Prescription (legend) drug
Regimen
Residue
Veterinarian–client–patient relationship
Withdrawal time

9. Discuss in basic terms the mechanisms by which drugs produce their effects in the body.
10. Discuss the mechanisms of clinically important drug interactions.
11. Discuss the different names that a particular drug is given.
12. List the items that should be included on a drug label.
13. List the steps and discuss the processes involved in gaining approval for a new drug.
14. List the government agencies involved in the regulation of animal health products.
15. Describe reasons for dispensing rather than prescribing drugs in veterinary medicine.
16. Discuss the primary methods of drug marketing.
17. List acceptable methods of drug disposal.

INTRODUCTION

Veterinary technicians are an essential component of the efficient health care delivery team in veterinary medicine. One of the important tasks that veterinary technicians carry out is administration of **drugs** to animals on the order of a veterinarian. Because this task may have serious consequences in terms of the outcome of a case, it is mandatory that technicians have a thorough knowledge of the types and actions of drugs used in veterinary medicine. They should have an understanding of the reasons for using drugs, called *indications,* and the reasons for not using drugs, called *contraindications* (pharmacotherapeutics). They also should know what happens to drugs once they enter the body (pharmacokinetics), how drugs exert their effects (pharmacodynamics), and how adverse drug reactions manifest themselves (toxicity). Because veterinarians dispense a large number of drugs, technicians also must be well versed in the components of a valid **veterinarian–client–patient relationship,** the importance of proper labeling of dispensed products, and methods of client education on the proper use of products to avoid toxic effects or residue. Finally, technicians should have a basic understanding of the laws that apply to drug use in veterinary medicine and the concept of the marketing of veterinary drugs. In short, veterinary technicians must have a working knowledge of the science of veterinary pharmacology.

DRUG SOURCES

Traditional sources of drugs are plants (botanical) and minerals. Plants have long been a source of drugs. The active components of plants that are useful as drugs include alkaloids, glycosides, gums, resins, and oils. The names of alkaloids usually end in *-ine,* and the names of glycosides end in *-in* (Williams and Baer, 1990). Examples of alkaloids include atropine, caffeine, and nicotine. Digoxin and digitoxin are examples of glycosides. Bacteria and molds (e.g., *Penicillium*) produce many of the antibiotics (penicillin) and anthelmintics (ivermectin) in use today. Animals once were important as a source of hormones such as insulin and as a source of anticoagulants such as heparin. Today, most hormones are synthesized in a laboratory. Mineral sources of drugs include electrolytes (sodium, potassium, and chloride), iron, selenium, and others. Laboratories are one of the most important sources of currently used drugs because chemists are finding methods of reproducing drugs previously obtained through plant and animal sources. Advances in recombinant deoxyribonucleic acid (DNA) technology have made it possible for animal and human products (e.g., insulin) in bacteria to be produced in large quantities.

INACTIVE INGREDIENTS

Veterinary pharmaceutic products and supplements may contain substances in addition to active ingredients. Inactive ingredients are classified as binders, coatings, coloring agents, disintegrants, emulsifiers, fillers, flavorings, flow agents, humectants, preservatives, sweeteners, and thickeners (Table 1-1).

PHARMACOTHERAPEUTICS

Veterinarians are challenged by the task of assessing a patient to determine a diagnosis and arrive at a plan of treatment. If the plan of treatment includes the use of drugs, the veterinarian must choose an appropriate drug and a drug regimen. The drug is selected through the use of one or more broadly defined methods called *diagnostic, empirical,* or *symptomatic.* The diagnostic method involves assessment of a patient, including a history, physical examination, laboratory tests, and other diagnostic procedures, to

TABLE 1-1 Inactive Ingredients

INACTIVE INGREDIENT	FUNCTION	EXAMPLES
Binder	Holds tablet together	Cellulose, lactose, methylcellulose, sorbitol, starch, xylitol, and others
Coating	Protects tablet from breaking, absorbing moisture, and early disintegration	Beeswax, carob extract, methylcellulose, cellulose acetate, acrylic resin, and others
Coloring agents	Provide color and enhance appearance	Yellow No. 5, annatto, caramel color, titanium oxide, FD&C Blue No. 1, FD&C Red No. 3, and others
Disintegrants	Expand when exposed to liquid, allowing tablets and capsules to dissolve and disperse their active ingredients	Cellulose products, crospovidone, sodium starch glycolate, and starch
Emulsifiers	Allow fat-soluble and water-soluble agents to mix so they do not separate	Stearic acid, xanthan gum, lethicin, and vegetable oils
Fillers/diluents	Increase bulk or volume	Calcium carbonate, calcium sulfate, cellulose lactose, mannitol, sorbitol, starch, sucrose, and vegetable oils
Flavor agents	Create a desired taste or mask an undesirable taste	Beeswax, carob extract, glyceryl triacetate, and natural orange
Flow agents	Prevent powders from sticking together	Calcium stearate, glyceryl triacetate, polyethylene glycol, silica, sodium benzoate, and talc
Humectants	Hold moisture in a product	Glycerin, glycerol, glycerol triacetate, and sorbitol
Preservatives	Prevent degradation and extend the shelf life of a product	Citric acid, glycerol, potassium benzoate, sodium benzoate, and others
Sweetening agents	Improve taste	Aspartate, fructose, glycerin, sorbitol, sucrose, and xylitol
Thickening agents	Increase the viscosity of a product	Methylcellulose, povidone, sorbitol, and others

Adapted from ConsumerLab.com: Review article: inactive ingredients in supplements (website). https://www.consumerlab.com/reviews/Inactive_Ingredients_in_Supplements/inactiveingredients. Accessed July 30, 2013.

arrive at a specific diagnosis. Once the diagnosis has been determined, the causative microorganism or altered physiologic state is revealed to allow selection of the appropriate drug. The empirical method calls on the use of practical experience and common sense when the drug choice is made. In other instances, drugs are chosen to treat the symptoms or signs of a disease if a specific diagnosis cannot be determined. In veterinary medicine, the comparative cost of a drug also may be an important consideration in selection of an appropriate drug. Once the drug to be used in treatment has been decided, the next step for the veterinarian is to design the plan for administering the drug. This plan, called a **regimen**, includes details about the following:

- The route of administration
- The total amount to be given (dose)
- How often the drug is to be given (frequency)
- How long the drug will be given (duration)

Every drug has the potential to cause harmful effects if it is given to the wrong patient or according to the wrong regimen. Some medications have greater potential than others for producing harmful outcomes. According to the U.S. Food and Drug Administration (FDA), when a drug has potential toxic effects or must be administered in a way that requires the services of trained personnel, that drug cannot be approved for animal use except when given under the supervision of a veterinarian. In such a case, the drug is classified as a **prescription drug** and must be labeled with the following statement: "Caution: Federal law restricts the use of this drug to use by or on the order of a licensed veterinarian." This statement sometimes is referred to as the *legend,* and the drug is called a *legend (prescription) drug.* Labels that state "For veterinary use only" or "Sold to veterinarians only" do not designate prescription drugs. Technicians should be aware that prescription drugs often have been approved by the FDA for use in specific species or for particular diseases or conditions. Veterinarians have some discretion to use a drug in ways not indicated by the label, if they take responsibility for the outcome of use. Use of a drug in a way not specified by the label is called **extralabel use.**

Federal law and sound medical practices dictate that prescription drugs should not be dispensed indiscriminately. Before prescription drugs are issued or extralabel use is undertaken, a valid veterinarian–client–patient relationship must exist. For this relationship to occur, several conditions must be met. These include but are not limited to the following:

- The veterinarian has assumed responsibility for making clinical judgments about the health of the animal(s) and the need for treatment, and the client has agreed to follow the veterinarian's instructions.
- The veterinarian has sufficient knowledge of the animal(s) to issue a diagnosis. The veterinarian must have seen the animal recently and must be acquainted with its husbandry.
- The veterinarian must be available for follow-up evaluation of the patient.

Drugs that do not have enough potential to be toxic or that do not require administration in special ways do not require the supervision of a veterinarian for administration. These drugs are called *over-the-counter* drugs because they may be purchased without a prescription. Drugs that have the potential for abuse or dependence have been classified as *controlled substances.* Careful records of the inventory and use of these drugs must be maintained, and some of them must be kept in a locked storage area.

When a drug and its regimen have been selected, veterinary technicians often are directed through verbal or written orders to administer the drug. Technicians have several important responsibilities in carrying out these orders:

1. Ensuring that the correct drug is being administered
2. Administering the drug by the correct route and at the correct time
3. Carefully observing the animal's response to the drug
4. Questioning any medication orders that are not clear
5. Creating and affixing labels to medication containers accurately
6. Explaining administration instructions to clients
7. Recording appropriate information in the medical record

Technicians should be aware that even when the correct drug is administered in a correct manner, an unexpected adverse reaction might occur in a patient. All adverse events or reactions should be reported immediately to the veterinarian.

PHARMACOKINETICS

Pharmacokinetics is the complex sequence of events that occurs after a drug is administered to a patient (Figure 1-1). Once a drug has been given, it is available for absorption into the bloodstream and delivery to the site where it will exert its action. After a drug is absorbed, it is distributed to various fluids and tissues in the body. It is not enough, however, for the drug simply to reach the desired area. It also must accumulate in that fluid or tissue at the required concentration to be effective. Because the body immediately begins to break down and excrete the drug, the amount available to the target tissue becomes less and less over time. The veterinarian then must administer the drug repeatedly and at fixed time intervals to maintain the drug at the site of action in the desired concentration. Some drugs are administered at a high dose (loading dose) until an appropriate blood level is reached. Then the dose is reduced to an amount that replaces the amount lost through elimination. Doses of other drugs are at the replacement level throughout the regimen. The point at which drug accumulation equals drug elimination is called the *steady state* or *distribution equilibrium.* This equilibrium represents the state where the amount of drug leaving the plasma for tissue equals the amount of drug leaving the tissue for the plasma. Underdosing leads to less-than-effective levels in tissue, and overdosing may result in toxic levels (Figure 1-2). Drug levels can be measured in blood, urine, cerebrospinal fluid, and other appropriate body fluids to help a veterinarian determine whether an appropriate level has been achieved. This procedure, which is called *therapeutic drug monitoring,* is being used increasingly in

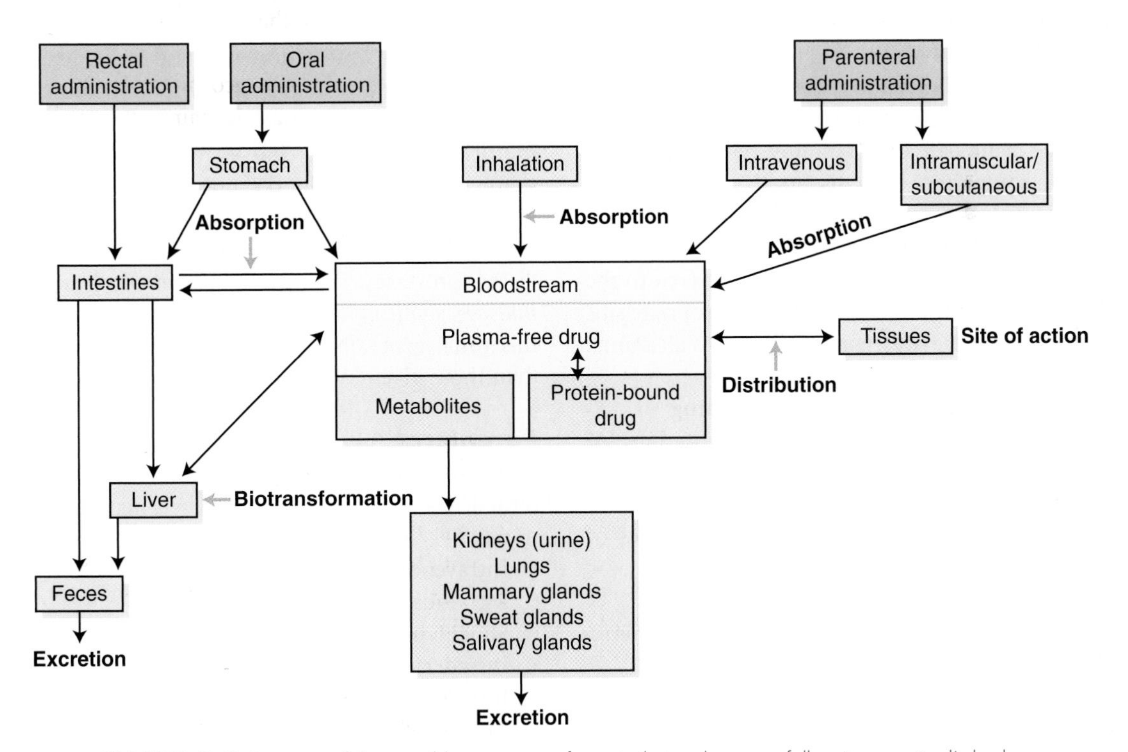

FIGURE 1-1 Diagram of the possible sequence of events that a drug may follow in an animal's body.

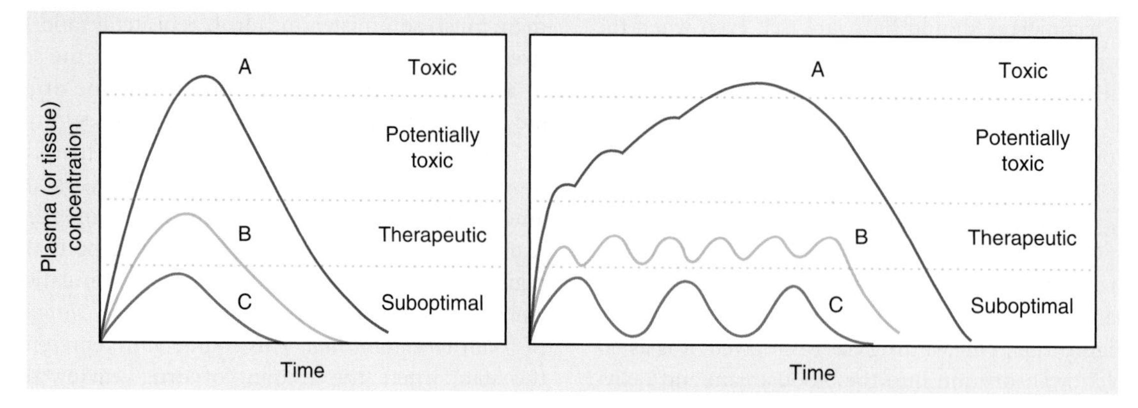

FIGURE 1-2 The effect of dose amounts on the effectiveness of a drug. (From Jenkins WL: Textbook of veterinary internal medicine, diseases of the dog and cat, St. Louis, 1983, WB Saunders.)

veterinary practice. Nonsteroidal antiinflammatory drugs (NSAIDs), cardiac drugs, anticonvulsants, and thyroid drugs are commonly monitored.

The primary factors that influence blood concentration levels of a drug and a patient's response to it include the following:

- Rate of drug absorption
- Amount of drug absorbed
- Distribution of the drug throughout the body
- Drug metabolism or biotransformation
- Rate and route of excretion

These factors are explored after the drug administration routes have been discussed.

Routes of Administration

A drug is of no use unless it can be delivered to the patient in an appropriate form at an appropriate site. The way in which a drug is administered to an animal patient is influenced by several factors:

- Available pharmaceutic form of the drug
- Physical or chemical properties (irritation) of the drug
- How quickly onset of action should occur
- Use of restraint or behavioral characteristics of the patient
- Nature of the condition being treated

The routes of administration of drugs to animal patients are as follows.

Oral

In veterinary medicine, drugs commonly are administered through the oral route. Medications given by this route may be placed directly in the mouth or may be given via a tube passed through the nasal passages (nasogastric tube) or through the mouth (orogastric tube). The mucosa of the digestive tract is a large absorptive surface area with a rich blood supply. Drugs given by this route, however, are not absorbed as quickly as drugs administered by injection, and their effects are subject to species (e.g., ruminants vs. animals with a simple stomach) and individual differences. Many factors may influence the absorption of drugs from the digestive tract, including the pH of the drug, its solubility (fat vs. water), the size and shape of the molecule, the presence or absence of food in the digestive tract, the degree of gastrointestinal (GI) motility, and the presence and nature of disease processes. *This route is not suitable for animals that are vomiting or have diarrhea.* Drugs given by this route generally produce a longer lasting effect than those given by injection.

Parenteral

Drugs that are given by injection are called **parenteral** drugs. A drug can be injected via many different routes:

- Intravenous (IV)
- Intramuscular (IM)
- Subcutaneous (SC)
- Intradermal (ID)
- Intraperitoneal (IP)
- Intraarterial (IA)
- Intraarticular
- Intracardiac

- Intramedullary
- Epidural/subdural

Drugs given by the intravenous route produce the most rapid onset of action, accompanied by the shortest duration. Medications that are irritating to tissue generally are given by this route because of the diluting effect of blood. Intravenous medications should be administered slowly to lessen the possibility of a toxic or allergic reaction. Unless a product is specifically labeled for intravenous use, it should never be given by this route. Oil-based drugs and those with suspended particles (i.e., those that look cloudy or thick) generally should not be given intravenously because of the possibility of an embolism. Special care should be taken to ensure that irritating drugs are injected into the vein and not around it, to avoid causing phlebitis.

The intramuscular route of administration produces a slower onset of action than the intravenous route but usually provides a longer duration of action. The onset of action by this route can be relatively fast with a water-based form (aqueous) and is slower with other diluents (vehicles) such as oil or with other forms such as microfine crystals. When an injectable drug is placed in a substance that delays its absorption, this may be referred to as a *depot* preparation. Altering the molecule of the drug itself can influence its onset or duration of action. Onset of action usually is inversely related to duration of action. Irritating drugs should not be given by the intramuscular route, and back pressure always should be applied to the syringe plunger before intramuscular administration of a drug to ensure that the injection is not directed into a blood vessel.

The subcutaneous route produces a slower onset of action but a slightly longer duration than the intramuscular route. Irritating or hyperosmotic solutions (i.e., those with a greater number of suspended particles than are found in body fluid) should not be given by this route. (See Chapter 15.)

Quantities of medications that are appropriate for the species or individual being treated should be used to prevent possible dissection of the skin from underlying tissue, which could lead to death or loss (sloughing) of surface skin.

The intradermal route involves injecting a drug into the skin. This route is used in veterinary medicine primarily for testing for tuberculosis and allergies.

The intraperitoneal route is used to deliver drugs into the abdominal cavity. The onset and duration of action of drugs given by this route are variable. This route is used to administer fluids, blood, and other medications when normal routes are not available or are not practical. Problems such as adhesions and puncture of abdominal organs may be caused by this method.

The intraarterial route involves injecting a drug directly into an artery. This route seldom is used intentionally, but this may happen by mistake. Administration of drugs into the jugular vein of a horse must be done with caution to avoid injection into the underlying carotid artery. Intracarotid injection results in delivery of a high concentration of the drug directly to the brain, and seizures or death may result.

Through the intraarticular route, a drug is injected directly into a joint. This method is used primarily to treat inflammatory conditions of the joint. Extreme care must be exercised to ensure that sterile technique is used when an intraarticular injection is given. Technicians usually do not use this route.

The intracardiac route is used to inject drugs through the chest wall directly into the chambers of the heart. This provides immediate access to the bloodstream and ensures that the drug is delivered quickly to all tissue in the body. This method is often used in cases of cardiopulmonary resuscitation and in euthanasia.

The intramedullary route is another route that is seldom used in veterinary medicine. It involves injection of the substance directly into the bone marrow. The bones used most often are the femur and the humerus. The intramedullary route usually is used to provide blood or fluids to animals with very small or damaged veins or for treatment of animals with very low blood pressure.

When spinal anesthesia is provided, drugs may be injected into the epidural or subdural space. The epidural space is outside the dura mater (meninges) but inside the spinal canal. The subdural space is inside the dura mater. Injection of drugs into the subdural space (cerebrospinal fluid) is also called the *intrathecal route.* A veterinarian usually carries out these methods of drug delivery.

Inhalation

Medications may be delivered to a patient in inspired air by converting a liquid form into a gaseous form through the use of a vaporizer or nebulizer. Examples of drugs that may be given by this route include anesthetics, antibiotics, bronchodilators, and mucolytics.

Topical

Drugs that are administered topically are placed on the skin or on mucous membranes. Drugs generally are absorbed more slowly through the skin than through other body membranes. The rate of absorption may be increased or absorption facilitated by placement of the drug in a vehicle such as dimethyl sulfoxide (DMSO). Medication also may be applied to the mucosa of the oral cavity (sublingual), the rectum (suppositories), the uterus, the vagina, the mammary glands, the eyes, and the ears. In horses, caustic materials may be applied topically to inhibit the growth of exuberant granulation tissue (proud flesh).

Transdermal drug administration is a form of topical administration that involves the use of a patch applied to the skin to deliver a drug through intact skin directly into the blood. This method is used most commonly to administer an analgesic in a slow, continuous manner or to administer compounded drugs to animals when oral administration may be difficult (e.g., cats).

Drug Absorption

Before drugs can reach their site of action, they must pass across a series of cellular membranes that make up the absorptive surfaces of the sites of administration. The degree to which a drug is absorbed and reaches the general circulation is called *bioavailability.*

The **manufacturing** process can have a significant effect on the physical and chemical characteristics of drug molecules that influence their bioavailability. Because of manufacturing differences, the generic equivalent form of a drug may differ somewhat from a trademark form in overall efficacy. Bioavailability often is demonstrated with the use of a blood level curve (Figure 1-3). Factors that may affect the absorption process include the following:

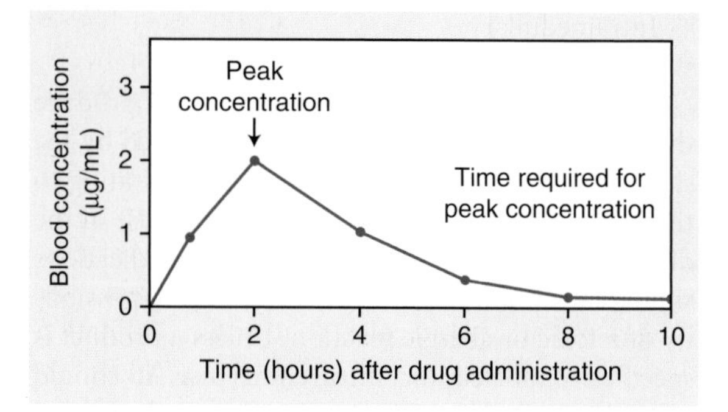

FIGURE 1-3 The blood level of a drug varies with the passage of time.

- Mechanism of absorption
- pH and ionization status of the drug
- Absorptive surface area
- Blood supply to the area
- Solubility of the drug
- Dosage form
- Status of the GI tract (motility, permeability, and thickness of the mucosal epithelium)
- Interaction with other medications

Drugs pass across cellular membranes through three common methods. Passive absorption (transport) occurs by simple diffusion of a drug molecule from an area of high concentration of drug on one side of the membrane to an area of lower concentration on the other side. This method requires no expenditure of energy by the cell. The drug may pass through small pores in the cell membrane or may dissolve into the cell membrane on one side, pass through the membrane, and exit on the other side. For example, a disintegrated tablet or capsule results in a high concentration of drug in the GI tract. This concentration then passes through the cellular membranes of intestinal villi and adjacent capillaries, and the drug then appears in lesser concentration in the bloodstream. Alternatively, a drug may cross a membrane passively with the help of a carrier.

Drug transporters also play a major role in drug absorption. The best described transporter is the P-glycoprotein (P-gp). P-gp is produced at the direction of the MDR1 (ABCB1) gene. It uses adenosine triphosphate (ATP) as an energy source to pump drugs from cells. It is found in most mammalian tissue and appears to act in a protective manner. It is useful in intestinal, renal, placental, liver, and brain tissue, where it helps to pump transported drugs out of the body or away from protected sites. The protection is achieved by pumping the drugs into the intestine, bile, or urine for elimination or away from the fetus or brain (Boothe, 2012).

Some small drug molecules such as electrolytes may simply move with fluid through pores in cell membranes. Active transport of drugs across cell membranes moves molecules from an area of lower concentration to an area of higher concentration and requires that the cell use energy. This is the usual mechanism for the absorption of sodium, potassium, and other electrolytes. In pinocytosis, a third method of passive transport, cells engulf drug molecules by invaginating their cell membrane to form a vesicle that then breaks off from the membrane in the interior of the cell. The method of absorption that occurs in a particular situation depends on whether the drug is fat soluble or water soluble, the size and shape of the drug molecule, and the degree of ionization of the drug.

Many drugs can pass through a cell membrane only if they are nonionized (i.e., not positively or negatively charged). Most drugs exist in the body in a state that consists of both ionized and nonionized forms. The pH of a drug and the pH of the area in which the drug is located can determine the degree to which a drug becomes ionized and thus is absorbed. Weakly acidic drugs in an acidic environment do not ionize readily and therefore are absorbed well. The absorption of basic drugs is more favorable in an alkaline environment. If a drug is placed in an environment in which it readily ionizes, such as a mildly acidic drug in an alkaline environment or a mildly alkaline drug in an acidic environment, it does not diffuse and may become trapped in that environment.

As the absorptive surface of the area of drug placement increases, so does the rate of absorption. One of the largest absorptive surfaces in the body is found in the small intestine because the efficient design of the villi maximizes the surface area.

At any site of drug administration, as the blood supply to an area increases, so does the rate of absorption of the drug. Drugs are absorbed from an intramuscular site at a faster rate than from a subcutaneous site because of the proportionately greater blood supply to the muscle. Initiating the fight-or-flight response increases blood flow to the muscle but decreases blood flow to the intestines. Heat and massage also increase blood flow to an area. Poor circulation, which may occur during shock or cardiac failure, decreases blood flow, as does cooling or elevation of a body part. These factors then can positively or negatively influence drug absorption.

Another important factor that determines the rate at which drugs pass across cell membranes is the solubility of the drug. The lipid (fat) solubility of a drug tends to be directly proportional to the degree of drug nonionization. As was stated previously, the nonionized form is the one that usually is absorbed. The degree of lipid solubility of a drug often is expressed as its lipid **partition coefficient.** A high lipid partition coefficient indicates enhanced drug absorption.

Drug absorption rates often depend on the formulation of the drug. Various inert ingredients, such as carriers (vehicles), binding agents, and coatings, are used to prepare dosage forms. These substances have major effects on the rate at which formulations dissolve. *Depot* and *spansule* are terms that are associated with prolonged- or sustained-release formulations in veterinary medicine. Subcutaneous implants that contain growth stimulants that break down slowly and release their products over prolonged periods are used in some situations.

When drugs are given orally, the condition of the GI tract can have a major influence on the rate and extent of drug absorption. Factors such as degree of intestinal motility, emptying time of the stomach, irritation or inflammation of the mucosa (e.g., gastritis, enteritis), damage to or loss of villi (e.g., viral diseases), composition and amount of food material, and changes in intestinal microorganisms can affect the rate and extent of absorbance of medications. Another consideration regarding drugs that are absorbed from the GI tract is the first-pass effect. This refers to the fact that substances are absorbed from the GI tract into the portal venous system, which delivers the drug to the liver before it enters the general circulation. In some instances, a drug then is metabolized in the liver to altered forms; this process may make the drug inactive or less active.

The process of combining some drugs with other drugs or with certain foods can negatively affect drug absorption. The availability of tetracycline is reduced if it is administered with milk or milk products. Antacids may reduce the absorption of phenylbutazone or iron products. Technicians always should consult appropriate references about potential interactions before administering new drugs.

Drug Distribution

Drug distribution is the process by which a drug is carried from its site of absorption to its site of action. Drugs move from the absorption site into the plasma of the bloodstream, from the plasma into the interstitial fluid that surrounds cells, and from the interstitial fluid into the cells, where they combine with cellular receptors to create an action. Equilibrium soon is established between these three compartments while the drug moves from the blood into the tissue and then from the tissue back into the blood (Figure 1-4). How well a drug is distributed throughout the body depends on several factors.

The rate of movement of drug molecules from one of the previously listed compartments to the other is proportional to the differences between the amounts of drug in all areas. The difference between the amounts of drug in two compartments is called the *concentration gradient,* and as the gradient increases (difference), so does the tendency of the drug to move from the area of higher concentration to the area of lower concentration.

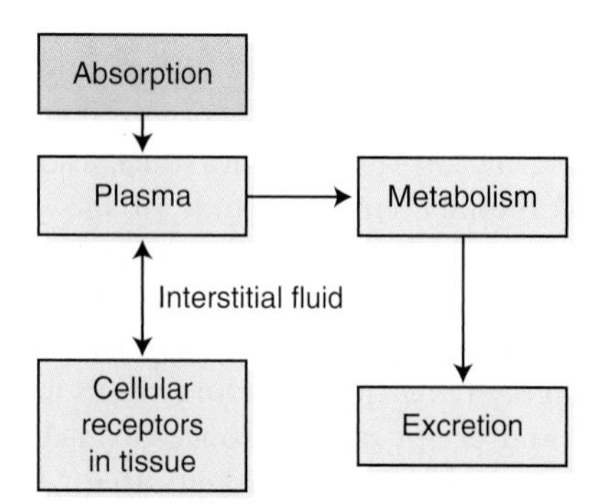

FIGURE 1-4 Drug distribution establishes an equilibrium between the amount of drug at the site of absorption, the amount in the plasma, and the amount at the cellular receptor sites.

A drug within the plasma comes into contact with various proteins (e.g., albumin) and binds with them or remains free. When a drug is bound to a protein, it becomes inactive and is unavailable for binding with cell receptors or for metabolism. A bound drug may be regarded as a temporary storage site of a drug because a bound drug eventually frees itself from the protein. Low levels of plasma proteins may occur in malnutrition or in certain diseases, and plasma binding may be reduced.

Drugs that are highly lipid soluble tend to move readily from the plasma into the interstitial fluid. Drugs in the nonionized form follow a similar pattern. Once a drug is present in a tissue, it may become bound or stored there. Tissues such as fat, liver, kidney, and bone may act as storage sites for drugs such as barbiturates, inhalation anesthetics, and others. When a drug moves from the storage tissue back into the blood and additional doses are given, an exaggerated or prolonged effect may result because of the additive effects.

Barriers that exist in particular tissues tend to retard the movement of all or certain classes of drugs into them. The exact nature of these barriers has not been well explained in the literature although the P-gp transporter may play an important role. The placenta acts as a barrier to some drugs that could be toxic to a fetus and permits the passage of others. Anesthetics that do not excessively depress a fetus must be chosen when a cesarean section is performed. The so-called blood–brain barrier is generally minimally permeable to all drugs, although it becomes relatively permeable to many antibiotics on inflammation. A defect in the P-gp drug transporter in the blood–brain barrier has been identified in individuals of several dog breeds, including collies, Old English sheepdogs, Australian shepherds, Shetland sheepdogs, and English shepherds and can result in potential toxicity to drugs like ivermectin. The eye also has a barrier that impedes some drugs from diffusing into its tissue.

Disease processes can interfere with drug distribution. Antibiotics usually do not diffuse well into abscesses or exudates. Heart failure and shock can reduce normal blood flow to tissue and thus impede drug distribution. Kidney failure (uremia) can alter the plasma binding of some drugs such as furosemide and phenylbutazone. Liver failure can cause a reduction in the amount of protein (albumin) available for protein binding.

Some clinicians believe that reptiles have a renal–portal system that can distribute potentially toxic levels of a drug to the kidney if the drug is injected into the posterior one third of the body.

Biotransformation

Biotransformation, or **metabolism,** is the body's ability to change a drug chemically from the form in which it was administered into a form that can be eliminated from the body. Most biotransformation occurs in the liver because of the action of microsomal enzymes called *cytochrome P450 enzymes* found in liver cells. These enzymes induce chemical reactions that change the drug chemically to allow elimination in the urine or bile. Once a drug has been biotransformed, it is called a *metabolite.* Metabolites are usually inactive, but in some cases, may have similar, less, or more activity. Some biotransformation does occur in other tissues such as the kidney, lung, and nervous system.

The following four chemical reactions are induced by microsomal enzymes in the liver to biotransform drugs:

1. Oxidation—loss of electrons
2. Reduction—gain of electrons
3. Hydrolysis—splitting of the drug molecule and addition of a water molecule to each of the split portions
4. Conjugation—the addition of glucuronic acid or similar compounds to the drug molecule; when these compounds are attached to a drug molecule, the drug becomes much more water soluble.

Biotransformation reactions involving oxidation, reduction, or hydrolysis are called phase I reactions, while reactions involving conjugation are called phase II reactions. Drugs may be processed through both phases or only phase II. As a rule, phase I reactions make drugs more water soluble and because of this more susceptible to phase II metabolism. Phase II reactions generally make the drugs water soluble enough for elimination by the kidneys (Boothe, 2012).

Many factors, including species, age, nutritional status, tissue storage, and health status, can alter drug metabolism. Cats have limited ability to metabolize aspirin, narcotics, phenols, and barbiturates because of their reduced ability to form glucuronic acid. Young animals usually have poor ability to biotransform drugs because their liver enzyme systems are not fully developed until around 3 months of age. Old animals have a decreased capacity to biotransform because their ability to synthesize needed liver enzymes may be impaired. Malnourished animals have fewer protein raw materials available for use in manufacturing enzymes for biotransformation, and animals with liver disease are not able to process the raw materials available for enzyme production. Drugs present in storage compartments such as fat or plasma proteins are not available to be metabolized.

Drug Excretion

Most drugs are metabolized by the liver and then are eliminated from the body by the kidneys via the urine. They can be excreted, however, by the liver (bile), mammary glands, lungs, intestinal tract, sweat glands, salivary glands, and skin. An understanding of the route of excretion of drugs is very important because alterations or diseases of a particular organ can cause a reduced capacity to excrete the drug, and toxic accumulation may result. For example, the anesthetic agent ketamine can cause serious central nervous system (CNS) depression in cats with urinary obstruction because the kidneys excrete this drug.

Kidneys excrete drugs by two principal mechanisms. The first method is called *glomerular filtration.* A glomerulus and its corresponding tubule make up the individual functional unit of the kidney, called a *nephron.* A glomerulus acts like a sieve to filter drug molecules (metabolites) from the blood into the glomerular filtrate, which is then eliminated as urine (Figure 1-5). The second mechanism that kidneys use to excrete drugs is called *tubular secretion.* Kidney tubule cells secrete metabolites from the capillaries surrounding the tubule and into the glomerular

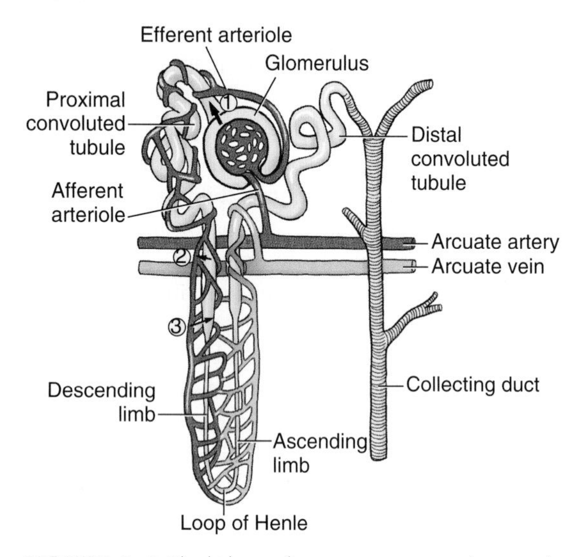

FIGURE 1-5 The kidneys eliminate or conserve drug metabolites by glomerular filtration *(1)*, tubular reabsorption *(2)*, and tubular secretion *(3)*.

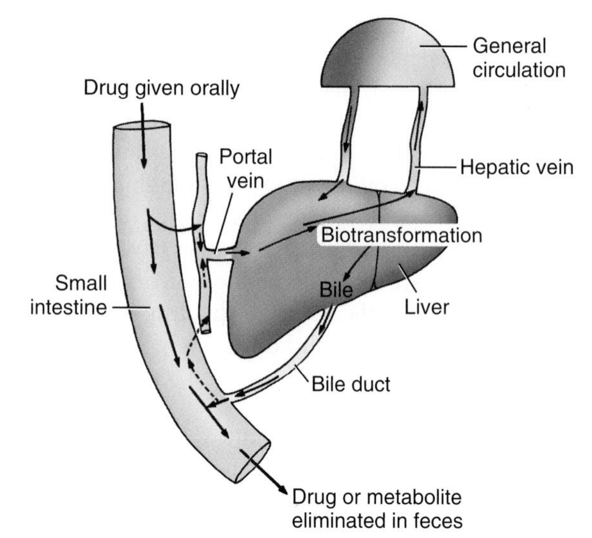

FIGURE 1-6 Drugs or their metabolites in the intestine may be eliminated in the feces or absorbed/reabsorbed for a pass through the liver.

filtrate, which becomes urine as it exits the kidneys. In some instances, drug molecules may be reabsorbed from the glomerular filtrate back into the blood through *tubular reabsorption.*

It is important that the nephrons (glomerulus and corresponding tubule) are healthy and that they have an adequate blood supply, so they can do an effective job of excreting metabolites. The lower urinary tract (bladder and urethra) also must be functioning normally, so filtered or secreted metabolites can be eliminated. If any part of this system from the glomerulus to the urethra is compromised or diseased, toxic levels of a drug may accumulate.

The liver excretes drugs by first incorporating them into bile, which is eliminated into the small intestine. In the small intestine, the drug then may become a part of the feces and be eliminated from the body, or it may be reabsorbed into the bloodstream (Figure 1-6).

Some drugs or their metabolites may pass directly from the blood and into the milk via the mammary glands. This is an important consideration because of the potential effects of the drug on nursing offspring or on people who drink the milk. Quantities of drug that remain in animal products when they are consumed are called *residues.* Residues found in milk, eggs, or meat products are potentially dangerous to people for the following reasons:

- People may be allergic to the drug.
- Prolonged exposure to antibiotic residues can result in resistant strains of bacteria.
- Residue of some drugs may cause cancer in humans.

Drugs that convert readily between a liquid and a gaseous state (gas anesthetics) may be eliminated from the blood via the lungs. These gas molecules move from the blood into the alveoli of the lungs to be eliminated in expired air.

Drugs that are given orally and are not absorbed readily from the intestinal tract may pass through the tract and be eliminated through feces. As was mentioned previously, some drugs are excreted through the bile into the intestinal tract, and a few may be actively secreted across the intestinal mucosa into the intestine for elimination.

Some drugs are eliminated through sweat and saliva, although these routes usually are not clinically important. The rate of drug loss from the body can be estimated by calculating the drug's **half-life.** The half-life is the time required for the amount of drug present in the body to be reduced by one half (Figure 1-7).

PHARMACODYNAMICS

Pharmacodynamics is the study of the mechanisms by which drugs produce physiologic changes in the body. Drugs may enhance or depress the physiologic activity of a cell or a tissue. Drug molecules combine with components of the cell membrane or with internal components of the cell to cause alterations in cell function. The way in which drugs combine with structures (receptors) on or in a cell can be compared with a lock-and-key model. The geometric match of a drug molecule and a cellular receptor must be exact for the appropriate action to occur (Figure 1-8). The tendency of a drug to combine with a receptor is called *affinity*, and the degree to which the drug binds

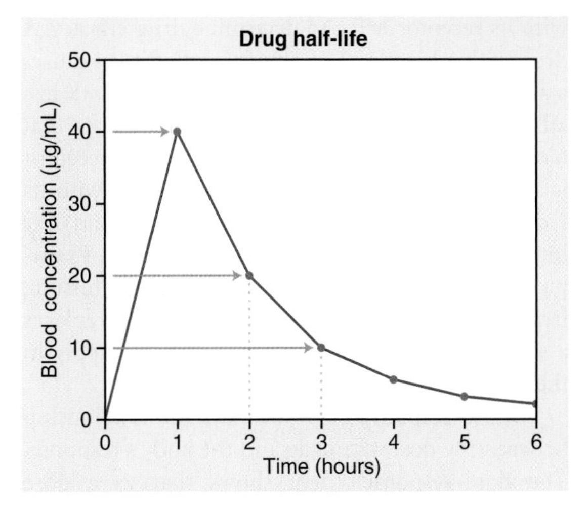

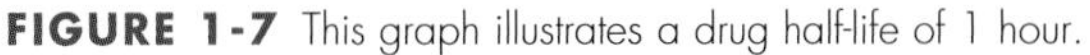
FIGURE 1-7 This graph illustrates a drug half-life of 1 hour.

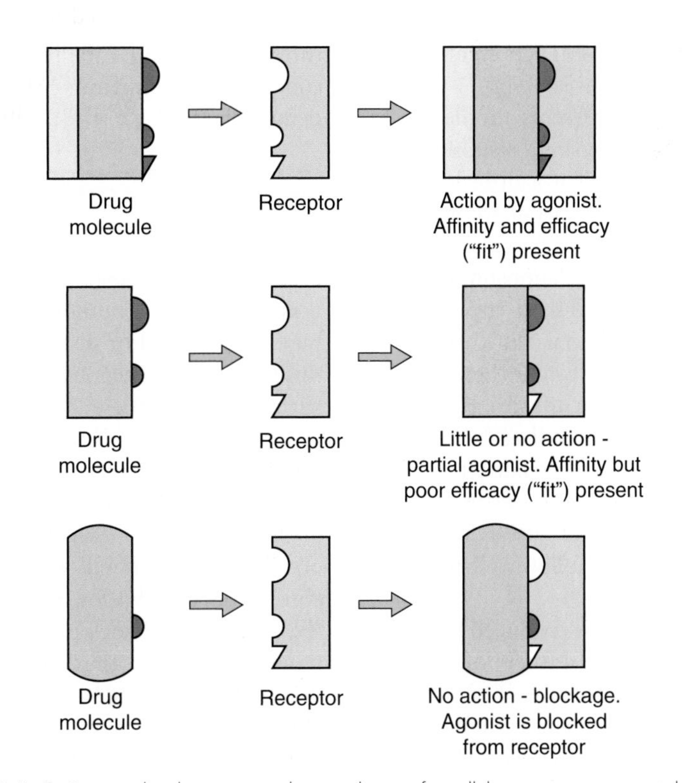

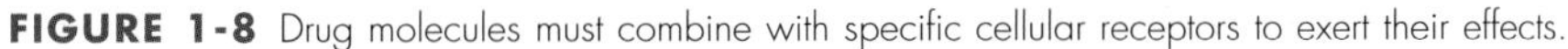
FIGURE 1-8 Drug molecules must combine with specific cellular receptors to exert their effects.

with its receptor helps to determine drug efficacy. A drug with a high level of affinity and efficacy causes a specific action and is an **agonist.** A drug with less affinity and efficacy is a partial agonist. A drug that blocks another drug from combining with a receptor is an **antagonist.** The combining of a drug with its receptor causes a particular drug action, and this interaction produces a particular drug effect. Examples of drug effects include stimulation, depression, irritation, and cell death. Sometimes, a drug replaces a substance that is missing or is in short supply in the body.

A dose–response curve displays the relationship between the dose of a drug and the body's response. The dose–response curve shows that as a dose increases, an increase in response occurs until a maximum response or plateau is achieved. *No drug produces a single effect.* Low doses of a narcotic may be used to treat patients with diarrhea. Higher doses may be used for pain relief, and even higher doses may depress the respiratory system. The *potency* of a drug is described as the amount of a drug needed to produce a desired response and is represented by a position along the dose–response curve.

The **efficacy** of a drug represents the degree to which a drug produces its desired response in a patient. Once the efficacy level of a drug has been reached, increasing the dose does not improve the effect.

The *therapeutic index* is the relationship between a drug's ability to achieve the desired effect and its tendency to produce toxic effects. The therapeutic index, which is expressed as the ratio between the LD_{50} and the ED_{50}, quantitates the drug's margin of safety. The LD_{50} is the dose of a drug that is lethal to 50% of the animals in a dose-related trial. The ED_{50} is the dose of a drug that produces the desired effect in 50% of the animals in a dose-related trial. The index is calculated as follows: therapeutic index = LD_{50}/ED_{50}.

The larger the number that is produced by dividing the LD_{50} by the ED_{50}, the greater the level of safety. Drugs with a narrow margin of safety (low therapeutic index) must be administered with caution to prevent toxic or fatal effects. The drugs used to treat cancer often have a low therapeutic index.

An **adverse drug event** is harm to a patient caused by administration of a drug for therapeutic or diagnostic reasons. It may be due to a medication error such as using the wrong drug, the wrong dose, or the wrong interval or administering the drug to the wrong patient. Another cause of an adverse event is the **adverse drug reaction.** An adverse reaction is due to the inherent properties of the drug itself. Adverse reactions may range from mild dermatitis to anaphylactic shock and death. Poor quality or purity of the drug may cause an adverse reaction. Some patients may react to carriers or binders of the drugs rather than the drug themselves. Aminoglycosides can cause harm to the kidney or eighth cranial nerve and impair hearing. Drugs can cause changes in the skin that make it more sensitive to light. This type of reaction is called *photosensitivity.*

Other types of adverse responses include abortion, liver or kidney damage, infertility, vomiting or diarrhea, and cancer. An unusual or unexpected reaction is called an *idiosyncratic drug reaction.* All adverse reactions should be reported to the drug manufacturer or the FDA. If the report is made to the drug company, the company is obligated to report the incident to the FDA.

DRUG INTERACTIONS

An altered pharmacologic response to a drug that is caused by the presence of a second drug is called a *drug interaction.* The normal response to the drug may be increased or decreased as a consequence of this interaction. The interaction may be beneficial or harmful to the patient.

Drug interactions can be classified as pharmacokinetic, pharmacodynamic, or pharmaceutic. A pharmacokinetic interaction is one in which plasma or tissue levels of a drug are altered by the presence of another. This alteration may be due to changes in absorption, distribution, metabolism, or excretion of the other drug. Metoclopramide hastens gastric emptying and promotes the delivery of a drug to the small intestine for absorption. When calcium and tetracycline are administered at the same time orally, calcium binds the tetracycline and the complex is not absorbed. Displacement of albumin-bound drugs by other drugs with a greater binding affinity may

TABLE 1-2 Drug Combinations That May Have Undesirable Consequences

PRECIPITANT DRUG	OBJECT DRUG	CONSEQUENCES
Antacids	Tetracycline	Reduced absorption of tetracycline
Ketoconazole	Digoxin, cyclosporine, tricyclic antidepressants	Decreased metabolism of object drugs
Sucralfate	Fluoroquinolones	Reduced absorption of quinolones
Fluoroquinolones	Theophylline	Decreased metabolism of theophylline
Omeprazole	Ketoconazole/itraconazole	Decreased oral absorption of object drugs
Phenobarbital	Theophylline, doxycycline, beta blockers	Increased metabolism of object drugs (cytochrome P-450 induction)
Cimetidine	Diazepam and theophylline	Decreased metabolism of object drugs (cytochrome P-450 inhibition)
MAO Inhibitors	Amitraz, selective serotonin reuptake inhibitors, tricyclic antidepressants, other MAOs	Dangerous accumulation of biogenic amines leading to serotonin syndrome or hypertensive state
Tetracyclines	Penicillins	Tetracyclines slow bacterial growth and inhibit penicillins that are most effective against rapidly growing bacteria

MAO, Monoamine oxidase.

result in an increase in the free drug, leading to an increased response. Many drugs are metabolized by the cytochrome P-450 enzyme system found in the liver, and several drugs can alter (increase or decrease) the activity of the P-450 system, causing drug interactions.

A pharmacodynamic interaction is one in which the action or effect of one drug is altered by another. These reactions occur at the site of drug action. These actions may be antagonistic (reversal of an alpha agonist with yohimbine), additive (CNS depression with combinations of preanesthetics), or synergistic (sulfonamide-trimethoprim combinations).

A pharmaceutic interaction occurs when physical or chemical reactions take place as a result of mixing of drugs in a syringe or other container. Amphotericin B may form a precipitate when mixed with electrolyte solutions other than 5% dextrose. Diazepam may precipitate if mixed with certain drugs. Furosemide may be chemically inactivated if mixed with an acid medium (Boothe, 2012).

Drug interactions are described as involving an object drug (the one being acted on) and a precipitant drug (the one that influences the other; Mealey, 2002). Table 1-2 lists selected drug combinations that may have undesirable consequences.

TECHNICIAN NOTES

- It generally is recommended that mixing of drugs in the same syringe or fluid administration system should be avoided unless the drugs are known to be compatible.
- When two drugs metabolized by the liver are given, one should anticipate a drug interaction.
- Concurrent use of drugs from the "behavior modifying" category can cause serious problems such as serotonin syndrome or hypertensive reactions.

DRUG NAMES

When a company completes the exhaustive research and development necessary to gain FDA approval to market a drug, it names this drug and has exclusive rights to the drug for the duration of the patent. During this time, no other company can manufacture the drug. This allows the original manufacturer time to recoup the cost of research and development and to earn a profit. On expiration of the patent, other companies may produce the drug. When other

TABLE 1-3 Drug Chemical, Generic, and Trade Names

CHEMICAL NAME	GENERIC NAME	TRADE NAME
22,23-dihydroavermectin B1a 22,23-dihydroavermectin B1b	Ivermectin	Heartguard Ivomec Eqvalan
dl 2-(o-chlorophenyl)-2-(methylamino) cyclohexanone hydrochloride	Ketamine hydrochloride	Ketaset Ketaject Vetalar
D(-)-α-amino-p-hydroxybenzyl-penicillin trihydrate	Amoxicillin	Amoxil Amoxi-Tabs Trimox

companies manufacture this previously developed product it is called a generic equivalent.

During the course of its testing, development, and marketing, a drug may be assigned several different names. These multiple names can be a source of confusion. For practical purposes, drugs are given the following types of names:

- Chemical—the name that describes the molecular structure of a drug. These names are scientifically very accurate, but they are complex and impractical for use in clinical settings.
- Code or laboratory—the name given to a drug by the research and development investigators. It is used for communication between research teams and consists of abbreviations and code numbers.
- Compendial—the name listed in the *United States Pharmacopoeia (USP)*. The *USP* is the legally accepted compendium that lists drugs and standards for their quality and purity.
- Official—usually the same as the compendial or generic name.
- Proprietary or trade—the name chosen by the manufacturing company. When it is registered, it is the exclusive property of the company. A name that is short and can be easily recalled is usually selected for the proprietary name. Federal copyright and trademark laws protect this name. On drug container labels, in package inserts, and in drug references, the proprietary name can be distinguished by a superscript R with a circle around it after the name.
- Generic—the common name chosen by the company. It is not the exclusive right of the company. It may be the same as the official or compendial name. These are drugs with patents that have expired, or they were never patented.

Table 1-3 provides chemical, generic, and proprietary names of three common drugs.

In textbooks and other scholarly works, generic names begin with a lowercase letter, and proprietary names begin with a capital letter. This practice is followed throughout this text (e.g., ketamine [Ketaset]).

DRUG LABELS

The Center for Veterinary Medicine (CVM) of the FDA requires that drug container labels list the following items (Webb and Aeschbacher, 1993):

- Drug names (both generic and trade names)
- Drug concentration and quantity
- Name and address of the manufacturer
- Controlled substance status (if applicable)
- Manufacturer's control or lot number
- Drug's expiration date

It is required that the label also list instructions for use of the drug and warnings of possible adverse effects of the drug. Because the label on the container usually has limited space, many manufacturers list this added information in an insert. An insert is a small folder that is placed inside the box with the drug container or is provided as a tear-off portion of the label.

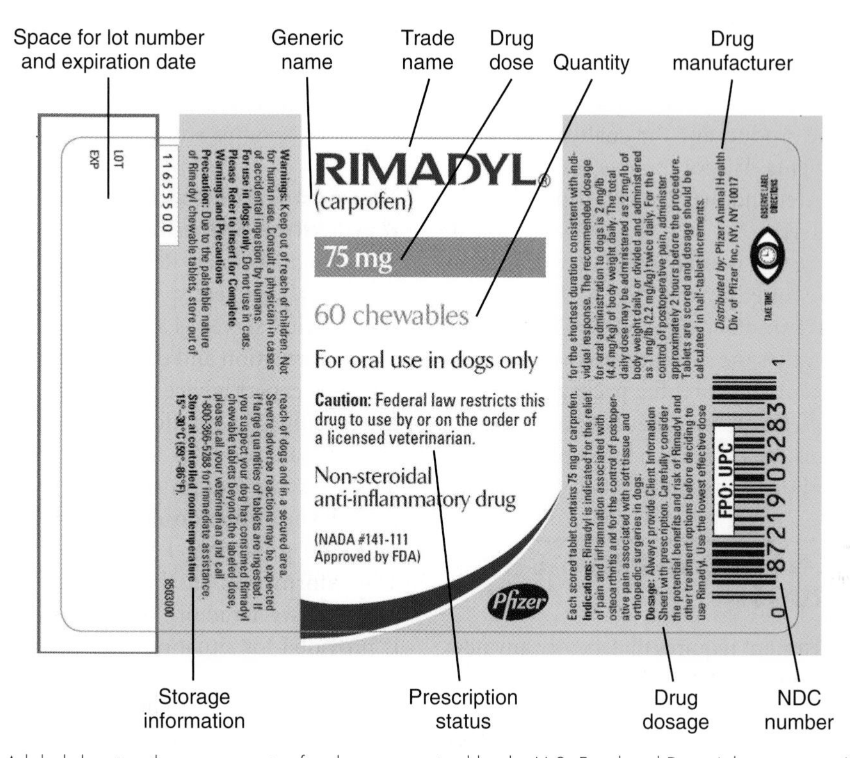

FIGURE 1-9 A label showing the components of a drug as required by the U.S. Food and Drug Administration. (Courtesy Zoetic, Inc., Exton, Pa.)

The trade name usually is placed first on a drug label and is scripted in bold letters (Figure 1-9). The generic name typically follows the trade name in smaller print. The label must display the concentration (strength) of a drug and the total quantity in the container. Drug strength often is expressed as milligrams or units per dosage unit (e.g., mg/mL or mg/capsule). Some drugs are sold in different concentrations with similar labels, and underdosing or overdosing can result. When the same drug is marketed in different strengths with similar labels, some companies use different sizes of bottles for the different strengths and display the concentrations in bold print. Atropine and xylazine are examples of drugs that are marketed in different concentrations for large and small animals.

The label must include the name and address of the manufacturer of the drug. This is important so that one can know whom to contact if adverse drug reactions occur or if other problems with the drug arise.

Drugs that have potential for abuse by humans are controlled under the Comprehensive Drug Abuse Prevention and Control Act of 1970. The Drug Enforcement Administration places drugs into categories or schedules according to their potential for abuse and requires that the label of a container for a controlled substance be identified with a capital C, followed by a Roman numeral that identifies which of the five categories is appropriate. This labeling must be placed on the upper right side of the container label.

Drug labels must list an expiration date for the product. This is to ensure that dispensed drugs have the intended safety and efficacy. Drugs are tested during development to determine the effective shelf life and proper storage conditions. Some drugs must be stored in refrigeration, and others must be stored in light-resistant (amber) containers to ensure that the shelf life is not shortened. *Storage instructions on the label should be followed carefully so as not to invalidate the expiration date.*

All drugs must have a lot or batch number on the label. The purpose of the lot number is to allow the manufacturer to know the exact time and date of production of the product and the quality and quantity of the ingredients. The lot number is determined by the manufacturer and may consist of numbers or numbers and letters.

Another feature that is often found on a drug label but that is not required by the FDA is the national drug code (NDC) number. The NDC is a 10-digit number that identifies the manufacturer or distributor, the drug formulation, and the package size.

Drugs intended for animals that may later be consumed by humans must have the appropriate withdrawal time listed on the insert or label.

DEVELOPMENT AND APPROVAL OF NEW DRUGS

The federal government requires that, before any new animal health product can be marketed, its safety and efficacy must be proved through rigorous testing. This testing requires the expenditure of much time and money. It has been estimated that, on average, it takes 10 years or more at a cost of millions of dollars to the manufacturer to place a new drug on the market. The steps in this process are outlined in Figure 1-10.

The development of new animal health products begins in the research and development department of the manufacturing company. The company wants to ensure that the drug not only is safe and effective for animals but also is safe for the environment and for the people who will consume products from animals treated with the drug. The company wants to be certain that a market is available for the product, that it will be produced at a cost that is reasonable for consumers, and that the product will be profitable for the company.

Regulatory Agencies

The three agencies of the U.S. government that regulate animal health products are the FDA, the Environmental Protection Agency (EPA), and the U.S. Department of Agriculture (USDA). The FDA regulates the development and approval of animal drugs and feed additives through its Center for Veterinary Medicine. The EPA regulates the development and approval of animal topical pesticides, and the USDA regulates the development and approval of biologics (vaccines, serums, antitoxins, and similar products).

The Food Animal Residue Avoidance Databank

The Food Animal Residue Avoidance Databank (FARAD), a project sponsored by the USDA Extension Service, serves as a repository of **residue** avoidance information and educational materials. FARAD provides expert advice concerning the avoidance of drug residues in an effort to achieve its goal of producing "safe foods of animal origin." FARAD produces a compendium of FDA-approved drugs and provides information about withholding times for milk and preslaughter **withdrawal times** for meat. The information in this compendium is available online (www.farad.org), and direct telephone access is provided for situations in which online information is not sufficient.

Steps in the Development of a New Drug

Preliminary Trials

When a new drug or product shows the potential for development by a company, it is first subjected to a series of preliminary trials. The company wants to know whether the product will actually perform as expected, whether it has potentially harmful adverse effects, and whether it will be profitable to market. If these concerns are satisfactorily answered, testing begins. First, the product is tested in a laboratory on simple organisms such as bacteria, yeasts, or molds. Computer models may be used to simulate animal models at this time.

Preclinical (Animal Safety) Trials

If preliminary trial findings prove satisfactory, the next step involves preclinical trials. These trials usually are carried out with the use of laboratory animals to gather information about appropriate doses of the drug. A few target (intended species) animals also may be used. If the results of the preclinical trials are satisfactory, the company then notifies the appropriate government agency that a new drug is under investigation. It does this by filing an

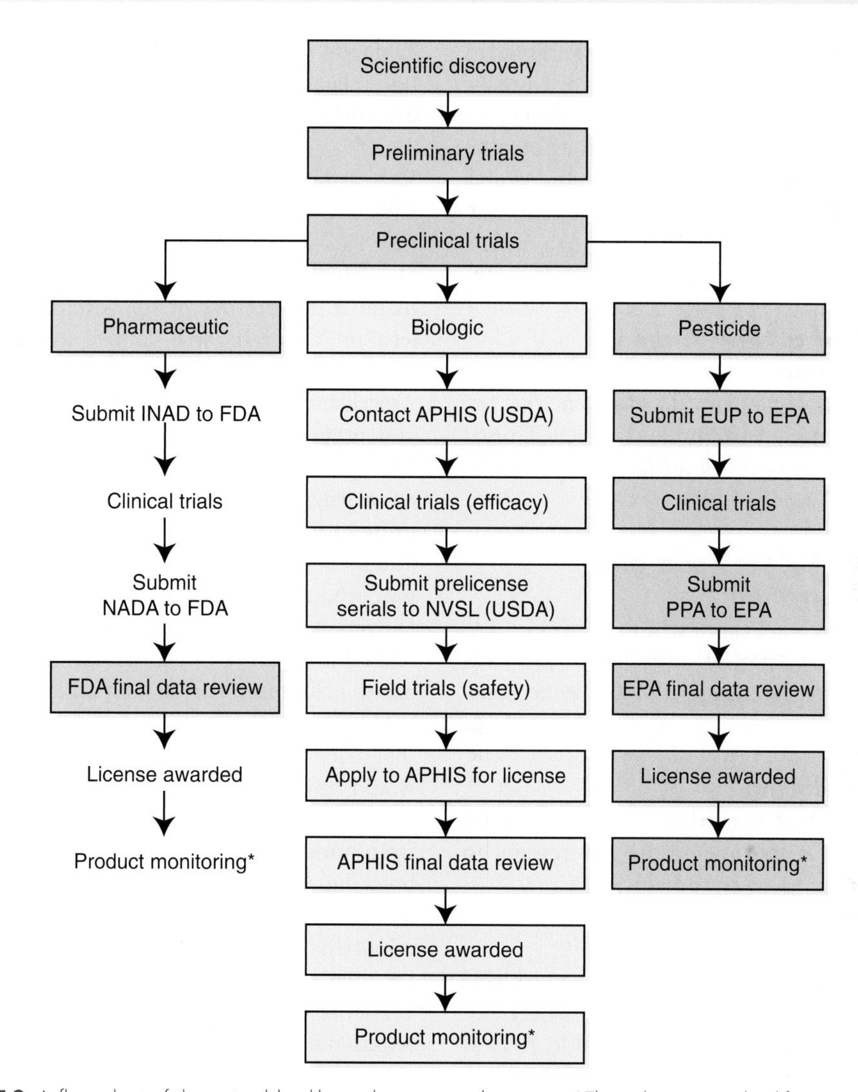

FIGURE 1-10 A flow chart of the animal health product approval process. *Throughout its market life,a product is monitored by the manufacturer and the appropriate government agency to ensure its continued safety. *APHIS*, Animal and Plant Health Inspection Service; *EPA*, Environmental Protection Agency; *EUP*, Experimental Use Permit; *FDA*, U.S. Food and Drug Administration; *INAD*, Investigational New Animal Drug; *NADA*, New Animal Drug Application; *NVSL*, National Veterinary Services Laboratory; *PPA*, Pesticide Permit Application; *USDA*, U.S. Department of Agriculture. (From Etchison K: The path to approval: how research discoveries become federally licensed products. Top Vet Med 4:13, 1993.)

Investigational New Animal Drug (INAD) application with the FDA. If the product is a pesticide, the company files for an Experimental Use Permit (EUP) from the EPA. If a biologic is involved, the company contacts the Animal and Plant Health Inspection Service of the USDA.

Clinical Trials

By this time, the manufacturer has compiled enough information to decide whether the product should be tested in the target species. These tests must prove that the drug is safe and effective. Potential toxic and adverse effects must be identified. Tissue residue and withdrawal time information must be accumulated if the product will be used in food-producing animals. Possible toxic effects on pregnant animals are explored, along with information about the potential for birth defects (teratogenesis). Shelf life studies also must be conducted to establish expiration date data. Results of these studies are validated through the use of statistical analysis.

Submission of a New Animal Drug Application

If the manufacturing company decides to market the drug, it then must file with the FDA a New Animal Drug Application (NADA). Procedures for pesticides and biologics are similar.

Final Review by the Food and Drug Administration

Volumes of research are submitted to the FDA, EPA, or USDA for review. Approval and a license for manufacture are granted if the appropriate agency validates the information.

Product Monitoring

As long as a product is marketed, it is monitored constantly by the company and the government to ensure its continuing safety and efficacy.

The Green Book

The Green Book is a list of all animal drug products that have been approved by the FDA for safety and effectiveness. This list was first published in 1989 as a cooperative, nonprofit effort between the USDA and Virginia Polytechnic Institute and State University. It is funded through an interagency agreement between the USDA and the FDA. Monthly updates are made to the list, and the entire list is published each January. *The Green Book* is available electronically at the FDA-CVM Web site (http://www.fda.gov/AnimalVeterinary/Products/ApprovedAnimalDrugProducts/default.htm).

FEDERAL LAWS RELATED TO DRUG DEVELOPMENT AND USE

In 1906, Congress passed the first legislation designed to regulate the manufacture, use, and sale of drugs. Table 1-4 provides a list of the major acts of legislation related to drug development and use and briefly describes the significance of each.

The Animal Medicinal Drug Use Clarification Act

In 1994, Congress passed the Animal Medicinal Drug Use Clarification Act (AMDUCA). This legislation made extralabel use of approved veterinary drugs legal under specific well-defined conditions. This act came about because of the lobbying efforts of the American Veterinary Medical Association (AVMA) and other groups in response to the FDA, which had tightened its policies on extralabel use of veterinary drugs. Previously, veterinarians had been permitted to use any drug as long as it could be legally obtained, was used according to sound professional practice, and left no residue in food products. However, public concerns over food safety issues related to residues of substances such as diethylstilbestrol, chloramphenicol, and antibiotics caused the FDA to issue compliance policy guidelines (CPGs) that made extralabel use illegal. Even though the FDA would not routinely prosecute veterinarians for extralabel use after issuance of the CPGs, practitioners nonetheless were placed in the position of breaking federal law to meet their obligations to animals and their owners. The AMDUCA allows veterinarians to legally select the most efficacious drugs for their patients. The AVMA issued an *AMDUCA Guidance Brochure* in 1998. This brochure outlines requirements of the act and provides an algorithm that can be used to determine when extralabel use is appropriate.

A section of the AMDUCA states that the FDA may prohibit or restrict extralabel use in animals if the agency finds that such use presents a risk to the public health. The following drugs and substances are prohibited or restricted for extralabel use in all food-producing animals.

Prohibited:

- Chloramphenicol
- Clenbuterol
- Crystal (Gentian) Violet
- Diethylstilbestrol or DES
- Dipyrone
- Fluoroquinolone-class antibiotics

TABLE 1-4 Federal Laws Regulating the Use of Pharmaceutics

DATE	LEGISLATION	SUMMARY
1958	Food additives amendment	Regulation of substances added to food for human consumption. Delaney clause specifies that no additive that causes cancer in humans or animals may be used.
1962	Kefauver-Harris amendment	Provided for safety and effectiveness of drugs by strict control of manufacturing for new animal drugs
1968	Animal drug amendment	Provided regulations for new animal drugs
1970	Comprehensive drug abuse and control act	Placed controlled substances into schedules according to their potential for abuse. Called for registration of veterinarians
1988	Generic Animal Drug and Patent Term Restoration Act	Allowed companies to produce and sell generic versions of animal drugs approved after October 1962 without duplicating original research
1994	Animal Medicinal Drug Use Clarification Act (AMDUCA)	Allows veterinarians under specific conditions to prescribe veterinary drugs in an off-label manner. It also allows human drugs to be used in animals under certain conditions.
1996	Animal Drug Availability Act	Created a new category of drugs, Animal Feed Drugs. Allows animal drugs to be added to animal feeds under the direction of a veterinarian. Supports flexible labeling of dosages on some products
2003	Animal Drug User Fee Act	Allows the FDA to collect fees from sponsoring companies for the review of certain animal drug applications
2004	Minor Use and Minor Species Health Act	Allows FDA-approved drugs to be used for treating minor species and for uncommon uses in major species
2008	Animal Generic Drug User Fee	Allows FDA to collect fees from sponsoring companies to study means of expediting the animal generic drug review process

FDA, U.S. Food and Drug Administration.

- Glycopeptides—all agents including vancomycin
- Nitroimidazoles—all agents, including dimetridazole, ipronidazole, metronidazole and others
- Medicated feeds
- Nitrofurans—all agents, including furazolidone, nitrofurazone and others.

Restricted:

- Antiviral agents
- Cephalosporin-class antibiotics except cephapirin (cattle, chickens, pigs, and turkeys)
- Phenylbutazone (all female dairy cattle 20 months of age or older)
- Sulfonamide-class antibiotics (lactating dairy cattle)
- Indexed drugs (legally marketed unapproved drugs)

Compounding of Veterinary Drugs

FDA-approved drugs are labeled for specific therapeutic uses in defined species. Because veterinarians must treat a variety of animal species that may vary greatly in size, it is not always possible to use an approved drug for every clinical situation; therefore, veterinarians may have to dilute or combine (**compound**) existing medications. For example, it may be in the best interest of a horse to combine more than one drug in a single syringe to minimize the number of injections. It also may be essential to dilute an injectable agent to obtain an appropriate concentration for a bird or mouse or to prepare an antidote (e.g., sodium sulfate) that is not commercially available. None of these activities would be permitted under a strict interpretation of FDA regulations, which traditionally have not distinguished the act of diluting or combining drugs from the act of manufacturing. Any alteration of a drug by a veterinarians or their employees that changes the concentration of the active ingredient, the preservatives, or the vehicles results in a new animal drug that is subject to the FDA approval process (Davidson, 1997). Recognizing the difficulties imposed by these regulations, the FDA issued a CPG (608.400) in 1996 to better define the conditions for which compounding is permitted. These conditions include but may not be limited to (1) identification of a legitimate veterinary medical need; (2) the need for an appropriate regimen for a particular species, size, gender, or medical condition; (3) lack of an approved animal or human drug that when used as labeled will treat the condition; and (4) too long a time interval for securing the drug to treat the condition.

The Veterinary Feed Directive

Congress established the Veterinary Feed Directive (VFD) as part of the Animal Drug Availability Act of 1996. The VFD established a new category of drugs "as an alternative to prescription status" for certain antimicrobial animal feed additives. Before this directive, all commercially available animal drugs for use in medicated feeds were available on an over-the-counter basis. The VFD therefore provides the FDA CVM greater control over the use of some new animal feed additives. The use of VFD drugs requires a valid veterinarian–client–patient relationship and the issuance of a VFD form by a veterinarian. The animal producer must secure the VFD form from the veterinarian and must present it to a feed mill to receive the medicated feed. The FDA has on its website "Blue Bird" labels to guide feed mills when labeling feeds treated with medication premixes. These labels ensure the safe and appropriate use of these feeds.

The Minor Use and Minor Species Animal Health Act

There is a shortage in the United States of approved animal drugs intended for use in less common animal species or those with less common conditions. The drugs that do exist may not be used legally in the animals that need the treatment. The Minor Use and Minor Species (MUMS) Animal Health Act of 2004 is intended as a mechanism to provide FDA-authorized drugs for those less common species and indications, similar to the human Orphan Drug Act of 1983. MUMS specifically defines the provision of labeled drugs for minor species, including sheep, goats, game birds, emus, ranched deer, alpacas, llamas, deer, elk, rabbits, guinea pigs, pet birds, reptiles, ornamental and other fish, shellfish, wildlife, and zoo and aquarium animals. MUMS is also designed to provide major species (e.g., cats, dogs, horses, cattle, swine, turkeys, chickens) with needed drugs for uncommon indications (minor uses).

DISPENSING VERSUS PRESCRIBING DRUGS

Although most physicians prescribe drugs, most veterinarians prescribe and dispense them. The primary reason why veterinarians maintain a pharmacy in their hospitals is that drug sales represent an important source of income. Food animal practitioners in particular use profit from drug sales to supplement their income because it may be difficult for them to charge sufficiently for their time. Another reason why veterinarians dispense drugs from their hospitals is that human pharmacies usually do not stock veterinary drugs. A few drugs are available only from human pharmacies, and others are used so infrequently that veterinarians find it more practical and economical to write a prescription for them.

MARKETING OF DRUGS

Pharmaceutic products are purchased by veterinarians from various sources. Some products are purchased directly from the manufacturer by telephone or by mail; others are obtained from sales representatives (detail persons) who call on veterinary clinics. Distributors (wholesalers) are companies that buy products from many different manufacturers and then resell the products to veterinarians through sales representatives or by phone. Generic drug companies sell generic products under their own label, usually by mail order.

Most of the pharmaceutic manufacturers are large companies that have separate divisions. One division sells products to veterinarians only, and the other sells over-the-counter products. It should be noted that the statement "sold to graduate veterinarians only" on a drug label does not mean that the product is a prescription drug. It only indicates a sales policy of the company. In a few instances, the same product is sold under different labels to veterinarians only and to over-the-counter markets. Some feed stores and cooperatives are able to sell over-the-counter products (similar to products sold by veterinarians) to consumers at prices lower than veterinarians can charge because of the quantity purchasing power of the stores. This can be a source of tension between veterinarians and retail markets.

In recent years, Internet pharmacies have emerged on the marketing scene. Many clients attempt to use these resources because of the reduced cost of some products. The primary concern in the veterinary community is that some Internet pharmacies are supplying prescription drugs to consumers without the authorization of a veterinarian with a veterinarian–client–patient relationship. The prescription may be issued by an out-of-state veterinarian who responds to client questionnaire information rather than through actual patient and client contact. Solving these problems may be difficult because the FDA regulates the drug products themselves, not the practice of the pharmacy. The board of pharmacy in the individual states where the Internet pharmacy is located and registered regulates the practice of pharmacy. The board of pharmacy in states where consumers are given prescriptions enforces requirements for out-of-state pharmacies. A program called "Vet-VIPPS" may be used to help validate the legitimacy of online pharmacies. Vet-VIPPS is a voluntary certification program that was created by the National Association of Boards of Pharmacy (www.nabp.net). The Vet-VIPPS seal of approval validates that the online pharmacy is appropriately licensed and is conducting business legitimately. A related issue is the sale of "ethical products" by these Internet companies. These are products for which the manufacturer has voluntarily limited their sale to veterinarians as a marketing decision. Some flea and tick control products are ethical products registered with the EPA or the FDA in the over-the-counter category. Improper sale of these ethical products may then be an ethical rather than a legal issue. Another controversial issue involving Internet pharmacies is the alleged use of imported drugs that have not been approved by the FDA.

DISPOSAL OF UNWANTED DRUGS

Improper disposal of unused drugs can be a potential risk to people, animals, and the environment. When unwanted drugs are placed in the trash without placement in a secure container, accidental poisonings of people or animals are possible. Several studies have found pharmaceuticals in drinking water, lakes, and rivers. The AVMA recommends six basic practices for the disposal of unwanted pharmaceuticals to avoid potential risks of improper disposal of these products (Anonymous, 2012):

1. Incinerate unwanted drugs when possible. The drugs should be placed in leak-proof, tamper-resistant packing to prevent diversion. An absorbent such as kitty litter should be added to liquids. Liquids in syringes should be evacuated in an absorbent material and the material placed in a leak-proof container for disposal. Drugs in a labeled container should have all personal information blacked out; however the drug information should be visible. The drugs should be placed in a leak-proof, tamper resistant container. The containers with the drugs scheduled for disposal should be marked "For Incineration Only" and stored in a locked container until time for disposal. State and federal guidelines should be followed when incinerating unwanted pharmaceuticals.
2. Unused drugs should be sent to the landfill when incineration is not possible. Drugs should be prepared for sending to the landfill in a similar manner to those being incinerated. The containers should be marked for landfill disposal and kept locked until the time of disposal.
3. Never flush unwanted pharmaceuticals down the toilet or drain. Drugs flushed down the toilet or drain may show up in the water supply and may be a cause of potential danger to consumers similar to those caused by drug residues in animal products. Antibiotic resistance, allergic responses, and poisonings are some of the potential consequences.

4. Maintain close inventory control. Keeping a close watch over practice inventories can reduce the amount of expired and unused drugs. Prescriptions may be written for infrequently used drugs to prevent in-house expiration. Drugs nearing their expiration date should be returned to the distributor when feasible.
5. Always follow federal and state guidelines. While reverse distributors may be used to dispose of controlled substances held by veterinary clinics (Appendix F), the AVMA recommends that law enforcement agencies be used by clients for the disposal of unwanted controlled substances prescribed for their pets.
6. Educate clients on proper disposal.

REVIEW QUESTIONS

1. Define the following terms:
   a. Agonist ______________________
   b. Contraindication ______________________
   c. Efficacy ______________________
   d. Over-the-counter drug ______________________
   e. Prescription drug ______________________
   f. Receptor ______________________
   g. Therapeutic index ______________________
   h. Withdrawal time ______________________
   i. Veterinarian–client–patient relationship ______________________

2. List four sources of drugs used in veterinary medicine. ______________________ ______________________

3. What are four components of a drug regimen? ______________________

4. Discuss the conditions that must be met before a valid veterinarian–client–patient relationship can be shown to exist. ______________________ ______________________

5. Discuss the responsibilities of a veterinary technician in the administration of drug orders. ______________________

6. Describe the sequence of events that a drug undergoes from administration to excretion. ______________________

7. List 11 possible routes for administering a drug to a patient, and discuss the advantages and/or disadvantages of each. ______________________

8. List some of the factors that influence drug absorption. ______________________ ______________________ ______________________ ______________________

9. Most biotransformation of drugs occurs in which of the following?
   a. Kidney
   b. Liver
   c. Spleen
   d. Pancreas

10. Most drug excretion occurs via which of the following?
   a. Kidneys
   b. Liver
   c. Spleen
   d. Intestine

11. Drugs usually produce their effects by combining with specific cellular ______________________.

12. The drug name that is chosen by the manufacturer and that is the exclusive property of that company is called ______________________.

13. What are six items that must be included on a drug label? ______________________

14. What are three government agencies that regulate the development, approval, and use of animal health products? ______________________ ______________________ ______________________

15. Why do many veterinary clinics dispense rather than prescribe most of the drugs that they use? ______________________

16. Describe the marketing of animal health products. ______________________

17. All FDA-approved veterinary drugs are listed in the publication entitled ______________________ ______________________ ______________________.

18. What is the purpose of FARAD?

____

19. Extralabel veterinary drug use was made legal (under prescribed circumstances) by what act of Congress? ______________________

20. Define compounding. ______________________

21. What are the potential dangers of residues in animal products? ______________________

22. List three classes of drug interactions.

a. ______________________

b. ______________________

c. ______________________

23. Drug interaction can be anticipated when two drugs are given that are both metabolized by the ______________________.

24. Define "ethical product." ______________________

25. Once a drug has been biotransformed, it is called a ______________________.

26. An(a) ________ is a reason to use a drug.

a. contraindication
b. indication

27. The diagnostic method of choosing a drug is based on all of the following except ______.

a. practical experience
b. assessment of the patient
c. obtaining a history
d. performing laboratory tests

28. Extralabel use means ______________.

a. sold over the counter (OTC)
b. using a drug in a way not specified by the label
c. using a drug according to the empirical method
d. deciding how long the drug should be given

29. All the following are true about a veterinarian–client–patient relationship except:

a. The veterinarian has seen and treated all the client's pets except a dog for which the owner would like to buy heartworm preventative.
b. The veterinarian has assumed responsibility for making clinical judgments about the health of the animal(s) and the need for treatment, and the client has agreed to follow the veterinarian's instructions.
c. The veterinarian has sufficient knowledge of the animal(s) to issue a diagnosis. The veterinarian must have recently seen the animal and must be acquainted with its husbandry.
d. The veterinarian must be available for follow-up evaluation of the patient.

30. _______ is the complex sequence of events that occurs after a drug is administered to a patient.

a. Half-life
b. Metabolism (biotransformation)
c. Pharmacokinetics
d. Residue

31. Parenteral drugs are administered ____________.

a. orally
b. by injection
c. SC
d. ID

32. __________ is the body's ability to change a drug chemically from the form in which it was administered into a form that can be eliminated from the body.

a. Half-life
b. Metabolism (biotransformation)
c. Pharmacokinetics
d. Residue

33. The _____ of a drug represents the degree to which a drug produces its desired response in a patient.

a. pharmacodynamics
b. pharmacokinetics
c. efficacy
d. metabolism

34. An adverse drug reaction is always life threatening.

a. True.
b. False.

35. All the following agencies regulate animal health products except ____________.

a. FDA
b. EPA
c. AVMA
d. USDA

36. List the six practices recommended by the AVMA for the safe disposal of unwanted drugs

____

______________.

REFERENCES

American Veterinary Medical Association: Disposal of controlled substances (website). https://www.avma.org/Advocacy/National/Federal/Pages/Disposal-of-Controlled-Substances.aspx. Accessed January 31, 2012.

Anonymous: Partnership to promote proper vet drug disposal, J Am Vet Med Assoc 116:240, 2012.

Boothe DM: Principles of drug therapy. In Boothe DM, editor: Small animal clinical pharmacology, ed 2, Philadelphia, 2012, WB Saunders.

Davidson G: Pharmacy update: new FDA policy gives clear guidance for compounding, Vet Tech 18(3):195–201, 1997.

Mealey KL: Clinically significant drug interactions, Compend Contin Educ Proc Pract Vet 24(1):10–22, 2002.

Webb AI, Aeschbacher G: Animal drug container labels: a guide to the reader, J Am Vet Med Assoc 202:1591–1599, 1993.

Williams BR, Baer C: Introduction to pharmacology. In Williams BR, Baer C, editors: Essentials of clinical pharmacology in nursing, Springhouse, Pa, 1990, Springhouse Corp.

CHAPTER 2

Routes and Techniques of Drug Administration

OUTLINE

Introduction
Dosage Forms
Drug Preservatives and Solvents
Drug Administration
- Oral Medications
- Parenteral Medications
- Intramuscular Injections
- Subcutaneous Injections
- Inhalation Medications
- Topical Medications

Medication Orders
Dispensed Medication Labeling
Controlled Substances
Client Education

LEARNING OBJECTIVES

After studying this chapter, you should be able to

1. Discuss the many types of available drug forms.
2. List and explain the six rights of administering medication.
3. Name available types of syringes and needles, and describe their common uses.
4. Correctly read doses in a syringe.
5. Explain the techniques available for administering medications, the routes commonly used, and how the treatment should be documented.
6. Describe what is involved in preparing a prescription and explain how the prescription is posted to the medical record.
7. Describe proper labeling of dispensed medications.
8. Discuss some of the U.S. Drug Enforcement Administration (DEA) requirements for the use of controlled substances in a veterinary practice.

KEY TERMS

Cerumen
Counterirritant
Cream
Elixir
Emulsion
Liniment
Ointment
Parenteral administration
Speculum
Suspension

INTRODUCTION

In a busy veterinary practice, a veterinary technician often administers treatments ordered by the veterinarian. Proper administration techniques should be used along with accurate documentation on the medical record. Additionally, a veterinary technician must be knowledgeable about dosage forms, syringe construction, and hatch marks and must be able to draw correct amounts of medication within a syringe, know the six rights of drug administration, be capable of administering medication by all available routes, be knowledgeable in the area of client education regarding drugs, and know how to properly handle controlled substances. Proper documentation of administered treatments is of utmost importance and ensures that the same treatment is not repeated by other veterinary personnel. Knowledge of adverse reactions that animals may have to particular medications is also crucial. The veterinary technician is the veterinarian's most important employee in a busy practice. Through observation of the patient during treatments, the technician is able to provide the veterinarian with information regarding the patient's response. The doctor, thus informed, can easily reach decisions regarding adjustment of the treatment regimen. The technician who recognizes the importance of administering proper treatment to the patient and who uses observation skills in assessing patient response to that treatment is an invaluable asset to the practice.

DOSAGE FORMS

Pharmaceutic companies manufacture drugs in various forms. Some drugs are available in a variety of forms; others may be available for administration in only one form. Most pharmaceutic companies endeavor to provide comfort to the patient and ensure ease of administration when formulating their drugs. Some common drug preparations may be administered orally, parenterally, through inhalation, intrarectally, and topically. The most common type of preparation is an oral medication. Oral preparations are usually easy to administer, have extended expiration dates, and are manufactured uniformly with respect to the content of the drug.

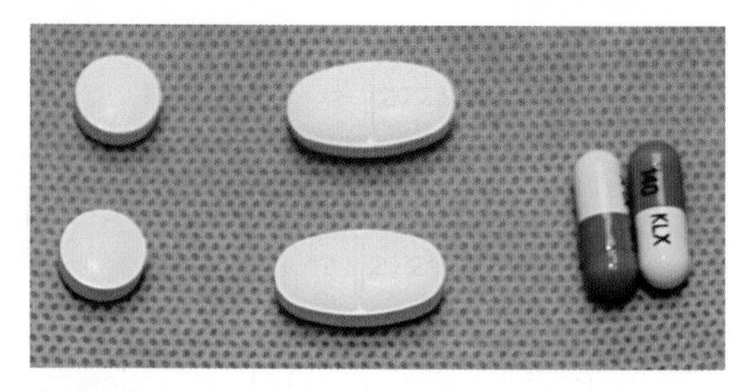

FIGURE 2-1 Tablets and capsules are the most common forms of oral medications.

Tablets are the most commonly used oral form (Figure 2-1). A tablet may be scored or unscored. A scored tablet has indentions that have been made into its surface, allowing it to be broken into halves or quarters. Therefore, a scored tablet provides a way of administering a smaller dose to the patient. A tablet that is unscored may be cut into a smaller size with the use of a pill cutter device. However, scored tablets break more readily and are less likely to fragment. Some tablets whose drug type may be irritating to the gastrointestinal tract may be enteric-coated. Capsules are containers that house medication. The capsule itself may be made of gelatin and glycerin. The contents of a capsule may be in powder or liquid form. Capsules may be advantageous to use because they allow a patient to be treated without an unpalatable taste coming into contact with the oral mucosa. Unfortunately, capsules cannot be broken down the way a scored tablet can to provide a smaller dose. Boluses are large rectangular tablets that may be scored or unscored. Boluses are used in the treatment of large animals (e.g., cattle, horses, sheep). Boluses usually are administered to bovines with the aid of a special instrument called a *balling gun.*

Liquid preparations for oral administration may be purchased in several different forms (e.g., mixtures, emulsions, syrups, or elixirs). Mixtures consist of aqueous solutions (i.e., water) and suspensions for oral administration. A **suspension** usually separates after long periods of shelf life and must be shaken well before it is used so that a uniform dose is provided. Syrups contain the drug and a flavoring in a concentrated solution of sugar water or other aqueous liquid. In veterinary medicine, an antibiotic (e.g., doxycycline) may be mixed with a liquid vitamin (e.g., Lixotinic) to ensure a more palatable taste for the patient. **Elixirs** usually consist of a hydroalcoholic liquid that contains sweeteners, flavoring, and a medicinal agent. **Emulsions** consist of oily substances dispersed in an aqueous medium with an additive that stabilizes the mixture. All liquid oral medications should be administered slowly to allow the patient to swallow before more liquid is given. Rapid administration of oral medication can result in aspiration into the lungs, thereby causing pulmonary problems.

> *TECHNICIAN NOTES* Rapid administration of oral medication can cause the liquid to be aspirated into the lungs, thereby causing pulmonary problems.

Two forms of parenteral injection that are available are injections and implants. Injections are available as single-dose vials, multidose vials, ampules, or large-volume bottles that may be used to administer intravenous (IV) infusions (Figure 2-2). A vial is a bottle that is sealed with a rubber diaphragm. A vial may contain a single dose or multiple doses. A single-dose vial must be discarded after one use (dose). Multidose vials usually contain preservatives that enable them to have a longer shelf life; thus they may be used for more than one dose. Ampules contain a single dose of medication in a small glass container with a thin neck, which is usually scored so that it can be snapped off easily. Some drugs may be unstable in solution and may require reconstitution with sterile water or another diluent; these may be used immediately for injection (Procedure 2-1).

> *TECHNICIAN NOTES* It is a good idea to place a paper towel over the neck of an ampule before breaking it, to protect the fingers from glass cuts.

Syringes and needles are used for parenteral administration of drugs (Box 2-1). This equipment must be sterile. Drugs should never be stored in syringes for a long time before administration occurs because some drugs may be absorbed into the plastic makeup of the syringe, resulting in an inadequate dose or inactivation of vaccines.

> *TECHNICIAN NOTES* All used needles should be discarded properly into a sharps container.

Implants are very hard sterile pellets that contain a chemical or a hormonal agent. Implants are inserted subcutaneously and are absorbed by the body over an extended time. Growth hormones are commonly manufactured in this form for use in cattle and are implanted in the subcutaneous dorsal aspect of the ear.

Topical medications are available in several forms. **Liniments** are medicinal preparations for use on the skin as a **counterirritant** or to relieve pain. Lotions are liquid suspensions or solutions with soothing substances that may be applied to the skin. An **ointment** is a semisolid preparation of oil and water,

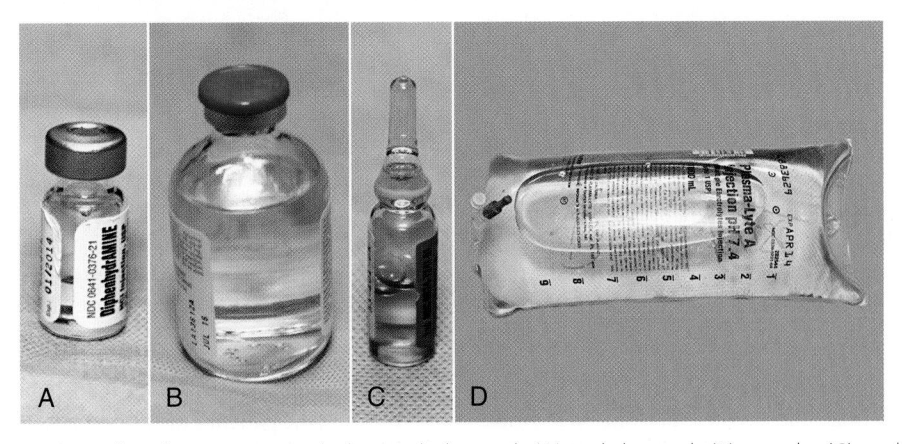

FIGURE 2-2 Parenteral medications are supplied in single-dose vials **(A)**, multidose vials **(B)**, ampules **(C)**, and large-volume bottles or bags used for intravenous administration **(D)**.

PROCEDURE 2-1

Reconstitution of a Medication

Materials Needed

Syringe of adequate size for the amount of diluent with a needle attached
70% isopropyl alcohol
Cotton swab

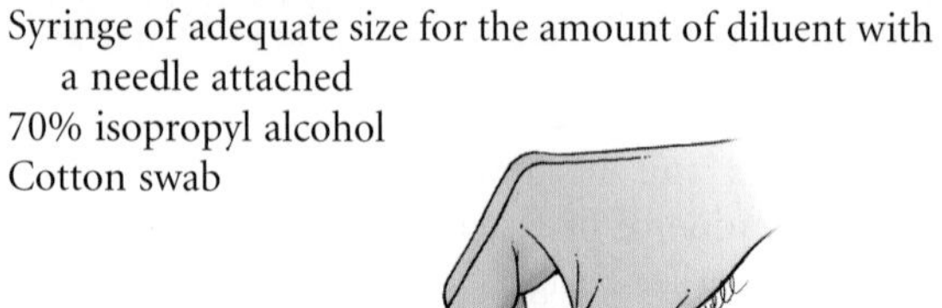

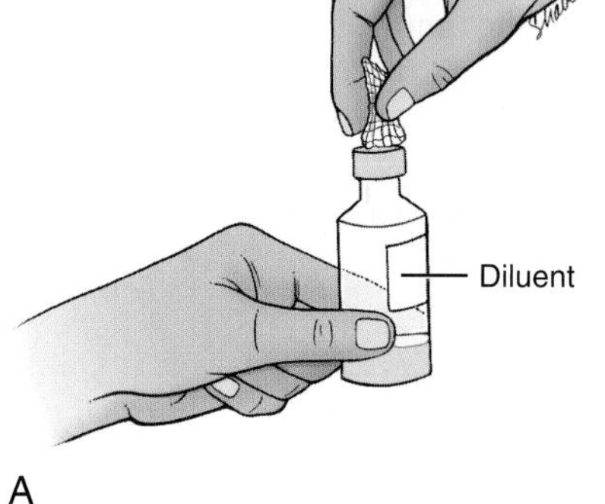

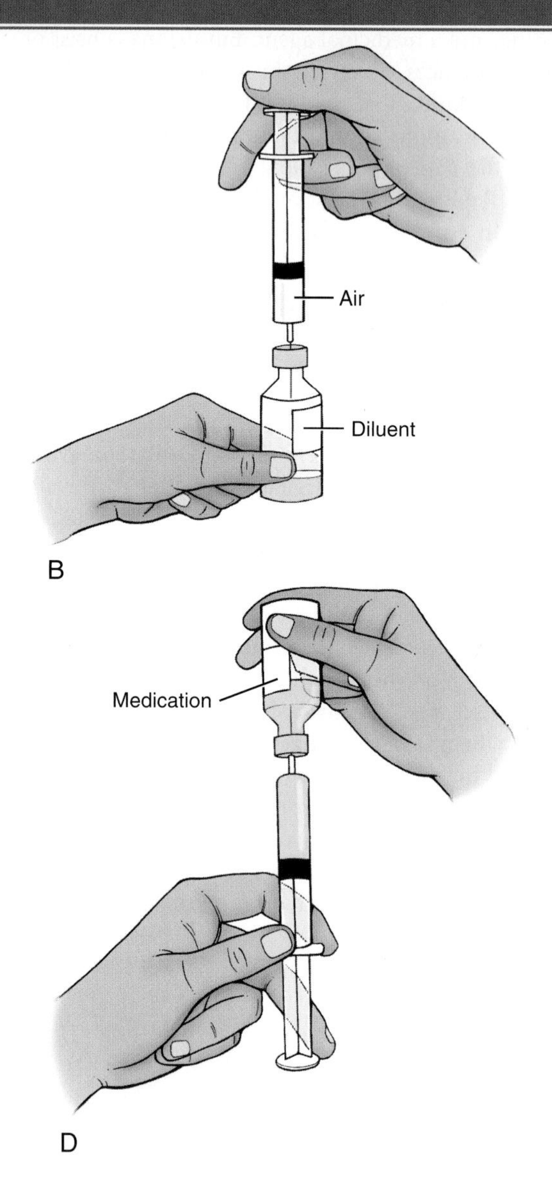

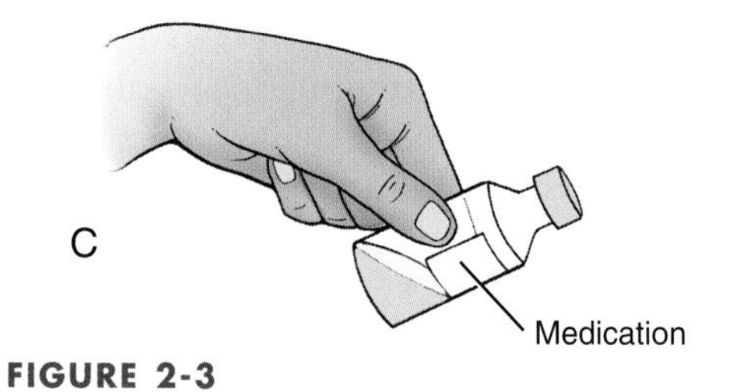

FIGURE 2-3

Procedure

1. Clean the rubber diaphragm of the medication vial and the diluent vial with an alcohol swab (Figure 2-3, *A*).
2. Remove the needle cap and pull back on the plunger to fill the barrel with air equal to the desired amount of diluent. Inject the air into the vial of diluent to create positive pressure and to ease withdrawal (Figure 2-3, *B*). Invert the diluent vial and withdraw the desired amount of diluent.
3. Inject the diluent into the medication vial and withdraw the syringe and needle. Shake the vial to mix well (Figure 2-3, *C*).
4. Positive pressure may be created in the freshly mixed medication vial before the desired amount of medication has been withdrawn. Once the medication has been withdrawn (Figure 2-3, *D*), label the syringe, and administer the drug to the patient. After withdrawing the patient's medication, dispose of the vial, or store it according to the label.

BOX 2-1 Syringes and Needles

Syringes

Syringes are available in various sizes and styles. The most commonly used sizes are 3 mL, 6 mL, 12 mL, 20 mL, 35 mL, and 60 mL. Syringes may be ordered from the manufacturer with or without an attached needle. The tip of the syringe, where the needle attaches, can be one of four types: Luer-Lok tip (Figure 2-4, *A*), slip tip (Figure 2-4, *B*), eccentric tip (Figure 2-4, *C*), or catheter tip (Figure 2-4, *D*). Each type of tip has its own advantages and disadvantages and is often chosen because of personal preference. A complete syringe consists of a plunger, barrel, hub, needle, and dead space (Figure 2-5). The area in which fluid remains when the plunger is completely depressed is called *dead space*.

Tuberculin syringe

A tuberculin syringe (Figure 2-6) holds up to 1 mL of medication. It usually is available with a 25-gauge or smaller attached needle. This syringe is commonly used for injections of less than 1 mL. Some tuberculin syringes have a dead space. Although the patient receives the proper amount of medicine, some liquid remains in this dead space, thus wasting the drug and costing the practice money. This is also important to remember when a tuberculin syringe is used to draw up controlled substances. The dead space will cause the controlled substance log book to reflect more controlled substance used than was actually administered from the vial. Thus, the dead space should be considered when amounts used are documented. Some tuberculin syringes are manufactured with low dead space or no dead space at all. In the case of syringes with no dead space, the needle screws into the tuberculin syringe instead of attaching to the tip.

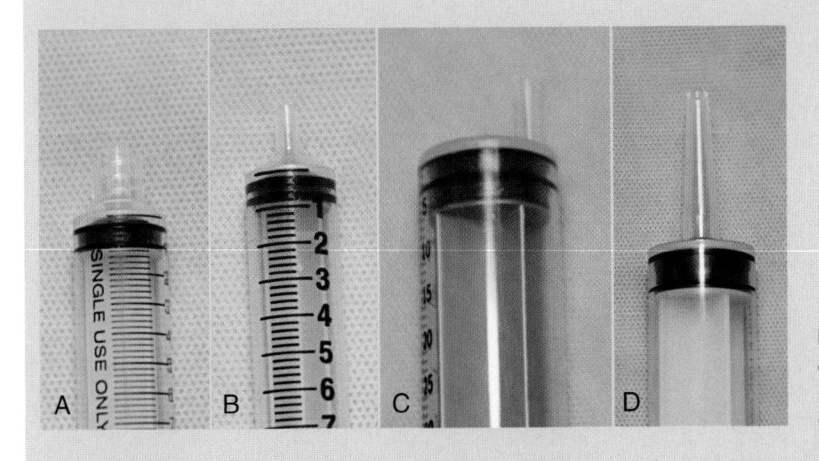

FIGURE 2-4 Syringes are available with different tips, such as Luer-Lok **(A)**, slip **(B)**, eccentric **(C)**, and catheter **(D)**.

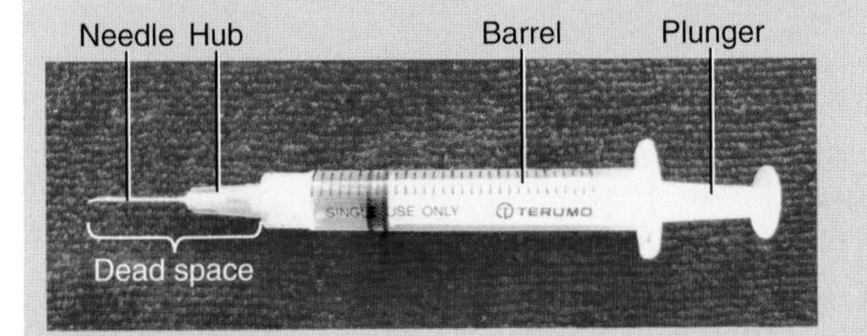

FIGURE 2-5 The parts of a needle and syringe. (From Sirois M: Elsevier's veterinary assisting textbook, St. Louis, 2013, Elsevier.)

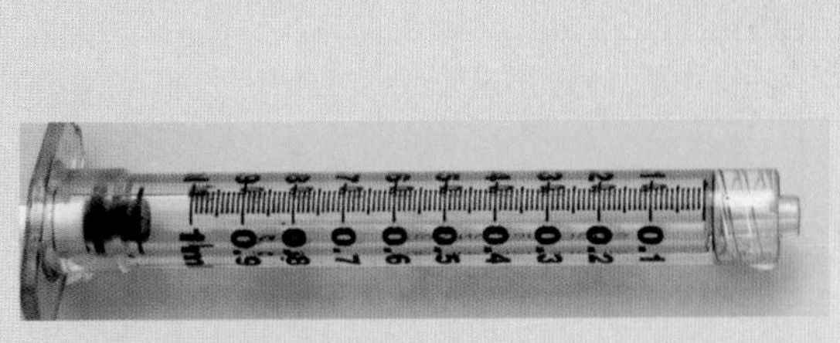

FIGURE 2-6 A tuberculin syringe. (From Mulholland J: The nurse, the math, the meds, St. Louis, 2011, Elsevier.)

Continued

BOX 2-1 Syringes and Needles—cont'd

Multidose syringe

A multidose syringe (Figure 2-7) is commonly used for large animals in cases when several animals require the same injection. It allows the user to set the dose and to give repeated injections until the barrel is empty of medication. This type of syringe may be disassembled and disinfected for reuse.

Insulin syringe

An insulin syringe (Figure 2-8) usually is supplied with a 25-gauge needle, and differing from other syringes, it has no dead space. The syringe is divided into units instead of milliliters and should be used only for insulin injection.

Figure 2-9 illustrates the importance of being familiar with the different types of syringes and the units of measurement found on each. This is necessary to ensure that one can draw up an accurate amount of medication.

FIGURE 2-7 A multidose syringe. (Courtesy Jorgensen Laboratories, Inc., Loveland, CO. In Sonsthagen T: Veterinary instruments and equipment, St. Louis, 2011, Elsevier.)

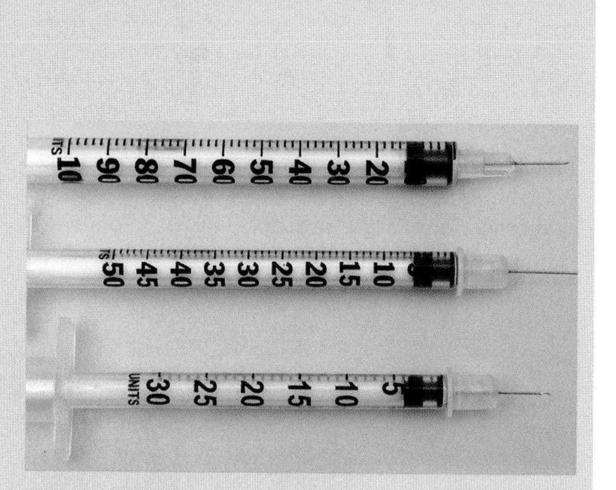

FIGURE 2-8 Insulin syringes. (From Mulholland J: The nurse, the math, the meds, St. Louis, 2011, Elsevier.)

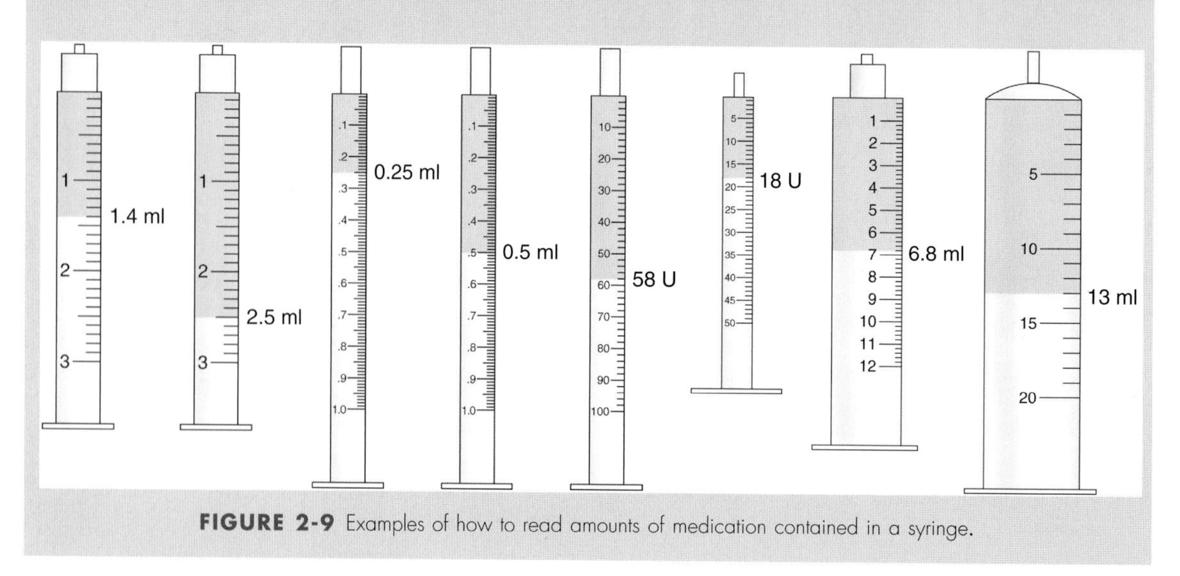

FIGURE 2-9 Examples of how to read amounts of medication contained in a syringe.

BOX 2-1 Syringes and Needles—cont'd

Needles

Needles are available in various sizes and styles, but all needles have the following three parts: hub, shaft, and bevel (Figure 2-10). Needle sizes vary by gauge and by length (Table 2-1/Figure 2-11). The gauge refers to the inside diameter of the shaft; the larger the gauge number, the smaller the diameter. The length of the needle is measured from the tip of the hub to the end of the shaft. Lengths longer than 1 inch usually are used in large animals and occasionally for biopsy. The bevel is the angle of the opening at the needle tip. It is often helpful when venipuncture is performed to have the beveled side of the needle facing up before the needle is inserted into the patient.

Bleeding needles (Figure 2-12) may be up to 3 inches long, are large gauge (14 to 16 gauge), and usually are used for obtaining blood from cattle and swine. These needles are made of stainless steel and are reusable after proper cleaning and disinfecting.

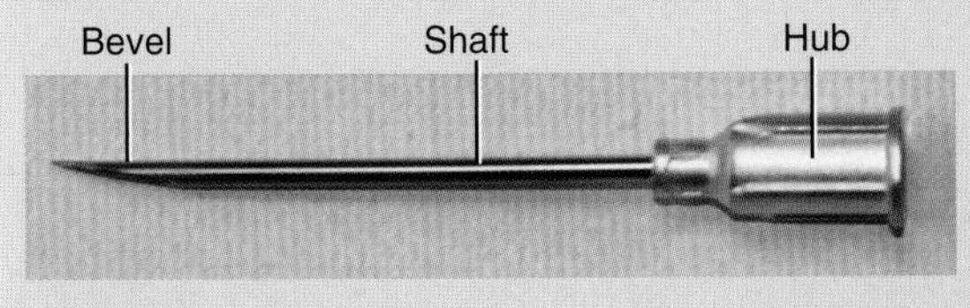

FIGURE 2-10 A needle consists of three parts: hub, shaft, and bevel.

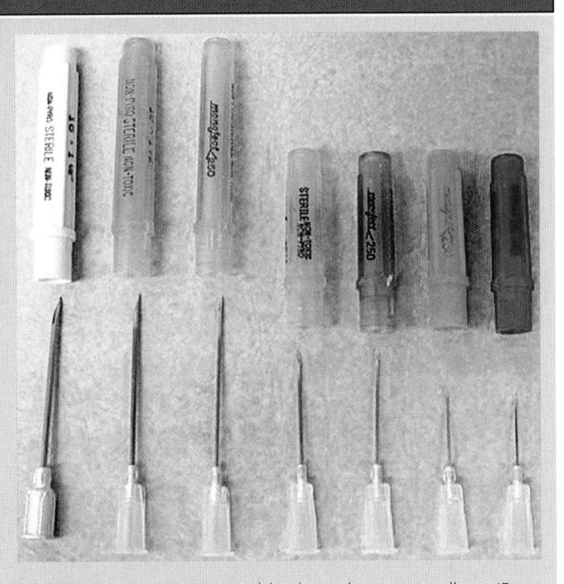

FIGURE 2-11 Disposable hypodermic needles. (From Sonsthagen T: Veterinary instruments and equipment, St. Louis, 2011, Elsevier.)

TABLE 2-1 Commonly Used Needle Gauges for Different Animals

ANIMAL	NEEDLE GAUGE
Swine	16, 18
Cattle	16, 18
Horses	16, 18, 20
Dogs	20, 21, 22, 25
Cats	22, 25
Small exotics	23, 25, 27

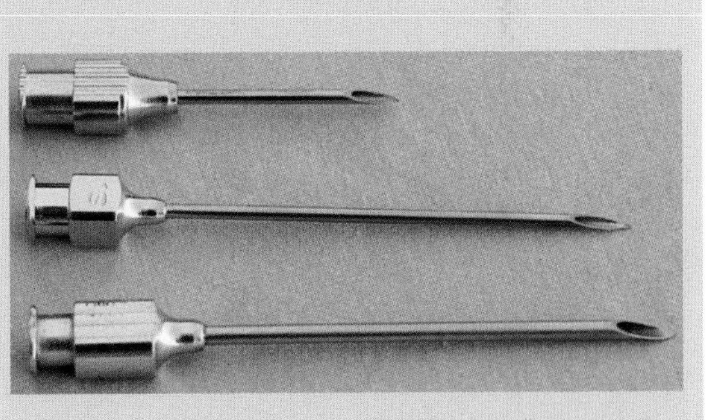

FIGURE 2-12 Stainless steel bleeding needles. (From Sonsthagen T: Veterinary instruments and equipment, St. Louis, 2011, Elsevier.)

plus a medicinal agent. The water in an ointment evaporates after application and leaves the drug behind on the skin's surface. Dusting powders (e.g., flea powder) are mixtures of drugs in powder form for topical application. Additionally, powders may have adsorbent (cornstarch) or lubricant (talcum) properties. Aerosols are drugs that have been incorporated into a suitable solvent and packaged under pressure with a propellant. Dusting powders and aerosols are common forms for some topical insecticides and wound dressings.

Microencapsulation is a drug form that stabilizes substances commonly considered unstable. Microencapsulation also may be used for drugs intended to be released slowly over a period of time (e.g., moxidectin [ProHeart injection]). When the drug's active ingredients are microencapsulated, a protective environment is formed against harmful substances and the stability of the product is improved. Microencapsulation completely masks the flavor of a drug and allows oral treatments to be administered with greater ease because the patient is unable to taste or smell the ingredients.

DRUG PRESERVATIVES AND SOLVENTS

In addition to the active ingredient, many drugs contain organic or inorganic agents as additives or pharmaceutic aids. These inactive (or inert) ingredients facilitate tablet administration, improve solubility, or increase stability. Although the quantity of inert ingredients is usually small, these ingredients can cause adverse effects, or a patient may be sensitive to or may smell the ingredients.

Parenterally administered drugs often contain chemical preservatives that are used to prevent destruction and loss of potency through oxidation or hydrolysis. The amount of preservative in the formulation of parenterally administered drugs is an optimal concentration, and the reconstituted medication should be used immediately to prevent the possibility of fungal or bacterial growth. Dilution of the drug reduces the effectiveness of the preservatives. Most drugs are water soluble, although some may need additives to increase solubility. Glycols are one example of additives used to increase solubility. Generally, propylene glycol and polyethylene glycols are preferred.

> **TECHNICIAN NOTES** Some vaccines may contain antibiotic preservatives. Care should be taken by personnel during reconstitution of these vaccines because liquid that escapes from the rubber seal of the vial could be sprayed inadvertently into an allergic person's eye (e.g., those persons with hypersensitivity to penicillin).

DRUG ADMINISTRATION

A veterinarian initiates administration of drugs for therapeutic purposes. (It is unlawful for a veterinary technician to prescribe drugs for an animal patient.) The role of the technician is to administer drugs to the patient on the order of a veterinarian. When doing this, a technician must always follow the *six rights:*

1. Right patient
2. Right drug—check label three times before administering the drug
3. Right dose
4. Right route
5. Right time and frequency
6. Right documentation

By following these rules, a technician will efficiently and effectively medicate a patient.

Oral Medications

The most common forms of drug therapy are tablets and capsules. These are easily administered (Procedure 2-2) and are sometimes used in conjunction with other drug forms.

In large animals, a balling gun (Figure 2-16) is used to administer boluses. Proper restraint and careful use of the instrument are necessary for proper administration and avoidance of injury to the patient.

Liquid oral medications may be administered to small animals through a syringe with the needle removed (Procedure 2-3 and Figure 2-17) or, in some instances, through an orogastric or nasogastric tube. Medications may be made more palatable for these patients by mixing with a vitamin mixture or food to ease administration. Oral liquid medications used in exotic animals may be administered through the drinking water or an orogastric tube. In large animals, a dose syringe (see Figure 2-16) is used to give small

PROCEDURE 2-2

Oral Administration of Tablets or Capsules for Dogs and Cats

Materials Needed

Medication in tablet or capsule form
Pilling gun (optional) (Figure 2-13)

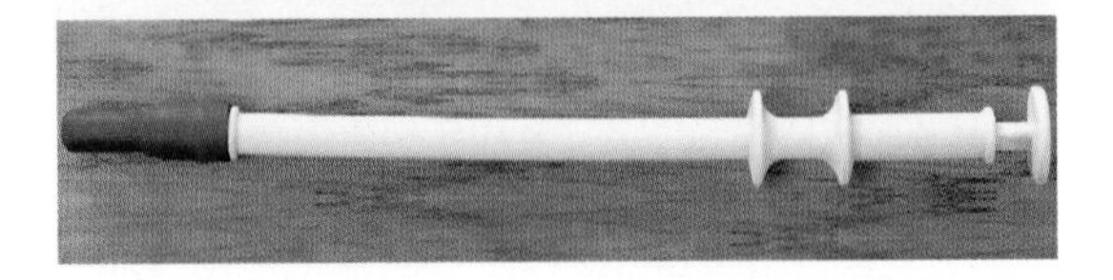

FIGURE 2-13 Example of a small-animal pilling gun. (From Sonsthagen T: Veterinary instruments and equipment, St. Louis, 2011, Elsevier.)

Procedure

1. Hold the animal's upper jaw with one hand and apply pressure against the upper premolars to cause the mouth to open.
2. Push the medication over the tongue of the animal with the other hand or with the pilling gun (Figure 2-14)
3. Close the animal's mouth.
4. Initiate swallowing by blowing into the animal's nose and/or rubbing its throat (Figure 2-15).

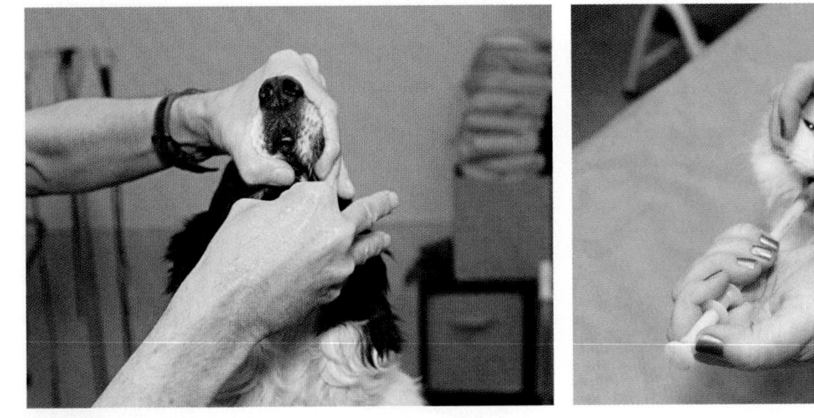

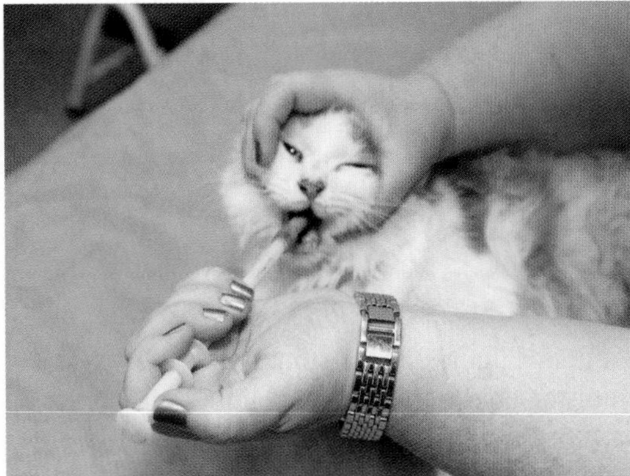

FIGURE 2-14

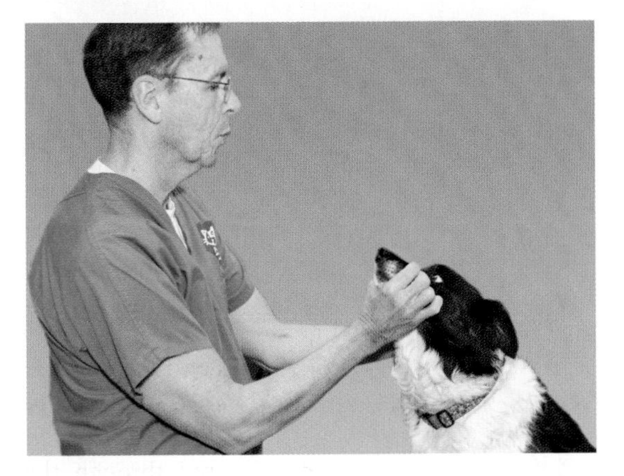

FIGURE 2-15

TECHNICIAN NOTES Coating the tablet or capsule with a palatable substance such as Cat Lax, peanut butter, or canned food may help in pilling difficult animals.

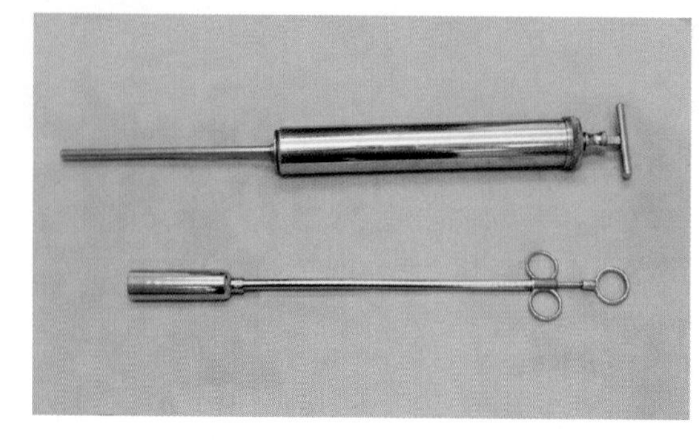

FIGURE 2-16 A balling gun used to administer a bolus to large animals and a dose syringe used to administer small volumes of liquids.

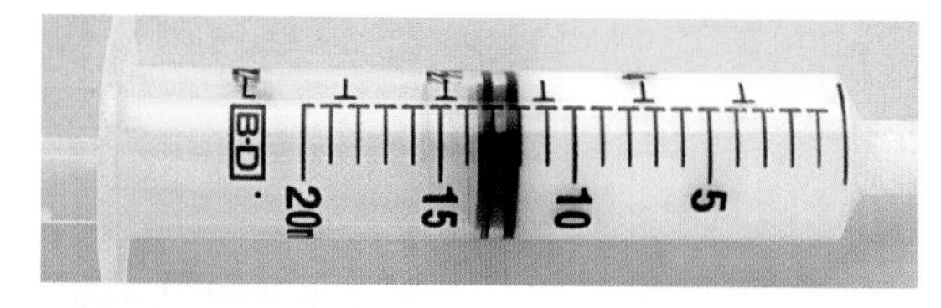

FIGURE 2-17 A syringe without a needle may be used to administer oral liquid medication. (From Macklin D, Chernecky C, Infortuna H: Math for clinical practice, 2nd edition, St. Louis, 2011, Mosby.)

amounts of liquids and a stomach tube is used to administer large amounts of oral liquid medications. In horses, the tube is passed via the nasogastric route (Figure 2-18, *A-C*). In cattle, the stomach tube is passed through a Frick **speculum** (Figure 2-19) via the orogastric route.

> **TECHNICIAN NOTES**
> - Remember when administering oral medications that it takes longer for a drug to be absorbed into the bloodstream by this route than by parenteral injection.
> - Do not use oral administration in animals that are vomiting.

Parenteral Medications

Parenteral administration (i.e., injection) of liquid medications may be used alone or in conjunction with other forms of medication. Some conditions are unfavorable for oral administration (e.g., in vomiting

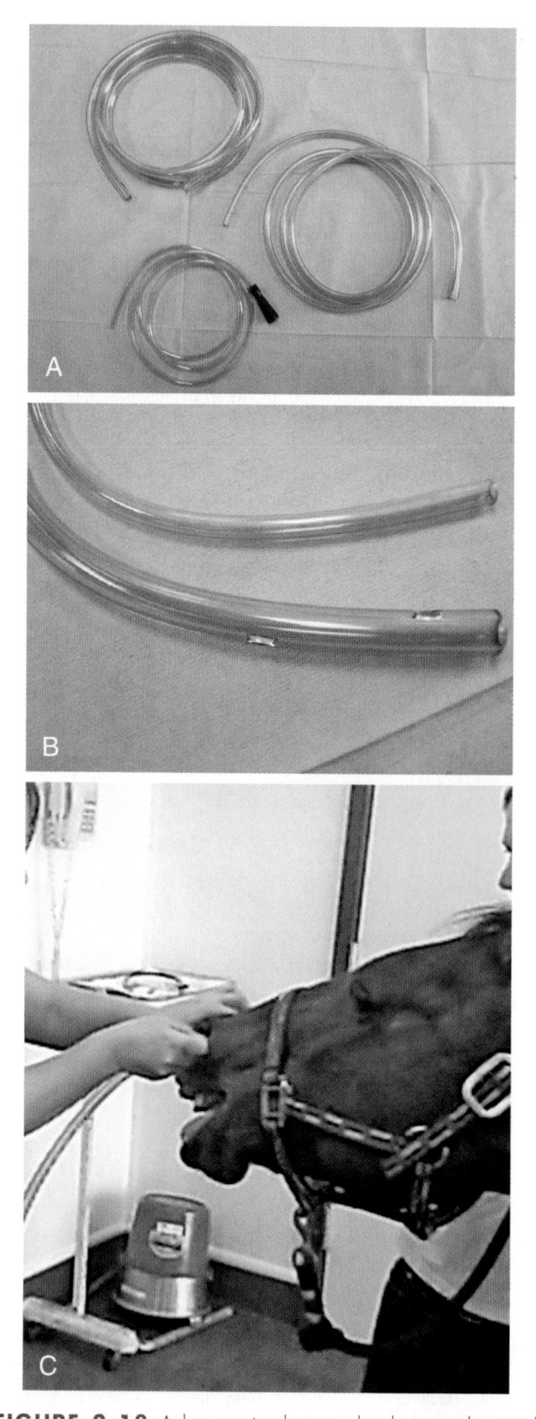

FIGURE 2-18 A large-animal stomach tube may be used to administer liquid medications to horses via the nasogastric route **(A-C)**. (A & B, from Hanie EA: Large animal clinical procedures for veterinary technicians, St. Louis, 2006, Mosby. C, from Sirois M: The principles and practices of veterinary technology, 2011, Elsevier.)

patients), and some drugs are available only for parenteral administration.

Approximately 10 routes are used commonly for **parenteral administration** of drugs; the most commonly used are the intramuscular, subcutaneous, and IV routes (Figures 2-21, 2-22, and 2-23). A veterinary technician must be aware of the proper route of administration for each drug. For those in doubt, the route of administration usually is listed on the drug label or the package insert. Sometimes, complications may result after parenteral administration of a drug. Common complications include irritation, necrosis, and infection of the injection site. Sometimes, allergic reactions to medications may occur. Clinical signs of an allergic reaction after a parenteral drug has been administered include swelling around the face or extremities, raised bumps or swellings on the skin's surface, edema, and salivation. If any complications are observed, these should be reported immediately to the veterinarian. Care should be exercised when an intramuscular injection is administered so that nerve damage or accidental injection into a vein or artery can be avoided. Negative pressure should be applied to the plunger of the syringe before an intramuscular (or subcutaneous) injection is performed. Should any blood be observed in the hub of the needle, the needle should be redirected or removed. Care should also be exercised when intraperitoneal injections are provided so that peritonitis does not develop and damage the abdominal viscera. Proper administration involves knowing (1) what equipment is needed, (2) how the

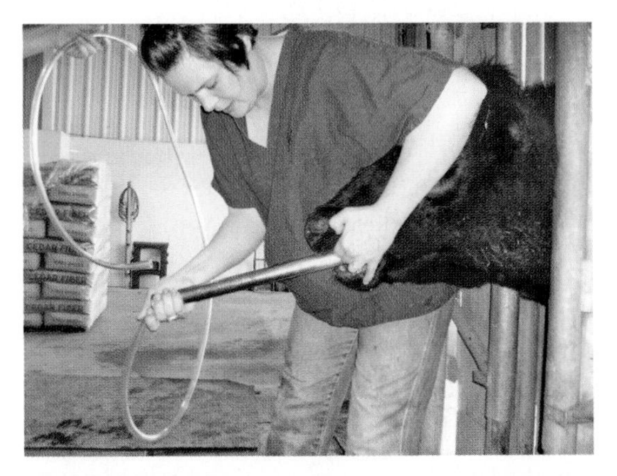

FIGURE 2-19 A Frick speculum can be used to facilitate passage of the stomach tube through the mouths of cattle. (Holtgrew-Bohling K: Large animal clinical techniques, 2011, Elsevier.)

PROCEDURE 2-3

Oral Administration of Liquid Medication With a Syringe for Dogs and Cats

Materials Needed

Syringe with the needle removed or oral dose syringe
Oral medication in liquid form

Procedure

1. Fill syringe with the calculated amount of medication.
2. Tilt the animal's head up slightly.
3. Insert the tip of the syringe into the animal's cheek pouch (Figure 2-20).
4. Administer the medication slowly.

TECHNICIAN NOTES Attachment of a J-12 Teat Infusion Cannula (Jorgensen Laboratories, Loveland, Colo) is helpful for administering oral liquid medications.

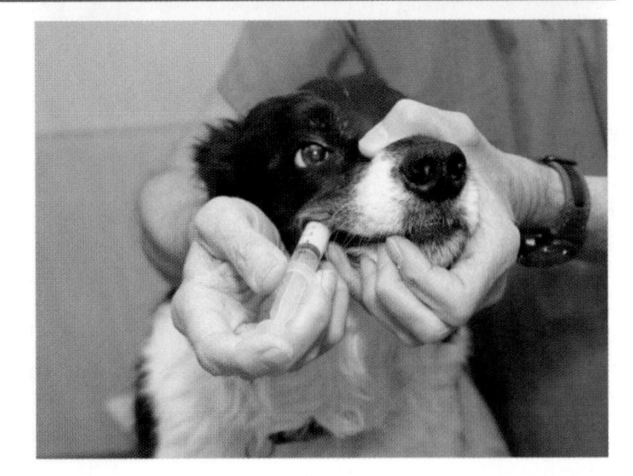

FIGURE 2-20

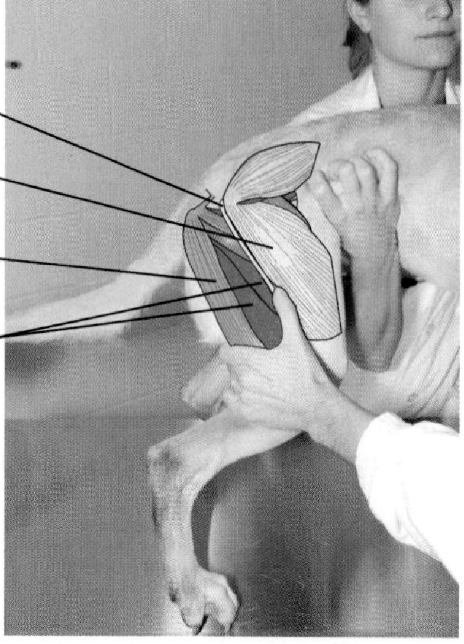

FIGURE 2-21 Intramuscular injections in the pelvic limb should be given in an area that avoids the large sciatic nerve. (Meric Taylor S: Small animal clinical techniques, 2009, Elsevier.)

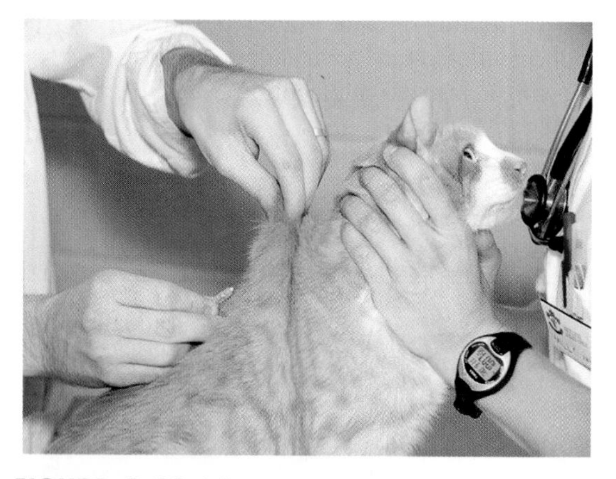

FIGURE 2-22 Subcutaneous injection. (Meric Taylor S: Small animal clinical techniques, 2009, Elsevier.)

dose should be calculated, and (3) the proper method for withdrawing and administering medication (Procedure 2-4).

IV administration allows the most rapid and effective drug administration (Procedure 2-5). IV therapy is used most commonly to maintain and restore fluid and electrolyte balance, to administer drugs, and to transfuse blood. IV administration

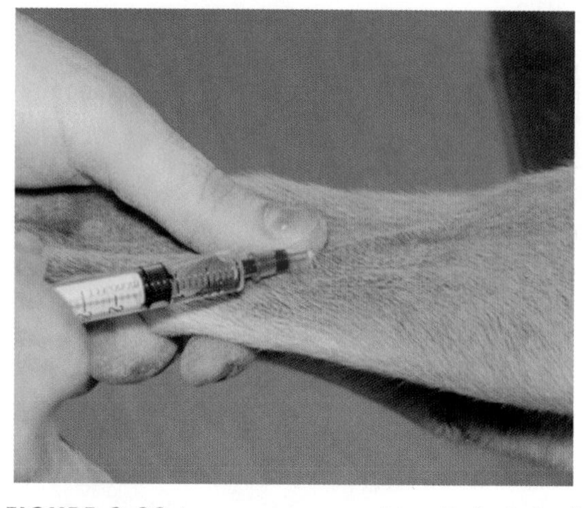

FIGURE 2-23 Intravenous injection. (Meric Taylor S: Small animal clinical techniques, 2009, Elsevier.)

also is used when the medication is contraindicated for other routes of administration. Sites for IV administration include the cephalic vein, the jugular vein, the lateral saphenous vein, and sometimes the femoral veins. Long-term IV therapy is best achieved with the cephalic or jugular veins.

In some cases, an animal may need repeated IV injections. The veterinarian may order the placement of an indwelling IV catheter in an effort to lessen vein damage and pain for the animal (Procedures 2-6 and 2-7).

> **TECHNICIAN NOTES** Intravenous (IV) catheters should be inspected frequently and changed if signs of phlebitis or other complications appear. Time of placement can be accounted for by writing (e.g., use a permanent marker) placement time on the adhesive bandage that secures the IV catheter in the animal's vein. IV and extension sets should be changed out on a schedule in accordance with clinic policy.

If the patient is receiving IV fluids, the Y-injection site (see Figure 2-28)—located on the IV tubing—may be used to administer medications by direct bolus (Procedure 2-8). When medications are to be administered continuously and for long periods, the IV tubing may be changed after a 48-hour to 72-hour

Text continued on page 43

PROCEDURE 2-4

Parenteral Administration of Medications—Intramuscular or Subcutaneous

Materials Needed

Syringe and needle (Figure 2-24)
Parenteral medication
Cotton swabs
70% isopropyl alcohol

Procedure

1. If the syringe is not supplied ready-to-use, firmly attach the needle to the syringe.
2. Swab the bottle's rubber diaphragm with cotton that is saturated with alcohol.
3. Remove the needle cap, insert the needle at an angle into the rubber diaphragm, and withdraw the calculated amount of the drug.
4. Hold the syringe with the needle pointing upward, and remove the large air bubbles by briskly tapping the barrel of the syringe.
5. Release the air bubbles by slightly pushing on the syringe plunger. Carefully replace the needle cap if the medication is not to be given immediately. Avoid contamination.
6. Swab the injection site with another cotton swab that is saturated with alcohol.
7. Insert the needle into the appropriate site and pull slightly on the plunger. If no blood is seen, inject the medication and remove the needle from the site. Blood indicates that a vessel has been entered. Withdraw the needle and continue with the same procedure at a different site.
8. Massage the injection site to aid distribution and decrease pain.
9. Properly dispose of the syringe and needle.

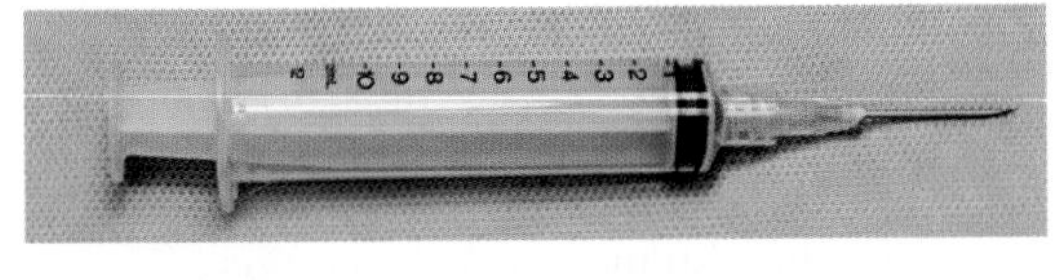

FIGURE 2-24

Guidelines for Parenteral Doses

- Round up to the nearest tenth if the amount is greater than 1 mL, and measure in a 3-mL syringe.
- Measure amounts less than 1 mL in a tuberculin syringe.
- In cats weighing less than 9 lb, 0.5 to 1 mL is an appropriate amount for intramuscular injection.
- In cats weighing more than 9 lb, 1 to 1.5 mL is an appropriate amount for intramuscular injection.
- In dogs weighing up to 10 lb, 0.5 to 1 mL is an appropriate amount for intramuscular injection.
- In dogs weighing 10 to 30 lb, 1 to 2 mL is an appropriate amount for intramuscular injection.
- In dogs weighing more than 30 lb, 2 to 4 mL is an appropriate amount for intramuscular injection.

TECHNICIAN NOTES Injecting multidose vials with air sometimes allows easier withdrawal of medication.

PROCEDURE 2-5

Parenteral Administration of Medication—Intravenous Direct Bolus

Materials Needed

Syringe containing calculated dose with needle attached
Cotton swabs
70% isopropyl alcohol or surgical scrub
Butterfly catheter (scalp vein needle, Figure 2-25)—optional
Syringe containing 3 mL of flushing solution (e.g., heparinized saline: 500 IU sodium heparin in 250 mL of normal saline)
Tape (optional)

Procedure Without Catheter

1. Clip the area over the venipuncture site, if desired.
2. Prepare the area with alcohol swabs or surgical scrub.
3. Have the restraint person hold pressure on the vein or use a tourniquet.
4. Perform venipuncture with the medication syringe and needle. If blood enters the hub of the needle, the venipuncture is successful.
5. Release pressure from the vein and inject the medication over the recommended time interval.
6. Remove the needle and apply pressure to the site to stop bleeding.
7. A bandage made of tape and cotton may be applied, if needed.

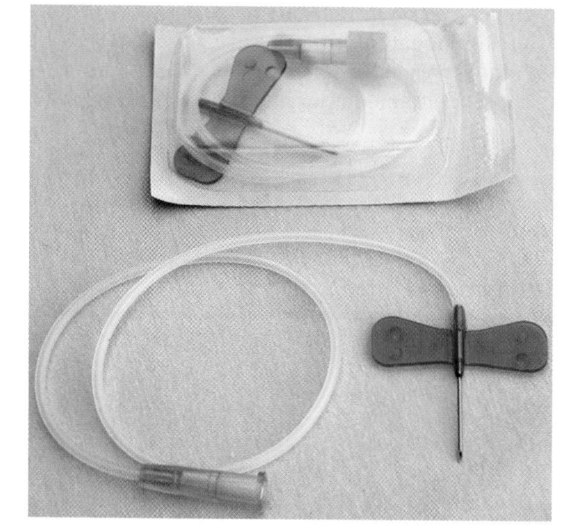

FIGURE 2-25 Butterfly catheter. (From Sonsthagen T: Veterinary instruments and equipment, 2011, Elsevier.)

Procedure With a Butterfly Catheter

Proceed with steps **1 through 3** as described in the previous section (McCurnin and Bassert, 2010).

4. Remove the cap from the catheter tubing and needle cover.
5. Perform venipuncture with the catheter. If this is successful, blood will return into the catheter tubing.
6. Release pressure from the vein, and allow the blood to fill the catheter tubing.
7. Remove the needle from the medication syringe and attach the syringe hub to the catheter tubing.
8. Administer the medication at the recommended time interval.
9. Remove the needle from the syringe containing the flushing solution. Remove the medication syringe from the catheter and attach the syringe containing the flushing solution.
10. Flush the catheter with 1 to 2 mL of solution to ensure administration of all medication.
11. Remove the catheter and apply pressure to the site to stop the bleeding.
12. A bandage may be applied as described earlier.
13. Properly dispose of all syringes and needles in an approved sharps container.

TECHNICIAN NOTES Watch for swelling at the injection site. Swelling may signal extravascular injection. Notify the veterinarian immediately if this should occur.

PROCEDURE 2-6

Administration by Bolus With an Indwelling Intravenous Catheter

Materials Needed

Syringe containing flushing solution (about 3 mL)
70% isopropyl alcohol
Cotton swabs
Syringe with medication and attached needle

Procedure

1. Clean the cap of the indwelling catheter with an alcohol swab.
2. Insert into the catheter cap the needle of the syringe containing the flushing solution. (Use the smallest gauge needle possible to help prevent a leak in the catheter cap.)
3. Gently aspirate to determine correct placement of the catheter (blood entering the hub shows proper placement).
4. Inject half the flushing solution into the catheter. Observe the area over the vein for swelling.
5. Remove the syringe and needle, and carefully replace the cap to prevent contamination.
6. Insert into the catheter cap the needle of the syringe containing the medication, and inject the medication over the recommended time interval.
7. Remove the syringe and needle from the catheter.
8. Flush the catheter with the remaining flushing solution.
9. Observe the area for swelling and look for signs of discomfort. Report any abnormal observations to the veterinarian.
10. Properly dispose of syringes and needles.

TECHNICIAN NOTES Some hospitals may require that, with flushing solution, two syringes should be used instead of the same syringe and needle for both flushes. Keep additional male adapter plugs (catheter caps) (Figure 2-26) in stock to replace a leaky cap.

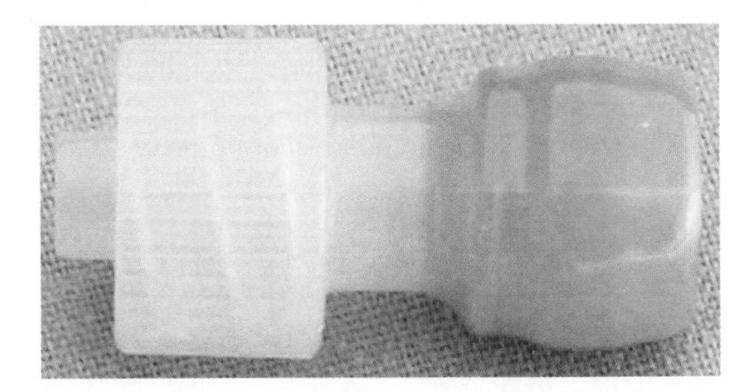

FIGURE 2-26 Example of a male adapter plug. (From Sonsthagen T: Veterinary instruments and equipment, 2011, Elsevier.)

PROCEDURE 2-7

Administration of Intravenous Fluids

Materials Needed

Indwelling catheter (Figure 2-27)
Tape
70% isopropyl alcohol or surgical scrub
Infusion set
Intravenous (IV) fluids
Clippers

Procedure

1. Remove the IV tubing from the container and the protective covering from the medication bottle or bag.
2. Remove the covering of the diaphragm of the medication bag or bottle.
3. Close the clamp on the IV tubing. Remove the cap of the IV tubing spike and insert it into the diaphragm of the medication bag or bottle.
4. Squeeze the drip chamber to allow fluid to collect in the chamber. Fill to the designated line or about half full.
5. Remove the protective cap from the end of the IV tubing and slowly open the roller clamp to allow the fluid to clear the tubing of air. Replace the protective cap and hang the medication bag or bottle on the IV pole near the patient.
6. Clip and scrub the chosen site for catheter placement.
7. After successful catheter placement, cap the catheter, wipe away any blood, and quickly tape in place. The time of placement should be recorded on the adhesive tape with a permanent marker.
8. Remove the catheter cap and the protective cap of the IV tubing and insert the end of the tubing directly into the end of the catheter. Or, if desired, a needle may be placed on the end of the tubing and inserted into the catheter cap.
9. Open the clamp to begin a slow drip and lower the medication bag or bottle to below the IV site to confirm correct placement.
10. Return the bottle or bag to the IV pole and set at desired flow rate.
11. Tape the tubing to the patient at the catheter site.

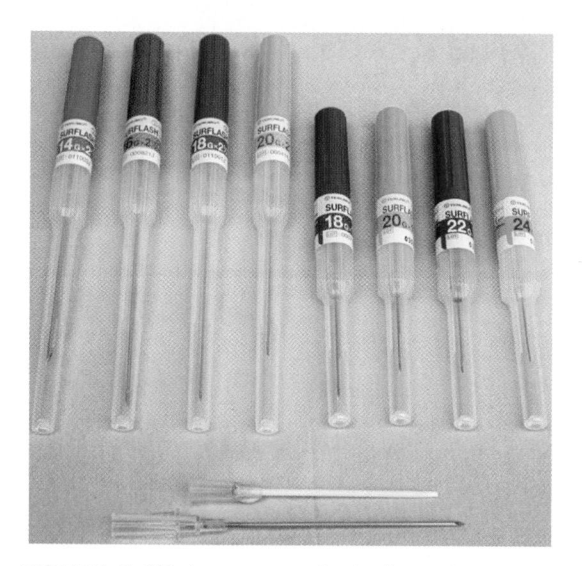

FIGURE 2-27 An assortment of indwelling catheters. (From Sonsthagen T: Veterinary instruments and equipment, 2011, Elsevier.)

TECHNICIAN NOTES

- Mark the fluid level and time on tape placed on the bag with a permanent marker (tape can be used on bottles). Use this procedure each time the patient is checked.
- If any medications are added to the fluids, write the medication, time, and amount on the medication bag or tape.
- Tape the catheter cap to the bag or bottle so that it will be ready when needed.

PROCEDURE 2-8

Administration by Bolus Using the Y-Injection Site

Materials Needed

Syringe with medication and the needle attached
Cotton swabs
70% isopropyl alcohol

Procedure

1. Close the clamp on the infusion set.
2. Clean the Y-injection site (Figure 2-28) with an alcohol swab.
3. Insert the needle of the medication syringe into the Y-injection site.
4. Inject the medication over the recommended time interval.
5. Remove the medication syringe and needle.
6. Open the clamp on the infusion set. Allow enough fluid to flow through the infusion set to ensure that all medication is received. Then return to the desired flow rate.
7. Properly dispose of the syringe and needle.
8. *Note:* No flushing solution is required for this procedure.

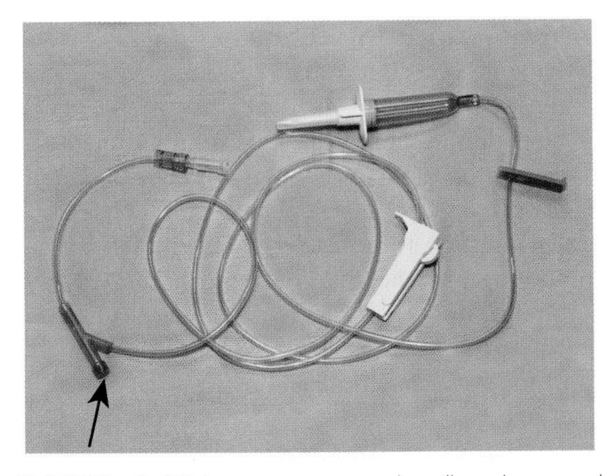

FIGURE 2-28 Intravenous set with roller clamp and Y-injection site.

TECHNICIAN NOTES To check for proper placement of the intravenous (IV) catheter, remove the bag of fluids from the IV pole and hold the bag and tubing below the level of the catheter (do not close the clamp on the infusion set). If blood returns into the tubing, the catheter is properly placed. Return the bag to the IV pole and continue fluid administration.

period (Veterinary Information Network Discussion Boards, 2013) or in accordance with clinic policy. Once the medication bottle or bag has been emptied, replacement is necessary to facilitate care of the patient. An indwelling catheter must be inspected frequently and changed if phlebitis or other complications occur. Recent studies have shown that catheter complications are related more to the lack of sterile technique in placement than the length of time it has been in place, although 72 to 96 hours generally should not be exceeded (Veterinary Information Network Discussion Boards, 2013). If the IV catheter is not used continuously, it should be flushed with saline every 8 to 12 hours. Some studies have shown that adding heparin to solutions used to flush catheters may not add any value over saline alone (Veterinary Information Network Discussion Boards, 2010).

A Simplex (i.e., gravity set) IV set may be used to administer medications or fluids intravenously to large animals (Figure 2-29). This administration set may be disinfected and reused. Disposable IV sets and large-volume fluid bags are available for large animals that require continuous IV therapy.

In pediatric patients and small exotics, IV medications may be administered by intraosseous cannulation. This route also may be used in larger patients when rapid administration of fluids or drugs is

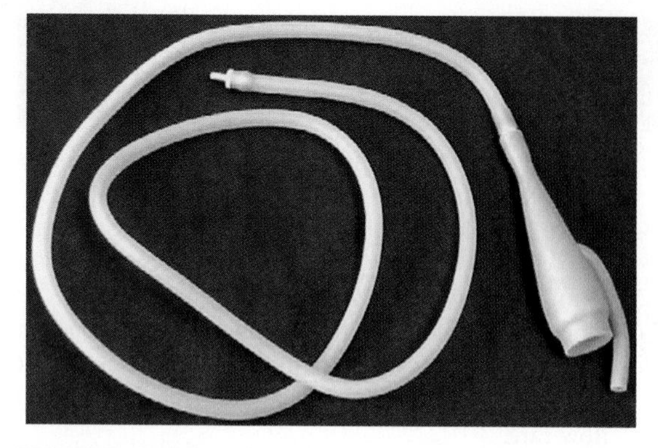

FIGURE 2-29 A large-animal intravenous set (Simplex). (Courtesy Jorgensen Laboratories, Inc., Loveland, CO. In Sonsthagen T: Veterinary instruments and equipment, 2011, Elsevier.)

necessary and a vein is not readily available. If needed, large volumes of fluid may be administered in this manner.

In some veterinary hospitals, the use of an infusion pump may facilitate continuous IV administration. Once the necessary flow rate is known (the rate is ordered by the veterinarian), the technician can set the infusion pump to deliver a constant amount of solution per minute or hour. To determine the pump settings, the technician considers the total amount of solution to be given and the time interval for infusion. The operating instructions for the infusion pump should be followed because each model may operate in a slightly different manner.

TECHNICIAN NOTES It should be remembered that any patient receiving IV fluid therapy should be monitored every 15 to 30 minutes.

Monitoring involves evaluating drip rate, ensuring that the IV catheter is properly placed in the vein, making sure the patient has not moved around in the cage to such an extent that the IV tubing has become kinked, and, most importantly, ensuring that the patient has not chewed on and thus dislodged the IV catheter. Animals can do surprising things, and it is up to the technician to provide an excellent level of nursing to ensure that no harm comes to the patient.

TECHNICIAN NOTES

- Some liquid medications for parenteral administration may "settle out" or precipitate (e.g., penicillin G procaine, triamcinolone acetonide [Vetalog]). Therefore these medications should be shaken gently to mix the solution before it is injected into the patient.
- Drugs that may cause tissue irritation are administered by the intravenous route (e.g., vincristine). Therefore, be sure to check the drug's package insert to identify the correct way to administer the drug.

Intramuscular Injections

- Ketamine (Ketaset) can be administered by intramuscular injection. Ketamine has a tendency to burn on injection, and careful restraint methods, along with rapid injection of this drug, should be used in cats.
- On insertion of the needle into the chosen muscle, always apply negative pressure to the syringe's plunger to be certain that the needle has not entered a blood vessel. If blood is seen in the hub of the syringe, remove and redirect the needle.

Subcutaneous Injections

- Most vaccines can be administered subcutaneously. However, the intrascapular area should always be avoided when subcutaneous injections are given.

Inhalation Medications

In veterinary medicine, inhalation is used primarily to produce anesthesia. The inhalant gas is placed into the anesthetic machine in liquid form and then is vaporized through the machine and delivered to the patient via an endotracheal tube, an anesthetic gas mask, or an induction chamber (Figures 2-30, 2-31, and 2-32). Medications occasionally may be nebulized to treat an upper respiratory tract problem, and oxygen may be delivered to a patient with dyspnea with the use of inhalation techniques.

Topical Medications

Topical administration of medicine involves application of drugs (**creams**, ointments, and drops) to the body's surface. Topical preparations usually provide

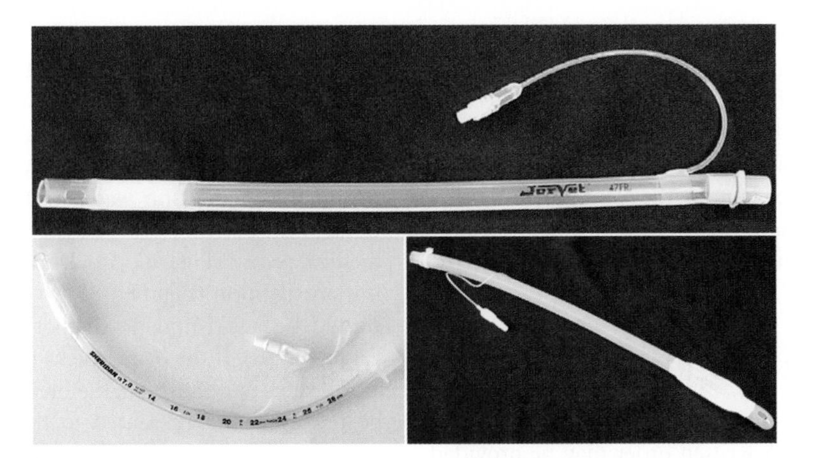

FIGURE 2-30 Endotracheal tube with cuff. (Courtesy Jorgensen Laboratories, Inc., Loveland, CO. In Sonsthagen T: Veterinary instruments and equipment, 2011, Elsevier.)

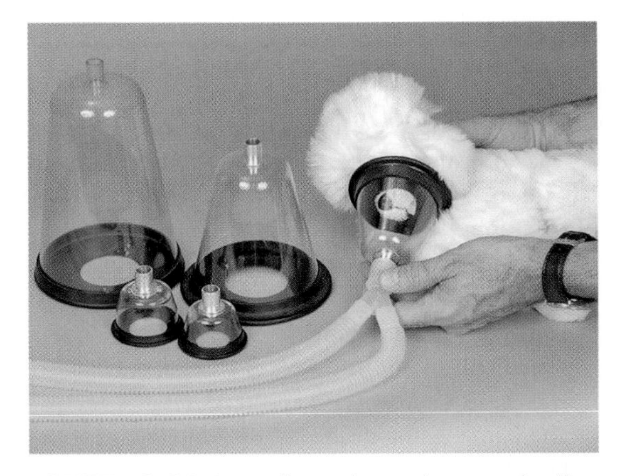

FIGURE 2-31 A small-animal anesthetic mask. (From Thomas J: Anesthesia and analgesia for veterinary technicians, 2011, Elsevier.)

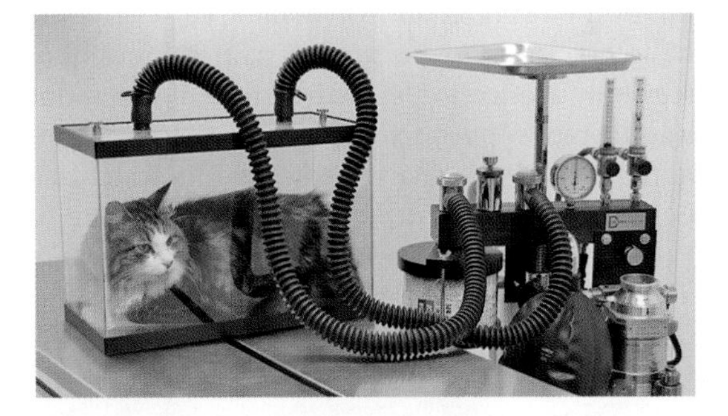

FIGURE 2-32 A small-animal induction chamber. (From Thomas J: Anesthesia and analgesia for veterinary technicians, 2011, Elsevier.)

local effects instead of systemic ones. Clipping hair from the affected area provides better visualization during treatment and makes application easier and absorption faster. The technician should observe the area after treatment and should report adverse reactions to the veterinarian. The technician should provide client education regarding skin medications, including information on frequency and number of applications. Many clients apply too much medication, which not only is unnecessary but also can be quite costly with some medications.

Ophthalmic drugs are supplied as an ointment or a solution. The eyes have the ability to remove foreign substances rapidly. Therefore, these preparations usually are applied several times a day. Application frequency depends on the disease or disorder, the drug, and the type of formulation. When ophthalmic preparations are applied, the hand that is holding the medication should rest on the animal's head above the affected eye (Figure 2-33). Drops should be placed at the inner canthus of the eye. If application of ointment is necessary, a small strip should be applied along the lower palpebral border; the applicator tip should not come into contact with the eye or conjunctiva. When you are demonstrating to a client how to apply eye medications, point out that the applicators have blunt tips. Therefore should the applicator tip inadvertently touch the eye, no harm should occur.

Drugs may be applied topically to the ears for local effect to soften **cerumen** and ease its removal or to treat a superficial infection or ear mites. Cleaning of the ears before otic medication is applied aids the effectiveness of treatment. The veterinary technician should provide instruction to the client regarding the correct ways to clean ears and to apply ear medication. By explaining the ear's anatomy, the technician can assure the client that it is difficult to reach the animal's eardrum when one is swabbing the ear clean.

MEDICATION ORDERS

In a veterinary hospital, most medication orders are written or verbal. A written order may be provided in prescription form or may be noted in the medical record. Verbal orders are given directly to the technician by the veterinarian. When filling a prescription, the technician must be familiar with abbreviations frequently applied to the medical record to describe drug therapy. Appendix A lists abbreviations commonly used in veterinary medicine. The technician must know the patient being treated, the route of administration used, and the frequency of administration. This information is described in the medication order. After the medication has been administered to the patient, a notation should be made in the medical record describing when, what, how, and by whom the medication was administered. Observations of the patient's progress should be noted in the medical record (Figure 2-34). If the medication order is a prescription (Figure 2-35) to be filled, the order should be dated and noted in the medical record (Figure 2-36). If the owner picks up the prescription at the veterinary hospital, the medical record should be retrieved and presented to the veterinarian for approval of the refill. The same procedure as described earlier should be followed for dispensing medication.

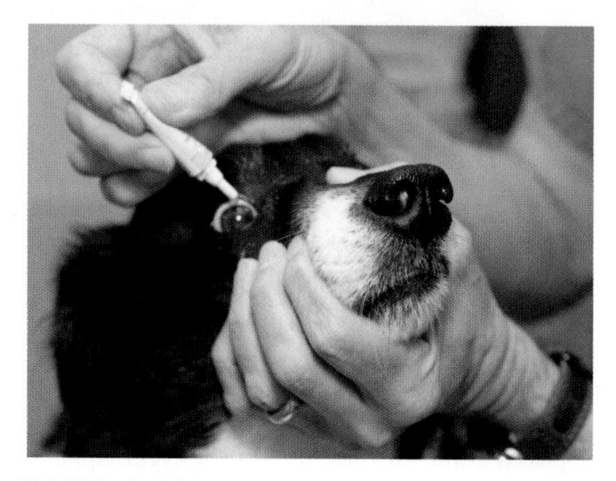

FIGURE 2-33 Ointment is applied to a dog's eye on the lower palpebral border.

DISPENSED MEDICATION LABELING

When a drug is prescribed for a patient, the drug label is an important part of the dispensing process. It is important that the label contain the following information:

- The veterinary facility's name, address, and telephone number.
- The veterinarian's name.
- The client's name and address.
- The patient's name and species.
- The name of the drug.
- The strength of the drug.
- The quantity being dispensed.
- Instructions to the client about how the drug should be administered.
    - The amount to be given for each dose.
    - The manner in which the drug should be administered.
    - How often the drug should be given.
    - Information that includes the duration of administration.

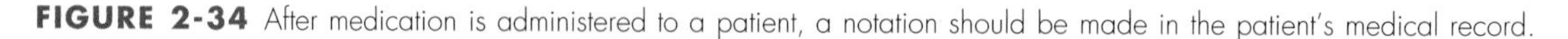

6-18-13 9:30 AM patient B&A
T-102°
250 mg Amoxicillin PO, flushed IV catheter
with 3 mL heparinized saline continue IV
lactated ringers at 15 gtt/min C. Smith, LVMT

FIGURE 2-34 After medication is administered to a patient, a notation should be made in the patient's medical record.

- The number of refills permitted.
- The expiration date of the drug being dispensed.
- The statement "for veterinary use only" should be included on the label.
- Optional statement to include is "keep out of reach of children."

CONTROLLED SUBSTANCES

Substances that have the ability to become habit-forming for humans are labeled as *controlled substances.* Every veterinarian who orders, dispenses, prescribes, or administers controlled substances must be registered with the Drug Enforcement Administration (DEA). This registration is valid for 3 years. The DEA further requires that the upper right corner of the original container of controlled substances should show a code containing a capital C (controlled), followed by a Roman numeral indicating one of the five schedules defined by the *Code of Federal Regulations* (Figure 2-37). Because some of these drugs may be misused, the DEA requires that they be kept in an unmovable locked area and that an inventory log be kept to report amounts used (administered or dispensed) and on hand (Figure 2-38). Records must also show the flow of controlled substances into and out of the practice including when drug are acquired, inventoried, stolen, lost, or distributed. These records must be readily retrievable and may be computerized. An inventory of all controlled substances must be completed at least every 2 years.

Each time a controlled drug is administered or dispensed to a patient, this event must be reported in the controlled substance inventory log, as well in the patient's medical record. This documentation should include the following: (1) date, (2) owner's name, (3) patient's name, (4) drug name, (5) amount administered or dispensed, and (6) the names of veterinary personnel who dispensed the drug.

Some of the common controlled substances used in veterinary clinics include analgesics and anesthetics like ketamine, tiletamine (Telazol), diazepam, pentobarbital, morphine, and butorphanol tartrate (Torbugesic). Others include diphenoxylate, hydrocodone, and phenobarbital. Anabolic steroids such as

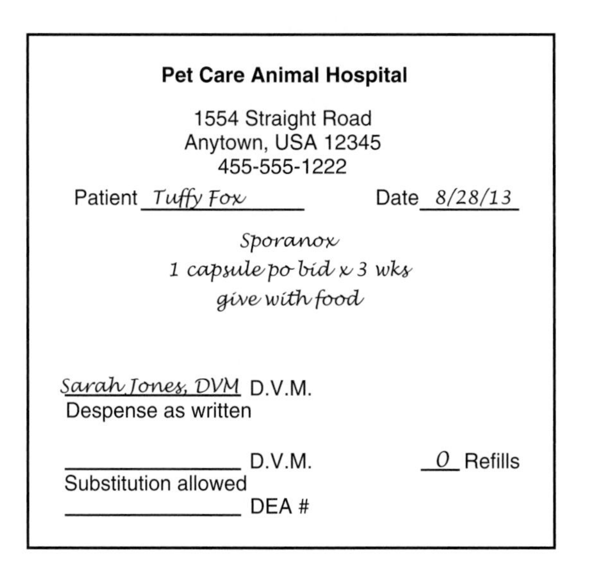

Pet Care Animal Hospital

1554 Straight Road
Anytown, USA 12345
455-555-1222

Patient Tuffy Fox Date 8/28/13

Sporanox
1 capsule po bid x 3 wks
give with food

Sarah Jones, DVM D.V.M.
Despense as written

______ D.V.M. 0 Refills
Substitution allowed
______ DEA #

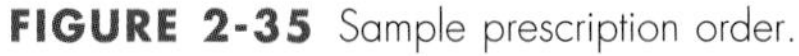
FIGURE 2-35 Sample prescription order.

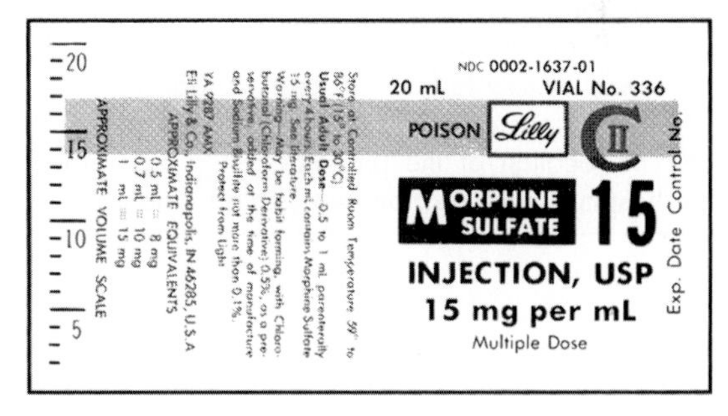

FIGURE 2-37 Label showing schedule II controlled substance designation. (From Mulholland J: The nurse, the math, the meds, 2011, Elsevier.)

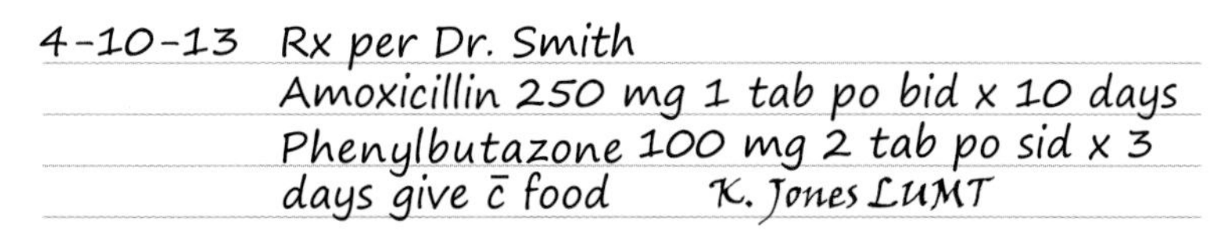

FIGURE 2-36 Prescriptions should be written in the patient's medical record.

Record of controlled substances administered/dispensed

Name of controlled substance: Ketamine Form: Injection Strength: 100 mg/mL Size: 10mL

Date	Patient/Animal name and address	Species of Animal	Initials of Person Administering/ Dispensing	Previous Balance	Amount Administered/ Dispensed (or purchased)	New Balance
1/10/13	Tim Smith / Toby	K-9	BD	10.0mL	1mL	9mL
1/15/13	Bill Potts / Prissy	Feline	LW	9mL	0.5mL	8.5mL
2/3/13	Chris Pettes / Gilbert	K-9	KM	8.5mL	2mL	6.5mL
2/8/13	Elaine Curtis / TJ	Feline	BD	6.5mL	0.4mL	6.1mL

FIGURE 2-38 Example of a controlled substance log.

stanozolol, testosterone, mibolerone, and boldenone are also controlled.

See Appendix F for more details on DEA regulations.

TECHNICIAN NOTES

Drug Storage

- The manufacturer's instructions should be followed closely to facilitate safe storage.
- Some drugs are sensitive to light and humidity.
- The location of the pharmacy in a veterinary hospital should not be accessible to the public.

CLIENT EDUCATION

Veterinary technicians should make themselves familiar with all administered and dispensed drugs. Often, it is the technician's duty to educate clients about how a medication should be administered, why it has been prescribed, and what adverse reactions may occur, if any. Technicians should consult the veterinarian to gather information about any questions that they cannot answer. If needed, written information about the medication should be available for the client's reference purposes.

REVIEW QUESTIONS

1. Name four common drug preparations.
   ____
2. Boluses are used in the treatment of ____________________ animals and are administered with a ____________________.
3. Name two types of parenteral injection forms.
   ____
4. Vials may be either ____________________ dose or ____________________ dose.
5. All used needles should be discarded in a ____________________.
6. Name the six rights of drug administration.
   ____________________.
7. Oral drugs should never be administered in animals that are ____________________.
8. Intravenous administration of drugs allows the most ____________________ and effective drug administration.
9. An indwelling catheter should be replaced with a new one every ____________________ hours.
10. A Simplex (i.e., gravity set) IV system is used to administer fluids to ____________________ animals.
11. Name six items that should be recorded in the controlled substance log ______.
12. Why should drugs given by injection not be stored in syringes for any length of time before administration? ____________________.
13. List four types of syringe tips that are available for use. ____________________
14. A tuberculin syringe holds up to ____________________ mL of medication.
15. What type of syringe is divided into units rather than milliliters?
16. A(n) ____________________ is an agent that produces superficial irritation that is intended to relieve some other irritation.
    a. elixir
    b. emulsion
    c. liniment
    d. counterirritant
17. A(n) ________ will usually separate after long periods of shelf life and must be shaken well before use to provide a uniform dose.
    a. elixir
    b. antimicrobial
    c. suspension
    d. anthelmintic
18. This type of syringe is constructed in such a way that the needle screws onto the tip of the syringe.
    a. Slip tip
    b. Eccentric tip
    c. Catheter tip
    d. Luer-Lok tip
19. All the following are sites for IV administration in small animals, except ______.
    a. jugular vein
    b. carotid artery
    c. lateral saphenous vein
    d. phalic vein
20. An indwelling catheter must be replaced every ___ hours.
    a. 48
    b. 24
    c. 60
    d. 72
21. If an IV catheter is not used continuously, it should be flushed with heparinized saline every __ to ___ hours.
    a. 6; 12
    b. 4; 18
    c. 8; 12
    d. 8; 10
22. Cerumen is a substance that is commonly found in what anatomic part of the body?
    a. Urinary bladder
    b. Ear
    c. Rectum
    d. Crown of the tooth
23. Any patient receiving IV fluid therapy should be monitored every ___ to ___ minutes.
    a. 1; 2
    b. 15; 30
    c. 90; 120
    d. 60; 120

24. IV tubing should be changed after a ___ to ___ hour period.
a. 12; 24
b. 12; 48
c. 12; 36
d. 48; 72

25. When an intramuscular injection is given in the pelvic limb of a dog or cat, the area near the _____ nerve should be avoided.
a. radial
b. sciatic
c. median
d. both b and c

REFERENCES

McCurnin DM, Bassert JM, editors: Clinical textbook for veterinary technicians, ed 6, Philadelphia, 2010, Elsevier Saunders.

Veterinary Information Network: Is flushing with heparinized saline still recommended to maintain catheter patency (website)? http://www.vin.com/Members/Boards/DiscussionViewer.aspx?documentid=4446868&ViewFirst=1. Accessed February 9, 2010.

Veterinary Information Network: Reuse of intravenous extension tubing or giving sets (website). http://www.vin.com/Members/Boards/DiscussionViewer.aspx?documentid=3995391&ViewFirst=1. Accessed February 9, 2013.

CHAPTER

3

Practical Calculations

KEY TERMS

Dosage rate
Dose
Equivalent weight
Milliequivalent
Percent concentration
Ratio concentration
Solution
Stock solution

OUTLINE

Introduction
Mathematic Fundamentals
Systems of Measurement
Metric System
Conversion Between Metric Units
Apothecary and Household Systems
Dosage Calculations
Solutions
Percent Concentrations
Calculations Involving Concentrations
MillieQuivalents
Calculations Involving Intravenous Fluid Administration
Calculations for Constant Rate Infusion Problems

LEARNING OBJECTIVES

After studying this chapter, you should be able to

1. Exhibit an understanding of the systems of measurement.
2. Explain how to perform conversions while using the metric system and other systems of measurement.
3. Demonstrate how to perform dosage calculations.
4. Explain how percent concentrations are prepared.

INTRODUCTION

Veterinary technicians often are asked to prepare and administer medications to animal patients. A veterinarian's orders may ask for administration of a specific number of milligrams or units of medication (dose). The technician then must determine the quantity (e.g., in milliliters or tablets) of the preparation that contains the appropriate dose. In other instances, the technician may be asked to calculate the dose on the basis of a dosage rate (found in the insert or in reference books) and the animal's weight. In either case, an error in calculation can seriously affect the health of a patient. This chapter provides the background information and applications needed by the veterinary technician to accurately carry out a veterinarian's medication orders.

MATHEMATIC FUNDAMENTALS

It is assumed that the student who uses this text has a basic understanding of fractions and decimals. With these fundamentals as a background, the concepts of percent, ratio, and proportion should be reviewed before the practice problems are solved.

Percent is defined as parts per hundred. Percent is a fraction with the percent as the numerator and 100 the denominator (e.g., 5% = 5/100). Percents may be written as decimals, fractions, or whole numbers.

Example 1: Decimal: 0.3%
(three-tenths percent [3/10 ÷ 100])
Fraction: 1/5%
(one-fifth percent [1/5 ÷ 100])
Whole number: 5%
(five percent [5 ÷ 100])

Percent may be changed to fractions or decimals.

Example 2: Change to a fraction:

$$5\% = 5/100 = 1/20$$

Change to a decimal:

$$5\% = 5/100 = 0.05$$

Note that a percent can be changed to a decimal quickly by dropping the percent sign and moving the decimal two places to the left.

Example 3:

$$5\% = 0.05$$

A *ratio* is a way of expressing the relationship of a number, quantity, substance, or degree between two components. In reality, ratios are fractions, with the first number in the ratio the numerator and the second number the denominator. The numbers may be placed side by side, separated by a colon, or they may be set up as a numerator/denominator (e.g., 1:5, 1/5). In mathematics, a ratio may be expressed as a quotient, a fraction, or a decimal, per the following:

Example 4:

$$1 \div 5, 1/5, 5\overline{)1.0} = 0.2$$

A *proportion* shows the relationship between two ratios. When a proportion is set up, the two ratios usually are separated by an = (equals) sign.

Example 5:

$$8:16 \text{ as } 1:2 \text{ or } \frac{8}{16} = \frac{1}{2}$$

The proportions above read "8 is to 16 as 1 is to 2." The two inner numbers in the first example (16 and 1) are called the *means,* and the two outer numbers (8 and 2) are called the *extremes.* In a true proportion, the product of the means equals the product of the extremes (16 × 1 = 16; 8 × 2 = 16). This fact makes the proportion a useful mathematical tool. When a part of the problem is unknown, *X* can be substituted for the unknown part in the proportion and the equation solved for *X*. Care must be taken to ensure that the proportion is set up correctly, and that the same unit of measure is used on both sides of the equation.

Example 6:

$$8:16 = 1:X \text{ or } \frac{8}{16} = \frac{1}{X}$$

$$8X = 16$$

$$X = 2$$

Example 7: To convert 0.2 g to milligrams, calculate the following:

$$1000\ \text{mg} : 1\ \text{g} = \text{X mg} : 0.2\ \text{g or } \frac{1000\ \text{mg}}{1\text{g}} = \frac{\text{X mg}}{0.2\text{g}}$$

$$\text{X} = 200(1000 \times 0.2)$$

SYSTEMS OF MEASUREMENT

The first step in the successful calculation of doses is to develop an understanding of the units of measure used to carry out the calculations. These units are components of the following three separate systems:

1. Metric system
2. Apothecary system
3. Household system

All three systems are expressed in the fundamental units of weight, volume, and length. Technicians should be able to convert values within each system and between the three systems.

Metric System

The fundamental units of measurement in the metric system are the gram (weight), the liter (volume), and the meter (length). Gram is abbreviated *g* or *gm,* liter is abbreviated *L* or *l,* and meter is abbreviated *m.* The usefulness of the metric system is that all units are powers of the fundamental units. Prefixes are used in combination with fundamental units to denote smaller or larger quantities. Table 3-1 illustrates the units of measurement used in the biologic sciences.

The units that are used most commonly in dosage calculations include the gram, the kilogram (kg; 1000 g), the milligram (mg; 1/1000 g), and the milliliter (mL; 1/1000 L). It should be noted that a milliliter is equivalent to the quantity of water contained in 1 cubic centimeter (cc), which is also equivalent to 1 g of weight. Therefore, for practical purposes, it may be said that 1 mL = 1 cc = 1 g.

On occasion, the microgram (μg) may be used. (It should be noted that this unit also may be abbreviated as *mcg.*) Care should be taken to differentiate this abbreviation from *mg,* which looks very similar when written orders are used.

Conversion Between Metric Units

The most fundamental way to convert between metric units is to multiply the units given by the conversion factor involving the units desired. If the desired conversion is from milligrams (mg) to grams (g), the number of milligrams given should be multiplied by the factor 1 g/1000 mg because 1 g = 1000 mg. The following steps would be involved in this conversion:

1. Write down the number of milligrams to be converted to grams.
2. To the right of that number, write down the number of milligrams in 1 g, with the milligrams as the denominator. (The numerator should always contain the unit to which you wish to convert.)
3. Multiply the two numbers together.

Example 1: Convert 3000 mg to grams.

Step 1. $3000\ \text{mg}$

Step 2. $3000\ \text{mg}\ \frac{1\text{g}}{1000\ \text{mg}}$

Step 3. $3000\ \text{mg} \times \frac{1\text{g}}{1000\ \text{mg}} = 3\ \text{g}$

TABLE 3-1 Units of Measure for the Biologic Sciences

WEIGHT	VOLUME	LENGTH	MULTIPLE POWER OF 10
Gram (g)	Liter (L)	Meter (m)	1
Kilogram (kg)	Kiloliter (kL)	Kilometer (km)	1000
Decigram (dg)	Deciliter (dL)	Decimeter (dm)	1/10
Centigram (cg)	Centiliter (cL)	Centimeter (cm)	1/100
Milligram (mg)	Milliliter (mL)	Millimeter (mm)	1/1000
Microgram (μg)	Microliter (μL)	Micrometer (μm)	1/1,000,000
Nanogram (ng)	Nanoliter (nL)	Nanometer (nm)	1/1,000,000,000
Picogram (pg)	Picoliter (pL)	Picometer (pm)	1/1,000,000,000,000

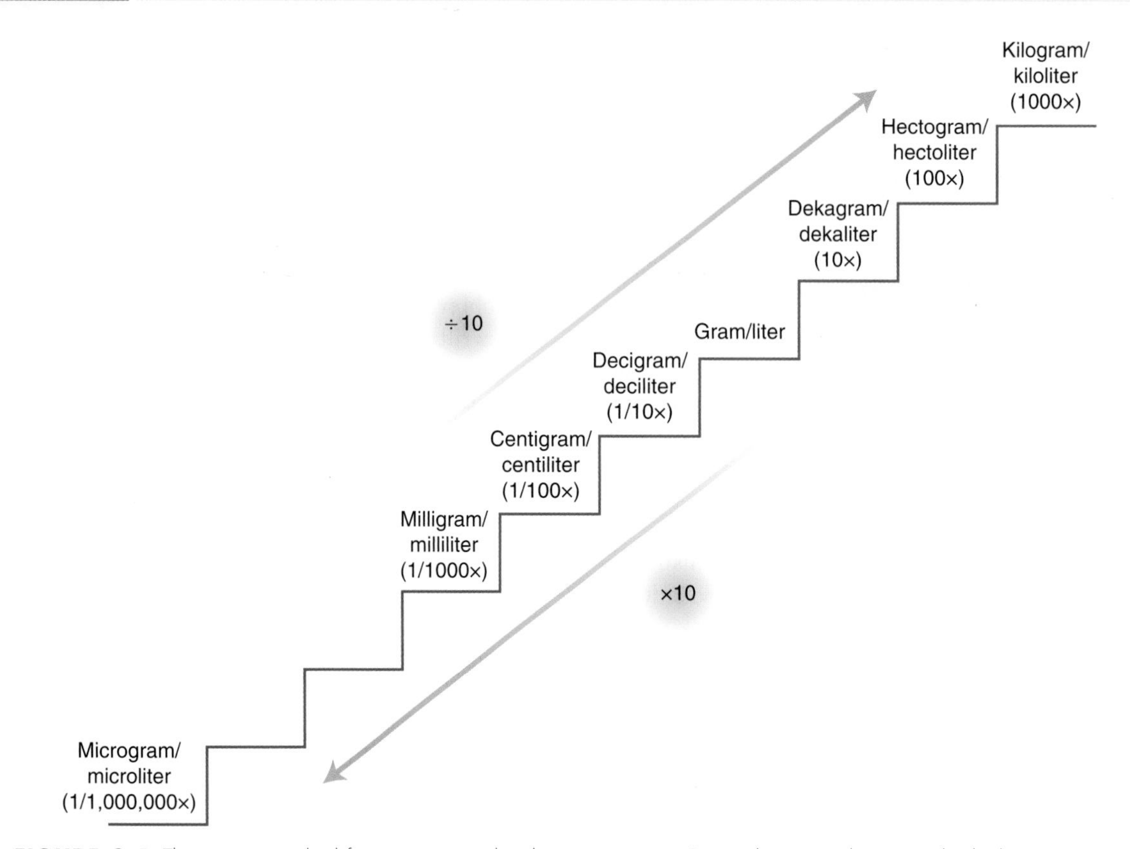

FIGURE 3-1 The stairstep method for converting within the metric system. For each step up the stairs, divide the given amount by 10. For each step down the stairs, multiply the given amount by 10.

Figure 3-1 illustrates the stairstep method of converting from one unit to another within the metric system. When converting measurements in the metric system via the stairstep method, divide by 10 for each step up to the desired measurement, and multiply by 10 for each step down to the desired measurement.

You also may think of converting measurements with this method by remembering that for each step up, the decimal point is moved one place to the left. For each step down, the decimal point is moved one place to the right.

Example 2:

$$500 \text{ mL} = \_\_\_\_\_ \text{ L}$$

Conversion of milliliters to liters requires three steps upward. Therefore, divide 500 by 10 three times (or 500 ÷ 1000). This moves the decimal point three places to the left, and the answer is 500 mL = 0.5 L.

Example 3:

$$2 \text{ g} = \_\_\_\_\_ \text{ mg}$$

To convert grams to milligrams, go down three steps. Multiply 2 by 10 three times (or 2 × 1000). This moves the decimal point three places to the right, and the answer is 2 g = 2000 mg.

A second method for performing conversions in the metric system can be called the *arrow method.* When this method is used, it is paramount to remember which units of measure are larger. Conversions between the commonly used units of kilograms, grams, milligrams, and micrograms are illustrated in the following text.

A kilogram is 1000 times larger than a gram (g), a gram is 1000 times larger than a milligram (mg), and a milligram is 1000 times larger than a microgram (mcg). This relationship can be abbreviated as follows with the use of the "greater than" symbol (>):

$$\text{kg} > \text{g} > \text{mg} > \text{mcg}$$

Many times, the technician will have to calculate the amount of drug to be given when the supply on hand is not measured in the same units as the order calls for. For example, the order is for 0.3 g of drug A, and the supply on hand is 150-mg tablets. Before it can be determined how many tablets should be given, 0.3 g must be converted to milligrams. Because it is known that 1 g = 1000 mg, 0.3 g can be changed to milligrams by multiplying 0.3 g by 1000 mg/g ($0.3 \times 1000 = 300$ mg). The decimal point is moved three places to the right ($0.3 \rightarrow 3_{\uparrow 1}\, 0_{\uparrow 2}\, 0_{\uparrow 3}$).

The conversion could have been made very quickly by simply moving the decimal point three places to the right. To know which direction to move the decimal, one should determine which way the arrow is pointing (e.g., kg > g > mg > mcg).

Any time the conversion is made between two adjacent units in the relationship of kg > g > mg > mcg, the decimal point will be moved three places.

The steps for converting grams to milligrams with the use of this method are as follows:

1. Write down the order first, using the units called for (0.3 g).
2. Write down the equivalent units (on hand) needed next to the order units (0.3 g = __ mg).
3. Place an arrow between the two units, with the closed part of the arrow pointing toward the smaller unit (g > mg)
4. Move the decimal point three places in the direction the arrow points ($0.3\ \text{g} \rightarrow 3_{\uparrow 1}\, 0_{\uparrow 2}\, 0_{\uparrow 3}$).

In the previous problem, it would take two 150-mg tablets to fill the 300-mg order.

If the order had been for 300,000 mcg of drug A, and the supply on hand had consisted of 150-mg tablets, micrograms would have to be converted to milligrams through the following steps:

1. Write the order (300,000 mcg).
2. Write down the equivalent units needed next to the order units (300,000 mcg = ___ mg).
3. Place an arrow between the two units, with the closed part of the arrow pointing toward the smaller units (mcg < mg).
4. Move the decimal three places in the direction the arrow points ($300\ \text{mg} \leftarrow 300_{\uparrow 3}\, 0_{\uparrow 2}\, 0_{\uparrow 1}\, 0.$ mcg).

In this problem, it would take two 150-mg (150,000 mcg) tablets to fill the 300,000-mcg order.

Additional problems for converting within the metric system are provided at the end of this chapter.

Apothecary and Household Systems

The apothecary and household systems of measurement are older systems than the metric system. The apothecary system is seldom used, but the household system is used for giving clients instructions about dosage.

The units most often encountered in the apothecary system are the minim, abbreviated *m* or *min;* the dram, abbreviated *dr;* the ounce, abbreviated *oz;* and the grain, abbreviated *gr.* A minim is equal to 1 drop, a dram is equal to 4 mL, an ounce is equal to 30 mL, and a grain is equal to 65 mg (64.8, sometimes rounded to 65). When quantities related to grains are written, the symbol *gr* should be placed before the number, and common fractions are used when appropriate (e.g., gr 1/50). The apothecary pound (12 oz) is not used when doses are calculated. Instead, the avoirdupois pound (16 oz) is used.

Units commonly used in the household system include the drop, abbreviated *gtt;* the tablespoon, abbreviated *T* or *Tbsp;* and the teaspoon, abbreviated *t* or *tsp.* One drop is equivalent to 1 min, 1 Tbsp is equivalent to 15 mL, and 1 tsp is equivalent to 5 mL. The pint, quart, and gallon are other units that are sometimes encountered. Boxes 3-1 and 3-2 illustrate equivalent values that are useful in dosage calculations. Practice problems for converting within and between the apothecary and household systems are found at the end of this chapter.

DOSAGE CALCULATIONS

The quantity of drug to be delivered to a patient is called the ***dose.*** A **dosage rate** expressed in milligrams per kilogram (or milligrams per pound) is multiplied by the animal's weight in kilograms (or

BOX 3-1 Weight Equivalents

1 kg = 1000 g = 2.2 lb
1 g = 1000 mg
1 mg = 1000 μg = 0.001 g
65 mg = 1 gr
1 μg = 0.001 mg = 0.000001 g
1 lb = 453.6 g = 0.4536 kg = 16 oz
1 oz = 28.35 g

BOX 3-2 Volume Equivalents

1 L = 1000 mL = 1 qt (946.4 mL)
500 mL = 1 pt (473 mL) = 2 cups (equivalent to 1 lb of water)
15 mL = 1 Tbsp
5 mL = 1 tsp
30 mL = 1 oz
240 mL = 1 cup/glass
4 mL = 1 dram
1 mL = 15 gtt/min*

*The number of drops/minim in 1 mL depends on the size of the dropper. With a standard-size dropper, 1 mL equals 15 drops.

pounds) to determine the dose. The dose then is divided by the amount (concentration) of the drug in the pharmaceutic form (e.g., tablet or solution) to determine the actual amount of the pharmaceutic form to be administered. The formula for dosage calculation, which should be committed to memory, is as follows:

$$\text{Dose} = \frac{\text{Animal's weight} \times \text{dosage rate}}{\text{Concentration of drug}}$$

Example 1: If a 20-kg dog is to be given amoxicillin at the rate of 10 mg/kg and injectable amoxicillin at a concentration of 100 mg/mL is available, the dosage calculation would be as follows:

$$\text{Dose} = \frac{20\text{ kg} \times 10\text{ mg/kg}}{100\text{ mg/mL}} = \frac{200\text{ mg}}{100\text{ mg/mL}} = 2\text{ mL}$$

Note that in the first step of the calculation, kilograms cancel out and leave only milligrams in the numerator. In the second step, milligrams cancel out and leave milliliters. If 100-mg amoxicillin tablets are available, the formula becomes as follows:

$$\text{Dose} = \frac{20\text{ kg} \times 10\text{ mg/kg}}{100\text{ mg/tablet}} = \frac{200\text{ mg}}{100\text{ mg/tablet}} = 2\text{ tablets}$$

Because most scales used to weigh animals for drug dosage calculation provide the weight in pounds, a conversion must be made from pounds to kilograms. To do this, divide the weight in pounds by 2.2.

Example 2: The dog in the previous problem weighed 44 lb, and 44 divided by 2.2 equals 20 kg. To convert kilograms to pounds (if the dose is provided in milligrams per pound), multiply the weight in kilograms by 2.2 (e.g., 20 kg × 2.2 = 44 lb).

If the order to the technician is to "give a dog 300 mg of amoxicillin," then the ordered amount is simply divided by the concentration of the drug to determine the amount to be administered.

Example 3: If the order is to give a dog 300 mg of amoxicillin (concentration 100 mg/mL), the calculation would be as follows:

$$\frac{300\text{ mg}}{100\text{ mg/mL}} = 3\text{ mL}$$

TECHNICIAN NOTES Because drugs are manufactured in different concentrations, always record the dose (milligrams, units, mEq) of active ingredient in the medical record rather than the number of milliliters, tablets, etc.

It should be noted that the dose of most drugs used to treat neoplasms is calculated according to the total body surface area of the patient. Body surface area is correlated with the weight of the animal. A table is available in Chapter 16 (see Table 16-2) for converting an animal's weight to surface area in square meters (sq M or m^2). In these cases, the formula for dosage calculation becomes the following:

$$\text{Dose} = \text{mg/m}^2(\text{from insert}) \times \text{m}^2(\text{from table})$$

Dosage calculation problems are provided at the end of this chapter.

SOLUTIONS

To understand dosage calculation problems and how to prepare dilutions of substances (e.g., allergy injections and disinfectants), a technician must have a basic understanding of solutions. ***Solutions*** are mixtures of substances that usually are not chemically combined with each other. In most cases the solvent will be a liquid, but it can be a solid. Solutions are made up of a dissolving substance, called the *solvent,* and a dissolved substance, called the *solute.* Not all substances form solutions with each other. Those that form solutions are called *miscible,* and those that do not are called *immiscible.* A solution is referred to as *saturated* if it contains the maximum amount of solute at a particular temperature and pressure. Under some circumstances, a solution can become supersaturated. Mixtures of substances in which the solute is made up of very large particles are called *suspensions.* The particles in suspensions settle on standing, and the mixture must be agitated before it is administered. True solutions do not settle and remain mixed without agitation. All parts of solutions contain equal parts of the solute.

When working with solutions, it is important to know the amount of solute in the solvent or to be able to measure it. The amount of solute dissolved in the solvent is referred to as the *concentration (strength)* of the substance. Concentrations may be expressed in a number of ways, including the following:

- Parts ratio
- Weight per volume (w/v) for liquids
- Volume per volume (v/v) for liquids
- Weight per weight (w/w) for solids

Solutions can be described in terms of parts without any reference to units of measurement. The parts simply refer to the relationship between the solvent and the solute. For example, instructions may call for a 1-to-32 (1:32) dilution of a disinfectant. The first number of the ratio refers to the amount of the disinfectant and the second number refers to the amounts of solvent and disinfectant combined. This strength of the mixture is expressed as a parts ratio or **ratio concentration**.

> *TECHNICIAN NOTES* A 1:32 dilution means that 1 mL of the drug is added to 31 mL of the solvent to produce 32 total mL of the solution.

Another unit that describes the relationship of parts (parts ratio) is called *parts per million* (ppm). Parts per million is equal to 1 mg of a solute in a kilogram or liter of solvent. One part per million is also equivalent to 1 µg in a gram or milliliter. Upson (1988) reports that 1 ppm is equivalent to 1 minute in approximately 2 years or 1 oz of sand in approximately 31 tons of cement. Parts per billion is a ratio unit that is used occasionally. It is equivalent to 1 µg in a kilogram or liter, or 1 nanogram in a gram or milliliter.

A ratio concentration can be converted to a percentage concentration by using a ratio and proportion equation:

Example 1: Express 1:32 as a percent concentration (parts per hundred).

Answer:

$$1:32 = Y:100 \text{ or } \frac{1}{32} = \frac{Y}{100}$$

$$32Y = 100$$

$$Y = 3.1\%$$

PERCENT CONCENTRATIONS

The term ***percent concentration*** may be used when w/v, w/w, or v/v concentrations are described. Percent (percentage) means parts of solute per 100 parts of the solution. Percent w/v means the number of grams of solute in 100 mL of solution; percent w/w describes the number of grams of solute in 100 g of diluent (liquid or solid); and v/v expresses the number of milliliters of solute in 100 mL of the solution.

A 100% solution (w/v) contains 100 g of solute per 100 mL of solution. Another way to say this is that it contains 1 g (1000 mg) of solute per 1 mL of solution (1000 mg/mL). To convert from a percent solution to mg/mL, multiply the percentage by 10 (e.g., a 5% Lasix solution contains 50 mg/mL). To convert milligrams per milliliter to a percent, divide the milligrams per milliliter by 10 (e.g., a Lasix solution containing 50 mg/mL is a 5% solution). Sometimes, the term *milligrams percent* (mg%) is encountered. This term is used to refer to the number of milligrams in 100 mL of solution. It is an expression of concentration but not of percent concentration (g/100 mL). A more accurate description of mg% would be milligrams per deciliter (mg/dL) because a deciliter is equal to 100 mL.

A 100% solution (w/w) contains 100 g of solute in 100 g of solid or liquid. A 5% solution (w/w) of sodium chloride would contain 5 g of sodium in 100 g of solution. To make this preparation, weigh out 5 g of sodium chloride and mix it with 95 g of water.

A 100% solution (v/v) would simply be pure drug or chemical. A 10% solution would contain 10 mL of the chemical in 100 mL of solution. When a w/v solution or a v/v solution is prepared, the desired amount of solute is added to a container, and enough solvent is added to create the desired volume. This process is called *diluting up*, or it may be said that you *q.s.* to the desired volume. The abbreviation *q.s.* means to add a "quantity sufficient" to arrive at the desired volume. For example, to make 100 mL of a 10% formalin solution, place 10 mL of formaldehyde (100% formalin) in a container and q.s. (quantity sufficient) to 100 mL (10 mL formalin, 90 mL distilled water.

The most common way of expressing drug concentration when the solute is a solid and the solvent is a liquid is weight per volume (w/v). For example, the concentration of most pharmaceutic preparations is expressed as milligrams per milliliter (mg/mL); the concentration for ketamine (Ketaset) for example is 100 mg/mL.

To convert a percent concentration to a ratio concentration, set up a ratio and proportion equation:

Example 1: Convert a 3.1% (parts per 100) solution to a ratio concentration.

Answer:

$$3.1:100 = 1:\text{Y or } \frac{3.1}{100} = \frac{1}{\text{Y}}$$

$$3.1\,\text{Y} = 100$$

$$\text{Y} = 32$$

Calculations Involving Concentrations

To determine the amount of solute needed to make a desired amount of solution, you may use the following formula:

$$\text{Grams of solute to q.s. to desired volume} = \frac{\% \times \text{desired volume}}{100}$$

Example 1: How many grams of sodium chloride are needed to make 1 L of 0.9% sodium chloride?

Answer:

$$\text{Grams needed} = \frac{0.9 \times 1000\ \text{mL}}{100} = 9\ \text{g}$$

Nine grams of sodium chloride are added to a container and is diluted up to 1000 mL.

When the amount of solute and the volume of solution are known, the percent solution may be calculated as follows:

$$\text{Percent solution} = \frac{\text{grams of solute} \times 100}{\text{volume of solution}}$$

Example 2: What percentage is a solution that contains 9 g of sodium chloride?

Answer:

$$\text{Percent solution} = \frac{9 \times 100}{1000} = \frac{900}{1000} = 0.9\%$$

To solve problems involving a change in concentration of the solution, the following formula may be used:

$$\text{Volume one(V1)} \times \text{Concentration one(C1)} = \text{Volume two(V2)} \times \text{Concentration two(C2)}$$

In these problems, let volume one (V1) be the volume of the **stock solution** used to prepare the new volume, let concentration one (C1) be the concentration of the stock solution, let volume two (V2) be the desired volume of the new solution, and let concentration two (C2) be the desired concentration of the new solution. The problem is solved for volume one, and this volume is diluted (q.s.) up to the desired volume. The formula then looks like this:

$$\text{Volume of stock}(V1) \times \text{Stock conc}\,(C1)$$
$$= \text{Desired volume}\,(V2) \times \text{Desired conc}(C2)$$

Example 3: How would you prepare 100 mL of a 5% dextrose solution from a 50% dextrose solution?

Answer:

$$V1 \times C1 = V2 \times C2$$
$$V1 \times 50 = 100 \times 5$$
$$V1 \times 50 = 500$$
$$V1 = 10$$

This formula demonstrates that you would take 10 mL of the 50% dextrose solution and q.s. to 100 mL (10 mL stock + 90 diluent) to prepare the 5% solution.

Another formula that may be used to solve problems in which a change in concentration is involved is as follows:

$$\{\text{Desired concentration/Stock concentration}\}$$
$$= \{\text{Amount of stock to use/Total amount to make}\}$$

Example 4: In solving the foregoing problem, the desired concentration is 5%, the available (stock) concentration is 50%, the amount to make is 100 mL, and the amount of stock to use is the unknown.

Answer:

$$\frac{5}{50} = \frac{X}{100}$$
$$50X = 500$$
$$X = 10\text{ mL}$$

MILLIEQUIVALENTS

When electrolytes are involved, the concentration of a solution is often expressed in terms of **milliequivalents** (mEq). One milliequivalent is equal to 1/1000 of an equivalent. An **equivalent weight** is equal to (for practical applications) 1 g molecular weight divided by the total positive valence of the material in question (Blankenship and Campbell, 1976). The concentration of an electrolyte solution is expressed as milliequivalents per liter (mEq/L), which can be calculated when the concentration of the solution is known by using the following formula:

$$\text{mEq/L} = \frac{\text{mg/dL} \times 10}{\text{eq wt}}$$

Example 1: How many milliequivalents per liter is found in a sodium chloride solution that contains 700 mg/dL?

$$\text{NaCl eq wt: } 23(\text{Na}) + 35.5(\text{Cl}) = 58.5$$
$$\text{mEq/L} = \frac{700 \times 10}{58.5} = 119.66$$

The number of milligrams per deciliter also can be calculated when the number of milliequivalents per liter is known by manipulating the previous formula as follows:

$$\text{mg/dL} = \frac{\text{mEq/L} \times \text{eq wt}}{10}$$

Example 2: How many milligrams per deciliter is contained in a solution that has 119.66 mEq/L?

Answer:

$$\text{mg/dL} = \frac{119.66 \times 58.5}{10} = \frac{7000}{10} = 700\text{ mg/dL}$$

CALCULATIONS INVOLVING INTRAVENOUS FLUID ADMINISTRATION

Calculations for determining the volume of fluid to administer are covered in Chapter 15. The rate at which to run intravenous fluids (in drops per minute) can be determined by dividing the volume of fluids to be given by the time in minutes during administration, and then multiplying that number by the drops per milliliter delivered by the administration set.

$$\frac{\text{Volume of infusion (mL)}}{\text{Time of infusion (min)}} \times \text{drop factor (gtt/mL)}$$
$$= \text{drops per minute}$$

The drip rate in drops per minute can be divided by 60 to determine the rate in drops per second—a number that is easier to work with when one is actually adjusting the flow.

Example 1: Give 480 mL of lactated Ringer's solution to Dog A over a 4-hour period using a standard 15 gtt/mL administration set.

$$\frac{480\text{ mL}}{240\text{ min}} = \frac{2\text{ mL}}{\text{min}} \times \frac{15\text{ gtt}}{\text{mL}} = \frac{30\text{ gtt}}{\text{min}} \times \frac{1\text{ min}}{60\text{ sec}} = \frac{1\text{ gtt}}{2\text{ sec}}$$

Giving one drop every 2 seconds will deliver 30 drops in a minute.

Calculations for Constant Rate Infusion Problems

Sometimes, medications given by intravenous infusion have to be administered at a dose delivered at a constant rate over a specified period of time. The dosage is often ordered in micrograms per kilogram per minute.

This dosage can be confusing because most drugs are available in a concentration expressed as milligrams/milliliter (mg/mL) and are delivered through infusion pumps at a rate expressed as milliliters/hour (mL/h). The following example problem illustrates a method for solving these problems without the use of an infusion pump.

Example 1: A 44-lb dog with acute heart failure is ordered to receive 10 mcg/kg/min of dopamine. You will add a 200-mg vial of dopamine to a 1-L bag of D_5W (dextrose 5% in water) solution (0.2 mg/mL). At what rate in drops per minute will you administer this solution to deliver the correct dosage?

Step 1: Convert to the same units. The dose is expressed in mcg/kg, so the patient's weight must be converted from pounds to kilograms, and the drug concentration must be expressed in mcg/mL.

$$44\text{ lbs} \times \frac{1\text{ kg}}{2.2\text{ lbs}} = \frac{44\text{ kg}}{2.2} = 20\text{ kg}$$

$$\frac{0.2\text{ mg}}{1\text{ mL}} \times \frac{1000\text{ mcg}}{1\text{ mg}} = \frac{200\text{ mcg}}{1\text{ mL}}$$

Step 2: Determine the number of micrograms per minute.

$$20\text{ kg} \times \frac{10\text{ mcg}}{\text{kg/min}} = \frac{200\text{ mcg}}{\text{min}}$$

Step 3: Determine the number of milliliters per minute.

$$\frac{200\text{ mcg}}{1\text{ min}} \times \frac{1\text{ mL}}{200\text{ mcg}} = \frac{1\text{ mL}}{1\text{ min}}$$

Step 4: Determine the number of drops per minute using a minidrip (60 gtt/mL) administration set.

$$\frac{1\text{ mL}}{\text{min}} \times \frac{60\text{ gtt}}{1\text{ mL}} = \frac{60\text{ gtt}}{1\text{ min}} \text{ or 1gtt/sec}$$

Formulas and recipes have been devised to simplify the constant rate infusion (CRI) calculations (Macintire and Tefend, 2004). The following formula can be used to determine the number of milligrams of drug that must be added to a bag of fluids to deliver a predetermined dosage rate to a patient. A volume of the delivery fluid equal to the volume of the drug added should be removed before the drug is added, to keep the dose and volume accurate.

$$M = \frac{(D)(W)(V)}{(R)(16.67)}$$

M = number of milligrams of drug to add to delivery fluid
D = dosage of drug in micrograms per kilogram per minute
W = patient body weight in kilograms
V = volume in milliliters of delivery fluid
R = rate of delivery in milliliters per hour
16.67 = conversion factor

The next formula can be used to adjust the dosage (mcg/kg/min) in accordance with the response of the animal.

$$R = \frac{(D)(W)(V)}{(M)(16.67)}$$

Another formula allows rapid calculation of the amount of drug to be added to a standard volume of 250 mL of fluid at a standard delivery rate of 15 mL/h.

Drug dosage (mcg/kg/min) × Body weight (kg) = milligrams of drug to add to 250 mL fluid and run at 15 mL/h.

Some CRI drugs are dosed in milligrams per kilogram per hour rather than micrograms per kilogram per minute. The following formula determines the amount of drug (mg) to be added to 250 mL of fluid for a delivery rate of 10 mL/h.

$$\frac{\text{Dose (mg/kg/h)} \times \text{Body weight (BW)(kg)} \times 25\text{ h}}{\text{Drug concentration (mg/mL)}} =$$

Number of milliliters of drug to add to 250 mL delivery fluid and administer at 10 mL/h

A combination of morphine and ketamine (MK) sometimes is delivered as a CRI for pain control in dogs and cats. A recipe (Ortel, 2006) for this combination calls for adding to a single 500-mL bag of fluids the following:

60 mg of ketamine (100 mg/mL)
60 mg of morphine (15 mg/mL)

When the two drugs are added, the patient's weight in kilograms becomes the infusion rate in milliliters per hour that is set on the infusion pump. The delivery dose is 1 mL/kg/h or 2 mcg/kg/min ketamine and 2 mcg/kg/min morphine.

For dogs, lidocaine (500 mg of a 20 mg/mL concentration) can be added to the MK recipe previously mentioned to make the MLK mixture. The MLK mixture also is run at a delivery rate of 1 mL/kg/h, delivering 17 mcg/kg/min of lidocaine, in addition to the ketamine and morphine.

REVIEW QUESTIONS

PROBLEMS USING RATIOS AND PROPORTIONS

Ratios

1. Express 1/4 as a ratio and as a decimal.
2. Express 0.75 as a ratio and as a fraction.
3. Express 0.004 as a ratio and as a fraction.
4. Express 1:80 as a fraction and as a decimal.
5. Express 9/1000 as a ratio and as a decimal.
6. Express 1:32 as a fraction and as a decimal.
7. Express 1/3 as a ratio and as a decimal.
8. Express 0.50 as a ratio and a fraction.
9. Express 2:3 as a fraction and decimal.
10. Express 0.01 as a ratio and as a fraction.

Proportions (Solve for X.)

1. $25:X = 5:10$
2. $\frac{4}{5} = \frac{X}{10}$
3. $\frac{1}{2}:100 = X:500$
4. $\frac{1/4}{X} = \frac{20}{400}$
5. Convert 0.2 g to milligrams using a proportion.

$$\frac{1000\text{ mg}}{1\text{ g}} = \frac{X\text{ mg}}{0.2\text{ g}}$$

6. If a drug concentration is labeled 5 mL = 250 mg, how many milligrams are in three fourths of a milliliter?

$$\frac{250\text{ mg}}{5\text{ mL}} = \frac{X}{3/4\text{ mL}}$$

7. How much bleach would you use to prepare 1000 mL of a 1:32 solution?

$$1:32 = X:1000$$

8. How much bleach would you use to prepare 1 gallon (3784 mL) of a 1:32 solution?

$$1:32 = X:3784$$

9. If you were to give a horse 1 mL per 250 lb of body weight of an anthelmintic, how many milliliters would you give to a horse that weighs 1250 lb?

$$\frac{1}{250} = \frac{X}{1250}$$

10. If a 10-lb dog gets one fourth of a tablet of an antibiotic, how many tablets will a 50-lb dog get?

$$\frac{1}{4}:10 = X:50$$

11. What is the percentage concentration of a 1/5000 solution?

$$\frac{1}{5000} = \frac{X}{100}$$

12. What is the ratio strength of a 5% solution?

$$5:100 = 1:X$$

13. If you mix 9 g of NaCl in 500 mL of sterile water, what is the percent concentration?

$$9:500 = X:100$$

14. If a 10-lb dog gets 0.5 mL of an anthelmintic, how many milliliters does a 60-lb dog get?

$$0.5:10 = X:60$$

15. How many grams of a drug should be used to prepare 200 mL of a 5% solution?

$$\frac{5}{100} = \frac{X}{200}$$

PROBLEMS USING THE METRIC SYSTEM

1. 150 mg = ______ g
2. 2 L = ______ mL
3. 2250 mg = ______ g
4. 5 g = ______ mg
5. 3000 mL = ______ L
6. 2 kg = ______ g
7. 0.5 kg = ______ g
8. 5000 mg = ______ kg
9. 1.25 mg = ______ g
10. 0.004 g = ______ mg
11. 2050 μg = ______ mg
12. How many grams would you administer if the veterinarian ordered 10 mg of acepromazine?

    ______
13. If the medical order is for 0.5 L of sodium chloride 0.9%, how many milliliters would be administered? ______
14. How many liters would you give to the patient if the order called for 750 mL to be administered? ______
15. If the veterinarian orders 300 μg of vitamin B_{12}, how much is this in milligrams?

    ______
16. If the order is for 2.5 mg of vitamin B_{12}, how many micrograms are administered?

    ______
17. A 1% solution of ivermectin contains how many micrograms per milliliter?

    ______
18. How many millimeters wide is a lesion 0.5 cm in diameter? ______
19. What is the weight in grams of a parrot weighing 0.9 kg? ______
20. How many kilograms does a 20-gm mouse weigh? ______

PROBLEMS USING THE APOTHECARY AND HOUSEHOLD SYSTEMS

1. 1.5 qt = ______ pt
2. 12 pt = ______ gal
3. 3 tsp = ______ Tbsp
4. 3 qt = ______ cups
5. 12 cups = ______ pt
6. 2 oz = ______ Tbsp
7. 1 gal = ______ oz
8. 1 pt = ______ oz
9. 6 pt = ______ qt
10. 48 oz = ______ lb

PROBLEMS COMBINING THE TWO SYSTEMS

1. 1 pt = ______ mL
2. 2 Tbsp = ______ mL
3. 15 mL = ______ cc
4. 2 cups = ______ oz
5. 6.5 mL = ______ pt
6. 125 mL = ______ tsp
7. 1.5 oz = ______ mL
8. 15 kg = ______ lb
9. 250 mL = ______ pt
10. 5 oz = ______ mL
11. 35 lb = ______ kg
12. 3 cups = ______ mL
13. 4 Tbsp = ______ oz
14. 90 mL = ______ oz
15. 260 mg = ______ gr

PROBLEMS MEASURING ORAL MEDICATIONS

1. The order is for 500 mg of amoxicillin, and tablets on hand are 250 mg. How many tablets will be administered? ______

2. The order is for 15 mg of prednisone, and 10-mg (scored) tablets are on hand. How many tablets will be administered?

____

3. The order is for 960 mg of sulfamethoxazole/trimethoprim (SMZ-TMP). Tablets on hand are 240 mg. How many tablets will be administered? _______________

4. The order is for enrofloxacin to be given once daily at 5 mg/kg to a 10-lb cat for 7 days. How many 22.7-mg tablets should be dispensed to the client?

____

5. The veterinarian prescribes 15 mg of prednisone every other day for 10 days. The tablets on hand are 10 mg.
How many tablets per dose will be administered? _______________
How many tablets will be dispensed?

____

6. The veterinarian prescribes 100 mg of cephalexin twice a day (b.i.d.) for 10 days. You have 100-mg tablets on hand.
How many will be dispensed?

____

7. The veterinarian prescribes sulfadimethoxine (Albon) for Coccidia. Your patient is a puppy that weighs 8 lbs and needs treatment for 21 days. The dose for Albon is a 25-mg/lb loading dose and 12.5-mg/lb maintenance dose to be given once daily (s.i.d.).The drug is supplied at 250 mg/5 mL.
How many milligrams does your patient need for a loading dose? _______________
A maintenance dose?

____

How many milligrams per milliliter are there in Albon? _______________
How many milliliters will be dispensed?

____

8. The veterinarian orders 4.4 mg/kg of carprofen for pain control divided into two equal daily doses for a 50-lb dog. On hand are 100-mg scored tablets. How many tablets are administered each morning and afternoon?

____

9. The order is for 0.5 mg/kg enalapril twice daily for a 20-kg dog for 30 days. On hand are 10-mg scored tablets. How many tablets should be dispensed? _______________

10. The veterinarian prescribes 2.5 mg of acepromazine three times a day (t.i.d.) for 3 days, and tablets on hand are 5 mg (scored).
How many tablets will be administered?

____

How many will be dispensed?

____

11. The veterinarian prescribes aminophylline to be given three times daily for 14 days to a 15-lb dog. The dose for aminophylline is 10 mg/kg.
How many kilograms does your patient weigh?

____

How many milligrams have to be administered to your patient?

____

Because the tablets on hand are 100 mg (scored), how many tablets per dose will you give to the patient?

____

How many tablets will be dispensed?

____

12. The veterinarian has ordered 5 mg/kg ponazuril once daily for a 1200-lb horse for 28 days. Tubes of 127 g of ponazuril paste are available; these contain 150 mg ponazuril per gram. How many tubes of the medication are needed for the 28-day treatment?

____

13. A farmer has 10 calves that weigh approximately 100 lbs each. A microscopic fecal examination reveals Coccidia. The veterinarian chooses to treat all 10 calves with Corid powder (20% amprolium) by drenching daily for 10 days. To make a drench solution, mix 3 oz of Corid powder in 1 qt of water (1 oz of powder = 3.5 Tbsp). The dose of Corid for drenching is 1 oz of solution per 100 lb of body weight.
How much solution should be mixed to drench these 10 calves for 10 days?

____

14. Doxycycline has been chosen as a treatment for a 1-kg Amazon parrot at the rate of 25 mg/kg b.i.d. for 7 days. The tablets on hand are 50 mg (scored).
How many tablets will be given for each treatment? ____________
How many tablets will be dispensed?
____
15. The veterinarian orders clenbuterol syrup for a 200-lb foal. The dosage is 0.8 mcg/kg twice daily for 3 days. The syrup contains 72.5 mcg/mL. How many milliliters is given at each dose? ____________

PROBLEMS MEASURING PARENTERAL MEDICATIONS

1. The veterinarian orders prednisone, 20 mg intramuscularly (IM). The vial is labeled 50 mg/mL. How many milliliters will be administered? ____________
2. The veterinarian orders an injection of desoxycorticosterone pivalate (Percorten-V) for a 20-lb dog at the dosage rate of 2.2 mg/kg. The concentration of desoxycorticosterone pivalate is 25 mg/mL. How much of the drug should be injected? ____________
3. The veterinarian orders phenylbutazone to be administered to a 1500-lb horse at a dose of 5 mg/kg intravenously. The vial is labeled 200 mg/mL. How many milliliters will be administered? ____________
4. The veterinarian orders penicillin G procaine for a 25-lb dog to be administered at a dose of 40,000 U/kg IM. The vial is labeled 300,000 U/mL. How many milliliters will be administered? ____________
5. The veterinarian orders cefazolin to be given to a 23-lb dog at a dosage of 20 mg/kg IV for surgical prophylaxis. The concentration of cefazolin on hand is 100 mg/mL. How much (mL) of the drug should be given?
____
6. A 78-lb dog is to be administered ampicillin trihydrate at a dose of 5 mg/lb subcutaneously. The antibiotic has been reconstituted, and the concentration is 200 mg/mL. How many milliliters will be administered to the patient?
____
7. A microscopic fecal examination reveals a *Giardia* infection in a 500-g African gray parrot. The veterinarian chooses to treat the infection with injectable metronidazole at a dosage of 30 mg/kg daily for 3 days. How many milligrams will the parrot receive at each treatment? ____________
8. A 45-lb dog is to be treated for lymphosarcoma with vincristine sulfate, 1 mg/mL. The dose is 0.5 mg/m^2.
How many square meters of body surface area does this patient have?
____
How many milligrams will be given to the patient? ____________
How many milliliters?
____
9. The veterinarian orders lincomycin HCl for a 500-lb Yorkshire boar. The dosage to be administered is 5 mg/lb/day IM for 5 days. The medication on hand is 100 mg/mL in a 50-mL multidose vial.
How many milligrams will be administered to the boar each day? ____________
How many milliliters will be administered to the boar each day? ____________
How many bottles of medication does the owner have to purchase to treat the boar for 5 days? ____________
10. A cat weighing 8 lb that has a small laceration on its left hip is to be administered ketamine HCl to produce anesthesia. The veterinarian orders 15 mg/kg IM. The vial is labeled 100 mg/mL.
How many milligrams will be administered to the cat? ____________
How many milliliters will be administered?
____
11. The veterinarian orders 7 mEq of potassium chloride to be added to the IV fluids. The vial is labeled 20 mEq in 10 mL. How many milliliters will be added to the fluids?
____
12. The veterinarian orders 4 U of regular insulin to be administered to a diabetic cat. The regular insulin is labeled 40 U/mL. How many milliliters will be administered?
____

13. The veterinarian orders testosterone propionate for a 475-lb Landrace boar. The dose to be administered is 1 mg/10 lb. The label on the vial is 25 mg/mL.
How many milligrams will be administered?
____
How many milliliters will be administered?
____
14. The veterinarian orders dexamethasone 60 mg IV to be given to a patient. The vial is labeled 2 mg/mL. How many milliliters will be administered? ______________
15. The veterinarian orders 15 mg of vitamin K_1. The vial is labeled 10 mg/mL. How many milliliters will be administered?
____
16. The order is for meloxicam at 0.2 mg/kg to control postsurgical pain in a 4.5-kg cat. The concentration of the drug is 5 mg/mL. What volume of the drug should be given?
____
17. A rabbit weighing 12 lb is to be given 0.02 mg/kg of buprenorphine subcutaneously for pain control. The concentration of the drug is 0.3 mg/mL. How much of the drug should be given?
____
18. Atropine (0.5 mg/mL) is ordered at 0.01 mg/lb to control bradycardia in a 75-lb dog. How much of the drug should be given?
____
19. The veterinarian orders enrofloxacin at 5 mg/kg IM for a 7-kg python with respiratory disease. The product contains 100 mg/mL. How much should be injected?
____
20. The order is for an injection of metoclopramide at 0.4 mg/kg for a 15-kg dog. The concentration of available product is 5 mg/mL. How much should be injected?
____

INJECTION PROBLEMS

Order	Give	Stock
1.	0.5 g IM	250 mg/mL
2.	20 mEq IV	40 mEq/10 mL
3.	0.75 mg IM	0.50 mg/mL
4.	150 mg IM	0.2 g/5 mL
5.	25 mg IM	100 mg/mL
6.	0.5 mg IM	0.5 mg/2 mL
7.	0.3 mg IV	0.4 mg/mL
8.	300,000 U SC	40,000 U/mL
9.	0.3 mg IM	0.5 mg/mL
10.	55 mg SC	250 mg/mL

PREPARING SOLUTIONS

1. Order: 100 mL of 10% formalin solution
On hand: formaldehyde 37% (considered as 100% formalin) and water
Amount needed: ______________
2. Order: 1000 mL 0.9% NaCl and 5% dextrose
On hand: 1000 mL 0.9% NaCl and 500 mL 50% dextrose
Amount of each needed: ______________
3. Order:100 mL 5% dextrose
On hand: 500 mL 50% dextrose and 250 mL sterile water for injection
Amount needed: ______________
4. Order: 500 mL 0.45% NaCl and 5% dextrose
On hand: 500 mL 0.9% NaCl and 500 mL 5% dextrose
Amount of each needed: ______________
5. Order: 2000 mL lactated Ringer's solution and 2.5% dextrose
On hand: 2 containers of 1000 mL lactated Ringer's solution and 250 mL 50% dextrose
Amount of each needed: ______________
6. Order: 50 mL 5% dextrose
On hand: 1000 mL sterile water for injection and 250 mL 50% dextrose
Amount of each needed: ______________
7. Order: 500 mL 2.5% dextrose and 0.45% NaCl
On hand: 1000 mL 0.45% NaCl and 500 mL 50% dextrose
Amount of each needed: ______________

8. Order: 1000 mL of 10% glyceryl guaiacolate solution
   On hand: packets containing 50 g guaifenesin (GG) powder and 1000 mL sterile water for injection
   Amount of each needed: ___________
9. Order: 8% thiamylal sodium solution
   On hand: One 5-g vial of powder and sterile water for injection
   Amount of sterile water needed:
   ____
10. Order: 5 mL of 2% cyclosporine ophthalmic solution
    On hand: 50 mL cyclosporine (Sandimmune Oral Solution) 100 mg/mL and 16 oz of extra virgin olive oil
    Amount of each needed: ___________
11. Order: 50 mL of 2% formalin for Knott's heartworm test
    On hand: 37% formaldehyde and water
    Amount of each needed: ___________
12. Order: Prepare 1 L of a 1:32 sodium hypochlorite solution
    On hand: Distilled water and 5% sodium hypochlorite
    Amount of each needed:
    ____
13. Order: Prepare 50 mL of a 0.5 mEq/mL KCl solution.
    On hand: Sterile water for injection and KCl (2 mEq/mL)
    Amount of each needed:
    ____
14. Order: Prepare 10 mL of a 5 mg/mL xylazine solution.
    On hand: 20 mg/mL xylazine and sterile water
    Amount of each needed:
    ____
15. Order: Prepare 15 mL of a 5 mg/mL enrofloxacin solution.
    On hand: 22.7 mg/mL enrofloxacin and sterile water for injection.
    Amount of each needed:
    ____

PROBLEMS CALCULATING INTRAVENOUS (IV) DRIP RATES

1. What drip rate will you use to administer 500 mL of lactated Ringer's solution over a 3-hour period with a standard (15 gtt/mL) administration set?
   ____
2. What drip rate would you use to deliver 120 mL 0.9% NaCl over a 2-hour period using a microdrip (60 gtt/mL) administration set?
   ____
3. What drip rate would you use to deliver 1.2 L of Normosol over a 10-hour period using a standard (15 gtt/mL) administration set?
   ____
4. What drip rate would you use to deliver 8 mcg/kg/min of drug C (500 mg/250 mL) to an 83-lb dog using a microdrip (60 gtt/mL) administration set?
   ____
5. What drip rate would you use to deliver 10 mcg/kg/min of dopamine (0.2 mg/mL) to a 22-lb dog using the microdrip (60 gtt/mL) administration set?
   ____
6. Using the formula

   $$M = \frac{(D)(W)(V)}{R(16.67)}$$

   how much nitroprusside (25 mg/mL) would you add to 1000 mL of 5% dextrose to deliver 2 mcg/kg/min of nitroprusside at a delivery rate of 12 mL/h to a 3.8-kg dog?
   ____
7. Using the formula

   $$R = \frac{(D)(W)(V)}{M(16.67)}$$

   calculate the new fluid delivery rate needed to increase the dosage of nitroprusside in problem 6 to 3 mcg/kg/min.
   ____

8. Using the formula

$$M = \frac{(D)(W)(V)}{R(16.67)}$$

how much dobutamine (12.5 mg/mL) would you add to 100 mL of a 5% dextrose solution to administer 15 mcg/kg/min to a 28-kg dog at a delivery rate of 10 mL/h?

____

9. How much furosemide (10 mg/mL) would you add to a 250-mL fluid bag to deliver 3 mcg/kg/min to a 5-kg patient with the fluid pump set at 15 mL/h? ______________________

10. How much morphine (15 mg/kg) would you add to a 250-mL fluid bag to deliver 0.2 mg/kg/h to a 10-kg animal with the pump set on 10 mL/h? ______________________

REFERENCES

Blankenship J, Campbell JB: Solutions. In Blankenship J, Campbell JB, editors: Laboratory mathematics: medical and biological applications, St. Louis, 1976, Mosby.

Macintire DK, Tefend M: Constant rate infusions: practical use, N Am Vet Conf Clinician's Brief, Orlando, Florida, April:25–28, 2004.

Ortel SO: Constant-rate infusions, Vet Tech 27(1):47–50, 2006.

Upson DW: General principles. In Upson DW, editor: Handbook of clinical veterinary pharmacology, ed 3, Manhattan, Kansas, 1988, Dan Upson Enterprises.

CHAPTER

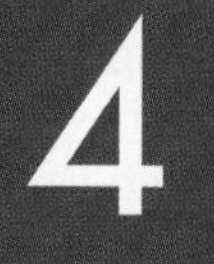

Drugs Used in Nervous System Disorders

KEY TERMS

Acetylcholine
Acetylcholinesterase
Adrenergic
Analgesia
Anesthesia
Autonomic nervous system
Catalepsy
Catecholamine
Cholinergic
Effector
Ganglionic synapse
Muscarinic receptors
Nicotinic receptors
Parasympathetic nervous system
Parasympathomimetic
Sympathetic nervous system
Sympathomimetic

OUTLINE

LEARNING OBJECTIVES

After studying this chapter, you should be able to

1. Define terms related to the pharmacology of the nervous system.
2. Develop a basic understanding of the anatomy and physiology of the nervous system.
3. Describe the subdivisions, functions, and primary neurotransmitters of the autonomic nervous system (ANS).
4. Describe how drugs affect the ANS.
5. List the different classes of ANS drugs.
6. List the two major classification schemes of barbiturates.
7. List indications and precautions for the use of barbiturates.
8. Describe dissociative anesthesia, and list three dissociative agents.
9. List the opiate receptors and the basic function of each.
10. List the indications for the use of narcotics.
11. List potential side effects of narcotic use or overdose.
12. Describe how opioid antagonists exert their effects, and list three examples of this category of drug.
13. Define *neuroleptanalgesic* and give an example.
14. List examples of drugs used to control seizures.
15. List commonly used inhalant anesthetic agents and compare their characteristics.
16. Describe the primary uses of central nervous system (CNS) stimulants.
17. List drugs used in behavioral pharmacotherapy.
18. Describe the characteristics of a good euthanasia agent.

INTRODUCTION

The nervous system is the body's primary communication and control center. It functions in harmony with the endocrine system to allow an animal to respond and adapt to its environment and to maintain a relatively constant internal environment (homeostasis) through control of the many internal organ systems. In broad terms, the nervous system serves three functions: (1) sensory, (2) integrative (analysis), and (3) motor (action). It senses changes within the environment and within the body, interprets the information, and responds to the interpretation by bringing about an appropriate action. The nervous system carries out this complex activity very rapidly by sending electric-like messages over a network of nerve fibers. The endocrine system works much more slowly by sending chemical messengers (hormones) through the bloodstream to target structures. The two systems are very closely interrelated functionally and anatomically. The nervous system exerts control over the endocrine system through the influence of the hypothalamus (brain) on the pituitary gland.

ANATOMY AND PHYSIOLOGY

The nervous system has two main divisions, the central nervous system (CNS) and the peripheral nervous system, as well as their related subdivisions

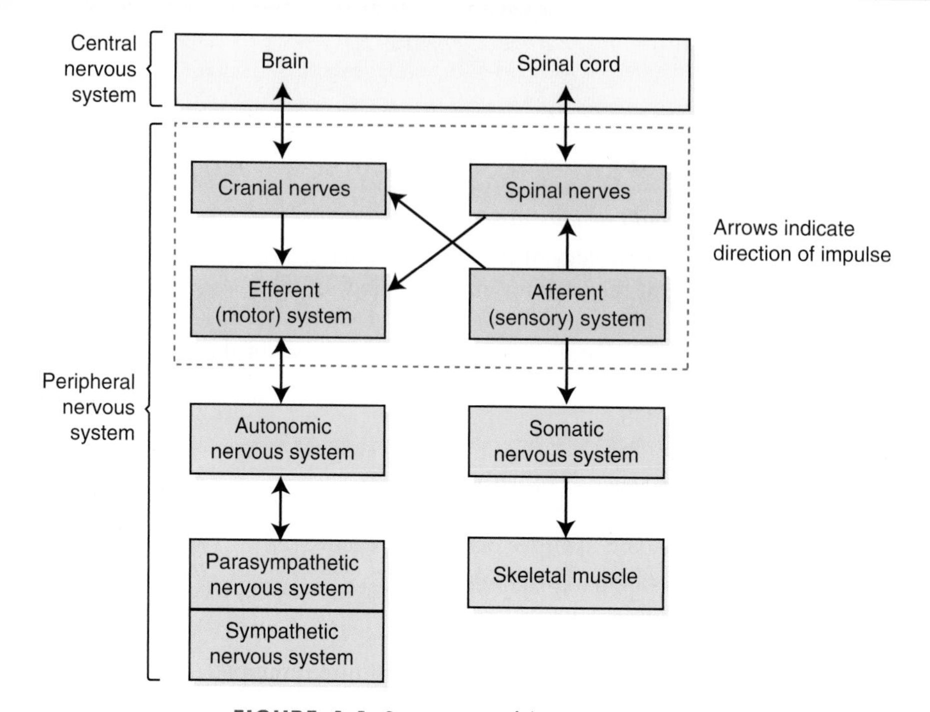

FIGURE 4-1 Organization of the nervous system.

(Figure 4-1). The CNS is composed of the brain and the spinal cord and serves as the control center of the entire nervous system. All sensory information must be relayed to the CNS before it can be interpreted and acted on. Most impulses that stimulate glands to act and muscles to contract originate in the CNS.

The nerve processes that connect the CNS with the various glands, muscles, and receptors in the body make up the peripheral nervous system. Functionally, the peripheral nervous system is divided into afferent and efferent portions. The afferent portion is composed of nerve cells that carry information from receptors in the periphery of the body to the CNS. The efferent system consists of nerve cells that carry impulses from the CNS to muscles and glands. Anatomically, the peripheral nervous system is composed of cranial nerves and spinal nerves.

The peripheral nervous system is also subdivided into a somatic nervous system and an **autonomic nervous system (ANS).** The somatic nervous system consists of efferent nerves that carry impulses from the CNS to skeletal muscle tissue. It is under conscious control and is therefore called *voluntary.* The ANS consists of efferent nerve cells that carry information from the CNS to cardiac muscle, glands, and smooth muscle. It is under unconscious control and is called *involuntary.* The ANS has two subdivisions, the **sympathetic nervous system** and the **parasympathetic nervous system.** Most tissues innervated by the ANS receive both sympathetic and parasympathetic fibers. In general, one division stimulates an activity by a receptor and the other inhibits the activity to serve as a method of checks and balances.

The fundamental unit of all branches and divisions of the nervous system is the neuron (nerve cell). Neurons have the amazing ability to transmit information from point to point. The second point may be nearby or at a great distance. Similar to all cells in the body, neurons have a nucleus surrounded by cytoplasm. Different from other cells, however, neurons have cellular extensions or processes called *axons* and *dendrites.* Axons carry electric-like messages away from the nerve cell, and dendrites carry electric-like messages toward the nerve cell (Figure 4-2). Transmission of these messages along nerve fibers occurs through a wave of charge reversal that

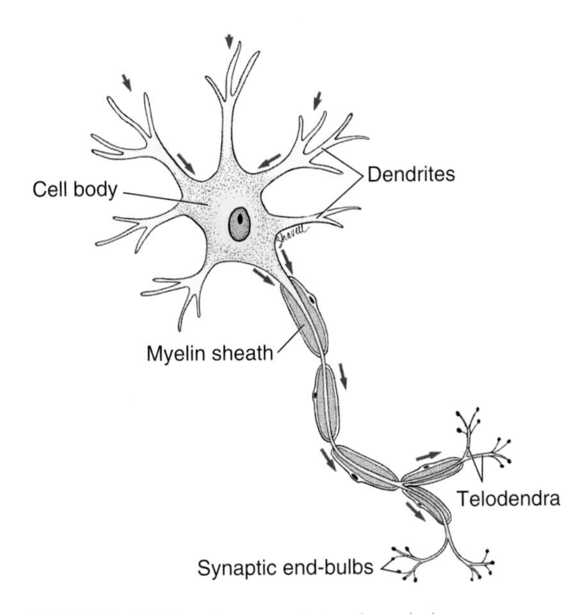

FIGURE 4-2 Impulse transmission through the neuron.

moves down the fiber (Figure 4-3). The resting (polarized) fiber has positive charges lined up on the outside of its membrane and negative charges lined up on the inside of its membrane. When a stimulus of sufficient magnitude reaches the fiber, depolarization or charge reversal (positive in, negative out) occurs in a progressive wave down the fiber toward the synapse. Repolarization is the movement of charges back to their original positions.

Axons may be short or long (up to 4 feet in humans), and they terminate, or end, in as many as 10,000 nerve endings called *telodendra* (Snyder, 1986). The large number of nerve endings allows for great variety in the number and type of connections made with other neurons. The synaptic end-bulbs of the telodendra pass nerve impulses to an adjacent structure (another neuron, gland, or muscle) by emitting a chemical messenger called a *neurotransmitter* into the gap or junction (synapse) between the nerve ending and the adjacent structure (Figure 4-4). Neurotransmitters then combine with receptors on the dendritic side of the synapse and cause a stimulatory or inhibitory effect. Dendrites may respond to

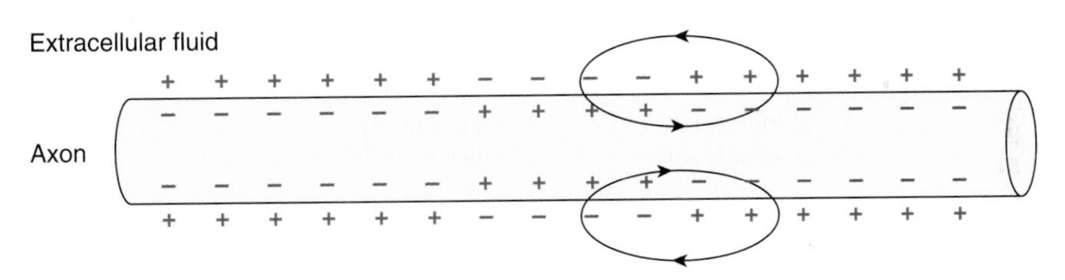

FIGURE 4-3 Electric impulse transmission along a nerve fiber.

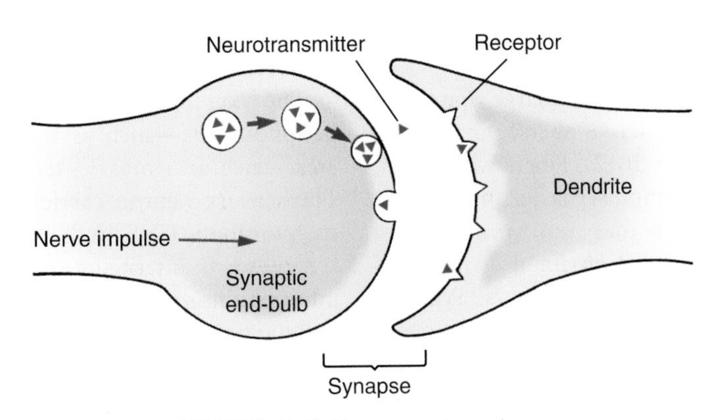

FIGURE 4-4 Neurotransmitter release.

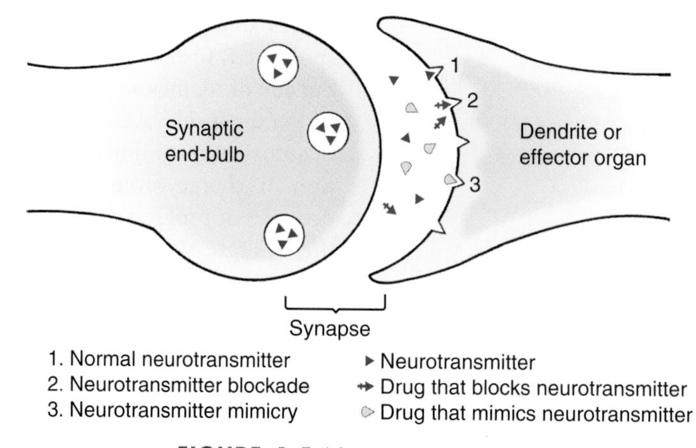

FIGURE 4-5 Neurotransmitter activity.

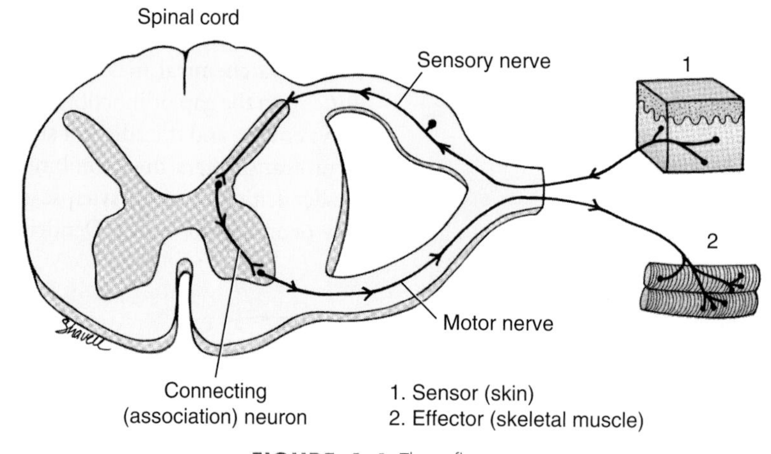

FIGURE 4-6 The reflex arc.

neurotransmitters by generating a nerve impulse, which is conducted via the axon to the adjacent structure (neuron, gland, or muscle). Neurotransmitters can be mimicked or blocked by the use of appropriate drugs (Figure 4-5).

Nerve fibers (nerves) may have a large diameter (A fibers), a medium diameter (B fibers), or a small diameter (C fibers; Boothe, 2012). Fibers with large diameters conduct nerve impulses faster than those with small diameters. Fibers that are surrounded by the insulating substance called *myelin* also transmit impulses faster than nonmyelinated fibers. Type A and B fibers are generally myelinated fibers.

The most basic impulse conduction system through the nervous system is the reflex arc (Figure 4-6). The reflex arc is composed of the following:

- A receptor
- A sensory neuron
- A center in the CNS for a synapse
- A motor neuron
- An effector

The receptor of the reflex arc may be located in a peripheral site—such as the skin—or in a central area—such as a muscle, tendon, or visceral organ. The sensory neuron carries the impulse from the receptor to the CNS. In the CNS, the sensory neuron synapses with interneurons in the spinal cord. These interneurons send the impulse to the brain for interpretation or send the impulse to a motor neuron. The motor neuron carries the message to an effector organ. If the impulse travels around the arc without going to the brain for analysis, the sequence of events

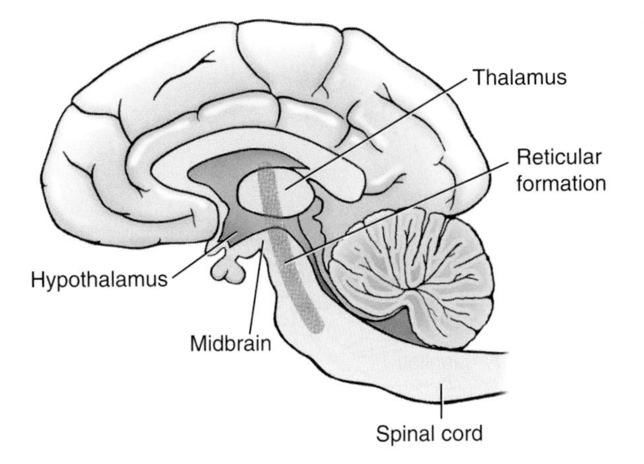

FIGURE 4-7 Pharmacologically important areas of the brain.

is called a *spinal reflex* (see Figure 4-6). A spinal reflex can occur even if the spinal cord is completely severed. For example, a hemostat applied to the toe of a dog with a severed cord can cause the dog to withdraw its leg by means of the spinal reflex.

Areas of the brain that have importance to an understanding of the pharmacology of the CNS are illustrated in Figure 4-7. The cerebrum is responsible for higher functions of the brain, such as learning, memory, and interpretation of sensory input (e.g., vision and pain recognition). The thalamus serves as a relay center for sensory impulses from the spinal cord, brainstem, and cerebellum to the cerebrum. The thalamus also may be involved in pain interpretation. The hypothalamus serves as the primary mediator between the nervous system and the endocrine system through its control of the pituitary gland. The hypothalamus also controls and regulates the ANS. The medulla carries both sensory and motor impulses between the spinal cord and the brain. It contains centers that control vital physiologic activities, such as breathing, heartbeat, blood pressure, vomiting, swallowing, coughing, body temperature, hunger, and thirst. The reticular formation is a network of nerve cells scattered through bundles of fibers that begin in the medulla and extend upward through the brainstem. The reticular activating system is a part of the reticular formation, which functions to arouse the cerebral cortex and is responsible for consciousness, sleep, and wakefulness (DeLahunta, 1983).

In summary, nerve activity is usually described as the generation of nerve impulses that occurs in a dendrite or cell body and then travels down an axon by electric-like activity, which is similar to the passage of an electric current down a wire. When this current reaches a synapse, a chemical "bridge" or neurotransmitter allows the message to be passed to one or as many as thousands of other neurons. Neurotransmitter substances include acetylcholine, norepinephrine, dopamine, serotonin, and gamma-aminobutyric acid (GABA). These other neurons then carry the message to an interpretation center or a structure that takes appropriate action. CNS drugs act by mimicking or blocking the effects of neurotransmitters.

AUTONOMIC NERVOUS SYSTEM

The ANS is that portion of the nervous system that controls unconscious body activities. ANS fibers innervate smooth muscle, heart muscle, salivary glands, and other viscera. This system operates automatically and involuntarily to control visceral functions, such as gastrointestinal (GI) motility, rate and force of the heartbeat, secretion by glands, sizes of the pupils, and various other involuntary functions and characteristics. In contrast to the somatic nervous system, the ANS has two subdivisions: parasympathetic **(cholinergic)** and sympathetic **(adrenergic).** The sympathetic division regulates energy-expending activities (fight-or-flight responses), and the parasympathetic division regulates energy-conserving activities.

The ANS has two neurons that carry impulses to target structures (in contrast to the somatic nervous system, which has only one). The cell body of the first neuron arises in the CNS—in the thoracolumbar cord for the sympathetic nervous system and in the craniosacral cord for the parasympathetic nervous system (Figure 4-8). The axon of the first neuron leaves the CNS and travels to a ganglion, where it synapses with dendrites of the second neuron. This second neuron then travels to the target structure (Figure 4-9). Axons of the first neuron are called *preganglionic,* and those of the second are called

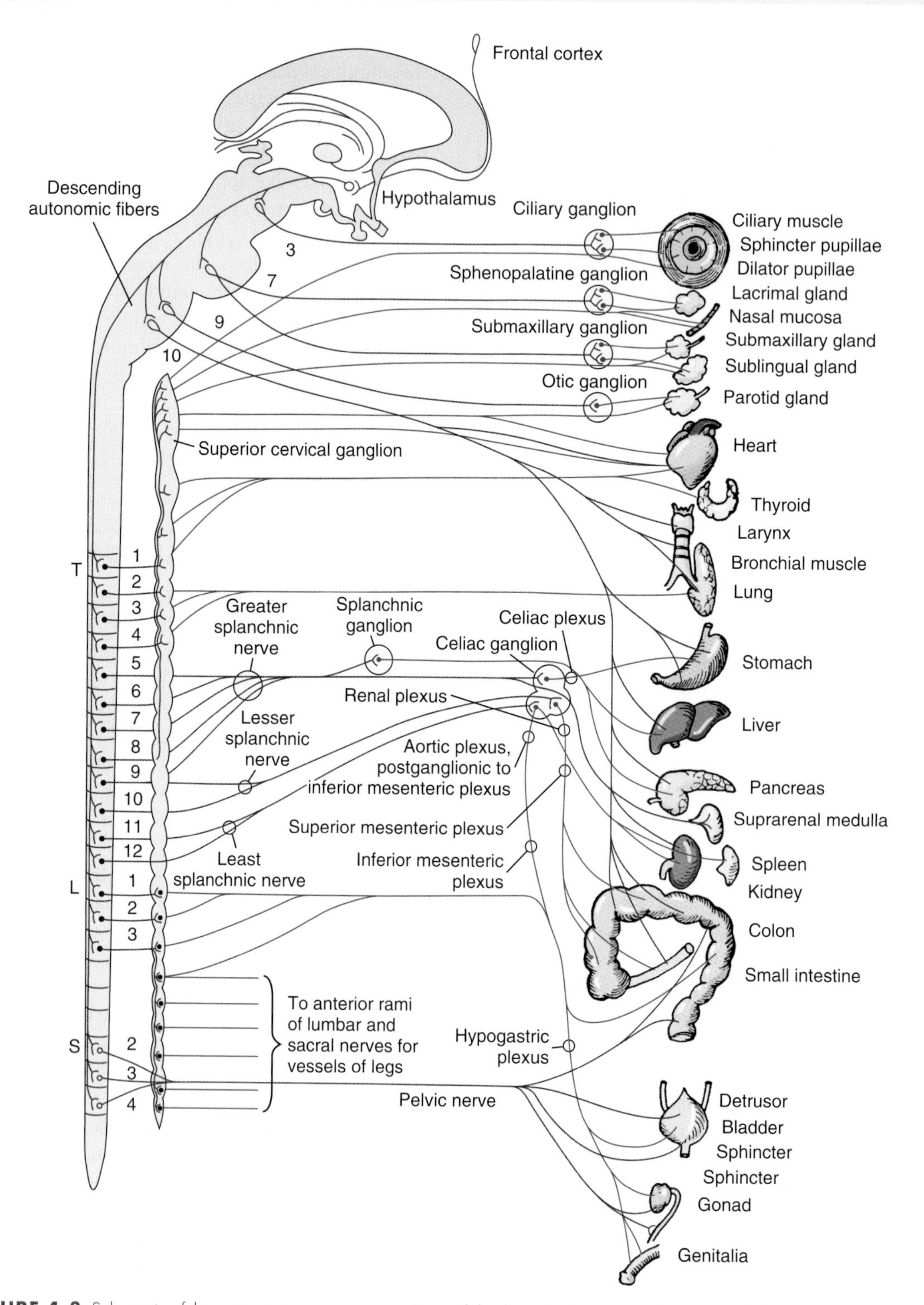

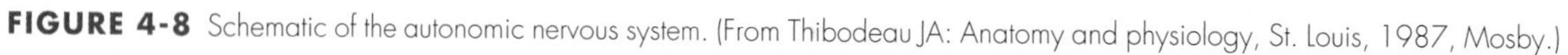
FIGURE 4-8 Schematic of the autonomic nervous system. (From Thibodeau JA: Anatomy and physiology, St. Louis, 1987, Mosby.)

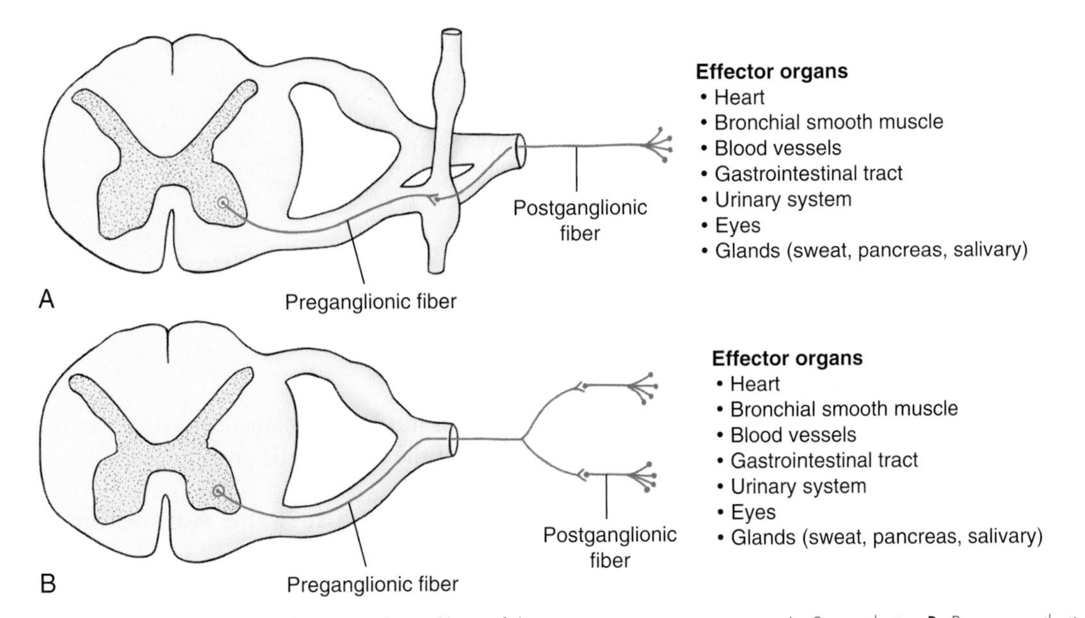

FIGURE 4-9 Preganglionic and postganglionic fibers of the autonomic nervous system. **A**, Sympathetic. **B**, Parasympathetic.

postganglionic. The synapse between the preganglionic neuron and the postganglionic neuron is called the **ganglionic synapse.**

Preganglionic fibers of the sympathetic nervous system are short. They end in ganglia adjacent to the spinal cord. The only exception is the preganglionic fiber to the adrenal medulla. The adrenal medulla itself is analogous to a postganglionic fiber because it releases epinephrine and norepinephrine directly into the bloodstream when stimulated by preganglionic fibers. Postganglionic sympathetic fibers are long.

Preganglionic fibers of the parasympathetic nervous system are generally long. They travel to ganglia located in the wall of the target organ. Postganglionic fibers are consequently short.

Normally, target sites of the ANS have both sympathetic and parasympathetic innervation. The physiologic functions of the two systems usually oppose each other, thereby bringing about a state of balance. When this balance is disrupted, drug therapy may be indicated to restore the balance. The adrenal medulla, sweat glands, and hair follicles have only sympathetic fibers.

Stimulation of the sympathetic nervous system causes an increase in heart rate and respiratory rate, a decrease in GI activity, dilation of the pupils, constriction of blood vessels in smooth muscle, dilation of blood vessels in skeletal muscle, dilation of bronchioles, and an increase in blood glucose levels. These actions prepare an animal to fight or to flee. On the other hand, stimulation of the parasympathetic nervous system causes a decrease in heart rate and respiratory rate, an increase in GI activity, constriction of the pupils, and constriction of the bronchioles.

Receptors of the sympathetic (adrenergic) nervous system are subdivided as follows (Figure 4-10):

- Alpha-1
- Alpha-2
- Beta-1
- Beta-2
- Dopaminergic

Generally, alpha receptors are stimulatory and beta receptors are inhibitory (Table 4-1). The parasympathetic (cholinergic) nervous system has **nicotinic** and **muscarinic receptors. Effector** organs have one or a combination of these receptors. A drug's effect is determined by the number of receptors in the effector and the drug's specificity for the receptor (Williams and Baer, 1990).

The primary neurotransmitters for adrenergic sites are norepinephrine, epinephrine, and dopamine. Epinephrine equally stimulates alpha and beta

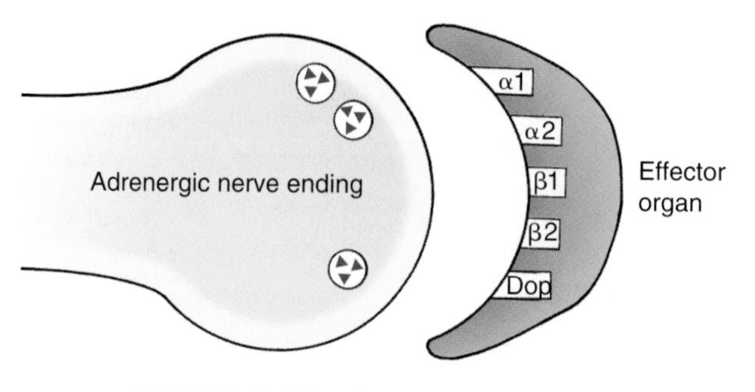

FIGURE 4-10 Adrenergic receptor types.

TABLE 4-1 Adrenergic Receptor Responses

RECEPTOR	TARGET ORGAN	RESPONSE
Alpha-1	Arterioles	Constriction
	Urethra	Increased tone
	Eye	Dilation of pupil
Alpha-2	Skeletal muscle	Constriction
Beta-1	Heart	Increased rate, conduction, and contractility
	Kidneys	Renin release
Beta-2	Skeletal blood vessels	Dilation
	Bronchioles	Dilation
Dopaminergic	Kidneys	Dilation of blood vessels
	Heart	Dilation of coronary vessels
	Mesenteric blood vessels	Dilation

receptors and is therefore a potent stimulator of the heart and an equally powerful dilator of bronchioles. Acetylcholine is the neurotransmitter at sympathetic postganglionic fibers to sweat glands and the smooth muscle of blood vessels (muscarinic sites).

The neurotransmitter for cholinergic sites is **acetylcholine.** Acetylcholine combines with both nicotinic and muscarinic receptors.

Cholinergic sites are found in both the sympathetic and parasympathetic nervous systems. Nicotinic receptors are found in all autonomic ganglia, in the adrenal medulla, and at the neuromuscular junction of the somatic nervous system. Muscarinic receptors are found at the synapse of postganglionic fibers of the parasympathetic nervous system and at a few of the sympathetic postganglionic fibers.

How Drugs Affect the Autonomic Nervous System

Autonomic drugs bring about their effects by influencing the sequence of events that involve neurotransmitters. Most autonomic drugs bring about this alteration of events by doing the following:

- Mimicking neurotransmitters
- Interfering with neurotransmitter release
- Blocking the attachment of neurotransmitters to receptors
- Interfering with the breakdown or reuptake of neurotransmitters at the synapse

CLASSES OF AUTONOMIC NERVOUS SYSTEM AGENTS

CHOLINERGIC AGENTS

Cholinergic agents are drugs that stimulate receptor sites mediated by acetylcholine. They achieve these effects by mimicking the action of acetylcholine (direct-acting) or by inhibiting its breakdown (indirect-acting). Cholinergic agents are also called **parasympathomimetic** because their effects resemble those produced by stimulating parasympathetic nerves.

Clinical Uses

Cholinergic agents do the following:

- Aid in the diagnosis of myasthenia gravis
- Reduce the intraocular pressure of glaucoma

- Stimulate GI motility
- Treat urinary retention
- Control vomiting
- Act as an antidote for neuromuscular blockers

Direct-Acting Cholinergics

- Acetylcholine. Acetylcholine is seldom used clinically because it is broken down so rapidly by **acetylcholinesterase.**
- Carbamylcholine. This product has been used to treat atony of the GI tract and to stimulate uterine contractions in swine.
- Bethanechol (Urecholine). Bethanechol is used to treat GI and urinary tract atony.
- Pilocarpine (Isopto Carpine, Akarpine, Pilocar). Pilocarpine reduces intraocular pressure associated with glaucoma.
- Metoclopramide (Reglan). Metoclopramide is used to control vomiting and to promote gastric tract emptying.

Indirect-Acting Cholinergic (Anticholinesterase) Agents

- Edrophonium (Tensilon). Edrophonium is used to diagnose myasthenia gravis.
- Neostigmine (Prostigmine, Stiglyn). These products are used to treat urine retention and GI atony and are used as an antidote to neuromuscular blocking agents.
- Physostigmine (Antilirium, Eserine). Uses of this product are similar to those of neostigmine.
- Organophosphate compounds. These are commonly used as insecticide dips and may result in toxicity if used inappropriately. See pralidoxime under Dosage Forms for Cholinergic Blocking Agents later in this chapter.
- Demecarium (Humorsol). This drug is used in the preventive management of glaucoma.
- Pyridostigmine (Mestinon). This drug is used for the treatment of myasthenia gravis.

Adverse Side Effects

Adverse side effects of the cholinergic drugs may include bradycardia, hypotension, heart block, lacrimation, diarrhea, vomiting, increased intestinal activity, intestinal rupture, and increased bronchial secretions.

CHOLINERGIC BLOCKING AGENTS (ANTICHOLINERGIC)

Cholinergic blocking agents are drugs that block the action of acetylcholine at muscarinic receptors of the parasympathetic nervous system.

Clinical Uses

Clinical uses of these drugs include the following:

- Treatment of diarrhea and vomiting via a decrease in GI motility
- Drying of secretions and prevention of bradycardia before anesthesia
- Dilation of the pupils for ophthalmic examination
- Relief of ciliary spasm of the eye
- Treatment of sinus bradycardia

The belladonna alkaloids of the deadly nightshade family of plants have been used as drugs for centuries and represent the prototype for this category of agents.

Dosage Forms

- Atropine. Numerous generic and trade name products are available for parenteral or ophthalmic administration. Atropine is used as a preanesthetic to dry secretions and prevent bradycardia; to counteract organophosphate poisoning; to dilate the pupils for ophthalmic examination; to control ciliary spasms of the eye; to treat sinus bradycardia; and to slow a hypermotile gut.
- Methscopolamine is an ingredient of Biosol-M. Methscopolamine is used to control diarrhea.
- Glycopyrrolate (Robinul-V). Glycopyrrolate is a quaternary ammonium compound with actions similar to atropine. It provides longer duration of action than atropine and is used primarily as a preanesthetic.
- Aminopentamide (Centrine). Aminopentamide is used to control vomiting and diarrhea in dogs and cats.
- Propantheline (Pro-Banthine). Propantheline is used to treat diarrhea, urinary incontinence, and bradycardia and to reduce colonic peristalsis in horses to allow rectal examination. Propantheline, similar to glycopyrrolate, is a quaternary ammonium compound.

- Pralidoxime (Protopam, 2-PAM). Pralidoxime is a cholinesterase reactivator used to treat organophosphate intoxication.

Adverse Side Effects

Adverse side effects of the cholinergic blockers are dose related. Overdoses can cause drowsiness, disorientation, tachycardia, photophobia, constipation, anxiety, and burning at the injection site.

> TECHNICIAN NOTES
> - Atropine administered as a preanesthetic causes dilation of the pupils. It dries secretions and prevents bradycardia.
> - Atropine is packaged in small-animal and large-animal concentrations. Care should be taken not to confuse the two preparations.

ADRENERGIC (SYMPATHOMIMETIC) AGENTS

Adrenergic (**sympathomimetic**) agents bring about action at receptors mediated by epinephrine or norepinephrine. Adrenergic agents may be classified as **catecholamines** or noncatecholamines, and either category can also be classified according to the specific receptor types activated (alpha-1, alpha-2, beta-1, beta-2). In most cases, alpha receptor activity causes an excitatory response (except in the GI tract), and beta stimulation causes an inhibitory response (except in the heart). Adrenergic activity is a complex subject, and more advanced texts should be consulted for a thorough explanation.

Clinical Uses

Adrenergic agents are used for the following purposes:

- To stimulate the heart to beat during cardiac arrest
- To reverse the hypotension and bronchoconstriction of anaphylactic shock
- To strengthen the heart during congestive heart failure
- To correct hypotension through vasoconstriction
- To reduce capillary bleeding through vasoconstriction
- To treat urinary incontinence
- To reduce mucous membrane congestion (vasoconstriction) in allergic conditions
- To prolong the effects of local anesthetic agents by causing vasoconstriction of blood vessels at the injection site, thereby prolonging their absorption
- To treat glaucoma (alpha stimulation increases the outflow of and beta stimulation decreases the production of aqueous humor)

Dosage Forms

- Epinephrine (Adrenalin). Epinephrine stimulates all receptors to cause an increase in heart rate and cardiac output, constriction of the blood vessels in the skin, dilation of the blood vessels in muscle, dilation of the bronchioles, and an increase in metabolic rate.
- Norepinephrine (Levophed). Norepinephrine is mostly an alpha stimulator with some beta stimulation. Its primary influence is that of a vasopressor (to raise blood pressure).
- Isoproterenol (Isuprel). Isoproterenol is a pure beta stimulator. Its primary use is for bronchodilation.
- Phenylephrine (Neo-Synephrine). Phenylephrine is an alpha stimulator that is used as a nasal vasoconstrictor.
- Dopamine (Intropin). Dopamine is a precursor of epinephrine and norepinephrine. Its action is dose dependent. It is used to treat shock and congestive heart failure and to increase renal perfusion.
- Phenylpropanolamine (Proin). Phenylpropanolamine is used to treat urinary incontinence in dogs.
- Dobutamine (Dobutrex). Dobutamine is a beta-1 agonist that is used for short-term treatment of heart failure.
- Albuterol [Proventil]. These products are beta agonists and their main use is bronchodilation.

Adverse Side Effects

These may include tachycardia, hypertension, nervousness, and cardiac arrhythmias. Hypertension, arrhythmia, and pulmonary edema may occur with an overdose.

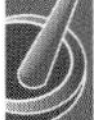

TECHNICIAN NOTES Epinephrine is normally packaged as a 1 : 1000 dilution. Many clinicians prefer a 1 : 10,000 dilution for treating cardiac arrest. Mix 1 mL of the original dilution with 9 mL of sterile water to prepare a 1 : 10,000 dilution. Epinephrine is stored under refrigeration. A note should be placed in the emergency crash cart specifying the location of this drug.

ADRENERGIC BLOCKING AGENTS

Adrenergic blocking agents are used to disrupt the activity of the sympathetic nervous system. They are classified according to the site of their action as an alpha blocker, beta blocker, or ganglionic blocker. Drugs usually block only one category of receptor.

Alpha Blockers

Alpha blockers have had limited use in veterinary medicine. Phenoxybenzamine has been advocated by some clinicians for the treatment of laminitis in horses and urethral obstruction in cats. Yohimbine is used for xylazine antagonism.

Clinical Uses

See section, Dosage Forms.

Dosage Forms

- Phenoxybenzamine (Dibenyline). Phenoxybenzamine is a hypotensive (vasodilator) agent.
- Aacepromazine. This tranquilizer acts as an alpha blocker and causes vasodilation.
- Prazosin (Minipress). Prazosin is a hypotensive agent.
- Yohimbine (Yobine). Yohimbine is used as an antidote for xylazine toxicity.
- Atipamezole (Antisedan). Atipamezole is a reversal agent for dexmedetomidine.

Adverse Side Effects

Adverse side effects may include hypotension (phenoxybenzamine, tranquilizers, prazosin), tachycardia (phenoxybenzamine), muscle tremors (yohimbine), and seizures (acepromazine).

Beta Blockers

Beta blockers are used to treat glaucoma, arrhythmias, and hypertrophic cardiomyopathy.

Clinical Uses

See section, Dosage Forms.

Dosage Forms

- Propranolol (Inderal). Propranolol is used to treat cardiac arrhythmias and hypertrophic cardiomyopathy.
- Timolol (Timoptic). Timolol is an ophthalmic preparation used to treat glaucoma.
- Atenolol (Tenormin). Used in a similar way to propranolol.
- Carteolol (Ocupress). Carteolol is a human labeled antiglaucoma medication.
- Levobunolol (Betagan). Levobunolol is a human labeled antiglaucoma medication.
- Metipranolol (OptiPranolol). Similar to the previous two products.

Adverse Side Effects

These include bradycardia, hypotension, worsening of heart failure, bronchoconstriction, heart block, and syncope.

Ganglionic Blockers

Ganglionic blockers are seldom used in veterinary medicine.

CENTRAL NERVOUS SYSTEM

CNS drugs have various uses in veterinary medicine. Depressant drugs are used to tranquilize or sedate animals to facilitate restraint or anesthetic procedures. They are also used to control pain, to induce **anesthesia**, and to prevent or control seizures. CNS drugs are also available to antagonize (reverse) the effects of some depressant drugs. Another group of CNS agents is used to stimulate the CNS to treat cardiac or respiratory depression or arrest. Euthanasia drugs allow veterinarians to provide a quick and painless end to hopeless medical situations.

Drugs that affect the CNS generally cause depression or stimulation. They are thought to generate these changes by altering nerve impulse transmissions between the spinal cord and the brain or within the brain itself. Altering impulse transmissions within the thalamus could prevent messages regarding painful stimuli from reaching interpretation centers within the cerebrum. Interfering with impulses within the reticular activating system could alter levels of consciousness or wakefulness (Ganong, 2003). The changes that occur in the transmission of nerve impulses as a result of administration of CNS drugs are probably brought about by altered neurotransmitter activity.

The categories of CNS drugs that are covered in this chapter include the following:

- Tranquilizers
- Barbiturates
- Dissociatives
- Opioid/antagonists
- Neuroleptanalgesics/antagonists
- Drugs to prevent or control seizures
- Inhalants
- Miscellaneous CNS drugs
- CNS stimulants
- Euthanasia agents

TRANQUILIZERS

Phenothiazine Derivatives

The mechanism of action of the phenothiazine derivatives on the CNS is not well understood. However, it has been proposed that they are dopamine blockers (Muir and Hubbell, 2007). The effects on the cardiovascular system are a result of alpha-adrenergic blockade.

Phenothiazine derivative tranquilizers produce sedation and allay fear and anxiety without producing significant **analgesia**. Sudden painful stimuli arouse the animal. Phenothiazine derivative tranquilizers produce an antiemetic effect by depressing the chemoreceptor trigger zone in the brain and have a mild antipruritic effect. These agents also reduce the tendency of epinephrine to induce cardiac arrhythmias.

Clinical Uses

Phenothiazine derivatives are used for prevention or treatment of vomiting, relief of mild pruritus, and sedation/tranquilization.

Dosage Forms

- Acepromazine maleate (PromAce)
- Chlorpromazine hydrochloride (Thorazine-human label)
- Promazine HCl (Sparine-human label)
- Prochlorperazine (Compazine-human label)

Adverse Side Effects

Phenothiazine derivative tranquilizers can cause hypotension and hypothermia through their vasodilator effects (alpha blockade). They also can induce seizures (by lowering the seizure threshold) in epileptic animals.

> *TECHNICIAN NOTES*
> - Phenothiazine derivatives should not be used within 1 month of worming with an organophosphate anthelmintic.
> - The tranquilizing effect may be reduced in an excited animal.

Phenothiazine derivative tranquilizers are approved for use in a wide variety of animals and for administration by almost any route. They generally are relatively safe drugs to use when administered appropriately. They should be given with care when used with other CNS depressants because of the additive effect. Most phenothiazine derivative tranquilizers are metabolized by the liver and excreted by the kidneys.

Benzodiazepine Derivatives

The mechanism of action of diazepam occurs through depression of the thalamic and hypothalamic areas of the brain. This drug produces sedation, muscle relaxation, appetite stimulation (especially in cats), and anticonvulsant activity. Diazepam also produces minimal depression of the cardiovascular and respiratory systems when compared with other CNS depressants. It sometimes is used in combination with ketamine to induce short-term anesthesia. Diazepam is very useful for treating seizures in progress.

Several potential drug interactions can occur when diazepam is administered simultaneously with other drugs, and appropriate references should be consulted.

Clinical Uses

Clinical uses include sedation, relief of anxiety and behavioral disorders, treatment of seizures, and appetite stimulation. All of the benzodiazepines are human-label products. Diazepam can be used as an injectable anesthetic.

Dosage Forms

- Diazepam (Valium, Diastat)
- Midazolam (Versed)
- Alprazolam (Xanax)

Adverse Side Effects

These are limited when used as directed. Dogs can exhibit excitement. An overdose may cause excessive CNS depression.

> *TECHNICIAN NOTES*
> - Diazepam should be stored at room temperature and protected from light.
> - Diazepam should not be stored in plastic syringes or in solution bags because it can be absorbed into the plastic.
> - Manufacturers recommend that it not be mixed with other medications or solutions.
> - Diazepam is metabolized by the liver and eliminated by the kidneys.
> - Alprazolam is also used as an appetite stimulant.

Xylazine Hydrochloride

Xylazine is an alpha-2 agonist with sedative, analgesic, and muscle relaxant properties. It is approved for use in dogs, cats, horses, deer, and elk. This agent causes vomiting in a large percentage of cats and in some dogs. Xylazine is antagonized by yohimbine. It produces effective analgesia in horses and is often used for treating the pain associated with colic and for sedation for minor procedures. It is also used in combination with ketamine for short-term field procedures in horses, such as castration and suturing of extensive wounds, because this combination usually produces 15 to 20 minutes of recumbency. Extralabel use of xylazine for cesarean sections in cattle and other surgical procedures is common. Xylazine is used in cats and dogs as a tranquilizer and in combination with other injectable agents for surgical procedures.

Clinical Uses

Clinical uses include sedation, analgesia, short-term anesthesia (when combined with other agents), and induction of vomiting.

Dosage Forms

- Rompun
- AnaSed
- Gemini
- Sedazine
- Cervizine (labeled for deer and elk)

Adverse Side Effects

These include bradycardia, hypotension, respiratory depression, and increased sensitivity to epinephrine, resulting in cardiac arrhythmias. An overdose increases the potential for these effects.

> *TECHNICIAN NOTES*
> - Because of the potential of xylazine to cause bradycardia or heart block in dogs, atropine should be used as a premedicant in this species.
> - Xylazine is used in cattle at one tenth of the equine dose.
> - Horses may appear heavily sedated with xylazine and still respond to painful stimuli by kicking.
> - Small-animal (20 mg/mL) and large-animal (100 mg/mL) concentrations are available. Care should be taken not to confuse them when administering a drug dose to an animal.

Detomidine Hydrochloride

Detomidine, similar to xylazine, is an alpha-2 agonist. It is approved as a sedative/analgesic for horses, and some clinicians report excellent analgesic properties in their patients when using this product. Some animals may respond to stimuli by kicking even when they appear heavily sedated with this drug.

Clinical Uses

Detomidine is used for sedation and analgesia in horses.

Dosage Form

- Dormosedan injectable
- Dormosedan Gel (for sublingual administration)

Adverse Side Effects

These may include sweating, muscle tremors, penile prolapse, bradycardia, and heart block.

> **TECHNICIAN NOTES** The manufacturer warns that detomidine should be used very carefully with other sedative drugs and that it should not be used with potentiated sulfa drugs such as trimethoprim/sulfamethoxazole.

Medetomidine

Medetomidine is an alpha-2-adrenergic agonist labeled for use as a sedative and analgesic in dogs older than 12 weeks. Atipamezole (Antisedan) is the reversal agent for this drug.

Clinical Uses

Uses include facilitating clinical examination, minor surgical procedures, and minor dental procedures that do not require intubation.

Dosage Form

- Domitor (not currently available in the U.S. market)

Adverse Side Effects

Side effects include bradycardia (product insert states that hemodynamics are maintained), atrioventricular heart block, decreased respirations, hypothermia, urination, vomiting, hyperglycemia, and pain at the injection site.

Dexmedetomidine

Dexmedetomidine is an alpha-2-adrenergic agonist labeled for use as a sedative and analgesic in dogs and cats. It is a "right-handed" enantiomer (isomer) of medetomidine (Plumb, 2011). It is considered to be more potent than medetomidine.

Clinical Uses

Dexmedetomidine is used as a sedative, preanesthetic, and analgesic in dogs and cats. It may be combined with other agents such as opioids and ketamine to produce surgical anesthetic levels. A combination of these three products for cats is sometimes called "kitty magic."

Dosage Form

- Dexdomitor

Adverse Side Effects

These include bradycardia, hypertension, vomiting, atrioventricular block, muscle tremors, and others.

> **TECHNICIAN NOTES**
> - Dexmedetomidine should not be used in dogs or cats with cardiovascular, respiratory, kidney, or liver disease or in patients with shock or severe debilitation or stress due to heat, cold, or fatigue.
> - Atipamezole may be used for treatment of dexmedetomidine-induced effects (Plumb, 2011).
> - Before the use of dexmedetomidine in combination with other sedatives is attempted, references should be consulted for potential side effects and dosages.

Romifidine

Romifidine is an alpha-2-adrenergic agonist labeled for use in horses.

Clinical Uses

Romifidine is used as a sedative to facilitate handling, examination, and treatment and as premedication before general anesthesia.

Dosage Form

- Sedivet

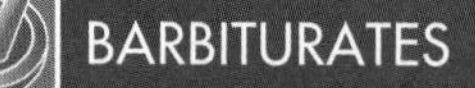

BARBITURATES

The barbiturates are one of the oldest categories of CNS depressants used in veterinary medicine. They are derived from the parent compound barbituric acid and cause various responses ranging from sedation to death, depending on the dose and the circumstances of use. Barbiturates are used in veterinary medicine as sedatives, anticonvulsants, general anesthetics, and euthanasia agents. They are easy and cheap to administer. They have great potential for

TABLE 4-2 Barbiturate Classifications

GENERIC NAME	PROPRIETARY NAME	CLASSIFICATION	DURATION OF ACTION
Phenobarbital	Luminal	Long-acting oxybarbiturate	4 to 8 hours
Pentobarbital	Nembutal	Short-acting oxybarbiturate	½ to 2 hours
Thiopental	Pentothal	Ultrashort-acting thiobarbiturate	10 to 30 minutes

complications because of their potent depressing effects on the cardiac and pulmonary systems (especially in cats) and because they are nonreversible and must be metabolized by the liver before elimination can occur. Individual patients with poor liver function, little body fat, or preexisting illnesses that cause acidosis may be at risk when receiving barbiturates. Because of their alkalinity, the ultrashort-acting barbiturates can cause necrosis of the tissue if administered outside the vein in the subcutaneous space. Barbiturates are metabolized by the liver and are potent depressors of the respiratory system.

Barbiturates are classified according to their duration of action as long-acting, short-acting, and ultrashort-acting. Alternatively, they are classified according to the chemical side chain on the barbituric acid molecule as an oxybarbiturate or a thiobarbiturate (Table 4-2). The long- and short-acting barbiturates have a side chain that is connected by oxygen; they are therefore called *oxybarbiturates.* The thiobarbiturates have a side chain connected by a sulfur. The thiobarbiturates are highly soluble in fat and tend to move rapidly out of the CNS into the fat stores of the body, thus accounting for their ultrashort activity.

Clinical Uses

Clinical uses include the prevention and treatment of seizures, as well as sedation, anesthesia, and euthanasia.

Long-Acting Barbiturates (Oxybarbiturates, 8 to 12 Hours)

Phenobarbital's proprietary and generic products are numerous. Phenobarbital is used primarily as an anticonvulsant to prevent epileptic seizures. It is administered by the oral route. Phenobarbital is a Class IV controlled substance.

Short-Acting Barbiturates (Oxybarbiturates, 45 Minutes to 1.5 Hours)

Pentobarbital sodium has numerous generic products, and Nembutal is a proprietary product. Pentobarbital is given by intravenous injection (the intraperitoneal route also may be used) and provides 1 to 2 hours of general anesthesia. In the early days of veterinary anesthesia, it was the general anesthetic that was routinely used in dogs. Today, pentobarbital is used primarily for controlling seizures in progress and as a euthanasia agent. Intravenous administration of glucose or concurrent use of chloramphenicol may prolong the recovery period. Pentobarbital is a Class II controlled substance.

Ultrashort-Acting Barbiturates (Thiobarbiturates, 5 to 30 Minutes)

Thiobarbiturates are very alkaline (especially at the higher concentrations) and must be given intravenously to avoid necrosis and subsequent sloughing of tissue. Thiobarbiturates are redistributed into the fat stores of the body within 5 to 30 minutes.

Extreme care should be taken when a thiobarbiturate is administered to a thin animal because of the lack of fat stores. Thiobarbiturates are prepared as a sterile powder in vials for dilution up to the desired concentration. They are stable for long periods in undiluted form. Sterile water for injection should be used as the diluent because solutions with electrolytes hasten precipitate formation. Solutions should not be administered if precipitates are present.

Thiobarbiturates can cause a period of apnea when they are rapidly administered intravenously. If spontaneous respirations do not resume in a short time, controlled respirations should be started. Barbiturates can also cause a period of CNS excitement when administered intravenously if they are given too slowly. It is often recommended to give one third to one half of the calculated dose rapidly to avoid the excitement phase. The remainder of the dose is administered in increments until the desired effect is achieved.

Dosage Forms

At this time (2013) thiobarbiturates are not available in the U.S. market.

Adverse Side Effects

These include excessive CNS depression, paradoxical CNS excitement, severe respiratory depression, and cardiovascular depression. Tissue irritation may occur when barbiturates are injected perivascularly.

> **TECHNICIAN NOTES**
> - Recovery from pentobarbital is often prolonged, and dogs exhibit padding limb movements during this time.
> - Thiobarbiturates should not be used in sighthounds or in any very thin animal.
> - Giving additional doses of thiobarbiturates may prolong recovery.
> - Barbiturates are potent depressors of the respiratory system.

DISSOCIATIVE AGENTS

The dissociative agents belong to the cyclohexylamine family, which includes phencyclidine, ketamine, and tiletamine. Involuntary muscle rigidity **(catalepsy),** amnesia, and analgesia characterize dissociative anesthesia. Pharyngeal/laryngeal reflexes are maintained, and muscle tone is increased. Because deep abdominal pain is not eliminated (surgical stage III is not usually reached) with dissociative anesthesia, it is recommended only for restraint, diagnostic procedures, and minor surgery. Dissociative agents, however, often are combined with other agents for abdominal surgery. Dissociative drugs produce minor cardiac stimulation, and respiratory depression can occur with higher doses. These agents act by altering neurotransmitter activity, causing depression of the thalamus and cerebral cortex, and activating the limbic system (Plumb, 2011).

Some species are often ataxic and hyperresponsive during induction and recovery with dissociative agents (Muir and Hubbell, 2007). Tremors, spasticity, and convulsions can occur at higher doses. Hallucinations have been reported in humans and are suspected in cats.

Clinical Uses

Dissociative agents are used for sedation, restraint, analgesia, and anesthesia.

Dosage Forms

- Ketamine HCl (Ketaset, Vetalar, Ketalar). Ketamine is approved for use in humans, primates, and cats but has extralabel uses in various species, including dogs, horses, birds, small ruminants, and reptiles. Tranquilizers, such as acepromazine, dexmedetomidine, xylazine, and diazepam, are often used concurrently with ketamine to enhance muscle relaxation and to deepen the level of anesthesia. Oral, ocular, and laryngeal reflexes are maintained when ketamine is used alone (except at high doses). Occasional spastic jerking movements can occur in cats that are administered ketamine. Ketamine also produces analgesic effects by acting as an N-Methyl-D-aspartate (NMDA) receptor antagonist (see Chapter 14).
- Increased salivation may accompany administration of this drug and can be controlled or prevented with the use of atropine or glycopyrrolate. An ophthalmic lubricant should be used because cats' eyes remain open after administration of ketamine. Ketamine is a Class III controlled substance.
- Tiletamine HCl (Telazol [tiletamine plus zolazepam HC]). Telazol is an injectable anesthetic that consists of a combination of tiletamine (chemically related to ketamine) and zolazepam (a benzodiazepine). Telazol is approved for use in dogs and cats. The pharmacokinetics and pharmacotherapeutics of tiletamine are similar to those of ketamine. Because of the zolazepam in this product, additional agents are not needed for muscle relaxation. Ocular lubrication should be used in cats receiving Telazol. Telazol is a Class III controlled substance.

- Phencyclidine (Sernylan). This dissociative agent is no longer available. It was originally used as an immobilizing agent for nonhuman primates. Its street name is "PCP" or "angel dust" (Upson, 1988).

Adverse Side Effects

These are usually associated with high doses and include spastic jerking movement, convulsions, respiratory depression, burning at the intramuscular injection site, and drying of the cornea.

> *TECHNICIAN NOTES*
> - Both ketamine and tiletamine may cause burning at the injection site. Adequate restraint should be used to ensure injection of all medication.
> - Metabolites of the dissociative agents are excreted through the kidneys. These drugs may be contraindicated in animals with compromised kidney function.
> - Use in animals with certain cardiac conditions (potentially hypertensive) may be dangerous.

OPIOID AGONISTS

An opioid is any compound derived from opium poppy alkaloids and synthetic drugs with similar pharmacologic properties. These drugs produce analgesia and sedation (hypnosis) while reducing anxiety and fear. Narcotic effects are produced in combination with opiate receptors at deep levels of the brain (e.g., thalamus, hypothalamus, limbic system). Opioid receptors are grouped into the following four classes (Paddleford, 1999):

1. Mu—found in pain-regulating areas of the brain; contribute to analgesia, euphoria, respiratory depression, physical dependence, and hypothermic actions
2. Kappa—found in the cerebral cortex and spinal cord; contribute to analgesia, sedation, and miosis
3. Sigma—may be responsible for struggling, whining, hallucinations, and mydriatic effects
4. Delta—modify mu receptor activity

Opioids are used as preanesthetics or postanesthetics because of their sedative and analgesic properties. Sedation is more pronounced at higher doses. They are sometimes used alone or in combination with tranquilizers as anesthetics for surgical procedures, for relief of colic pain in horses, and for restraint/capture of wild/zoo animals. At low doses, the opioids have antitussive (cough suppression) properties because of depression of the cough center in the brain; they also have antidiarrheal action because of a reduction in peristalsis or segmental contractions. Several potential adverse side effects are associated with narcotics. Opioids are potent respiratory depressants and because they affect the thermoregulatory centers in the brain (the body's thermostat), they may cause panting. They may also cause defecation, flatulence, vomiting or sound sensitivity. Excitement may occur in dogs if the narcotic is rapidly given intravenously. Cats and horses are reported to be sensitive to the opioids and may exhibit excitatory effects at high doses. Because opioids cross the placenta fairly slowly and their effects can be antagonized, they can be useful when cesarean section is performed. The liver metabolizes opioids, and resultant metabolites are eliminated in the urine. Many opioid preparations are Class II controlled substances, and narcotic-antagonists can block their effects.

Clinical Uses

Opioid agonists are used for analgesia, sedation, restraint, anesthesia, treatment of coughing, and treatment of diarrhea.

Naturally Occurring Narcotics

- Opium (laudanum—10% opium), paregoric. Opium is derived from the seed capsule of the opium poppy. Paregoric, also called *camphorated tincture of opium,* has been used for longer than 100 years for the treatment of diarrhea. It has been used in veterinary medicine for treating diarrhea, primarily in calves and foals.
- Morphine sulfate (Duramorph). Morphine is an opium derivative used to treat severe pain. Occasionally, it is used as a preanesthetic or anesthetic agent (e.g., cesarean section in dogs). It is also used to relieve anxiety associated with acute congestive heart failure. It exerts its effects primarily on mu receptors. Morphine is a Class II controlled substance that should be used under strict

supervision because of its potential for abuse. It is the standard opioid with which all others are compared in terms of analgesic effect.

Synthetic Narcotics

- Meperidine (Demerol). Meperidine is a mu agonist that is approximately one eighth as potent an analgesic as morphine. It is used for relief of acute pain, such as that occurring after orthopedic procedures. It also may be combined with a tranquilizer for use as an anesthetic agent (neurolept-analgesic). No meperidine products carry a veterinary label. However, human products often have extralabel uses in animals. Naloxone is the preferred antagonist.
- Oxymorphone (Numorphan and Opana). Oxymorphone is a semisynthetic opioid that is a mu agonist. It is approximately 10 times more potent an analgesic than morphine. This drug is used primarily in dogs for restraint, for diagnostic procedures, and for minor surgical procedures. It may be combined with tranquilizers to produce neuroleptanalgesia; naloxone is the antagonist.
- Butorphanol tartrate (Torbutrol, Torbugesic). Butorphanol is a synthetic, opioid agonist/antagonist. Its opioid agonist activity is exerted on kappa and sigma receptors while its antagonist activity occurs at the mu receptor. It is a Class IV controlled substance. Butorphanol has four to seven times the analgesic properties of morphine and significant antitussive effects (Plumb, 2011). Torbutrol is a product that is approved as an antitussive agent in dogs. It is also used in dogs and cats as an analgesic and preanesthetic. Torbugesic is approved for the treatment of pain associated with colic in horses. It is also used in combination with other sedatives/tranquilizers in horses, dogs, and cats as a preanesthetic or for minor surgical procedures. Butorphanol should not be used as the only analgesic agent (Claude, 2013).
- Fentanyl (Recuvrya, Sublimaze and Duragesic-human labels). Fentanyl is an opioid agonist that has approximately 100 times the analgesic properties of morphine. Fentanyl is a Class II controlled substance. Fentanyl transdermal patches are sometimes used in animals to control chronic pain (see Chapter 14).
- Hydrocodone bitartrate (Hycodan, Tussigon). Hydrocodone is an opioid agonist that is used as an antitussive agent in dogs. It is a Class III controlled substance.
- Etorphine (M-99). Etorphine is an opioid that produces analgesic effects 1000 times those of morphine. It is restricted to use by veterinarians in zoo or exotic animal practice (Upson, 1988). It is lethal to people who accidentally inject themselves (it also can be absorbed through intact skin) if the antagonist (diprenorphine) is not administered immediately. Etorphine is a Class II controlled substance.
- Pentazocine (Talwin). Pentazocine is a partial opioid agonist that is approved for pain relief in horses and dogs. It is a Class IV controlled substance.
- Diphenoxylate (Lomotil). Diphenoxylate is a synthetic opioid agonist that is combined with atropine for use as an antidiarrheal agent. This drug is a Class V controlled substance.
- Apomorphine (Apokyn-human label and generic products). Apomorphine is a dopamine agonist derived from morphine with the principal effect of inducing vomiting by stimulating the chemoreceptor trigger zone in the brain. This drug is often administered by placing a portion of a tablet in the conjunctival sac for absorption (see Chapter 8).
- Methadone (Dolophine). Methadone is a synthetic opioid that was developed as a treatment for morphine and heroin addiction in humans. Its primary use in veterinary medicine is in the treatment of colic pain in horses. Methadone is a Class II controlled substance.
- Codeine—generic labeling or in combination. Codeine is an opioid that is available in human label products for use as an antitussive in dogs. Codeine is a Class II agent when used alone but a Class III or Class V when used in combination products.
- Carfentanil (Wildnil). Carfentanil is used to induce wildlife anesthesia. It has 10,000 times the potency of morphine and is a Class II agent that should be used with care to avoid accidental exposure to the users.

- Buprenorphine (Buprenex). Buprenorphine is a human label, partial mu agonist–antagonist. It is a potent analgesic that is used in several small animal species with especially good results in the cat.
- Tramadol (see Chapter 14).

Adverse Side Effects

These can include respiratory depression, excitement (cats and horses), nausea, vomiting, diarrhea, defecation, panting, and convulsions. Overdose causes profound respiratory depression.

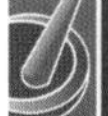

OPIOID ANTAGONISTS

Opioid antagonists block the effects of opioids by binding with opiate receptors, displacing narcotic molecules already present, and preventing further narcotic binding at the sites. These antagonists are classified as pure antagonists or as partial antagonists. The partial antagonists may have some agonist activity (analgesic and respiratory depressant effects).

These drugs usually are administered by the intravenous route and exert their effects very rapidly (15 to 60 seconds).

Clinical Uses

Opioid antagonists are used to antagonize the effects of opioid agonists.

Dosage Forms

- Naloxone (naloxone HCl injection, Narcan). Naloxone is a pure opioid antagonist that is chemically similar to oxymorphone, with high affinity for mu receptors. It has no agonist activity.
- Nalorphine (Nalline). Nalorphine is a partial antagonist that may produce untoward analgesic and respiratory depressant effects.
- Butorphanol-mu antagonist used primarily as a sedative or analgesic. It is rarely used as an antagonist.

Adverse Side Effects

Nalorphine may induce respiratory depression. Naloxone usually has few adverse effects if given in the correct dose.

NEUROLEPTANALGESICS

A neuroleptanalgesic agent consists of an opioid and a tranquilizer. Animals that receive neuroleptanalgesics may or may not remain conscious (Muir and Hubbell, 2007). They often defecate and are highly responsive to sound stimuli. The opioid effects of the neuroleptanalgesics can be antagonized with the opioid antagonists.

Clinical Uses

Neuroleptanalgesics are used for sedation, restraint, and anesthesia.

Dosage Forms

- Fentanyl and droperidol (Innovar-Vet). Innovar-Vet is no longer commercially available although its components are available; therefore a similar compounded product could be formulated.
- Other neuroleptanalgesics may be prepared by a clinician and include the following:
  - Acepromazine and morphine
  - Acepromazine and oxymorphone
  - Xylazine and butorphanol

Adverse Side Effects

These can include panting, flatulence, personality changes, increased sound sensitivity, and bradycardia. An overdose may cause severe depression of the CNS, respiratory system, and cardiovascular system.

DRUGS GIVEN TO PREVENT OR CONTROL SEIZURES

Seizures occur in animals for various reasons, which include but are not limited to unknown (idiopathic), infectious (postdistemper), traumatic (head injury), toxic (strychnine poisoning), and metabolic (heatstroke) factors. Prolonged seizures in progress require emergency action with intravenous therapy. Periodic, recurring seizures require preventive oral medication. Oral preventive therapy often must be titrated to the individual patient and reviewed regularly for the appropriate dose adjustment that controls seizure activity.

Clinical Uses

These drugs are used to prevent seizures or to control seizures in progress.

Dosage Forms

- Diazepam (Valium). Diazepam is a tranquilizer with potent antiseizure properties. It is administered intravenously and has a 3- to 4-hour duration of action.
- Pentobarbital (Nembutal and generic products). Pentobarbital is a short-acting barbiturate that is effective for controlling seizures. It is administered intravenously and has a 1- to 3-hour duration.
- Phenobarbital (Luminal, Solfoton, generic formulations). Phenobarbital is an effective antiseizure drug that is available in oral and parenteral formulations. The oral route is the usual means of administering this drug to dogs and cats. The injectable form is used in horses (foals) by some clinicians. Drowsiness is a potential side effect of phenobarbital. Phenobarbital is a Class IV controlled substance.
- Primidone (Mysoline-human label and Neurosyn-veterinary label). Primidone is similar chemically to phenobarbital, and a portion of the primidone dose is metabolized to phenobarbital by the liver. It is administered orally to dogs and cats, although its use in cats is controversial. Adverse side effects may include agitation, anxiety, polyuria, polydipsia, and dermatitis.
- Phenytoin sodium (Dilantin). The use of phenytoin has declined considerably through the years because of its variable pharmacokinetics in dogs and cats (Plumb, 2011). It may occasionally be used in combination with other antiseizure medications.
- Bromide is an old anticonvulsant that has sparked renewed interest, mainly as an adjunct to phenobarbital or primidone therapy.
- Clorazepate (Tranxene-SD). May be used as an adjunctive with other antiseizure agents.
- Felbamate (Felbatol). May be used for complex, partial seizures.
- Gabapentin(Neurontin). Gapapentin may be used as an adjunctive treatment of seizures that are difficult to control, as well as for partial complex seizures or pain control.
- Levetiracetam (Keppra). May be useful as an adjunct for refractory canine epilepsy.
- Zonisamide (Zonegran). Use is similar to levetiracetam.

Adverse Side Effects

These may include drowsiness, CNS depression, anxiety, agitation, polyuria, polydipsia, and hepatotoxicity (phenobarbital and primidone). Consult product inserts or appropriate references for specific effects.

TECHNICIAN NOTES

- Inadequate compliance is a frequent cause of failure of anticonvulsant therapy. Clients should be advised about the importance of following medication instructions carefully.
- Reserpine and phenothiazine drugs should not be given to epileptic animals.

INHALANT ANESTHETICS

Inhalant anesthetic agents are used to produce general anesthesia. They are converted from a liquid to a gaseous phase by an anesthetic vaporizer and are delivered to the lungs with the use of an oxygen source and a patient breathing circuit. From the alveoli of the lungs, they are absorbed into the bloodstream and delivered to the CNS, where they produce unconsciousness, analgesia, and muscle relaxation through mechanisms not fully understood.

Inhalants generally require little biotransformation for elimination from the body. They enter and exit the body through the lungs, and this facilitates a rapid induction and recovery from the effects of the agent compared with injectable anesthetic agents. It also permits a quicker alteration of the depth of anesthesia.

The amount (partial pressure) of inhalant anesthetic in the brain is proportionate to the alveolar concentration of the agent. Alveolar concentration depends on the amount of agent delivered to the lungs compared with the amount removed from the lungs. Delivery of the agent to the lungs can be increased by increasing the vaporizer setting, increasing the fresh gas (oxygen) flow, increasing minute ventilation, or decreasing mechanical and

TABLE 4-3 Physical Properties of Currently Used Inhalation Anesthetics

PROPERTY	SEVOFLURANE	DESFLURANE	ISOFLURANE	HALOTHANE	METHOXYFLURANE	NITROUS OXDE
Formula	F H F–C–F F–C–O–C–H H F–C–F F	F H F F–C–C–O–C–H F F F	F H F F–C–C–O–C–H F Cl F	Br F H–C–C–F Cl F	Cl F H H–C–C–O–C–H Cl F H	N O N
Molecular weight	200	168	184.5	197.4	165.3	44
Specific gravity (20°C)	1.52	1.47	1.49	1.86	1.41	–
Boiling point (°C)	59	23.5	48.5	50.2	104.7	–
Vapor pressure at 20°C (mm Hg)	160	664	239.5	244.1	22.8	–
mL Vapor/ mL liquid at 20°C	182.7	209.7	194.7	227	207	–
Preservative	None	None	None	0.01% thymol	0.01% butylhydroxytoluene	None
Stability soda lime	No?	Stable	Stable	Decomposes	Decomposes	Stable
UV light	–	–	Stable	Decomposes	Decomposes	–

From Paddleford RR: Manual of small animal anesthesia, ed 2, Philadelphia, 1999, WB Saunders.

physiologic dead space. Factors that influence removal of the agent from the lungs include the solubility (blood–gas partition coefficient) of the agent, the molecular weight of the agent, the partial pressure difference between the agent in the alveolus and the agent in the blood, the amount of alveolar surface available for exchange (absence of lung pathology), and cardiac output.

Uptake by tissue of an anesthetic agent depends mainly on the degree of tissue perfusion and the solubility of the agent in the tissue. Vessel-rich tissue (e.g., brain, heart, lungs, liver, kidneys, intestine, and endocrine glands) receives the greatest percentage of cardiac output and is consequently the first to reach equilibrium during uptake of an anesthetic gas and the first to download an agent. Lipid-rich cells, similar to brain cells, absorb more agent than do lipid-poor cells.

Characteristics important to the understanding of inhalant agents include the minimum alveolar concentration (MAC), partition coefficient, and vapor pressure (Table 4-3). The MAC value of an anesthetic agent is a measure of potency and is the alveolar concentration that prevents gross purposeful movement in 50% of patients in response to a standardized painful stimulus. Lower numbers indicate more potent agents, and values may vary slightly between species. The partition coefficient is the ratio of the number of molecules of an anesthetic gas that exist in two phases (blood/gas). It indicates the solubility of an agent in a tissue such as blood and correlates with the speed of induction and recovery. Lower numbers indicate faster agents. The vapor pressure of an agent indicates how volatile it is and the maximum concentration that can be achieved. Higher numbers indicate greater volatility and the need for a precision vaporizer.

Exposure to anesthetic waste gases can pose a health hazard to the veterinary technician if improper scavenging of waste is not performed. Reproductive, hepatic, and renal effects have been noted. Toxicity is likely due to the biotransformation of byproducts of the agents. Inhalant agents are biodegraded to various degrees (methoxyflurane, 50%; halothane, 25%; isoflurane, <0.2%; sevoflurane, 3%; nitrous oxide, 0.0004%).

Clinical Uses

Inhalant anesthetics are used to induce and maintain general anesthesia in animal patients.

Dosage Forms

- Isoflurane (Forane-human label, IsoFlo-veterinary label, Isothesia-veterinary label). Isoflurane was synthesized in 1968 and was used clinically in people by 1970. Isoflurane is a colorless liquid with a pungent odor. It is stable and does not require a preservative. A halogenated ether, it is one of the least soluble of the inhalant agents. It is less potent than halothane and methoxyflurane but has very rapid induction and recovery times. Isoflurane allows a stable heart rhythm and does not decrease cardiac output at clinically used levels. It is metabolized at a very low rate (<0.2%) This agent is used in a wide variety of species.
- Sevoflurane (Ultane-human label and SevoFlo-veterinary label). Sevoflurane is a halogenated ether with little odor, which makes it a good choice for mask induction. This agent is characterized by very rapid induction and recovery times. Its cardiovascular and respiratory effects are similar to those of isoflurane. Sevoflurane is often used in high-risk, small-animal patients because of its safety and rapid, smooth induction. Only 3% of sevoflurane is metabolized. The disadvantage of the use of this agent is its cost compared with that of isoflurane.
- Halothane (Fluothane). Halothane is a halogenated hydrocarbon that was first used clinically in human anesthesia in 1956. Halothane decomposes when exposed to ultraviolet light and for this reason has thymol added as an antioxidant. Halothane sensitizes the heart to the catecholamines; this may result in cardiac dysrhythmias. Similar to isoflurane and sevoflurane, halothane has a high vapor pressure and must be used in precision vaporizers. "Halothane hepatitis" has been reported in humans but is a very rare occurrence. This agent is metabolized at the rate of 25%, a considerably higher rate than that of the previous two agents.
- Methoxyflurane (Metofane). Methoxyflurane has been used since 1959. It is a methyl-ethyl-ether that is highly soluble in blood and other tissues. It consequently has a very slow induction and recovery time. Methoxyflurane is the most potent (MAC, 0.23% to 0.27%) of the agents considered in this section. It has a relatively low vapor pressure, making 3% the maximum level that can be vaporized. Also, because of this low vapor pressure, it can be used in nonprecison, in-circuit vaporizers or precision, out-of-circuit vaporizers. Methoxyflurane undergoes the greatest biotransformation (50%) of any of the inhalants. It has been associated with renal toxicity in human patients.
- Nitrous oxide. Nitrous oxide is a colorless inorganic gas. It was discovered to have anesthetic properties in the late 1700s. Nitrous oxide may be used as an adjunct to more potent agents during mask induction to speed the induction of anesthesia. General anesthesia cannot be produced with nitrous oxide alone. It is compressed to form a liquid and is supplied in blue cylinders. It has the lowest solubility coefficient of any of the inhalants, which means that it enters and exits the blood and tissue rapidly. Because nitrous oxide is 30 times more soluble than nitrogen, it displaces nitrogen from the alveoli, blood, and gas-filled cavities of the body. This means that it will diffuse into and potentially cause distention of the intestines and other gas-filled areas (e.g., pneumothorax). Nitrous oxide is delivered through a flowmeter and must always be given

with oxygen to prevent hypoxia. Oxygen should always be administered for several minutes after the nitrous oxide is turned off to prevent diffusion hypoxia. (The rapid exit of nitrous oxide from the blood will dilute the oxygen in the alveoli.)

MISCELLANEOUS CENTRAL NERVOUS SYSTEM DRUGS

Propofol

Propofol is a short-acting hypnotic that is unrelated to other general anesthetic agents. Its mechanism of action is not well understood. Chemically, it is an alkylphenol derivative. Propofol products are commercially available either as a milky white macroemulsion or as a clear microemulsion. Because most propofol products are white in color, some clinicians call these products "milk of amnesia." Propofol produces a rapid and smooth anesthetic induction in dogs when given slowly intravenously. It produces sedation, restraint, or unconsciousness, depending on the dose. A single bolus lasts 2 to 5 minutes, making it particularly useful when rapid recovery is important. Some of the products contain no preservative (Rapinovet, PropoFlo, Diprivan), must be refrigerated after opening, and should be discarded after 6 hours. PropoFlo-28 and PropoClear have labels indicating that they contain preservatives, need no refrigeration, and have a shelf life of 28 days.

Clinical Uses

Propofol is useful for anesthetic induction before administration of an inhalant anesthetic, for outpatient procedures, as a substitute for barbiturates in sighthounds, and for patients with preexisting cardiac arrhythmia. It is also useful as an anesthetic agent for dogs undergoing a cesarean section because it does not cross the placental barrier.

Dosage Forms

- Rapinovet, macroemulsion for dogs and cats
- PropoFlo, macroemulsion for dogs and cats
- Diprivan (human label)-macroemuslion
- PropoFlo-28, macroemulsion (with preservatives) for dogs.
- PropoClear, microemuslion with preservatives for dogs and cats.

Adverse Side Effects

Apnea may occur if propofol is given too rapidly intravenously. Occasional seizurelike signs may be seen. Prolonged recovery and/or Heinz body production may be seen in cats with repeated use.

Glyceryl Guaiacolate or Guaifenesin (Guailaxin, Gecolate)

Guaifenesin is a skeletal muscle relaxant that exerts its effects on the connecting neurons of the spinal cord and brainstem (Plumb, 2011). It is used primarily in equine medicine to induce general anesthesia, extend the anesthetic activity of other injectable field anesthetics, or enhance muscle relaxation of anesthetized patients. It may be used as a 5% or 10% solution in 5% dextrose. Some clinicians add other agents like ketamine and xylazine (GKX) to the solution before administering it intravenously. Relatively large amounts are required to induce general anesthesia, and small increments are given to maintain or extend the anesthetic effects of other agents.

Clinical Uses

These include induction or prolongation of general anesthesia in large animals and occasional use as an expectorant.

Dosage Forms

- Guaifenesin Injection
- GuaifenJect

Adverse Side Effects

Adverse side effects are limited. Hemolysis has been reported when greater than 5% solutions are used.

> **TECHNICIAN NOTES**
> - Guaifenesin is packaged as a soluble powder. It may be difficult to dissolve when the diluent is added. Warming 5% dextrose before mixing may aid solution preparation. It should be mixed only immediately before use because a precipitate forms if the solution is allowed to stand for several hours.
> - When increments of guaifenesin are administered to maintain or extend anesthesia, one should communicate thoroughly with the veterinarian to understand the quantity of this drug that should be administered.

Chloral Hydrate/Magnesium Sulfate

This combination has been used as an intravenous agent to produce anesthesia in large animals. Because of the potential for severe irritation of tissue if administered outside of the vein and because of the advent of more efficacious agents, this combination is seldom used.

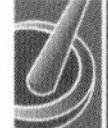

CENTRAL NERVOUS SYSTEM STIMULANTS

The primary medical use of the CNS stimulants is for treatment of respiratory depression or arrest. Many of the other uses of CNS stimulants are illegal or unethical (e.g., to enhance athletic performance).

Doxapram

Doxapram activates the respiratory system by stimulating respiratory centers in the medulla. It is labeled for use in dogs, cats, and horses. Its main indications are to stimulate respirations during or after general anesthesia; it is used in newborns and in cases of cardiopulmonary arrest. It is labeled for intravenous use, but it may be administered under the tongue (1 to 2 drops) or into the umbilical vein of the newborn.

Clinical Uses

These include use to stimulate respiration in newborns and use during or after anesthesia.

Dosage Forms

- Dopram-V
- Dopram. Approved for use in humans.

Adverse Side Effects

Adverse side effects are rare and usually are associated with overdoses. Hypertension, seizures, and hyperventilation may occur.

TECHNICIAN NOTES One to two drops of doxapram may be placed under the tongue or injected into the umbilical vein of the newborn to stimulate respirations.

Pentylenetetrazol (Metrazol)

Pentylenetetrazol is a generalized stimulant of the CNS that has been used to stimulate respirations and to hasten recovery from anesthesia. It has limited use in veterinary medicine.

Caffeine

Caffeine is a general CNS stimulant that promotes wakefulness.

Amphetamines

Amphetamines, which are potent stimulants of the cerebral cortex, are similar chemically to epinephrine. They have few legitimate medical indications in veterinary medicine.

NEUROMUSCULAR BLOCKING DRUGS

Neuromuscular blocking drugs, sometimes called *muscle relaxants,* interfere with neuromuscular transmission of impulses and are used as an adjunct to general anesthesia. These drugs provide no analgesia or sedation. However, they do stop ventilation, and this makes ventilation and constant patient monitoring necessary (Muir and Hubbell, 2007).

Neuromuscular blocking drugs are classified as depolarizing agents or nondepolarizing agents. Depolarizing agents act in a way that is similar to that of acetylcholine at the neuromuscular synapse, but the effects last longer, leading to muscle paralysis (Phase I block). These drugs are not broken down by acetylcholinesterase and have no antagonist. Nondepolarizing agents prevent (competitive inhibition) acetylcholine from binding to receptor sites (Phase II block). These drugs are not degraded by cholinesterase, but they can be antagonized by edrophonium or neostigmine.

Clinical Uses

Neuromuscular blocking agents are used as an adjunct to general anesthesia (e.g., ophthalmic/orthopedic surgery) and to facilitate endotracheal intubation.

Dosage Forms

- Depolarizing
    - Succinylcholine chloride (Anectine-human label)
    - Decamethonium (Syncurine)

- Nondepolarizing
  - d-Tubocurarine chloride (Curare)
  - Gallamine (Flaxedil)
  - Pancuronium bromide (Pavulon)
  - Vecuronium bromide (Norcuron)
  - Atracurium (Tracrium)

BEHAVIORAL PHARMACOTHERAPY

The use of drugs to treat behavioral problems in animals is a relatively new but rapidly growing area of veterinary medicine. Behavior problems—such as separation anxiety, fears and phobias, unruliness, hyperactivity, compulsive disorders, cognitive dysfunction in older dogs, and inappropriate elimination in cats—are being diagnosed in increasing numbers. Many animals with behavioral disorders are taken in desperation to animal shelters, but a growing number of clients are willing to attempt to correct these conditions with environmental management, behavior modification, and/or pharmacotherapy.

Informed consent should be obtained from the client before these drugs are used (Seibert, 2013) because many of the drugs used in behavioral pharmacotherapy are human psychiatric drugs that have not been approved for use in animals. The technician or veterinarian should explain to the animal owner the extralabel status of the drug, its possible side effects or precautions, and the medical effects to be expected in the pet. Owners should also be aware that pharmacotherapy may not be a cure-all for problems of behavior and that these problems may return after therapy is discontinued.

All drugs used in psychotherapy are thought to produce their effects through alteration of neurotransmitter activity in the brain (Simpson and Simpson, 1996a, 1996b). The five neurotransmitters of clinical importance in behavioral pharmacotherapy are acetylcholine, dopamine, norepinephrine, serotonin, and GABA.

Dopamine, norepinephrine, and serotonin are called *monoamine neurotransmitters* because they have similar chemical structures. Monoamines are found in large quantities in areas of the brain often associated with expression and control of emotions. The primary method by which monoamines are inactivated is through their reuptake from the synapse back into synaptic vesicles in nerve endings (see Figure 4-4). Drugs that block or inhibit their reuptake increase their activity. Acetylcholine is the most widely distributed neurotransmitter in the body. It is associated with a variety of behavioral effects and is inactivated by cholinesterase at the synapse. Some of the most common side effects of drugs used in behavioral psychotherapy are related to their anticholinergic effects, such as dry mouth, increased heart rate, urine retention, and constipation. GABA is considered to be an inhibitory neurotransmitter and is widely distributed in the brain.

Pharmacotherapeutic Agents

Drugs most commonly used in treating behavioral problems in veterinary medicine include antianxiety medications, antidepressants, and miscellaneous agents—such as synthetic progestins. All drugs listed in the following section carry a human label, except those that are otherwise indicated.

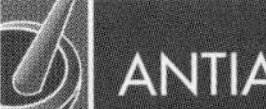

ANTIANXIETY MEDICATIONS

Benzodiazepines

The benzodiazepines most commonly used in veterinary medicine include diazepam, alprazolam, and lorazepam. All the benzodiazepines are similar in structure and mechanism of action. They are thought to bind with and promote GABA activity in the cerebral cortex and in subcortical areas, such as the limbic system.

Clinical Uses

Behavioral uses of benzodiazepines include the treatment of fears and phobias, separation anxiety, aggression, anxiety-induced stereotypes, urine marking in cats, and appetite stimulation.

Dosage Forms

- Diazepam (Valium)
- Alprazolam (Xanax)
- Lorazepam (Ativan)

Adverse Side Effects

These may include lethargy, ataxia, polyuria and polydipsia (PUPD), hyperexcitability, and hepatic necrosis (cats).

Azapirones

Buspirone is the azapirone agent that is used in behavioral pharmacotherapy. In contrast to the benzodiazepines, it possesses no muscle relaxant, anticonvulsant, or sedative effects. Its antianxiety effect is thought to be caused by blocking serotonin receptors.

Clinical Uses

Veterinary uses include the control of urine spraying/marking and the control of fearfulness and anxiety.

Dosage Form

- Buspirone (Buspar)

Adverse Side Effects

Few serious side effects appear to exist.

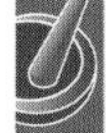

ANTIDEPRESSANTS

Tricyclics

Tricyclics used commonly in veterinary medicine include amitriptyline, imipramine, and clomipramine. These drugs are thought to exert their effects by preventing reuptake of norepinephrine and serotonin. Clomipramine is apparently a selective inhibitor of serotonin reuptake. The tricyclic group is often used on a long-term basis and may take several weeks of use to become effective. Some of the tricyclics are available in the generic form and are relatively inexpensive to use.

Clinical Uses

Uses include the treatment of separation anxiety, obsessive disorders (e.g., lick granuloma, tail chasing), fearful aggression, hyperactivity, hypervocalization, and urine marking.

Dosage Forms

- Amitriptyline (Elavil, generic forms)
- Imipramine (Tofranil)
- Clomipramine (Anafranil, Clomicalm-veterinary label)

Adverse Side Effects

Side effects may include sedation, tachycardia, heart block, mydriasis, dry mouth, reduced tear production, urine retention, and constipation.

Serotonin Reuptake Inhibitors

Serotonin reuptake inhibitors include fluoxetine, sertraline, paroxetine, and fluvoxamine. As their name indicates, these drugs increase the amount of serotonin in the synapse by inhibiting its reuptake back into the nerve terminal. Serotonin reuptake inhibitors have fewer potential side effects than the tricyclics but are usually more expensive.

Clinical Uses

These drugs are used for a variety of behavioral syndromes, including obsessive disorders, phobias, aggression, and separation anxiety.

Dosage Forms

- Fluoxetine (Prozac, human label) (Reconcile, labeled for use in dogs)
- Sertraline (Zoloft)
- Paroxetine (Paxil)
- Fluvoxamine (Luvox)

Adverse Side Effects

Side effects are relatively few but include anorexia, nausea, lethargy, anxiety, and diarrhea.

Monoamine Oxidase-B Inhibitors

The neurotransmitter dopamine is broken down by the enzyme monoamine oxidase-B (MAO-B). Substances such as selegiline (a MAO-B inhibitor) block or inhibit MAO-B and allow dopamine levels to increase. Decreased dopamine levels may be associated with certain types of dementia that are seen in older dogs (canine cognitive dysfunction). Canine cognitive dysfunction is characterized by disorientation, decreased activity level, abnormal sleep–wake cycles, loss of house training, decreased or altered responsiveness, and decreased or altered greeting behavior.

Clinical Uses

Uses include treatment of old-dog dementia and treatment of canine Cushing's disease.

Dosage Form
- Selegiline (Eldepryl, Zelapar, Anipryl-veterinary label)

Adverse Side Effects
Side effects include vomiting, diarrhea, anorexia, restlessness, lethargy, salivation, shaking, and deafness.

Synthetic Progestins
Synthetic progestins are sometimes used to treat behavioral problems through mechanisms associated with changing hormonal levels (reduced gonadotropins) or through some direct effect on the cerebral cortex.

Clinical Uses
Uses include the treatment of urine spraying/marking, intermale aggression, and dominance aggression.

Dosage Forms
- Megestrol acetate (Megace, Ovaban [veterinary label])
- Medroxyprogesterone (Depo-Provera)

Adverse Side Effects
Transient diabetes mellitus (cats), PUPD, increased weight gain, personality changes, endometritis, endometrial hyperplasia, mammary hypertrophy, mammary tumor, adrenal atrophy, and lactation are side effects.

Miscellaneous Behavioral Agents
- Gabapentin. Gabapentin may be used for anxiety or social phobias.
- Clorazepate (Tranxene-SD). Clorazepate is used for anxiety or social phobias; it is a Class IV controlled substance
- Methylphenidate (Ritalin). Methylphenidate has been used for hyperactivity in dogs; it is a Class II controlled substance

EUTHANASIA AGENTS

Euthanasia agents should have several properties that make them effective medically and aesthetically for this emotion-laden procedure. These drugs should rapidly produce unconsciousness without struggling, vocalizations, or excessive involuntary movement. Death should follow quickly as a result of the cessation of all vital functions, such as respiratory and cardiac functions.

The main component of most of the euthanasia agents is pentobarbital. Pentobarbital may also be combined with other agents, such as propylene glycol and alcohol. Pentobarbital alone is a Class II controlled substance, and pentobarbital combinations usually are Class III controlled substances.

Clinical Uses
These agents are used to produce a rapid, humane death.

Dosage Forms
- Pentobarbital sodium (Sleepaway, Socumb-6GR, Fatal Plus, pentobarbital generic). These products are Class II controlled substances for intravenous use.
- Pentobarbital sodium (Beuthanasia-D, Euthasol, SomnaSol). These drugs are Class III controlled substances for intravenous use. This product is different from the pentobarbital sodium described previously in that it contains rhodamine B, a bluish-red dye that helps to distinguish it from other parenteral pentobarbital solutions, as well as phenytoin and preservatives.

Adverse Side Effects
These may include muscle twitching; death may be delayed if the drug is injected outside the vein.

REVIEW QUESTIONS

1. Define the difference between an agonist and an opioid antagonist. ______________________
2. Define *neurotransmitter*.

   ____
3. The area of the brain that serves to relay information from the spinal cord and brainstem to the interpretation center in the cerebrum is the ______.
   a. cerebellum
   b. thalamus
   c. hypothalamus
   d. hippocampus
4. Most CNS drugs act by ______________________ or ______________________ the effects of neurotransmitters.
5. What are the primary neurotransmitters for adrenergic receptors? ______________________
6. List the four primary ways in which drugs affect the ANS. ______________________
7. List five indications for the use of cholinergic agents. ______________________
8. Atropine, scopolamine, glycopyrrolate, and aminopentamide are examples of what specific drug class?

   ____
9. What category of drug is used to treat cardiac arrest and anaphylactic shock?

   ____
10. Propranolol is an example of what category of drug?
    a. Alpha agonist
    b. Beta agonist
    c. Alpha blocker
    d. Beta blocker
11. What are some adverse side effects of xylazine, and what drug may be used to antagonize its effects? ______________________
12. Why would you be concerned about using a thiobarbiturate to induce anesthesia in a very thin dog? ______________________
13. What are some of the characteristics of a cat anesthetized with ketamine?

    ____
14. List some of the signs of a narcotic overdose.

    ____
15. List two narcotic antagonists.

    ____
16. Why should glyceryl guaiacolate not be mixed until just before use? ______________________
17. You are assisting in the delivery of a litter of puppies and you deliver one that is not breathing adequately. What drug would the veterinarian instruct to give, and by what route? ______________________
18. Why are euthanasia solutions that contain only pentobarbital classified as Class II controlled substances, whereas those that contain pentobarbital and other substances are classified as Class III controlled substances?

    ____
19. All psychotherapy drugs are thought to produce their effects by altering ______________________ activity in the brain.
20. Dissociative agents, such as ketamine and tiletamine, may cause ______________________ at the injection site.
21. A hypnotic (anesthetic) known for its very short duration and its white color is

    ______________________.
22. An inhibitory neurotransmitter that is widely distributed in the brain is

    ______________________.
23. A benzodiazepine that is used as an antianxiety medication and as an appetite stimulant in cats is ______________________.
24. An example of a tricyclic antidepressant used in veterinary medicine for separation anxiety in dogs is ______________________
25. ______________________ is used to treat old-dog dementia.
26. The nervous system carries out activity very rapidly by sending electric-like messages over a network of nerve fibers. The ______ system works much more slowly by sending chemical messengers through the bloodstream to target structures.
    a. hematopoietic
    b. endocrine
    c. exocrine
    d. cytokine

27. The ____ nervous system is under voluntary control.
   a. somatic
   b. autonomic

28. The ____ is the fundamental unit of the nervous system.
   a. hepatocyte
   b. nephron
   c. beta cell
   d. neuron

29. Axons carry electric-like messages ____ (from) the nerve cell, and dendrites carry electric-like messages _____ (from) the nerve cell.
   a. away; toward
   b. toward; away

30. Neurotransmitters cannot be mimicked or blocked by the use of appropriate drugs, and that is why patients with nervous system disorders do not have a very good prognosis.
   a. True
   b. False

31. The ANS is that portion of the nervous system that controls _____ body activities.
   a. conscious
   b. unconscious

32. The neurotransmitter for cholinergic sites is ______.
   a. atropine
   b. scopolamine
   c. pralidoxime
   d. acetylcholine

33. Epinephrine (adrenaline) is responsible for all of the following except _______.
   a. can cause an increase in metabolic rate
   b. can cause an increase in heart rate and cardiac output
   c. communication with stem cells in the bone marrow
   d. can constrict blood vessels in the skin

34. Xylazine is antagonized by _______.
   a. hemp
   b. detomidine HCl
   c. Valium
   d. yohimbine

35. All the following are benzodiazepines except ______.
   a. yohimbine
   b. diazepam
   c. alprazolam
   d. lorazepam

36. The direct-acting cholinergic metoclopramide is ordered for a 50 lb dog to control vomiting and promote gastric emptying. The dosage of metoclopramide is 0.25 mg/kg and the concentration of the drug is 5 mg/mL. How many milliliters would you prepare? ______.

37. A 12-year-old dog weighing 30 lb is experiencing urinary incontinence and will be treated with phenylpropanolamine at a dosage of 2 mg/kg. Proin tablets (25 mg) are available. How many tablets will you give? ______.

38. A 1000-lb horse will be treated with detomidine at a dosage of 10 mcg/kg IV for abdominal pain. The concentration of detomidine is 10 mg/mL. What quantity will you prepare? ______.

39. Dexmedetomidine will be given to an 8-lb cat as a preanesthetic at a dosage of 30 mcg/kg. The concentration of Dexdomitor is 0.5 mg/mL. What quantity would you draw up? ______.

40. A 12-lb cat will be given buprenorphine (0.3 mg/mL) squirted into the mouth at a dosage of 0.02 mg/kg for postsurgical pain. What quantity will you prepare? ______.

41. A 15-year-old dog with advanced osteosarcoma will be euthanized with a pentobarbital solution (Beuthanasia solution). The dog weighs 85 lbs and the dosage of Beuthanasia is 1 mL/10 pounds. How many milliliters will you prepare? ______.

REFERENCES

Boothe DM: Control of pain in small animals: opioid agonists and antagonists and other locally and centrally acting analgesics. In Boothe DM, editor: Small animal clinical pharmacology and therapeutics, Philadelphia, 2012, WB Saunders.

Claude A: Acute pain management in the small animal practice: pharmaceutical options, Music City Vet Conf, Murfreesboro, Tenn, 2013.

DeLahunta A: Diencephalon. In DeLahunta A, editor: Veterinary neuroanatomy and clinical neurology, Philadelphia, 1983, WB Saunders.

Ganong WF: Review of medical physiology, ed 21, New York, 2003, McGraw-Hill.

Muir WW, Hubbell JA: Handbook of veterinary anesthesia, ed 4, St. Louis, 2007, Mosby Elsevier.

Paddleford RR: Manual of small animal anesthesia, Philadelphia, 1999, WB Saunders.

Plumb DC: Veterinary drug handbook, ed 7, Ames, Iowa, 2011, Wiley-Blackwell.

Seibert LM: Behavior drug protocols, Music City Vet Conf, Murfreesboro, Tenn, 2013.

Simpson BS, Simpson DM: Behavioral pharmacotherapy part I: antipsychotics and antidepressants, Compend Contin Educ Pract Vet 18(10):1067–1081, 1996a.

Simpson BS, Simpson DM: Behavioral pharmacotherapy part II: anxiolytics and mood stabilizers, Compend Contin Educ Proc Vet 18(11):1203–1210, 1996b.

Snyder S: Mood modifiers. In Snyder S, editor: Drugs and the brain, New York, 1986, Scientific American Library.

Upson DW: Central nervous system. In Upson DW, editor: Handbook of clinical veterinary pharmacology, ed 3, Manhattan, Kansas, 1988, Dan Upson Enterprises.

Williams BR, Baer C: Drugs affecting the autonomic nervous system. In Williams BR, Baer C, editors: Essentials of clinical pharmacology in nursing, Springhouse, Pa, 1990, Springhouse Corp.

CHAPTER

5

Drugs Used in Respiratory System Disorders

KEY TERMS

Aerosolization
Antitussive
Bronchoconstriction
Bronchodilation
Decongestant
Expectorant
Humidification
IgA
Inspissated
Mucolytic
Nebulization
Nonproductive cough
Productive cough
Reverse sneeze
Surfactant
Viscid

OUTLINE

Introduction
Respiratory Anatomy and Physiology
Respiratory Defense Mechanisms
Principles of Respiratory Therapeutics
Inhalation Therapy for Respiratory Disease
Categories of Respiratory Drugs
EXPECTORANTS
- Guaifenesin
- Iodide Preparations
- Hypertonic Saline

MUCOLYTICS: ACETYLCYSTEINE
ANTITUSSIVES: CENTRALLY ACTING AGENTS
- Butorphanol Tartrate
- Hydrocodone Bitartrate
- Codeine
- Dextromethorphan
- Temaril-P

BRONCHODILATORS
- Cholinergic Blockers
- Antihistamines
- Beta$_2$-Adrenergic Agonists
- Methylxanthines

DECONGESTANTS
ANTIHISTAMINES
CORTICOSTEROIDS
MISCELLANEOUS RESPIRATORY DRUGS
- Respiratory Stimulants
- Mast Cell Stabilizers
- Leukotriene Antagonists

LEARNING OBJECTIVES

After studying this chapter, you should be able to

1. Describe the basic anatomy and physiology of the respiratory system.
2. List the protective mechanisms of the respiratory system.
3. Describe the fundamental principles of treatment of the respiratory system.
4. List the differences between the actions of expectorants, antitussives, and mucolytics.
5. Describe the action of bronchodilators.
6. Describe the use of antihistamines and decongestants in respiratory disease.
7. List potential uses for respiratory stimulants.
8. List the advantages and disadvantages of inhalant therapy.

INTRODUCTION

Veterinary references list a wide variety of diseases of the respiratory system. A partial listing of general origins includes the following:

- Allergies
- Aspiration
- Bacteria
- Congenital defects
- Fungi
- Immunologic factors
- Neoplasia
- Neurologic conditions
- Parasites
- Trauma
- Viruses

The respiratory system has a series of defense mechanisms by which it protects itself from disease. These natural defenses can be damaged by management practices such as those that cause a buildup of ammonia in enclosed, poorly ventilated housing. They can also be suppressed by inappropriate therapy, such as the use of cough suppressants for a productive cough. Because it is essential that these defense mechanisms function optimally for prompt recovery from respiratory disease, it is very important that technicians have a basic understanding of respiratory anatomy and physiology, respiratory defense mechanisms, and respiratory therapeutics.

RESPIRATORY ANATOMY AND PHYSIOLOGY

The respiratory system consists of the lungs and the passageways that carry air to and from the lungs (Figure 5-1). These passageways include the nostrils, nasal cavity, pharynx, larynx, trachea, bronchi, and bronchioles.

The passageways that lead to the lungs are referred to as the *upper respiratory system.* The upper respiratory system begins with the nostrils, which open into the nasal cavity. The nasal cavity contains turbinates that are covered with mucous membranes. These turbinates increase the surface area of the nasal cavity to allow **humidification** and warming of inspired air. Air that passes out of the nasal cavity moves, in turn, through the pharynx and the larynx into the trachea. The trachea bifurcates into right and left bronchi,

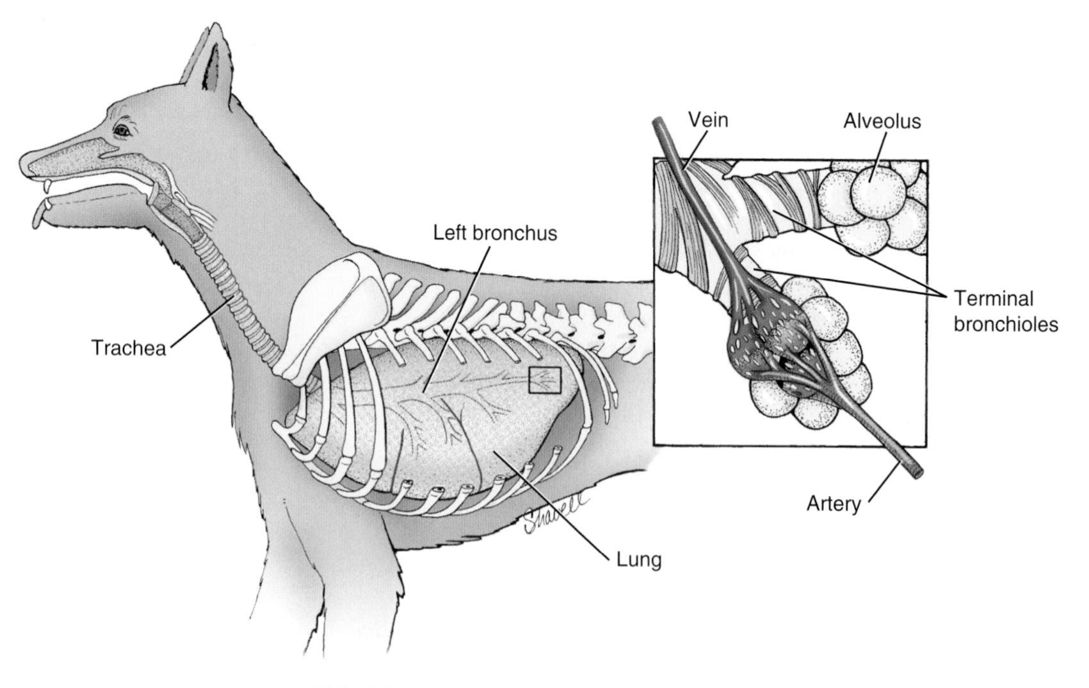

FIGURE 5-1 Anatomy of the respiratory system.

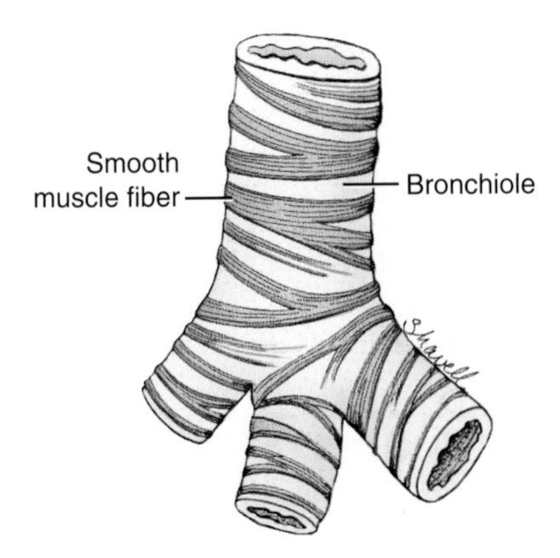

FIGURE 5-2 Smooth muscle fibers in the walls of the bronchioles relax to allow bronchodilation and contract to cause bronchoconstriction.

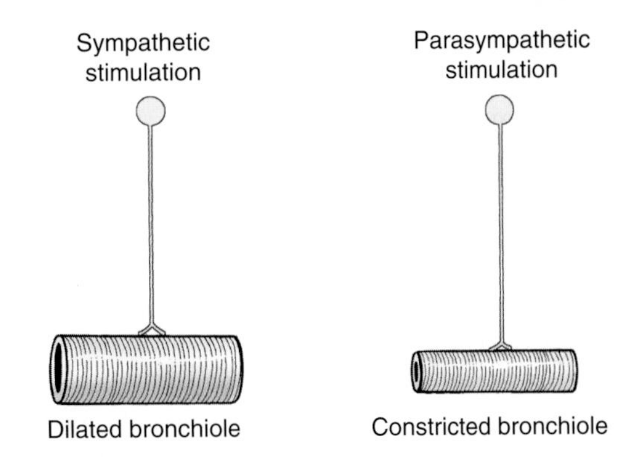

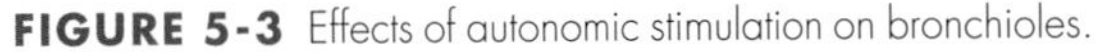

FIGURE 5-3 Effects of autonomic stimulation on bronchioles.

which lead to right and left lungs, respectively. Each bronchus then divides into a series of passageways of decreasing size, called *bronchioles*. Smooth muscle fibers are found in the walls of the bronchioles. Contraction of smooth muscle fibers decreases the diameter of the bronchioles, and relaxation of fibers allows the diameter to return to normal size (Figure 5-2).

The upper respiratory tract is lined with ciliated, pseudostratified columnar epithelial cells. Interspersed between the epithelial cells are goblet cells capable of secreting mucus. Mucus is secreted onto the surface of the epithelial cells and is moved toward the pharynx by movement of the cilia (mucociliary apparatus).

Sympathetic stimulation results in decreased production of mucus by the goblet cells and relaxation of smooth muscle in the walls of the bronchioles, leading to **bronchodilation.**

Parasympathetic stimulation causes increased secretion of mucus and constriction of smooth muscle **(bronchoconstriction)** (Figure 5-3).

The bronchioles terminate in small, saclike structures called *alveoli*. The alveoli are arranged in grapelike clusters and are lined with a chemical substance called **surfactant,** which reduces the surface tension of the alveoli and helps to keep them from collapsing. The alveoli are surrounded by capillaries; this makes it possible for the blood to unload its carbon dioxide into the alveoli and to pick up oxygen from the alveoli.

Functions that the respiratory system serves include the following:

- Oxygen–carbon dioxide exchange
- Regulation of acid–base balance
- Body temperature regulation
- Voice production

The work of the respiratory system can be divided into the following four parts:

1. Ventilation—movement of air into and out of the lungs. The inspiratory portion of ventilation is usually an active process, whereas expiration is usually a passive process. Forced inspiration may be associated with upper airway obstruction, and active expiration may be related to intrathoracic airway obstruction (Tilley and Smith, 2000).
2. Distribution—distributing of inspired gases throughout the lungs.
3. Diffusion—movement of gases across the alveolar membrane.
4. Perfusion—supply of blood to the alveoli. The ratio of perfusion to ventilation of the alveoli is normally close to 1:1.

RESPIRATORY DEFENSE MECHANISMS

The respiratory system has several effective methods of defense against disease processes, including the following:

- Nasal cavity: The turbinates of the nasal cavity provide a large surface area for warming and humidifying inspired air. Hair in the nasal passages also may help to filter out larger particulate matter.

- Protective reflexes: The cough, the sneeze, and perhaps the **reverse sneeze** respond to stimulation of receptors on the surfaces of air passageways to forcefully expel foreign material. Laryngospasm and bronchospasm also help to prevent introduction of materials into the lung tissue.
- Mucociliary clearance: The layer of mucus secreted onto the surface of the epithelial lining of the respiratory tract helps to trap foreign debris that enters the respiratory passages. Wavelike actions of the cilia then move the debris up the passages ("escalator" action) to the pharynx, where it can be swallowed or expelled. Macrophages and immunoglobulin **(IgA)** also contribute to the defensive qualities of the mucociliary apparatus by immobilizing or phagocytizing foreign material.

PRINCIPLES OF RESPIRATORY THERAPEUTICS

It is important that a specific diagnosis be made through radiology, cytology, or appropriate culture before treatment of respiratory disease is initiated because the correct treatment for one type of disease may be contraindicated for another. Once the diagnosis has been made, treatment for respiratory disease is divided into the following three general goals (McKiernan, 1988):

1. Control of secretions: Secretions may be reduced by decreasing their production or increasing their elimination. Removing the cause of the secretions by means of antibiotic, antifungal, antiparasitic, or other appropriate therapy is of vital concern. Methods are also aimed at making the secretions less **viscid** through the use of expectorants or through **nebulization** of **mucolytics** (aerosol therapy).
2. Control of reflexes: Coughing may be suppressed through the use of antitussives or bronchodilators if the cough is **nonproductive.** Sneezing is controlled by removal of the offending agent or through the use of vasoconstrictors. Bronchospasms may be controlled with bronchodilators and corticosteroids.
3. Maintaining normal airflow to the alveoli: Airflow to the alveoli may be maintained by reversing bronchoconstriction, by removing edema or mucus from alveoli and air passages, and by providing oxygen therapy. Intermittent positive-pressure ventilation and other ventilation strategies are often used in humans and may have application in selected animal cases.

INHALATION THERAPY FOR RESPIRATORY DISEASE

Although drugs used to treat respiratory disease are often administered by the oral or parenteral route, inhalation therapy may also be useful. **Aerosolization** (nebulization) of drugs allows their delivery at high concentrations directly into the airways while minimizing their blood levels—a feature that may reduce the chance of a toxic reaction. The efficacy of an inhaled drug depends on the dose and on how well it is distributed in the lungs. Distribution of an aerosol depends on several factors such as the size, shape, and pattern of the airways and the breathing pattern of the animal. The size of the inhaled particle plays a significant role in its distribution. The optimum particle size for entry into the peripheral airways is 1 to 5 microns (Lavoie, 2001). Particles smaller than 0.5 micron are likely to be exhaled, and those larger than 5 microns could be deposited in the upper airways. Airway pathology (e.g., excessive mucus or exudate) can interfere with distribution of the drug, causing some clinicians to assert that inhalation therapy should always be accompanied by systemic treatment (Boothe, 2012). Concurrent use of a bronchodilator and/or a mucolytic may be a helpful adjunct to inhalation therapy.

Two basic types of aerosol delivery systems are available for inhalation therapy: nebulizers and metered dose inhalers (MDI). Generally, nebulizers produce and deliver smaller particles that reach deep into the respiratory system whereas MDIs deliver particles to the upper airways. Nebulizers use compressors to create an aerosol that can be inhaled without the necessity of using positive pressure to force the aerosol into the airways. Nebulizers produce the aerosol using a jet or ultrasonic mechanism. In jet nebulizers, compressed air or oxygen is forced

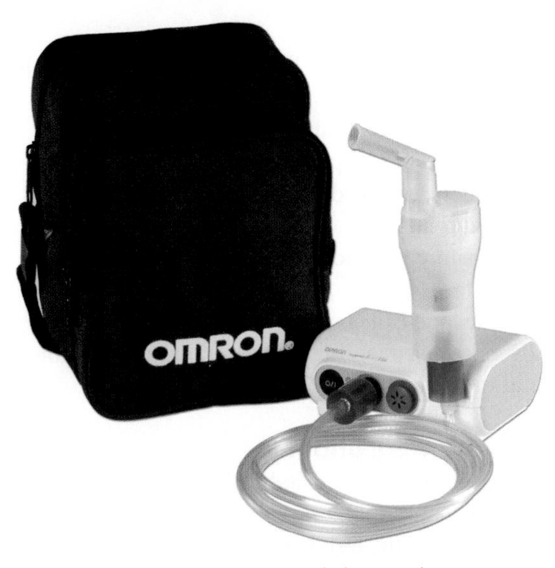

FIGURE 5-4 Omron nebulization device.

through a small orifice to create the aerosol. Drugs in solution are drawn from a fluid reservoir and shattered into droplets by the gas stream. Ultrasonic nebulizers use high-frequency vibrations from a piezoelectric crystal to create the aerosol. Ultrasonic nebulizers are more efficient at creating smaller aerosol droplets and are gentler on drug molecules than the jet nebulizers. Aerosolized drugs can be delivered to cats and dogs in a tentlike structure, closed container, or face mask, but a tight fitting face mask, endotracheal tube, or tracheostomy tube probably delivers the most efficient concentration of the drug to the patient (Reinero and Selting, 2013). Nebulizers must be kept meticulously clean to avoid iatrogenic infection of a patient already compromised with an airway pathology. Small inexpensive nebulizers are available for adaption for veterinary use (Omron) (Figure 5-4).

MDIs are designed for home use by animal owners. The aerosol of an MDI is driven by a propellant. Older MDIs used chlorofluorocarbons (CFCs) as the propellant, but CFCs are being replaced by hydrofluoroalkanes (HFAs), which contain no chlorine and do not affect the ozone. HFA propellants allow drugs to be delivered as a solution rather than a microsuspension, which, in turn, allows the production of a smaller particle that can reach deeper in the airways (Boothe, 2012). The use of spacers and holding chambers with the MDIs makes delivery to the patient more efficient and directed.

Clinical Uses

Nebulizers have been used primarily in the treatment of respiratory infections. Nebulizers are used to provide airway humidification (saline), mucolytics, bronchodilators, and antimicrobials. Mucolytics and saline can help treat pneumonia and other airway infections by decreasing the viscosity of airway secretions and improving their clearance from the airway. Bronchodilators increase flow through the airways, and antimicrobials counter infectious agents. A potential use of nebulizer therapy may be for inhaled chemotherapy, which would take advantage of the concept that high doses of the agents may be delivered to the lung while avoiding the potential side effects of intravenous use.

MDI therapy has been used primarily for feline lower airway disease (asthma), lower airway disease in horses (heaves or recurrent airway obstruction [RAO]), and, occasionally, in lower airway disease (bronchitis) in dogs. MDIs frequently contain bronchodilators like albuterol or clenbuterol and/or corticosteroids.

Box 5-1 lists drugs frequently used in inhalation therapy.

MDI units for inhalation therapy are available for use in small animals (Opti-Chamber, Aero-Chamber, AeroKat, AeroDawg) and in horses (Aero-Mask) (Figure 5-5).

CATEGORIES OF RESPIRATORY DRUGS

EXPECTORANTS

Expectorants are drugs that liquefy and dilute viscid secretions of the respiratory tract, thereby helping in evacuation of those secretions. Most expectorants are administered orally, although a few are given by inhalation or parenterally. Expectorants are thought to act directly on the mucus-secreting glands or by reducing the adhesiveness of mucus. Expectorants are indicated when a **productive cough** is present

BOX 5-1 Drugs Administered by Aerosolization

Bronchodilators
- Isoproterenol
- Isoetharine
- Albuterol
- Atropine
- Glycopyrrolate

Glucocorticoids
- Beclomethasone
- Triamcinolone

Mucokinetics
- Water
- Saline
- Bicarbonate
- *N*-Acetylcysteine

Antimicrobials
- Ceftriaxone (40 mg/mL in water or dimethyl sulfoxide)
- Chloramphenicol (13 mg/mL)
- Enrofloxacin (10 mg/mL)
- Gentamicin, amikacin (5 mg/mL)
- Kanamycin
- Polymyxin B (66,600 IU/mL)
- Amphotericin B (7 mg/mL in 5% dextrose)
- Nystatin
- Clotrimazole (10 mg/mL in polyethylene glycol)
- Enilconazole (10 mg/mL in water)

Other
- Alcohol

From Boothe D: Small animal clinical pharmacology and therapeutics, ed 2, St. Louis, 2012, Elsevier.

and are often combined with other substances, such as ammonium chloride, antihistamines, or dextromethorphan.

Guaifenesin

Guaifenesin is found in a few veterinary-label products and in many human-label over-the-counter cough preparations. Guaifenesin is more commonly used in equine practice to induce or maintain general anesthesia.

Clinical Uses

These include relief of cough symptoms related to upper respiratory tract conditions.

Dosage Forms

These are primarily liquid (syrup) and tablet preparations.

- Guaifenesin oral tablets
- Guaifenesin syrup/liquid
- Guaifenesin powder
- Robitussin-AC
- Triaminic expectorant

Adverse Side Effects

Adverse side effects of guaifenesin are rare, although mild drowsiness or nausea may occur.

Iodide Preparations

Ethylenediamine dihydriodide is an expectorant that may be useful in treating mild respiratory disease of horses and cattle. Iodide preparations should not be used in pregnant or hyperthyroid animals.

Hypertonic Saline

Aerosolized hypertonic saline has been used as an expectorant in humans and may have potential for use in veterinary patients. It is thought to work by exerting an osmotic pull of fluid into the airway lumen, which helps to liquefy the contents for easier removal.

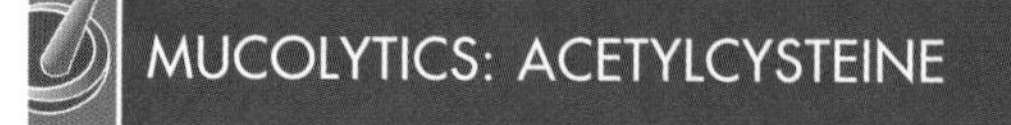

MUCOLYTICS: ACETYLCYSTEINE

Mucolytics, such as acetylcysteine, decrease the viscosity of respiratory secretions by altering the chemical composition of the mucus through the breakdown of chemical (disulfide) bonds. Acetylcysteine is the only mucolytic of clinical significance in veterinary medicine. It is administered by nebulization for pulmonary uses. This drug is also administered orally as an antidote for acetaminophen toxicity.

Clinical Uses

Acetylcysteine is used to break down thick or **inspissated** respiratory mucus and to treat acetaminophen toxicity.

Dosage Forms

Dosage forms with a human label include a 10% solution and a 20% solution in 4-mL, 10-mL, and 30-mL vials. A veterinary-labeled product for horses

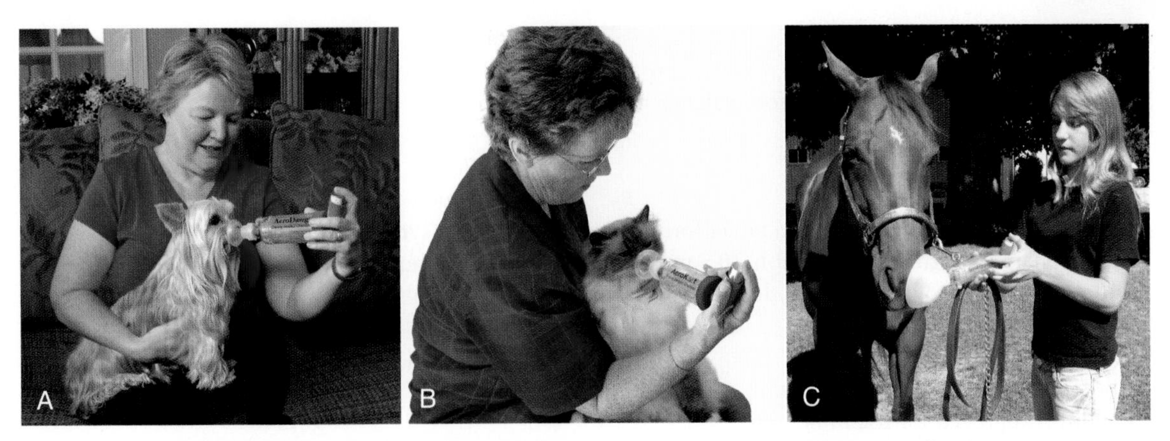

FIGURE 5-5 A, AeroDawg MDI device. B, AeroKat MDI device. C, AeroHippus chamber.

is available in powder form for oral administration in some countries.

- Mucomyst
- Acetadote
- ACC
- Dembrexine (Sputolysin)—veterinary label
- Bromhexine

Adverse Side Effects

Adverse side effects are few when acetylcysteine is nebulized. However, the drug may cause nausea or vomiting when administered orally.

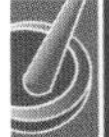

ANTITUSSIVES: CENTRALLY ACTING AGENTS

Antitussives are drugs that inhibit or suppress coughing. Antitussives are classified as centrally acting or peripherally acting (Figure 5-6). Centrally acting agents suppress coughing by depressing the cough center in the brain, whereas peripherally acting agents depress cough receptors in the airways. Peripherally acting antitussives are seldom used in veterinary medicine because they are usually prepared as cough drops or lozenges, which are not practical for administration to animal patients.

Butorphanol Tartrate

Butorphanol is a synthetic opiate, agonist/antagonist with significant antitussive activity. It is a Class IV controlled substance. It is also used as a preanesthetic and as an analgesic.

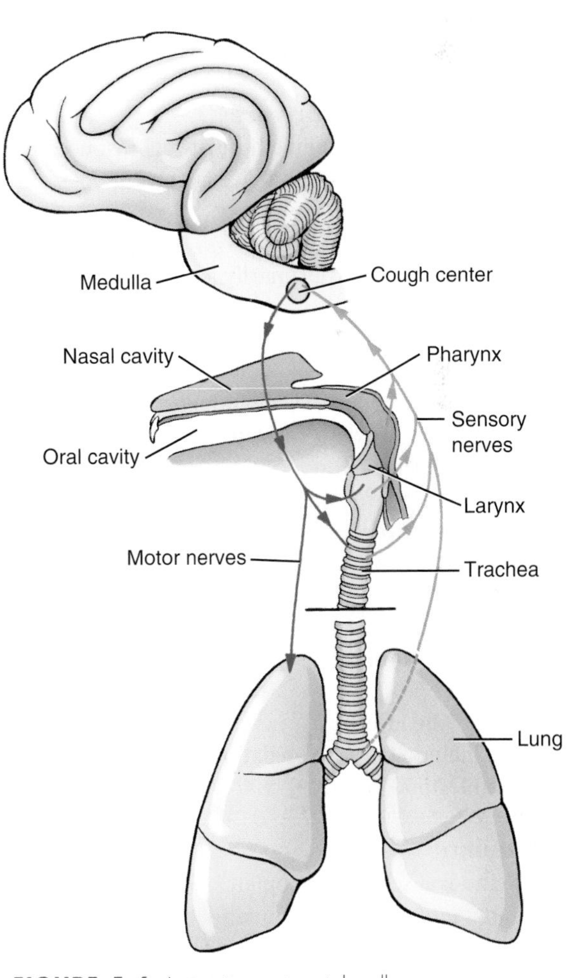

FIGURE 5-6 Antitussives act peripherally on sensory nerve endings or centrally on cough centers.

Clinical Uses
Butorphanol tartrate is used for the relief of chronic nonproductive coughs in dogs and for analgesia and preanesthesia in dogs and cats.

Dosage Forms
Dosage forms include injectable and tablet forms.
- Butorphanol (Torbutrol) injection (0.5 mg/mL, 10-mL vial); approved for use in dogs
- Butorphanol (Torbugesic-SA) (2.0 mg/mL); approved for use in cats
- Butorphanol (Torbugesic) injection (10 mg/mL, 50 mL); approved for use in horses
- Butorphanol (Torbutrol) tablets (1 mg, 5 mg, and 10 mg)

Adverse Side Effects
Adverse side effects may include sedation and ataxia.

Hydrocodone Bitartrate
Hydrocodone is a schedule II opiate agonist used for the treatment of nonproductive coughs in dogs.

Clinical Uses
Hydrocodone is used primarily as an antitussive for harsh, nonproductive coughs.

Dosage Forms
Dosage forms include several human-label combination products in syrup and tablet form.
- Hycodan (hydrocodone and homatropine) tablets
- Tussigon (hydrocodone and homatropine) tablets
- Hycodan (hydrocodone and homatropine) syrup
- Hydropane (hydrocodone and homatropine) syrup
- Hydrocodone/acetaminophen combination; contraindicated in cats

Adverse Side Effects
These include potential sedation, constipation, and gastrointestinal upset.

Codeine
Codeine is a schedule V opiate agonist that is used as an antitussive in human-label combination products.

Clinical Uses
Clinical uses of codeine are similar to those of hydrocodone.

Dosage Forms
These include combination human-label products primarily in syrup form.
- Codeine phosphate oral tablets, 30 mg and 60 mg
- Codeine sulfate oral tablets (15 mg, 30 mg, and 60 mg)
- Codeine phosphate with aspirin (Empirin with codeine)

Adverse Side Effects
Adverse side effects include sedation and constipation.

> **TECHNICIAN NOTES**
> - Codeine-only products are Class II (C-II).
> - Codeine with aspirin or acetaminophen is C-III.
> - Codeine syrups are C-III or C-V (by state).

Dextromethorphan
Dextromethorphan is a nonnarcotic antitussive that is chemically similar to codeine. It has no analgesic or addictive properties. It acts centrally and elevates the cough threshold. Similar to the two drugs previously mentioned, it is available primarily in human-label combination products. Dextromethorphan may be used in cats (Boothe, 2012).

Clinical Uses
Dextromethorphan is used to suppress a nonproductive cough.

Dosage Forms
The primary dosage form is the syrup product.
- Dimetapp DM (dextromethorphan, phenylpropanolamine, and brompheniramine)
- Robitussin DM (dextromethorphan and guaifenesin)

Adverse Side Effects
Adverse side effects are rare when this drug is given in the correct dose but can include drowsiness and gastrointestinal upset.

> TECHNICIAN NOTES Technicians who administer combination products to cats should take special precautions to ensure that the product does not contain acetaminophen.

Temaril-P

Temaril-P is a combination product that contains a centrally acting antitussive (trimeprazine tartrate) and a corticosteroid (prednisolone).

Clinical Uses

Temaril-P is used as an antitussive and as an antipruritic.

Dosage Forms

Dosage forms include tablets.

- Temaril-P tablets 5 mg trimeprazine tartrate, 2 mg prednisolone

Adverse Side Effects

These include sedation, depression, hypotension, and minor central nervous system signs.

BRONCHODILATORS

Contraction of the smooth muscle fibers that surround the bronchioles results in bronchoconstriction and often corresponding dyspnea. Contraction of these smooth muscle fibers can result from the following three basic mechanisms (Bill, 2006) (Figure 5-7):

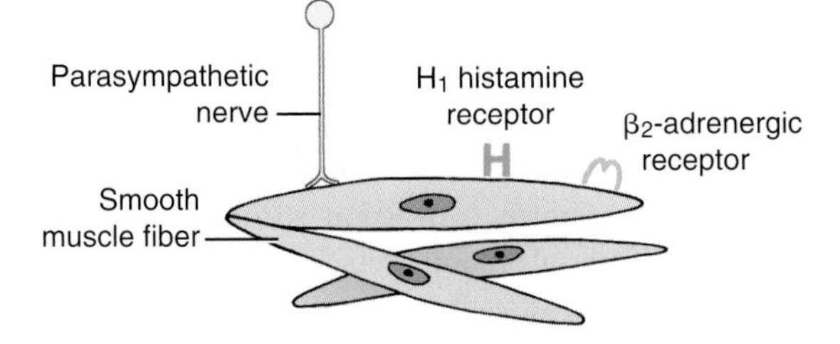

FIGURE 5-7 Bronchoconstriction may result from (1) acetylcholine release at parasympathetic nerve endings, (2) stimulation of H_1 histamine receptors, and (3) blockade of beta$_2$-adrenergic receptors.

1. Release of acetylcholine at parasympathetic nerve endings or inhibition of acetylcholinesterase. Increased acetylcholine levels also tend to increase secretions of the respiratory tract, thus reducing airflow and adding to the level of dyspnea.
2. Release of histamine through allergic or inflammatory mechanisms. Histamine combines with H_1 receptors on smooth muscle fibers to cause bronchoconstriction. Histamine also increases the inflammatory response in the airways, further leading to increased levels of secretion and viscosity.
3. Blockade of beta$_2$-adrenergic receptors by drugs such as propranolol results in bronchoconstriction. Stimulation of beta$_2$-adrenergic receptors, however, produces bronchodilation.

Drugs that cause bronchodilation are of four basic categories. Those categories include the cholinergic blockers, the antihistamines, the beta$_2$ adrenergics, and the methylxanthines.

Cholinergic Blockers

Cholinergic blockers produce bronchodilation by combining with acetylcholine receptors on smooth muscle fibers and preventing the bronchoconstrictive effects of acetylcholine. Cholinergic blockers such as atropine, aminopentamide (Centrine), and glycopyrrolate (Robinul-V) have limited use in treating bronchoconstriction, except in cases of organophosphate or carbamate toxicity. Ipratropium bromide, a synthetic anticholinergic, may be of some value in treating equine pulmonary obstructive disease (Hoffman, 2001) and may have potential for use in dogs and cats as an inhalant.

Antihistamines

Antihistamines are discussed later in this chapter.

Beta$_2$-Adrenergic Agonists

Beta$_2$-adrenergic agonists combine with appropriate receptors on the smooth muscle fibers and effect relaxation of those fibers. They also stabilize mast cells and reduce the amount of histamine released (Bill, 2006). It is preferred that these drugs have limited beta$_1$ activity because beta$_1$ stimulation can produce tachycardia.

Clinical Uses
$Beta_2$-adrenergic agonists are used as bronchodilators.

Dosage Forms
- Epinephrine. This drug is a potent bronchodilator that is used only in life-threatening situations (e.g., anaphylactic shock) because it also produces significant tachycardia.
- Pseudoephedrine/pyrilamine (EquiPhed) is approved for horses not intended for food.
- Isoproterenol (Isuprel). This drug also causes $beta_1$ stimulation and has limited use as a bronchodilator in veterinary medicine.
- Albuterol (salbutamol) (Ventolin, Proventil)
- Clenbuterol (Ventipulmin syrup and clenbuterol HCl oral syrup). Ventipulmin is approved for horses not intended for food.
- Terbutaline (Brethine)
- Metaproterenol (Alupent)
- Salmeterol (Serevent)

Adverse Side Effects
These include tachycardia and hypertension.

Methylxanthines
Methylxanthine derivatives that are used therapeutically include aminophylline and theophylline. These two products are very similar in their chemistry and pharmacologic effects. Both inhibit an enzyme in smooth muscle cells called *phosphodiesterase.* When $beta_2$ receptors are stimulated, a chemical messenger called *cyclic adenosine monophosphate (cyclic AMP)* that is released in the smooth muscle cell completes the relaxation response to allow dilation. Phosphodiesterase inhibits cyclic AMP in the cell, thereby tending to promote bronchoconstriction. By inhibiting the inhibitor (phosphodiesterase) and allowing cyclic AMP to accumulate, the methylxanthines tend to promote bronchodilation.

Methylxanthines also cause mild stimulation of the heart and respiratory muscles and minor diuresis.

Caffeine and theobromine (found in chocolate) are methylxanthines.

Aminophylline is an ethylenediamine salt of theophylline. It is available in various human-label products. One hundred milligrams of aminophylline contains approximately 79 mg of theophylline (Plumb, 2011). Injectable forms are available, as are immediate- and sustained-release oral forms.

Clinical Uses
Methylxanthines are used for bronchodilation in respiratory and cardiac conditions and for mild heart stimulation (positive inotropic effect).

Dosage Forms
- Theo-Dur
- Slo-bid
- Theophylline—timed release
- Aminophylline (generic)—injectable and tablets
- Aminophylline syrup

Adverse Side Effects
These may include gastrointestinal upset, central nervous system stimulation, tachycardia, ataxia, and arrhythmia.

TECHNICIAN NOTES Because theophylline may interact adversely with many drugs, including phenobarbital, cimetidine, erythromycin, thiabendazole, clindamycin, and lincomycin, appropriate precautions should be taken before this drug is administered.

DECONGESTANTS

Decongestants are drugs that reduce the congestion of nasal membranes by reducing associated swelling. Decongestants may be administered as a spray or as nose drops or may be given orally as a liquid or as a tablet. These drugs act directly or indirectly to reduce congestion through vasoconstriction of nasal blood vessels. These products have limited use in veterinary medicine but may be used to treat selected feline upper respiratory tract disease.

Many human label decongestants are available. Those that are given orally and act systemically include ephedrine and pseudoephedrine. Topically applied decongestants include oxymetazoline and phenylephrine.

ANTIHISTAMINES

Antihistamines are substances that are used to block the effects of histamine. Histamine is released from mast cells by the allergic response and combines with H_1 receptors on bronchiole smooth muscle to cause bronchoconstriction. Antihistamines may be useful in treating respiratory disease because they prevent mast cell degranulation and block H_1 receptors on smooth muscle. Antihistamines are thought to be more effective when used preventively because they apparently do not replace histamine that has already combined with receptors (Bill, 2006).

Respiratory conditions that may be treated with antihistamines include "heaves" in horses, pneumonia in cattle, feline asthma, and insect bites.

Generic names for antihistamines often are easily recognized because most end in the suffix "-amine" (e.g., pyrilamine, diphenhydramine, chlorpheniramine).

Veterinary-label antihistamines for treating respiratory conditions are available in injectable and oral preparations.

Clinical Uses

Antihistamines are used in the treatment of allergic and respiratory conditions. They also may be used for their antiemetic effects.

Dosage Forms

- Pyrilamine (Histagranules, Hist-Eq, Histall)
- Tripelennamine (Re-Covr)
- Probahist syrup
- Antihistamine injection
- Diphenhydramine; human-approved
- Doxylamine
- Hydroxyzine (Atarax)
- Clemastine (Tavist)
- Cyproheptadine (Periactin). May be used in cats to block bronchoconstriction and also as an appetite stimulant.
- Cetirizine (Xyrtec)
- Loratadine (Claritin)
- Fexofenadine (Allegra)

Adverse Side Effects

These include sedation and, occasionally, gastrointestinal effects.

CORTICOSTEROIDS

Corticosteroids are used primarily in the treatment of allergic respiratory conditions. They are considered the most effective drugs in the treatment of equine chronic obstructive pulmonary disease (Lavoie, 2001). Corticosteroids prepared for inhalation therapy have strong antiinflammatory effects locally in the lungs and are rapidly biodegraded when absorbed into the general circulation. Oral corticosteroids (prednisone or prednisolone) are considered the drugs of choice in the treatment of chronic airway inflammation in dogs and cats (Dowling, 2001). Corticosteroid therapy controls the signs of respiratory disease, not the cause; good short-term effects often ensue with few of the residual effects that may accompany long-term use.

Clinical Uses

Corticosteroids are used in the treatment of equine heaves, feline asthma, acute respiratory distress syndrome, and allergic pneumonia.

Dosage Forms

- Prednisolone sodium succinate (Solu-Delta-Cortef)
- Prednisolone (Delta Albaplex, Temaril-P, generic forms)
- Prednisone tablets and syrup
- Dexamethasone (Dexasone, Dexamethasone Solution, Azium)
- Beclomethasone dipropionate (Vanceril) (for inhalation)
- Fluticasone propionate (Flovent) (for inhalation)
- Triamcinolone (Vetalog)

Adverse Side Effects

Few adverse side effects are noted if these products are used according to recommendations.

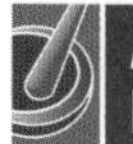

MISCELLANEOUS RESPIRATORY DRUGS

Many other drugs are used to treat respiratory disorders. These include antimicrobials, mast cell stabilizers, and diuretics. Antimicrobials are used in cases of bacterial infection of the respiratory tract and may be administered parenterally or by nebulization. Mast cell stabilizers, such as cromolyn, are most effective if used before inflammatory activation. Diuretics are used to treat respiratory disease in which pulmonary edema is a major problem.

Respiratory Stimulants

Doxapram Hydrochloride

Doxapram is a general central nervous system stimulant that is used primarily as a stimulant for the respiratory system.

Clinical Uses

Doxapram is used for stimulation of respiration during and after anesthesia and to speed awakening and restoration of reflexes after anesthesia. In neonatal animals, doxapram is used to stimulate respiration after dystocia or cesarean section.

Dosage Form

- Dopram-V for injection (20 mg/mL, 20-mL vial).

Adverse Side Effects

These include hypertension, arrhythmia, hyperventilation, central nervous system excitation, and seizures. These effects are most likely to occur at high doses (Plumb, 2011). The safety of doxapram in pregnant animals has not been established.

Mast Cell Stabilizers

Cromolyn (Cromolyn Sodium for Inhalation) is a substance that inhibits the release of histamine and leukotrienes from sensitized mast cells found in nasal and lung mucosa and in the eyes. It may also inhibit bronchospasm. It is used primarily in the treatment of horses with RAO (heaves).

Leukotriene Antagonists

Montelukast sodium (Singulair tablets) and zafirlukast (Accolate tablets) are leukotriene receptor antagonists. Leukotrienes are proinflammatory products of arachidonic acid released from mast cells and eosinophils. Montelukast has been used in veterinary medicine to treat feline asthma, inflammatory bowel disease (IBD), heartworm respiratory disease syndrome, and upper respiratory infection. Zafirlukast has been used to treat feline asthma, feline IBD, and canine atopic dermatitis. Both of these products have produced marginal efficacy (Plumb, 2011).

Naloxone

Naloxone is used to stimulate respirations in narcotic overdose.

Yobine

Yobine is used to stimulate respirations in xylazine overdose.

REVIEW QUESTIONS

1. What structures would a molecule of oxygen pass over or through as it travels from the environment to the alveoli?

   ____

2. What are the four primary functions of the respiratory system?

   ____

3. Describe the function of the three basic defense mechanisms of the respiratory system.

   ____

4. What are three important principles of respiratory therapeutics?

   ____

5. Expectorants are indicated when what type of cough is present? ______________________
6. Mucolytics decrease the viscosity of respiratory mucus by what mechanism?

   ____

7. Acetylcysteine is administered by what method for pulmonary uses? ______________________

8. What is the mechanism of action of most antitussives used in veterinary medicine?

____

9. Codeine is classified in what category of controlled substances?

____

10. List three mechanisms that can cause smooth muscle contraction in the bronchioles.

____

11. List two bronchodilators that are beta$_2$-adrenergic agonists.

____

12. The methylxanthines bring about bronchodilation by inhibiting what cellular enzyme?

____

13. List two potential uses for antihistamines in veterinary medicine.

____

14. What suffix is found at the end of many antihistamine names?

____

15. List two potential uses for Dopram.

____

16. Maxi Jones is being treated for canine infectious tracheobronchitis. Dr. Ladd has instructed you to dispense Hycodan tablets at 0.22 mg/kg b.i.d. for 7 days. Maxi weighs 50 lb and 5-mg tablets are available.
What dose of Hycodan does Maxi require?

____

How many tablets will you dispense?

____

17. List two uses of acetylcysteine in veterinary medicine. ______________________

18. Which of the following is *not* an example of a methylxanthine?
a. Aminophylline
b. Theophylline
c. Caffeine
d. Theobromine
e. These are all examples of methylxanthines.

19. Particles of what size are capable of reaching the alveoli? ______________________

20. Give an example of a beta$_2$-adrenergic agonist bronchodilator.

____

21. All of the following are functions of the respiratory system, except _______.
a. oxygen–carbon dioxide exchange
b. regulation of acid–base balance
c. production of sodium bicarbonate to aid in regulation of acid–base balance
d. body temperature regulation

22. ______ are drugs that liquefy and dilute viscid secretions of the respiratory tract, thereby helping to evacuate those secretions.
a. Antitussives
b. Decongestants
c. Bronchodilators
d. Expectorants

23. _____ are drugs that inhibit or suppress coughing.
a. Antitussives
b. Decongestants
c. Bronchodilators
d. Expectorants

24. ________ _______ is used for the relief of chronic nonproductive coughs in dogs and for analgesia and preanesthesia in dogs and cats.
a. Hydrocodone bitartrate
b. Butorphanol tartrate
c. Temaril P
d. Doxapram HCl

25. Drug products with codeine alone are in what schedule of controlled substances?
a. Class I
b. Class III
c. Class V
d. Class II

26. Temaril-P is a combination product that contains a centrally acting antitussive (trimeprazine tartrate) and _______.
a. prednisolone
b. aminophylline
c. furosemide
d. theophylline

27. Aminophylline and theophylline are _______ derivatives.
a. adrenergic
b. cholinergic
c. methylxanthine
d. acetylcysteine

28. _______ are drugs that reduce the congestion of nasal membranes by reducing associated swelling.
a. Antihistamines
b. Decongestants
c. Bronchodilators
d. Expectorants

29. _______ are substances that are used to block the effects of histamine.
a. Antihistamines
b. Decongestants
c. Bronchodilators
d. Expectorants

30. Solu-Delta-Cortef is a brand name for _______.
a. prednisolone
b. dexamethasone
c. prednisolone sodium succinate
d. fluticasone propionate

31. A 1200-lb horse with heaves (RAO) will be treated with Ventipulmin syrup (72.5 mcg/mL) at a dosage of 0.8 mcg/kg daily for 3 days. How many milliliters will you dispense?
____

32. A 25-lb dog with acute pulmonary edema will be treated with aminophylline at a dosage of 5 mg/kg three times a day for 5 days. There are 100-mg tablets available. How many will you dispense? _______________

33. A 40-lb dog will be treated with naloxone for respiratory depression due to morphine overdosage. The dosage for naloxone is 0.04 mg/kg and the concentration of the naloxone is 0.4 mg/mL. How many milliliters will you prepare?
____

34. An 8-lb cat with feline asthma will be treated with montelukast at a dosage of 0.5 mg daily for 3 days. Singulair tablets (4 mg) are available. How many tablets will you dispense? _______________

35. A shelter dog with mild canine infectious respiratory disease (CIRD) will receive two Temaril-P tablets twice a day for 4 days and then 1 tablet twice a day for 6 days. How many tablets will you prepare?
____

REFERENCES

Bill R: Drugs affecting the respiratory system. In Bill R, editor: Pharmacology for veterinary technicians, ed 3, St. Louis, 2006, Mosby.

Boothe DM: Drugs affecting the respiratory system. In Small animal clinical pharmacology and therapeutics, Philadelphia, 2012, WB Saunders.

Dowling PM: Respiratory drugs, in Proceedings. Annu Meet Am Vet Med Assoc, Boston, 2001.

Hoffman AM: What's new with aerosol medications in the horse, in Proceedings. Annu Meet Am Vet Med Assoc, Boston, 2001.

Lavoie JP: Inhalation therapy for equine heaves, Comp Contin Educ Pract Vet 23(5):475–477, 2001.

McKiernan B: Respiratory therapeutics, in Proceedings. 17th Semin for Vet Tech, West Vet Conf, Las Vegas, 1988.

Plumb DC: Veterinary drug handbook, ed 7, Ames, Iowa, 2011, Wiley-Blackwell.

Tilley LP, Smith WK: The 5-minute veterinary consult: canine and feline, ed 2, Baltimore, 2000, Lippincott Williams & Wilkins.

Veterinary Information Network. VIN Proceedings Library (website). Reinero CN, Selting KA: Inhalational therapies in dogs and cats, 2010. http://www.vin.com/members/proceedings.plx?CID=ACVIM2010&PID=559. Accessed March 19, 2013.

CHAPTER

6

Drugs Used in Renal and Urinary Tract Disorders

OUTLINE

LEARNING OBJECTIVES

After studying this chapter, you should be able to

1. Identify the anatomic features of the urinary system.
2. Discuss the formation of urine through glomerular filtration, tubular reabsorption, and tubular secretion.
3. Compare the different classes of drugs and describe the indications for each class.
4. Explain how renal dysfunction can affect the metabolism and excretion of many drugs and their metabolites.

KEY TERMS

Agonist
Antagonist
Atony
Catecholamine
Detrusor
Detrusor areflexia
Erythropoiesis
Erythropoietin
Hematuria
Hypertension
Hypertonus
Hypokalemia
Lower motor neurons
Nephrology
Nephron
Polydipsia
Polyuria
Retroperitoneal
Upper motor neurons
Uremia
Urinary incontinence
Urinary tract infection

INTRODUCTION

The urinary system (i.e., the renal system) is composed of two kidneys, two ureters, a urinary bladder, and a urethra (Figures 6-1 to 6-4). The medical study of the renal system is known as **nephrology** because the basic functional unit of the kidney is the **nephron.** The kidneys work in the body similar to the way in which a fish aquarium filter works. All the water in an aquarium is sent through the filter to capture waste products in the water so that the tank is kept clean. Thus, the kidneys filter all waste products from the bloodstream but allow those elements needed by the body to remain. The kidneys are bean shaped and lie on each side of the spine. They are also **retroperitoneal.**

The job of the nephron is to regulate water and soluble matter (especially electrolytes) in the body.

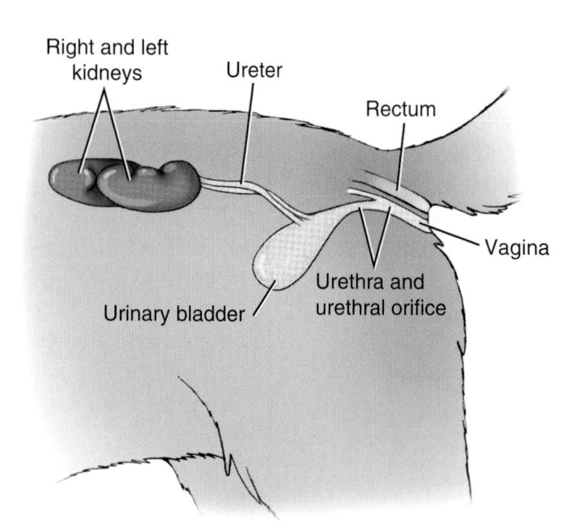

FIGURE 6-1 Side view of the urogenital system of a female dog.

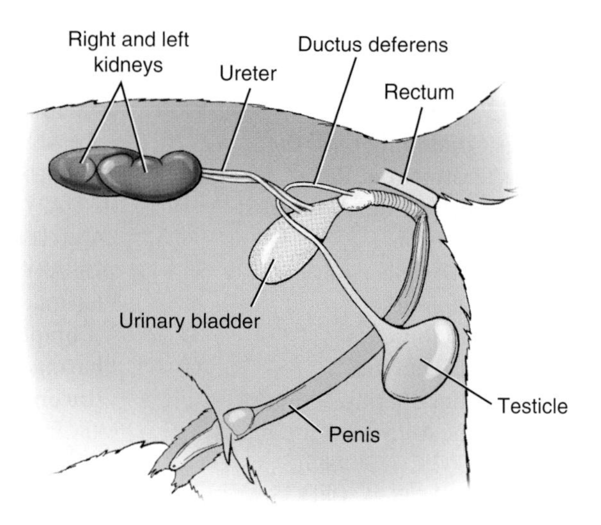

FIGURE 6-2 Side view of the urogenital system of a male dog.

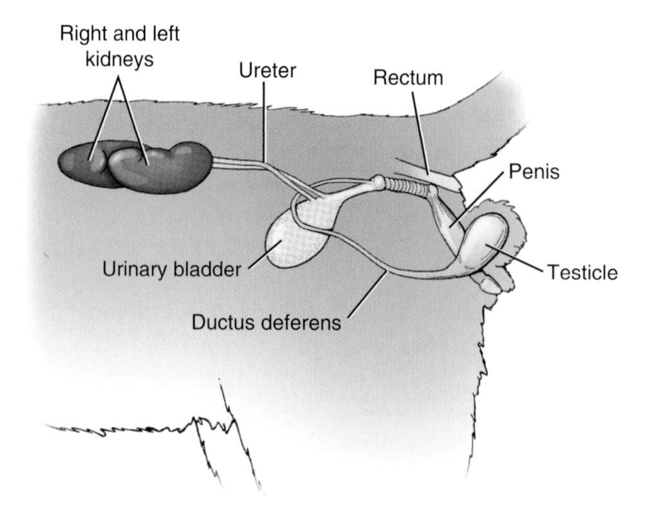

FIGURE 6-3 Side view of the urogenital system of a male cat.

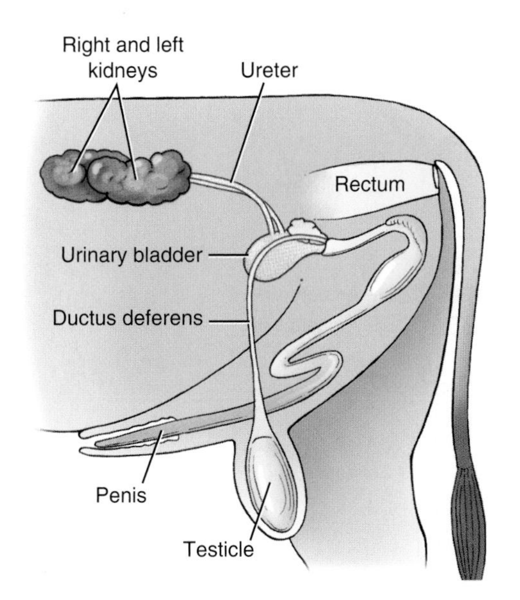

FIGURE 6-4 Side view of the urogenital system of a bull.

Nephrons filter the blood under pressure and then reabsorb necessary fluid and molecules back into the blood. The kidneys thus excrete a variety of waste products produced by metabolism such as urea, uric acid, and water. The kidneys are involved in factors of homeostasis such as acid–base balance, regulation of electrolyte concentrations, blood volume control, and regulation of blood pressure. The kidneys communicate with other organs in the body through hormones that are secreted into the bloodstream.

Veterinary technicians should educate clients about the importance of nutrition, especially in those dog breeds predisposed to developing urinary bladder stones (e.g., dalmatians, miniature schnauzers). Fresh water should be available for animals at all times. Companion animals observed straining to urinate or with bloody urine (i.e., **hematuria**) should be brought to the veterinary hospital immediately.

PHYSIOLOGIC PRINCIPLES

The formation of urine is a rather complex process that involves glomerular filtration, tubular reabsorption, and tubular secretion (Figure 6-5). The glomerular filtrate is composed of water and dissolved substances, which pass from the plasma into the glomerular capsule. The formation of glomerular filtrate is controlled by effective filtration pressure (EFP = arterial blood pressure − [plasma osmotic pressure + capsule pressure]). The amount of glomerular filtrate is directly proportional to the EFP (Figure 6-6). Changes in blood flow through the glomerulus, glomerular blood pressure, plasma osmotic pressure, and capsule pressure affect glomerular filtration.

The kidney tubules are responsible for the reabsorption or the secretion of specific substances. Substances needed by the body are reabsorbed from the filtrate, pass through the tubular cell wall, and reenter the plasma. This process filters needed substances and returns them to the body. Reabsorbed materials include water, glucose, amino acids, urea, and ions such as Na, K, Ca^{2+}, Cl^-, HCO_3^-, and HPO_4^{2-}. Any excess of these substances or of substances that are not useful remain in the filtrate and are excreted in the urine.

Tubular secretion occurs when substances are carried to the tubular lumen. This involves the active transport of certain endogenous substances and many exogenous substances. These secreted substances include potassium and hydrogen ions, ammonia, creatinine, and some drugs. The main effects of tubular secretion are to rid the body of certain materials and to help control blood pH (Figure 6-7). The kidneys are active in the metabolism and excretion of many drugs and their metabolites. Therefore, it is very important to remember that these actions may be inhibited in cases of renal failure or dysfunction. Drug therapy in animals with renal dysfunction has increased risks. Renal failure can impair a drug's absorption from an administration site, affect a drug's distribution in the body, and affect the elimination of the drug from the body.

If the kidneys' functionality is decreased, **erythropoiesis** may not occur correctly. Erythropoiesis is the formation of erythrocytes. **Erythropoietin** is a hormone secreted by the healthy kidney that communicates with the bone marrow to make more red blood cells. In diseased kidneys, this hormone is secreted in reduced amounts or not at

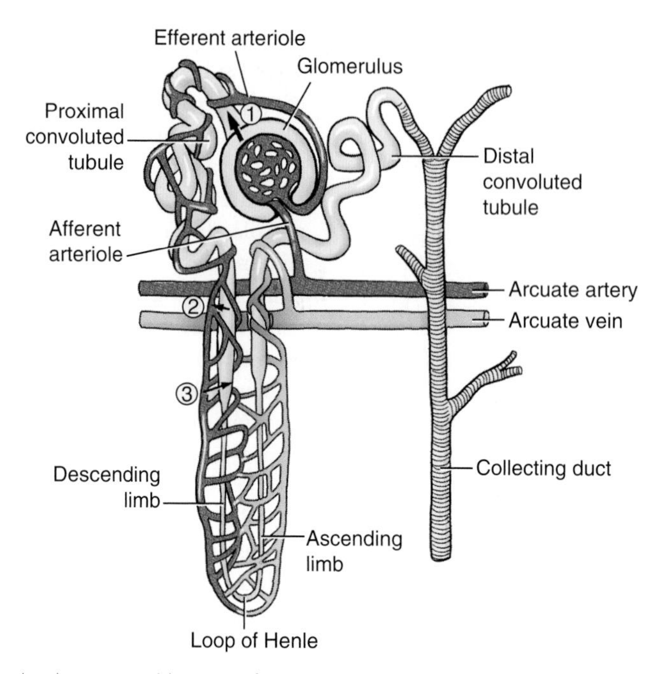

FIGURE 6-5 Shown are the direction and location of glomerular filtration: *1*, tubular reabsorption; *2*, tubular secretion; and *3*, as they would occur in the glomerulus and the proximal tubule.

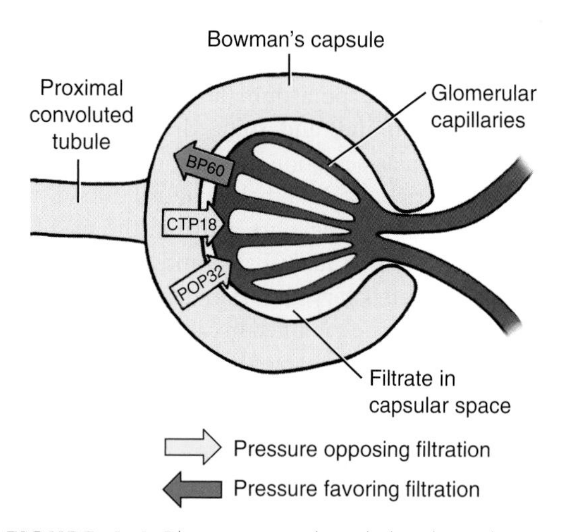

FIGURE 6-6 Filtration occurs through the glomerular membrane within Bowman's capsule. The amount of filtrate produced is determined by the difference between the pressures favoring filtration and those opposing filtration. This diagram shows that filtration occurs because 60 − (32 + 18) = 10 mm Hg. Values greater than or less than 10 mm Hg would correlate with more or less filtration, respectively. Pressure values (60, 32, 18) are measured in mm Hg. *BP*, Blood pressure; *CTP*, capsular tissue pressure; *POP*, plasma osmotic pressure.

all, and the animal may develop a nonregenerative anemia as a result. Injections of human recombinant erythropoietin may be given to animals to treat this anemia.

Uremia can increase the sensitivity of some tissues to certain drugs. For example, sensitivity to central nervous system depressants is increased; therefore the dose of opiates, barbiturates, and tranquilizers should be reduced in uremic patients. Xylazine (Rompun) and ketamine hydrochloride (Ketaset) are contraindicated in uremic patients. Impaired renal excretion or biotransformation causes delayed elimination of many drugs and enhances their toxicity and duration of action.

Box 6-1 lists drugs that commonly require dosage modification in renal insufficiency. Modifications can be made by measuring the plasma concentration of a drug and adjusting the dose accordingly. However, this is impractical in most clinical settings, so a veterinarian may use the normal dose but lengthen the time intervals at which it is administered or give a smaller dose at normal time intervals. Technicians may be responsible for administering

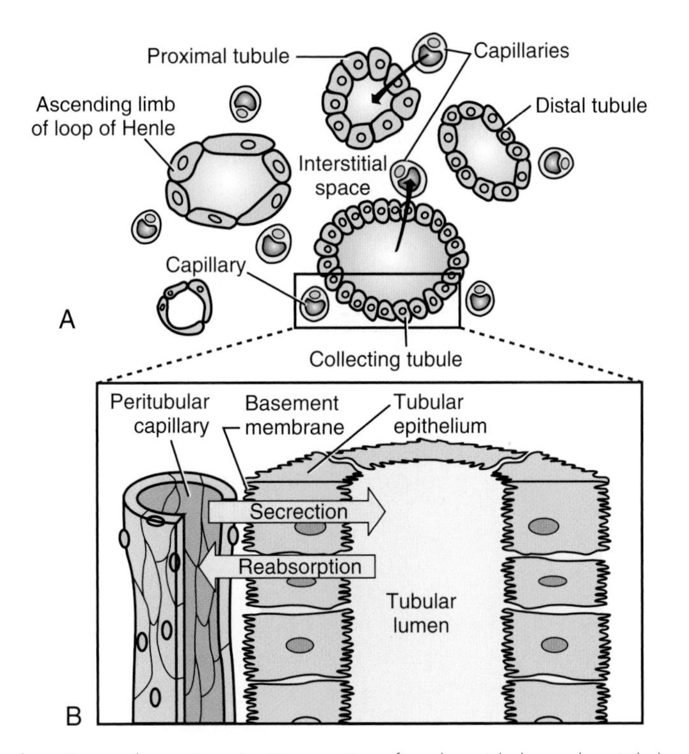

FIGURE 6-7 Tubular reabsorption and secretion. **A,** Cross-section of nephron tubules and peritubular capillaries. Interstitial fluid occupies the interstitial space. Reabsorption is represented by substance *X* going from tubule to capillary, and secretion is represented by substance *Y* going from capillary to tubule. **B,** Longitudinal section of nephron tubule. Shown is the relationship among the tubular lumen, epithelial cell, and capillary.

anesthesia, and it is important to remember that patients with renal failure are at greater anesthetic risk and require even closer monitoring than patients with normal renal function.

RENAL FAILURE

Renal failure is among the major causes of nonaccidental death in dogs and cats. Although the disease is most common in older animals, it may be diagnosed in younger animals. Renal damage may stem from many causes including: infectious disease, diabetes mellitus, toxins, neoplasia, congenital disorders, immunologic problems, and amyloidosis. Diets with excessive protein, phosphorus, and sodium are other factors that may cause renal damage. Renal damage may be categorized as prerenal, renal, or postrenal. Renal failure may be differentiated as acute, chronic, or end-stage, according to parameters common to each stage.

DRUGS COMMONLY USED FOR THE TREATMENT OF RENAL DYSFUNCTION AND ASSOCIATED HYPERTENSION

DIURETIC DRUGS

Diuretics are drugs used to remove excess extracellular fluid by increasing urine flow and sodium excretion and by reducing **hypertension.** A number of conditions may indicate the need for a diuretic drug. Classifications of commonly used diuretics include loop diuretics, osmotic diuretics, thiazide and thiazide-like diuretics, potassium-sparing diuretics, and carbonic anhydrase inhibitors.

Loop Diuretics

Loop diuretics are highly potent diuretics that inhibit the tubular reabsorption of sodium. Once these

BOX 6-1 Dosage Modifications in Renal Insufficiency

Drugs That Require Dosage Modification or That Are Contraindicated in Renal Insufficiency
Acetazolamide
Antimonials
Aspirin
Atropine
Barbital
Bendroflumethiazide
Cephalothin
Chelating agents
Chlorothiazide
Clindamycin
Colistin and polymyxin
Decamethonium
Digoxin
Erythromycin
Furosemide (increased dose)
Gentamicin
Iodide
Kanamycin
Lincomycin
Mannitol
Mercurials
Methenamine
Methotrexate
Neomycin
Neostigmine
Nitrofurantoin
Ouabain
Penicillins
Phenazopyridine
Procainamide
Spironolactone
Streptomycin
Sulfonamides
Tetracyclines
Tetraethylammonium
Tubocurarine, gallamine
Vancomycin

Drugs That Do Not Require Dosage Modification or That Are Not Contraindicated in Renal Insufficiency
Acetaminophen
Chloramphenicol
Diazepam
Narcotic analgesics
Novobiocin
Pentobarbital
Phenobarbital
Phenothiazine
Phenytoin
Procaine
Propranolol

From Kirk RW: Current veterinary therapy VII: small animal practice, Philadelphia, 1980, WB Saunders.

drugs are administered, their actions are generally rapid. Additionally, loop diuretics promote the excretion of chloride, potassium, and water. Some patients receiving long-term loop diuretic therapy may also need potassium supplementation.

Clinical Uses
Loop diuretics are useful in the treatment of congestive heart failure (CHF) in canines and felines, pulmonary edema, udder edema, hypercalcemic nephropathy, and uremia, as an adjunct in the treatment of hyperkalemia, and sometimes as an antihypertensive agent (Plumb, 2011).

Dosage Forms
- Furosemide (Lasix, Disal, Diuride)
- Torsemide (Demadex, Torasemide)

Adverse Side Effects
These include **hypokalemia** (because of the increased excretion of potassium), other fluid and electrolyte abnormalities, ototoxicity, gastrointestinal distress, hematologic effects, weakness, and restlessness (Plumb, 2011).

TECHNICIAN NOTES A potassium supplement may be given to patients who are receiving long-term potassium-depleting diuretic therapy to prevent hypokalemia.

Osmotic Diuretics
Osmotic diuretics can be administered intravenously to promote diuresis by exerting high osmotic pressure in the kidney tubules and limiting tubular

reabsorption. Water is drawn into the glomerular filtrate, which reduces its reabsorption rate and increases the excretion of water. These drugs may be used to treat oliguric acute renal failure and to reduce intracranial pressure.

Clinical Uses

These drugs are used for oliguric renal failure, reduction of intraocular and cerebrospinal fluid (intracerebral) pressure, and rapid reduction of edema or ascites (Plumb, 2011).

Dosage Forms

- Mannitol 20%
- Glycerine (oral)

Adverse Side Effects

These drugs should not be used in patients with anuria secondary to renal disease, in patients that are severely dehydrated, or in patients with pulmonary congestion or edema. Osmotic diuretics may cause fluid and electrolyte imbalances (Plumb, 2011).

Thiazide Diuretics

Thiazide diuretics reduce edema by inhibiting reabsorption of sodium, chloride, and water. Their duration of action is longer than that of loop diuretics.

Dosage Forms

- Chlorothiazide (Diuril—human label)
- Hydrochlorothiazide (HydroDIURIL—human label)

Clinical Uses

Chlorothiazide may be used for the treatment of nephrogenic diabetes insipidus and hypertension in dogs. Hydrochlorothiazide may be used in the treatment of calcium oxalate uroliths, hypoglycemia, and as a diuretic for patients with heart failure (Plumb, 2011).

Adverse Side Effects

These include hypokalemia if therapy is prolonged. Hypersensitivity may be a side effect in some individuals. These drugs should not be used during pregnancy or in patients with severe renal disease, preexisting electrolyte/water balance abnormalities, hepatic disease, or diabetes mellitus. The drugs may cause gastrointestinal upset (Plumb, 2011).

TECHNICIAN NOTES

- Similar to loop diuretics, thiazide diuretics cause an increase in potassium excretion. A potassium supplement may be necessary to prevent hypokalemia.
- These drugs cross the placental border.

Potassium-Sparing Diuretics

Potassium-sparing diuretics have weaker diuretic and antihypertensive effects than other diuretics; therefore they conserve potassium. These agents are also referred to as *aldosterone antagonists.* They work by antagonizing aldosterone, an adrenal mineralocorticoid. This action enhances the excretion of sodium and water and reduces the excretion of potassium. Aldosterone secretion may be a factor in edema associated with heart failure.

Dosage Forms

- Spironolactone (Aldactone—human label)
- Triamterene (Dyazide, Dyrenium—human label)

Adverse Side Effects

These are uncommon, but hyperkalemia may result if these drugs are administered concurrently with potassium supplements or angiotensin-converting enzyme (ACE) inhibitors, such as captopril or enalapril. They should not be prescribed for patients with hyperkalemia, Addison's disease, anuria, acute renal failure, or significant renal impairment (Plumb, 2011).

Carbonic Anhydrase Inhibitors

A carbonic anhydrase inhibitor is a substance that decreases the rate of carbonic acid and hydrogen production in the kidney, thereby promoting the excretion of solutes and increasing the rate of urinary output (Mosby, 1998). These drugs also reduce intraocular pressure by reducing the production of aqueous humor and may be used in the treatment of glaucoma.

Dosage Forms

- Acetazolamide (Diamox—human label)
- Dichlorphenamide (Daranide—human label)
- Methazolamide

Clinical Uses

Acetazolamide may be used in metabolic alkalosis, glaucoma, and hyperkalemic periodic paralysis (HYPP) in horses. Dichlorphenamide is used primarily for open angle glaucoma. Methazolamide is also used primarily for open angle glaucoma (Plumb, 2011).

Adverse Side Effects

These include the ability to cause hypokalemia. Acetazolamide is contraindicated in patients with hepatic, renal, pulmonary, or adrenocortical insufficiency; hyponatremia; hypokalemia; or electrolyte imbalances. Dichlorphenamide and methazolamide are contraindicated in patients with hyperchloremic acidosis (Plumb, 2011).

> *TECHNICIAN NOTES* Carbonic anhydrase inhibitors have the least efficacy when compared with the other tubular inhibitors and are not commonly used to treat edema.

CHOLINERGIC AGONISTS

Cholinergic agents act directly or indirectly to promote the function of acetylcholine. Cholinergic agents also may be referred to as *parasympathomimetic agents* because their effects mimic stimulation of the parasympathetic nervous system. Cholinergic **agonists** mimic the action of natural acetylcholine by directly stimulating cholinergic receptors. Once the cholinergic agonist binds with receptors on the cell membrane of smooth muscles, the permeability of the cell membrane changes, permitting calcium and sodium to enter into the cells. Depolarization of the cell membrane occurs, and muscle contraction is achieved.

Clinical Uses

These drugs are used primarily to increase the contractility of the urinary bladder.

Dosage Form

- Bethanechol (Urecholine—human label)

Adverse Side Effects

These include the potential for cholinergic toxicity. They should not be used in patients with gastrointestinal obstructions or if the integrity of the urinary bladder wall is unknown. Other side effects may include salivation, lacrimation, urination, and defecation (SLUD). A cholinergic crisis may occur if this drug is injected intravenously or subcutaneously, so atropine should be readily available (Plumb, 2011).

> *TECHNICIAN NOTES*
> - Observe the patient for signs of cholinergic toxicity (e.g., vomiting, defecation, dyspnea, and tremors).
> - Atropine is antidotal.

ANTICHOLINERGIC DRUGS

The action of anticholinergic drugs is the opposite of that of cholinergic agents. They block the action of acetylcholine at receptor sites in the parasympathetic nervous system. These drugs may also be described as parasympatholytic because of their ability to block the passage of impulses through the parasympathetic nerves. Their action produces muscle relaxation.

Clinical Uses

Anticholinergic drugs can be used for treating urge incontinence by promoting the retention of urine in the urinary bladder.

Dosage Forms

- Propantheline (Pro-Banthine—human label)
- Butylhyoscine (Buscopan)

Adverse Side Effects

These include decreased gastric motility and delayed gastric emptying, which may decrease the absorption of other medications.

ADRENERGIC ANTAGONISTS

Adrenergic blocking agents disrupt the sympathetic nervous system by blocking impulse transmission at adrenergic neurons, adrenergic receptor sites, or adrenergic ganglia. These agents also may be described as sympatholytic agents because of their ability to block sympathetic nervous system stimulation. The classification of adrenergic **antagonists** is based on their site of action (i.e., alpha blockers, beta blockers, or autonomic ganglionic blockers).

Alpha-Adrenergic Antagonists

Alpha-adrenergic antagonists relax vascular smooth muscle, enhance peripheral vasodilation, and decrease blood pressure by interrupting the actions of sympathomimetic agents at alpha-adrenergic receptor sites.

Clinical Uses

In the urinary system, these drugs reduce internal sphincter tone when the urethral sphincter is in **hypertonus.** This action is useful in the treatment of urinary retention because of **detrusor areflexia** or functional urethral obstruction. Prazosin is effective in controlling moderate to severe hypertension, which may be a complicating factor in chronic renal failure.

Dosage Forms

- Phenoxybenzamine (Dibenzyline—human label)
- Nicergoline (Sermion)
- Moxisylyte (Carlytene)
- Prazosin (Minipress—human label)

Adverse Side Effects

These include a rapid decrease in blood pressure, resulting in weakness or syncope after the first dose of prazosin. This is usually self-limiting. Phenoxybenzamine HCl should not be used in horses exhibiting clinical signs of colic. Phenoxybenzamine HCl may cause increased intraocular pressure, tachycardia, nasal congestion, inhibition of ejaculation, weakness/dizziness, gastrointestinal effects, and constipation in equines. Phenoxybenzamine HCl may have to be obtained through a compounding pharmacy (Plumb, 2011).

> **TECHNICIAN NOTES**
> - Prazosin may be used alone or combined with a diuretic to produce the desired effect.
> - Because the liver metabolizes alpha-adrenergic antagonists, dosage modification is not necessary in patients with renal dysfunction.

Beta-Adrenergic Antagonists

Beta-adrenergic antagonists inhibit the action of **catecholamines** and other sympathomimetic agents at beta-adrenergic receptor sites, thereby inhibiting stimulation of the sympathetic nervous system.

Clinical Uses

These include control of mild to moderate hypertension associated with chronic renal failure.

Dosage Form

- Propranolol (Inderal—human label)

Adverse Side Effects

These include decreased cardiac output and the promotion of bronchospasm. Therefore caution should be exercised with their use in patients with cardiac or pulmonary disease (Cowgill, 1991).

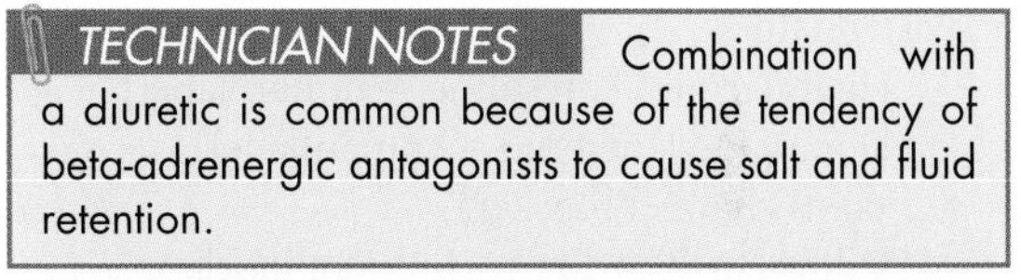

TECHNICIAN NOTES Combination with a diuretic is common because of the tendency of beta-adrenergic antagonists to cause salt and fluid retention.

ANGIOTENSIN-CONVERTING ENZYME INHIBITORS

ACE inhibitors block the conversion of angiotensin I to angiotensin II, decrease aldosterone secretion, reduce peripheral arterial resistance, and alleviate vasoconstriction.

Clinical Uses

ACE inhibitors are used to treat heart failure, hypertension, chronic renal failure, and protein-losing glomerulonephropathies in dogs and cats.

Dosage Forms

- Benazepril
  - Fortekor (veterinary label)
  - Benazepril (Lotensin—human label)

- Captopril (Capoten—human label)
- Enalapril (Enacard)
- Lisinopril
- Ramipril

Adverse Side Effects

These include complications in patients with renal insufficiency caused by excretion by the kidneys.

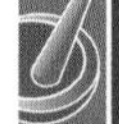

VASODILATORS AND CALCIUM CHANNEL BLOCKERS

A vasodilator or calcium channel blocker may be substituted for or used in combination with other medications if previous drug therapy to control hypertension fails.

Clinical Uses

These drugs are used to treat nonresponding hypertension. Dopamine may be used to promote diuresis in patients unresponsive to loop or osmotic diuretics.

Dosage Forms

- Vasodilators
  - Hydralazine (Apresoline—human label)
  - Dopamine (Intropin—human label)
- Calcium channel blockers
  - Diltiazem (Cardizem—human label)
  - Verapamil (Isoptin—human label)
  - Amlodipine (Norvasc—human label)

Adverse Side Effects

These include hypotension, edema, conduction disturbances, heart failure, and bradycardia (Cowgill, 1991). Hydralazine is excreted by the kidneys and requires dosage modification when used to treat hypertension in patients with renal failure.

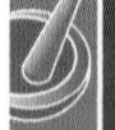

ANTIDIURETIC HORMONE

Antidiuretic hormone (ADH) is normally secreted by the posterior pituitary gland. This secretion regulates fluid balance in the body. In some conditions, such as pituitary diabetes insipidus, this hormone fails to be synthesized or excreted properly, and **polyuria** and **polydipsia** may occur.

Clinical Uses

ADH is used to treat diabetes insipidus.

Dosage Form

- Vasopressin (Pitressin—human label)

Adverse Side Effects

These are uncommon.

> *TECHNICIAN NOTES* Chlorpropamide (Diabinese, Glucamide) is a human product that is used to control type II diabetes mellitus. It potentiates the action of ADH and may be used to treat mild diabetes insipidus.

URINARY ACIDIFIERS

Urinary acidifiers are used to produce acid urine, which assists in dissolving and preventing formation of struvite uroliths. Since the introduction of urinary acidifying diets, urinary acidifiers have not been routinely prescribed.

Dosage Forms

- Methionine (Methigel, Methio-Tabs)
- Ammonium chloride (Uroeze)

Adverse Side Effects

These include gastrointestinal disturbances. These products should not be administered to patients with severe liver, kidney, or pancreatic disease or to those who exhibit acidosis.

> *TECHNICIAN NOTES* It is very important to inform clients who may change from using an acidifier to one of the available acidifying diets that while the diet is being administered, no acidifiers, salt, vitamin or mineral supplements, or any other food items—other than what is allowed in the diet—should be given to the patient.

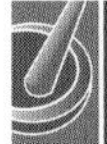

XANTHINE OXIDASE INHIBITORS

Xanthine oxidase inhibitors decrease the production of uric acid and are used in combination with a urate calculolytic diet for the dissolution of ammonium acid urate uroliths. Once dissolution occurs, a urine-alkalizing, low-protein, low-purine, low-oxalate diet is usually prescribed to prevent recurrence of uroliths.

Dosage Form
- Allopurinol (Zyloprim—human label)

Clinical Uses
These are used as a uric acid reducer in dogs, cats, reptiles, and birds.

Adverse Side Effects
These are uncommon, but because excretion occurs via the kidneys, the dosage may be altered in patients with renal insufficiency. Xanthine oxidase inhibitors should not be used in red-tailed hawks (Plumb, 2011). Hypersensitivity and hepatic and renal effects can occur.

> *TECHNICIAN NOTES* In cases of recurrence, allopurinol may once again be prescribed.

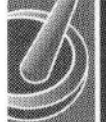

URINARY ALKALIZERS

Urinary alkalizers may be used in the management of ammonium acid urate, calcium oxalate, and cystine urolithiasis.

Dosage Forms
- Potassium citrate (Urocit-K—human label)
- Sodium bicarbonate, administered orally
- Tiopronin tablets (Thiola—human label)

Adverse Side Effects
These include possible fluid and electrolyte imbalance with the use of sodium bicarbonate.

PHARMACOTHERAPY OF RENAL FAILURE COMPLICATIONS

Because the renal cortex produces erythropoietin, chronic renal failure can cause an absolute or relative deficiency in its production. The resultant complication is normocytic, normochromic anemia that is classified as nonregenerative. Parenteral androgens, such as nandrolone (Durabolin) and testosterone enanthate, are capable of stimulating the production of red blood cell precursors and may increase the level of erythropoietin. Injections of recombinant human erythropoietin (Epogen, Procrit) have been shown to correct anemia associated with chronic renal failure (Ettinger, 2000). Human recombinant erythropoietin (rHuEPO) has been used to treat dogs and cats for anemia associated with chronic renal failure. Because of the expense of the drug and the potential risk of the formation of antibodies to erythropoietin, this drug is considered today to be a "last ditch effort" and the hematocrit level (i.e., packed cell volume [PCV]) should be in the "teens" before its therapy is considered. Hopefully, canine and feline recombinants will be developed in the future to reduce autoantibody formation. In addition, it is hoped that in the future, EPO may be demonstrated to have benefits in reducing the number of blood transfusions (Plumb, 2011).

Epoetin Alpha (Epogen, Procrit)

Adverse Side Effects
These include local or systemic allergic reactions in animals and pain occurring at the injection site. Headaches, along with seizures, have occurred in humans.

PHARMACOTHERAPY OF URINARY INCONTINENCE

Ettinger (2000) states: "Pharmacologic agents are selected for management of **urinary incontinence** when **urinary tract infection,** morphologic abnormalities, and mechanical types of excessive outlet resistance have been excluded as possible causes of the problem." Urinary incontinence may be described as a neurogenic disorder or a nonneurogenic disorder. A neurogenic disorder is evidenced by a neurologic lesion that affects the **upper motor neuron** segments or the **lower motor neuron** segments. When upper motor neuron segments are affected, the result is a spastic neuropathic urinary bladder.

Detrusor muscle contractions are normal, but bladder and urethral functions are abnormal. Therefore, as the bladder fills with urine, contractions occur more frequently (hypercontractility) and bladder capacity decreases. In addition, contraction of the detrusor muscle and relaxation of the urethral sphincter often are not coordinated. This results in interrupted, incomplete, and involuntary urination.

Functional urinary obstruction and urinary retention may also be present. When lower motor neuron segments are affected, the result is an **atonic,** neuropathic urinary bladder. With this disorder, detrusor muscle contractions are abnormal and the sensation of fullness is absent when the urinary bladder fills (hypocontractility). This causes the urinary bladder to distend, and eventually capacity increases. Urinary bladder distention may cause damage to the tight junctions between smooth muscle fibers. Urination eventually occurs when pressure inside the urinary bladder exceeds urethral outlet resistance.

Nonneurogenic disorders occur as a result of some type of anatomic anomaly of the lower urinary tract. In the young dog, this is usually a congenital anomaly. A congenital anomaly seen in young female dogs is ectopic ureter, which causes constant dribbling of urine. This occurs when the ureters end in abnormal places rather than at normal sphincters. In the older dog, acquired anatomic anomalies are usually responsible for nonneurogenic disorders. Conditions that commonly cause such problems include chronic cystitis, chronic urethritis, neoplasia, urolithiasis, and postsurgical adhesions. Other nonneurogenic disorders include functional abnormalities such as urethral incompetence and partial urethral obstruction. One type of nonneurogenic urethral incompetence is often seen in spayed female dogs and is usually responsive to hormonal therapy. Once the cause of the urinary incontinence has been identified, medical or surgical management begins. If a morphologic abnormality is causing urinary incontinence, surgical correction of the problem is necessary.

Medical management may include treatment for infection, if present, and treatment for the cause of the urinary incontinence (e.g., urethral incompetence, urinary bladder hypercontractility or hypocontractility). Drugs used in the medical management of urinary incontinence include the previously mentioned cholinergic agonists, anticholinergics, alpha-adrenergic antagonists, smooth muscle relaxants, skeletal muscle relaxants, tranquilizers, alpha-adrenergic agonists, and hormones such as estrogen and testosterone. Table 6-1 outlines these drugs for easy reference.

Dosage Forms

- Baclofen (Lioresal)
- Ephedrine sulfate
- Flavoxate HCl (Urispas—human label)
- Imipramine (Tofranil)
- Oxybutynin (Ditropan, Oxytrol)
- Phenylpropanolamine (PPA)

Clinical Uses

Baclofen is used as a muscle relaxant for treating urinary retention in dogs. Ephedrine is a sympathomimetic used for the treatment of urinary incontinence. Flavoxate is a medication used to treat hyperactive urinary bladder and urge incontinence in dogs. Imipramine is a tricyclic antidepressant used to treat urinary incontinence in dogs and cats. Oxybutynin chloride is a genitourinary smooth muscle relaxant used as a urinary antispasmodic in dogs or cats. Phenylpropanolamine HCl is a sympathomimetic used primarily for urethral sphincter hypotonus (Plumb, 2011).

Adverse Side Effects

Baclofen should not be used in cats. It may cause sedation, weakness, pruritis, salivation, and gastrointestinal upset. Ephedrine sulfate is contraindicated in patients with severe cardiovascular disease, glaucoma, prostatic hypertrophy, hyperthyroidism, diabetes mellitus, and hypertension. Flavoxate HCl is not commonly used in veterinary medicine, but the most likely adverse effect is weakness. Imipramine HCl may cause tachycardia, hyperexcitability, and tremors. Phenylpropanolamine HCl should be used cautiously in patients with glaucoma, prostatic

TABLE 6-1 Pharmacotherapy of Urinary Incontinence

DRUG	ACTION	EXAMPLES OF INDICATIONS
Bethanechol (Urecholine)	Cholinergic agonist	Bladder hypocontractility
Propantheline (Pro-Banthine)	Anticholinergic agent	Urge incontinence, bladder hypercontractility
Butylhyoscine (Buscopan)	Anticholinergic agent	Urge incontinence, bladder hypercontractility
Phenoxybenzamine (Dibenzyline)	Alpha-adrenergic antagonist	Urethral hyperreflexia
Nicergoline (Sermion)	Alpha-adrenergic antagonist	Urethral hyperreflexia
Moxisylyte (Carlytene)	Alpha-adrenergic antagonist	Urethral hyperreflexia
Aminopropazine (Jenotone)	Smooth muscle relaxant	Urge incontinence, bladder hypercontractility
Dantrolene (Dantrium)	Skeletal muscle relaxant	Urethral hyperreflexia
Diazepam (Valium)	Tranquilizer/skeletal muscle relaxant	Urethral hyperreflexia
Phenylpropanolamine	Alpha-adrenergic agonist	Urethral incompetence
Diethylstilbestrol (DES)	Antineoplastic, estrogen (hormone)	Hormone-responsive urethral incompetence
Testosterone cypionate	Hormone	Hormone-responsive urethral incompetence
Testosterone propionate	Hormone	Hormone-responsive urethral incompetence

hypertrophy, hyperthyroidism, diabetes mellitus, cardiovascular disorders, or hypertension (Plumb, 2011).

MISCELLANEOUS RENAL DRUGS

Urinary Tract Analgesics

Phenazopyridine

Phenazopyridine is used in humans as a urinary tract analgesic. It can be bought over-the-counter. It can be used alone or with sulfa drugs. Its use is contraindicated in felines because they are quite susceptible to dose-related methemoglobinemia, and oxidative changes in hemoglobin may be irreversible, causing formation of Heinz bodies and anemia (Osborne, 2001).

Tricyclic Antidepressants

Amitriptyline

Amitriptyline (Elavil)

Amitriptyline has many properties and has been used in treating interstitial cystitis in humans. Its mechanism is not fully understood. Amitriptyline is a tricyclic antidepressant and anxiolytic drug with anticholinergic, antihistaminic, anti–alpha-adrenergic, antiinflammatory, and analgesic properties. It has been used extensively for the treatment of interstitial cystitis in humans. Although it is a popular drug, its exact mechanism of action and therapeutic value in managing patients with interstitial cystitis remain unknown. This drug has been used recently for symptomatic treatment of idiopathic feline lower urinary tract disease (FLUTD) (Plumb, 2011).

Adverse Side Effects

Many side effects such as dry mouth, rapid heart rate, and sedation (i.e., antihistamine effects) are associated with this drug. High doses can cause heart toxicity. Sometimes it may cause cats to be less interested in grooming themselves. Additionally, weight gain may occur (Papich, 2002).

Glycosaminoglycans

Glycosaminoglycans (GAGs) are found covering the transitional epithelium of the urinary tract. These urothelial GAGs have the ability to keep microorganisms and crystals from adhering to the urinary bladder wall and limit the transepithelial movement of urine proteins and solutes (ionic or nonionic). Defects in surface GAGs and subsequent urothelial permeability are believed to be a factor in the pathogenesis of idiopathic FLUTD (Osborne, 2001).

Pentosan Polysulfate Sodium (Elmiron)

Clinical Uses

This drug is often used to manage human interstitial cystitis and has been used to reinforce urothelial GAGs and to reduce transitional cell injury. It has been used in the adjunctive treatment of feline interstitial cystitis or FLUTD. However, studies using pentosan for FLUTD have shown that it is not effective for short-term acute FLUTD (Plumb, 2011).

Adverse Side Effects

The safety and efficacy of pentosan polysulfate or other GAGs for the treatment of FLUTD have not been reported. In canines, vomiting, anorexia, lethargy, or mild depression are possible. Pentosan has some anticoagulant effects, so bleeding is possible in any species (Plumb, 2011).

Other Agents

Epakitin

Epakitin is a chitosan-based nutritional supplement made from a polysaccharide extracted from crab and shrimp shells.

Clinical Uses

The product information states that Epakitin binds phosphorus in the intestine, causing phosphorus to be eliminated through the intestinal tract. Reducing the amount of phosphorus absorbed then helps to lower the elevated levels of phosphorus noted in renal failure.

Azodyl

Azodyl product information claims that this product has the potential to reduce the azotemia of renal failure through "enteric dialysis."

TECHNICIAN'S ROLE

Veterinary technicians have a vital role in the care of patients with problems that affect the urinary system. This role includes providing client support and education, carrying out patient nursing care, performing necessary laboratory or radiologic examinations, providing surgical assistance, and understanding the various drugs and diets available for the treatment of renal disease.

REVIEW QUESTIONS

1. What structures constitute the urinary system?

   ____

2. Name two drugs that are contraindicated in uremic patients.

   ____

3. Renal damage may be categorized as

   ____________________,

   ____________________, or

   ____________________.

4. Explain how diuretics work.

   ____________________.

5. What supplement may be administered in conjunction with loop diuretics?

   ____________________.

6. ACE inhibitors block the conversion of angiotensin I to ____________________.
7. Urinary acidifiers are used to produce acid urine, which assists in dissolving and preventing the formation of ____________________ uroliths.
8. The renal cortex produces ____________________; thus chronic renal failure can cause an absolute or relative ____________________ in its production.
9. Why is furosemide referred to as a loop diuretic? ____________________.
10. Where is ADH secreted? ____________________
11. The ureters _____.
    a. originate from the urinary bladder and lead to the outside of the body
    b. originate from the kidneys and connect with the urinary bladder
    c. are found inside the nephrons
    d. are found inside the glomerulus
12. Persistently high blood pressure is known as _____.
    a. hypertonus
    b. hyperkalemia
    c. hypertension
    d. atony

13. Diuretics are used to remove ____ fluid.
    a. intracellular
    b. extracellular
14. Antidiuretic hormone (ADH) is normally secreted by the _______ pituitary gland.
    a. anterior
    b. posterior
15. What supplement may be administered in conjunction with loop diuretics?
    a. Calcium
    b. Phosphorus
    c. Aluminum hydrochloride
    d. Potassium
16. Urinary acidifiers are used to produce acid urine, which assists in dissolving and preventing the formation of ____.
    a. calcium
    b. uroliths
    c. urinary casts
    d. bacteria
17. _____ is a medical term for bloody urine.
    a. Hematuria
    b. Hemolysis
    c. Hematopoiesis
    d. Uremia
18. What part of the kidney is responsible for the reabsorption, or the secretion, of certain substances?
    a. Nephrons
    b. Tubules
    c. Glomerular filtrate
    d. Extracellular fluid
19. Patients with renal failure are at a lesser anesthetic risk than patients with normal renal function.
    a. True
    b. False
20. Loop diuretics inhibit the tubular reabsorption of ______.
    a. calcium
    b. phosphorus
    c. sodium
    d. potassium
21. A border collie named Sam is presented to the veterinarian and diagnosed with CHF, chronic kidney failure, and clinical signs of pulmonary edema. Sam weighs 40 lb and the veterinarian prescribes furosemide at 3.5 mg/kg once a day for a month. The pharmacy has on hand 50-mg, 20-mg, and 12.5-mg furosemide tablets. What is the dose that Sam should receive each day? What milligram tablets should be dispensed and how many?
    a. 63 mg/day; furosemide (50 mg × 30 tablets) and furosemide (12.5 mg × 30 tablets)
    b. 140 mg/day; furosemide (50 mg × 90 tablets)
    c. 70 mg/day; furosemide (50 mg × 30 tablets) and furosemide (20 mg × 30 tablets)
    d. 35 mg/day; furosemide (20 mg × 30 tablets) and furosemide (12.5 mg × 30 tablets) and furosemide (12.5 mg × 7.5 tablets [cut in quarter-size tablets])
22. A miniature schnauzer named Miss Peepers is presented to the veterinarian with reports from the client that she is straining to urinate and that blood is present in the urine. The veterinarian suspects possible infection-induced struvite uroliths in the urinary bladder and prescribes methionine for the dog at 100 mg/kg q12h, with the hope that the drug will help to dissolve any forming or formed uroliths. The client cannot afford radiography or ultrasonography on this particular office visit. Miss Peepers weighs 13.5 lb. In the pharmacy, there are methionine (200-mg tablets) and methionine (500-mg tablets). What is the dose the dog should receive q12h? How many tablets of each dosage need to be dispensed for a month's supply if the 500-mg tablets cost $0.50/each and the 200-mg tablets cost $0.25/each?
    a. 1350 mg q12h; methionine (500 mg × 90 tablets)
    b. 675 mg q12h; methionine (500 mg × 90 tablets)
    c. 900 mg q12h; methionine (500 mg × 60 tablets)
    d. 613 mg q12h; methionine (500 mg × 60 tablets and 200 mg tablets × 30 cut in halves)

23. Spironolactone is prescribed at 1.5 mg/kg q12h for a Labrador Retriever weighing 65 lb. What is the dose this dog should receive?
a. 13 mg q12h
b. 64.99 mg q12h
c. 48.75 mg q12h
d. 44.13 mg q12h

24. The veterinarian orders a prescription of furosemide at 2.5 mg/kg b.i.d. for a patient that weighs 55 lb. How many milligrams should the patient receive for one dose?
a. 25 mg
b. 62.5 mg
c. 61.5 mg
d. 18.3 mg

25. A dog weighing 33 lb with protein-losing nephropathy is presented to the veterinarian who orders enalapril 0.5 mg/kg PO once daily. What is the dose this dog requires?
a. 5.5 mg daily
b. 7.5 mg daily
c. 9.5 mg daily
d. 2.5 mg daily

REFERENCES

Cowgill LD: Clinical significance, diagnosis, and management of systemic hypertension in dogs and cats. In Cowgill LD, editor: Managing renal disease and hypertension, Kansas City, 1991, Harmon-Smith.

Ettinger SJ: Textbook of veterinary internal medicine, vol I and II, ed 5, Philadelphia, 2000, WB Saunders.

Mosby's pocket dictionary of medicine, nursing and allied health, ed 3, St. Louis, 1998, Mosby.

Osborne CA: Idiopathic lower urinary tract diseases: therapeutic rights and wrongs, in Proceedings. Annu Meet Am Vet Med Assoc, Boston, 2001.

Papich MG: Saunders handbook of veterinary drugs, Philadelphia, 2002, WB Saunders.

Plumb DC: Veterinary drug handbook, ed 7, Ames, Iowa, 2011, Wiley-Blackwell.

CHAPTER 7

Drugs Used in Cardiovascular System Disorders

KEY TERMS

Afterload
Arrhythmia (Dysrhythmia)
Automaticity
Bradyarrhythmia
Bradycardia
Cardiac remodeling
Chronotropic
Depolarization
Inotropic
Preload
Premature ventricular contraction
Repolarization
Stroke volume
Tachyarrhythmia
Tachycardia

OUTLINE

LEARNING OBJECTIVES

After studying this chapter, you should be able to

1. Describe the basic anatomy and physiology of the cardiovascular system.
2. List four compensatory mechanisms of the cardiovascular system.
3. List five basic objectives of the treatment of cardiovascular disease.
4. Differentiate between an inotropic and a chronotropic drug.
5. List and describe the indications, physiologic effects, and toxic side effects of the cardiac glycosides.
6. List the four categories of antiarrhythmic drugs and give an example from each category.
7. List potential adverse side effects of the antiarrhythmic drugs.
8. Describe the actions and potential side effects of the vasodilator drugs.
9. Describe the actions and potential side effects of the angiotensin-converting enzyme (ACE) inhibitors.

10. Describe the actions and potential side effects of the diuretics used to treat cardiovascular disease.
11. Describe the purpose of dietary sodium restriction in the therapy of cardiovascular disease.
12. List ancillary drugs or procedures that may be used in the treatment of cardiovascular disease.

INTRODUCTION

Heart disease has a relatively high incidence in veterinary medicine. Studies have found that approximately 11% of all dogs presented to veterinary clinics exhibited some degree of heart disease (Roudebush et al, 2000). Heart disease may be congenital or acquired. However, the acquired form accounts for most cases. The incidence and cause may vary from location to location. Heartworm disease accounts for a large percentage of heart disease in some parts of the country, whereas acquired disease of the atrioventricular valves or myocardium has a more uniform distribution. Acquired disease is encountered more often in older animals, and congenital disease is more prevalent in younger ones.

Whatever the cause, treatment of heart disease is often individualized to the particular patient according to cause, degree of progression, and owner cooperation. The response to treatment must be monitored carefully and adjusted while the disease progresses, which may cause poor liver or kidney function, or while toxic side effects develop. Some cardiovascular drugs have a narrow margin of safety (i.e., they are potentially toxic at low doses), and failing liver and kidney function may reduce the body's ability to metabolize or eliminate these drugs.

Because veterinary technicians are often the persons who monitor the progress of hospitalized patients, they must be aware of the signs of cardiovascular disease and of normal and abnormal responses to drugs used to treat this disease.

ANATOMY AND PHYSIOLOGY OF THE HEART

The heart is a four-chambered pump that is responsible for moving blood through the vascular system. The two dorsal chambers are called *atria,* and the two ventral chambers are called *ventricles* (Figure 7-1). Each of the chambers is composed primarily of strong muscle tissue called *myocardium,* which contracts to eject the blood. Even though the heart is considered one organ, it functions as two pumps (Spinelli and Enos, 1978).

The right atrium and ventricle constitute the "right-side pump," and the left atrium and ventricle make up the "left-side pump." Blood from the general circulation returns by way of the vena cava to the right atrium, enters the right ventricle through the right atrioventricular valve (tricuspid valve), and is pumped through the pulmonary artery to the lungs. In the lungs, the blood gives up carbon dioxide and picks up oxygen. The oxygenated blood returns to the heart via the pulmonary veins, where it fills the left atrium, passes through the left atrioventricular valve (mitral valve), and enters the left ventricle. The mitral and tricuspid valves swing open when the atria contract and snap shut when the ventricles contract. The closing of the valves as the ventricles contract prevents blood from flowing back into the atria. The left ventricle then contracts and ejects the oxygenated blood through the aorta into the branching arteries. These arteries divide into arterioles and end in the thin-walled capillaries throughout the body, where

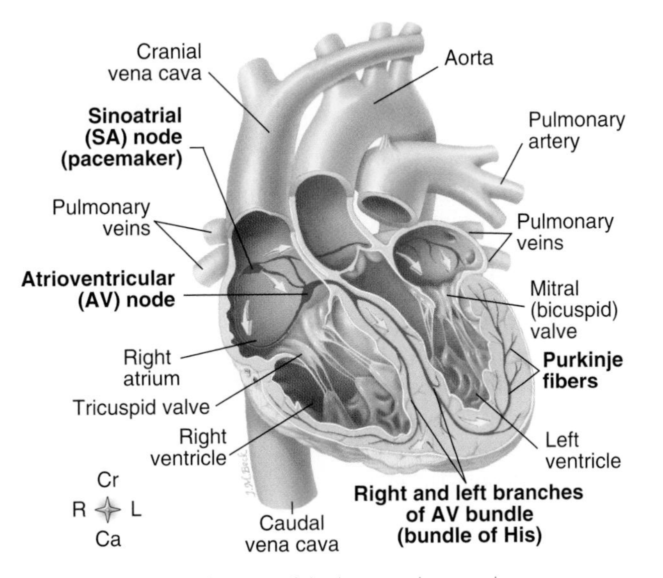

FIGURE 7-1 Schematic of the heart and its conduction system.

carbon dioxide is loaded to the blood and oxygen is unloaded to the tissue. Because the left ventricle must work harder to pump blood throughout the body than the right ventricle must work to pump blood to the lungs, the left ventricular wall is thicker than the right ventricular wall.

The pumping action of the heart is divided into two phases—systole and diastole. Systole is the period of contraction of the chambers, and diastole represents the relaxation phase when the chambers are filling with blood. Because each cell in the heart is capable of contracting spontaneously, the interaction of these two phases must be carefully coordinated to create an efficient pumping action. Diastolic time must be adequate to allow the atria to fill completely, and atrial systole must occur shortly before ventricular systole to allow the ventricles to fill maximally. Coordination of these two phases is achieved primarily through a wave of electric activity that arises in a specialized group of cells in the right atrium and then is conducted throughout the myocardium by a special conduction system.

The structures that make up the cardiac conduction system (see Figure 7-1) include the sinoatrial node, the atrioventricular node, the bundle of His and its branches, and the Purkinje system. Under abnormal conditions, parts of the myocardium and conduction system are capable of spontaneous discharge. Normally, however, the sinoatrial node discharges most rapidly and spreads a wave of depolarization over remaining areas of the heart before they can depolarize spontaneously. The rate of discharge of this node therefore controls the heart rate and is called the *cardiac pacemaker.* Impulses generated by the sinoatrial node travel over the atria to the atrioventricular node, face a brief delay (about 0.1 second) in the atrioventricular node, travel down the bundle of His to its left and right branches, and pass into the ventricular muscle via the Purkinje fibers. Myocardial cells are joined together by structures called *intercalated disks* and by fusing of cell membranes into an interconnected mass of cells called a *syncytium.* The syncytium of cells in the atria is separate and is insulated from the syncytium in the ventricles (Ganong, 2003). An electric stimulus from the sinoatrial node is transmitted over the entire atrial mass by the syncytial arrangement of cells. The impulse is not, however, transmitted directly into the ventricular syncytium. The impulse first must be picked up and transmitted by the atrioventricular node through its conduction system to the ventricular syncytium. Stimulation of a single atrial or ventricular muscle fiber causes the entire atrial or ventricular muscle mass to contract as a unit. When situations cause spontaneous depolarization of cardiac muscle or abnormalities of the conduction system, **arrhythmias** may occur.

When a cardiac cell is stimulated by electric activity that arises in the sinoatrial node, it undergoes depolarization and contracts. **Depolarization** is characterized by the rapid influx of sodium ions into the cell through channels or "gates," the slower influx of calcium ions, and the outflow of potassium ions (Figure 7-2). Until the sodium, potassium, and calcium ions have returned to the positions they had before depolarization, the cell is in a refractory period (Figure 7-3). A cell in an absolute refractory state cannot normally depolarize. In a relative refractory period, however, a cardiac cell can depolarize again, but the stimulus must be stronger than normal. A refractory period is essential for a cardiac cell to prevent it from remaining in a constant state of contraction as the result of stimulation by recycling impulses. The return of the ions to their original positions is brought about in part by the sodium–potassium pump and is an essential part of the **repolarization** process. Summed electric activity arising from the contraction of all heart cells represents the electrocardiogram (Figure 7-4), and each of its waves signifies activity in a particular area.

Even though the heart establishes its own inherent rate of beating, this rate is subject to outside influences through the autonomic nervous system. The sympathetic portion of the autonomic nervous system, through $beta_1$ receptors, produces positive **chronotropic** and **inotropic** effects on the heart. The parasympathetic branch of the autonomic nervous system causes negative chronotropic effects through cholinergic receptors.

The heart pumps blood through a series of arteries (arterial tree) to deliver it to the tissues. The larger of these arteries have elastic properties, which allow

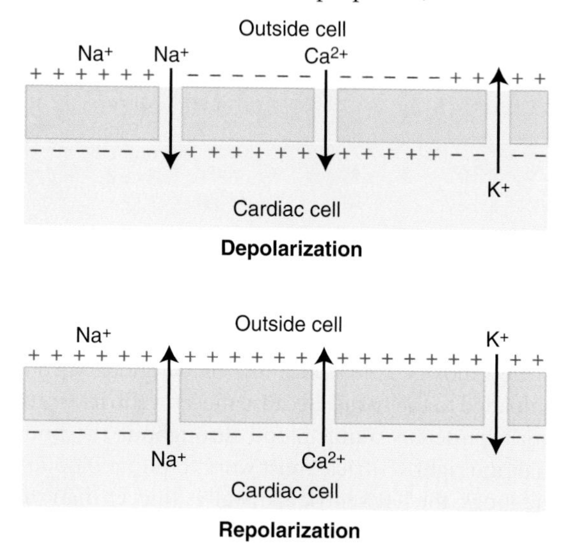

FIGURE 7-2 Depolarization and repolarization of a cardiac cell. Repolarization: the sodium–potassium–adenosine triphosphate (ATP) pump restores electrolytes to their resting sites.

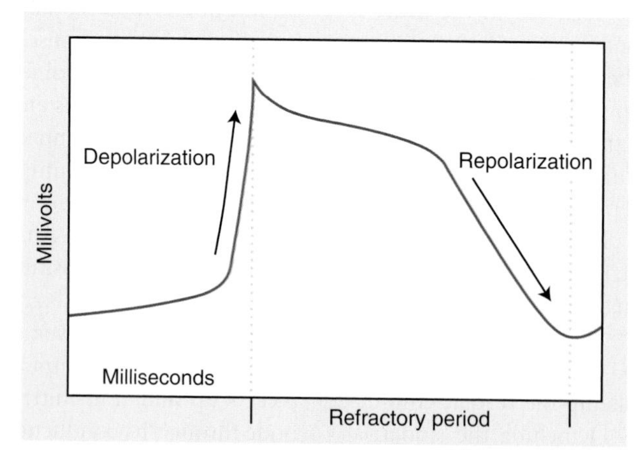

FIGURE 7-3 Schematic of the refractory period of a cardiac cell. After depolarization (contraction), cardiac muscle cells are unable to contract again until they have undergone repolarization. The time during which they are unable to contract is the refractory period.

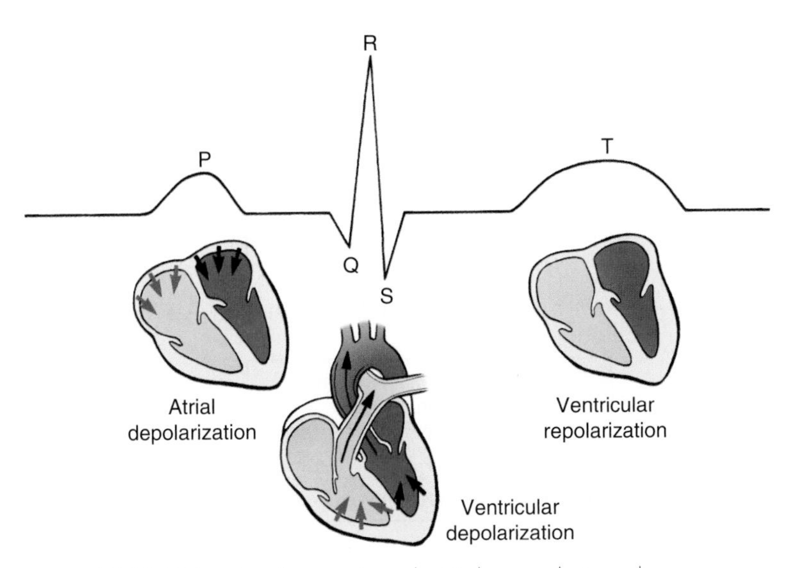

FIGURE 7-4 Cardiac events as depicted on an electrocardiogram.

them to stretch and recover when blood is pumped into them, thereby serving as a second pump (Upson, 1988). The smaller arteries are capable of changing their diameter (constricting or dilating) through the action of smooth muscle in their walls to increase or decrease the resistance against which the heart must pump. Stimulation of alpha-1 receptors causes vessels to constrict, and stimulation of $beta_2$ receptors causes vessels to dilate.

The amount of blood that the heart is capable of pumping per minute is called *cardiac output;* this value is calculated by multiplying the heart rate by the stroke volume. The **stroke volume** is determined in part by the amount of blood that fills the ventricle during diastole, called the ***preload,*** and the arterial resistance that the ventricle must pump against, called the ***afterload.***

COMPENSATORY MECHANISMS OF THE CARDIOVASCULAR SYSTEM

The cardiovascular system has a built-in reserve capacity, which allows it to increase its output during times of need (e.g., athletic performance) and to compensate for cardiac disease. The four basic factors of cardiac reserve or compensation are described as follows:

1. Increasing the heart rate. Increasing the rate of contraction increases cardiac output up to the point at which the rate is so fast that there is inadequate time for ventricular filling.
2. Increasing the stroke volume. Up to a point, an increased force of contraction results in an increase in the amount of blood that is pumped.
3. Increasing the efficiency of the heart muscle.
4. **Cardiac remodeling**. The heart is composed of muscle that responds to work by increasing its size and becoming stronger. This change usually precedes the development of heart failure signs by months or years.

Many disorders can result in cardiac disease. However, most that respond to pharmacologic therapy fall into one of the following categories:

- Valvular disease. Valvular insufficiency, a backflow or leakage of blood backward through the valve, is a relatively common acquired heart disorder of dogs. If the tricuspid valve is affected, ascites may occur. If the mitral valve is involved, pulmonary edema may result. Valvular disease may result from progressive bacterial endocarditis. Inadequate opening of valves may also occur and cause disease. Insufficiency or stenosis may be accompanied by a murmur.

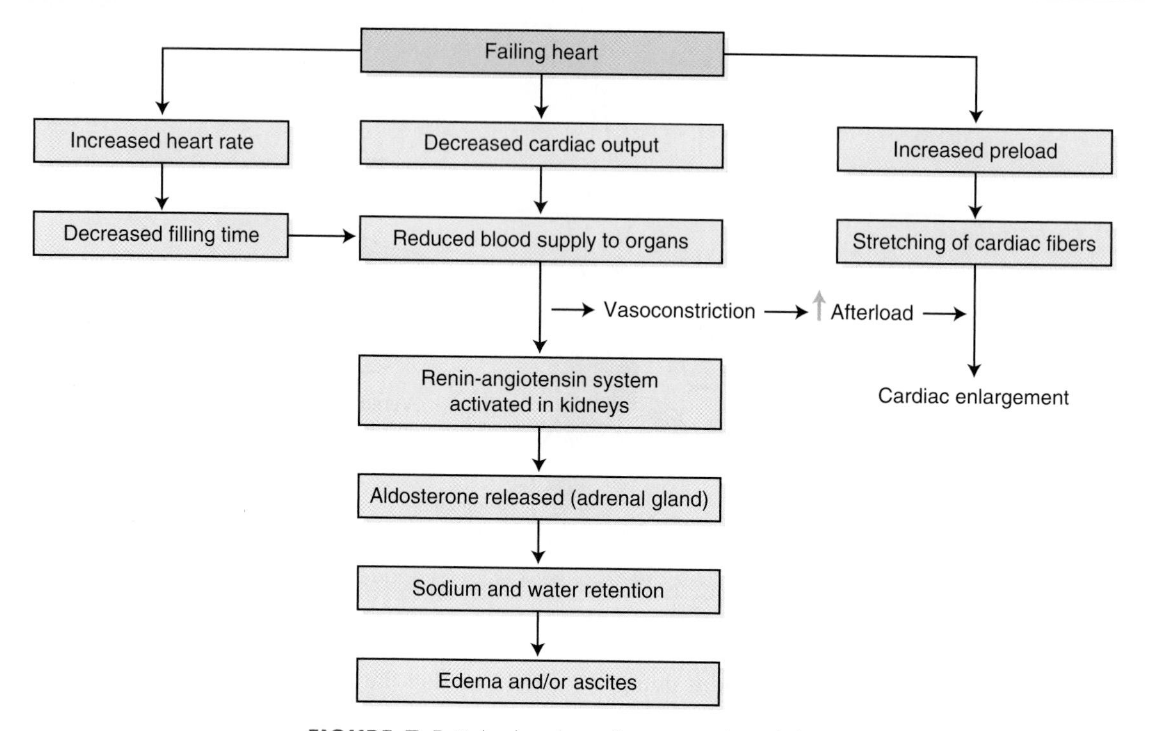

FIGURE 7-5 Pathophysiology of congestive heart failure.

- Cardiac arrhythmias. If a focus of cardiac tissue depolarizes out of sequence with the sinoatrial node, an arrhythmia may result. Various types of arrhythmias, including **tachyarrhythmias** (arrhythmias with a rapid rate) and **bradyarrhythmias** (arrhythmias with a slow rate), may occur. Arrhythmias may occur in the atria (supraventricular) or in the ventricles (ventricular). Several categories of drugs (e.g., catecholamines, xylazine, digoxin, and others) predispose the heart to arrhythmias.
- Myocardial disease. Cardiomyopathy, a disease of the myocardium, primarily affects dogs and cats. It may be classified as congestive (the myocardium becomes thin and ineffective in its pumping action) or hypertrophic (the myocardium becomes thickened and restricts ventricular filling). Each type is often accompanied by various arrhythmias.
- Other potential causes of cardiac disease include congenital defects (right-to-left shunts), abnormalities of cardiac innervation, vascular disease (hypertension), and heartworm disease.

Cardiovascular diseases with the greatest prevalence include mitral disease in dogs, hypertrophic cardiomyopathy in cats, dilated cardiomyopathy in dogs, "Boxer" cardiomyopathy, and heartworm disease (Hamlin, 2003).

Congestive heart failure (CHF) (Figure 7-5) occurs when the pumping ability of the heart is impaired to the extent that sodium and water are retained in an effort to compensate for inadequate cardiac output. It is associated with exercise intolerance, pulmonary edema, and ascites. The heart usually becomes structurally remodeled in this condition.

Because cardiac disease is a progressive condition in which structural changes occur before clinical signs appear, a classification scheme has been adapted from human medicine to categorize veterinary patients into four categories according to the course of the disease and the treatment for each stage (DeFrancesco, 2013). Table 7-1 lists these stages and general treatment options for each.

TABLE 7-1 Stages and Treatment of Cardiac Disease

STAGE	DESCRIPTION/SIGNS	TREATMENT
A	High risk for development of heart failure but no structural abnormality of the heart	None
B	Structural abnormality present but no signs of heart failure	ACEI? Beta blockers? Restricted sodium diet?
C	Structural abnormality present and current or previous signs of heart failure/coughing, reduced exercise tolerance	Dog: diuretic, pimobendan ACEI, sodium restricted diet? Cat: diuretic, ACEI
D	End stage signs of heart failure resistant to standard treatment/ dyspnea at rest	Multimodal therapy

ACEI, Angiotensin-converting enzyme inhibitor.

BASIC OBJECTIVES IN THE TREATMENT OF CARDIOVASCULAR DISEASE

Basic objectives in the treatment of cardiovascular disease include the following (Ettinger, 2000):

- Control rhythm disturbances
- Maintain or increase cardiac output
    - Increase the strength of contraction
    - Decrease the afterload
        - Arteriolar dilator
        - Decrease the preload
        - Venodilator
        - Relieve fluid accumulations
    - Diuretics
    - Dietary salt restriction
- Increase the oxygenation of the blood
    - Bronchodilation
- Ancillary treatment
    - Narcotics/sedatives
    - Oxygen

CATEGORIES OF CARDIOVASCULAR DRUGS

POSITIVE INOTROPIC DRUGS

The general principle involved in the use of drugs that improve the strength of contraction is that the heart, even in the presence of disease, has reserve capacity for contraction that can be called on to improve cardiac output. Some clinicians advise cautious use of positive inotropic drugs because these can increase the oxygen demand of cardiac muscle, can potentially damage the contractile apparatus, and can increase the tendency for arrhythmias. Proof of clinical efficacy of positive inotropic drugs is lacking, and their use is controversial (Boothe, 2012). Their popularity has waxed and waned through the years as newer, more effective products have come into use.

Cardiac Glycosides (Digitalis)

The digitalis compounds (digoxin and digitoxin) are obtained from the dried leaves of the plant *Digitalis purpurea.* The beneficial effects of these compounds have been known for hundreds of years and include (1) improved cardiac contractility, (2) decreased heart rate, (3) antiarrhythmic effects, and (4) decreased signs of dyspnea.

Digitalis increases the strength of contraction by increasing the level of calcium ions available in the contractile filaments within cardiac muscle cells. This action occurs as a result of inhibition of sodium–potassium–adenosine triphosphatase (Figure 7-6). The heart rate is slowed by prolonging atrioventricular conduction time and by increasing parasympathetic, autonomic stimulation. The primary actions of the digitalis drugs are to (1) increase the force of contraction, (2) decrease the rate of contraction, and (3) improve baroreceptor function (Hamlin, 2003).

Digitalis use is indicated in patients with cardiac disease that results from impaired cardiac contraction or atrial arrhythmias as suggested by clinical signs such as exercise intolerance, weak peripheral pulses, pulmonary edema, and coughing—or by electrocardiographic diagnosis.

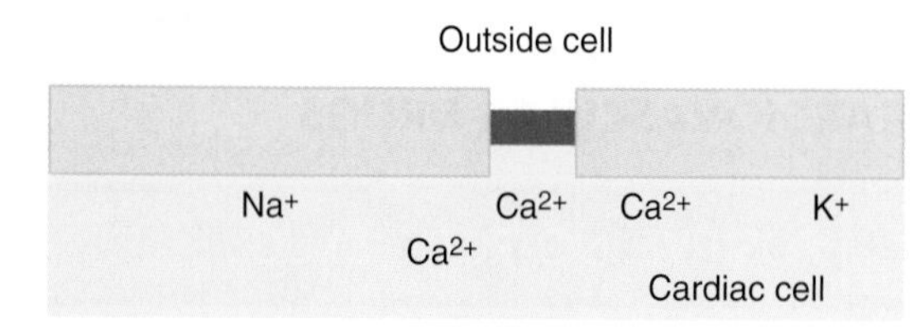

FIGURE 7-6 Effect of digitalis on the sodium–potassium–adenosine triphosphate (ATP)ase pump. Digitalis compounds block the sodium–potassium–ATPase enzyme, reduce the amount of Ca^{2+} pumped from the cell during repolarization, and increase the amount of Ca^{2+} available for depolarization.

Clinical Uses

Clinical uses of the digitalis compounds include the treatment of CHF, atrial fibrillation, and supraventricular **tachycardia.**

Dosage Forms

Dosage forms include tablets and elixirs.

- Veterinary approved products are no longer available.
- Human approved
    - Digoxin for injection (Lanoxin, 0.25 mg/mL or 0.1 mg/mL in ampules)
    - Digoxin tablets (Lanoxin, 0.125 mg, 0.25 mg)
    - Digoxin oral solution (Lanoxin, 0.05 mg/mL, 60-mL bottle)

Adverse Side Effects

Adverse side effects from the use of digitalis compounds are often associated with high or toxic serum levels of drugs and can include anorexia, vomiting, diarrhea, and various arrhythmias. Cats are relatively more sensitive than dogs to toxic effects (Plumb, 2011). Digitalis compounds are adversely affected when given concurrently with many drugs (e.g., cimetidine, metoclopramide, diazepam, anticholinergics, and others). Consult appropriate references for suitability.

> **TECHNICIAN NOTES**
> - The bioavailability of digoxin varies from 60% in tablet form to 75% in elixir form, and adjustments are likely needed if the dosage form is changed.
> - Clients should be advised to monitor their pets carefully for signs of toxicity and to advise the veterinarian if any arise.

Catecholamines

Catecholamines include a group of sympathomimetic (adrenergic) compounds that (1) increase the force and rate of muscular contraction of the heart (increase in cardiac output), (2) constrict peripheral blood vessels (increase blood pressure), and (3) elevate blood glucose levels. Catecholamines increase cardiac contractility primarily by stimulating $beta_1$ receptors. Because of their short serum half-lives, catecholamines are used mainly for short-term management of severe heart failure.

Epinephrine

Epinephrine is the preferred drug for providing stimulation for contraction of the heart and for supporting the circulatory system after cardiac arrest. It may be administered by the intracardiac, intratracheal, or intravenous route, and a 1:10,000 solution is preferred. Most products provide a 1:1000 solution. Because epinephrine greatly increases the workload of the heart and increases the tendency for arrhythmias, it is not used for therapy of chronic heart failure.

Clinical Uses

Epinephrine is used in veterinary medicine for cardiac resuscitation and for the treatment of anaphylaxis.

Dosage Forms

Human label forms of epinephrine are used.

- Epinephrine HCl for injection, 0.1 mg/mL (1:10,000) in 10-mL syringes
- Epinephrine HCl for injection (Adrenalin Chloride, 1 mg/mL [1:1000] in ampules and vials)

Adverse Side Effects

These include hypertension, arrhythmias, anxiety, and excitability.

> **TECHNICIAN NOTES**
> - A 1:10,000 solution can be prepared from a 1:1000 solution by mixing 1 mL of the drug with 9 mL of sterile water for injection. Alternatively, 0.5 mL of drug can be mixed with 4.5 mL of sterile water for injection.
> - Epinephrine is stored under refrigeration.

Isoproterenol

Isoproterenol is seldom used in the treatment of cardiac disease. It is indicated in atropine-resistant **bradycardia.**

Dopamine

Dopamine is a biosynthetic precursor of norepinephrine. It stimulates dopaminergic receptors in coronary, mesenteric, renal, and cerebral vascular beds. It also is capable of stimulating alpha- and beta-adrenergic receptors to increase heart contractility, heart rate, and blood pressure. Dopamine use in cardiac cases is mainly limited to heart failure associated with anesthetic emergencies or after cardiac resuscitation.

Clinical Uses

Dopamine is used for adjunctive treatment of acute heart failure and oliguric renal failure and for the supportive treatment of shock.

Dosage Forms

- Dopamine HCl—40 mg/mL, 80 mg/mL, 160 mg/mL
- Dopamine HCl in 5% dextrose—0.8 mg/mL, 1.6 mg/mL, 3.2 mg/mL

Adverse Side Effects

These include vomiting, tachycardia, dyspnea, and blood pressure variations (hypotension or hypertension).

Dobutamine

Dobutamine is a synthetic inotropic agent related structurally to dopamine. It causes increased cardiac contractility, as does dopamine, but does not produce dilation of selected vascular beds. Dobutamine is a direct $beta_1$-adrenergic agent. It produces increased cardiac output with little tendency to cause arrhythmias or increased heart rate. It is available only as a human label product and is administered in diluted form by intravenous infusion. Consult the *Veterinary Drug Handbook* (Plumb, 2011) for directions on preparation of the solution for infusion.

Bipyridine Derivatives

Amrinone and milrinone are representatives of a new class of positive inotropic drugs that appear to work by inhibiting enzymes that ultimately lead to an increase in cellular calcium. Amrinone (Inocor) is given intravenously and is limited to short-term inpatient use, whereas milrinone is given orally and has potential for long-term use.

Inotropic, Mixed Dilator
Pimobendan

Pimobendan was approved for use in veterinary medicine in April 2007. It is a positive inotropic drug that increases the calcium sensitivity of cardiac myofilaments and inhibits the enzyme phosphodiesterase.

Clinical Uses

Pimobendan is labeled for the treatment of atrioventricular insufficiency or dilated cardiomyopathy in dogs.

Dosage Form

- Vetmedin Chewable Tablets in 1.25-mg, 2.5-mg, or 5-mg sizes

Adverse Side Effects

Side effects may include anorexia, lethargy, diarrhea, and others.

Contraindication

Pimobendan is contraindicated in cases of hypertrophic cardiomyopathy, aortic stenosis, or any other condition when cardiac augmentation is inappropriate for anatomic reasons.

ANTIARRHYTHMIC DRUGS

An arrhythmia is a variation from the normal rhythm of the heart. Such a variation may result from an abnormality of impulse generation (increased **automaticity**) or from abnormalities of impulse conduction. Many arrhythmias arise when a local group of cells begins to depolarize faster than the sinoatrial node (pacemaker), which causes disruption of the normal depolarization pattern of the heart. The location of this group of cells is called an *ectopic focus* (foci if more than one location is involved). Arrhythmias usually result in reduced cardiac output caused by poorly coordinated pumping activity. Some arrhythmias may be auscultated by an experienced ear, but arrhythmias more often are diagnosed through their production of abnormal waveforms seen on an electrocardiogram.

Factors that may cause or predispose the heart to arrhythmias include the following:

- Conditions that cause hypoxemia
- Electrolyte imbalances
- Increased levels of or increased sensitivity to catecholamines
- Drugs such as digitalis compounds, xylazine, and others
- Cardiac trauma or disease that results in altered cardiac cells

Arrhythmias are classified in relation to heart rate as tachyarrhythmias or bradyarrhythmias. Tachyarrhythmias are further classified into ventricular or atrial, depending on their location, and can lead to rapid contraction rates in corresponding chambers. At these rapid rates, pumping efficiency is greatly reduced because of decreased filling time. Rapid, uncoordinated activity called *flutter* or *fibrillation* may also result.

Pharmacologists classify antiarrhythmic drugs into the following four basic categories (Boothe, 2012):

1. Class IA includes quinidine, procainamide, and others.
   Class IB includes lidocaine, tocainide, and mexiletine.
   Class IC includes flecainide and encainide.
2. Class II includes the beta-adrenergic blockers (propranolol).
3. Class III includes bretylium and amiodarone.
4. Class IV includes the calcium channel blockers (verapamil, nifedipine, amlodipine, and diltiazem).

Class IA

Drugs in Class IA depress myocardial excitability, prolong the refractory period, decrease automaticity, and increase conduction times. Class IA drugs are used to treat atrial and ventricular arrhythmias and may be given orally on a long-term basis.

Quinidine

Quinidine is an alkaloid that is obtained from cinchona plants or is prepared from quinine (Plumb, 2011).

Clinical Uses

Quinidine is used to treat ventricular arrhythmias and atrial fibrillation in small animals and horses.

Dosage Forms

Human label forms are used.

- Quinidine sulfate
  - Tablets, 100, 200, and 300 mg
  - Sustained-release tablets, 300 mg
- Quinidine gluconate
  - Sustained-release tablets, 324 mg
  - Injection, 80 mg/mL
- Quinidine polygalacturonate (Cardioquin)

Adverse Side Effects

These include anorexia, vomiting, diarrhea, weakness, and laminitis (horses).

> **TECHNICIAN NOTES** Do not allow animals to chew or crush quinidine oral dosage forms.

Procainamide

Procainamide is an antiarrhythmic that is chemically related to procaine.

Clinical Uses

Procainamide is used to treat **premature ventricular contractions (PVCs),** ventricular tachycardia, and some forms of atrial tachycardia.

Dosage Forms

Human label procainamide hydrochloride is used.

- Injection, 100 mg/mL in 10-mL vials and 500 mg/mL in 2-mL vials, generic

Adverse Side Effects

These include anorexia, vomiting, diarrhea, hypotension, and others. However, these effects are generally dose related.

Class IB

Drugs in this category exert their influence by stabilizing myocardial cell membranes. By blocking the influx of sodium into the cell, these drugs prevent depolarization and decrease cell automaticity

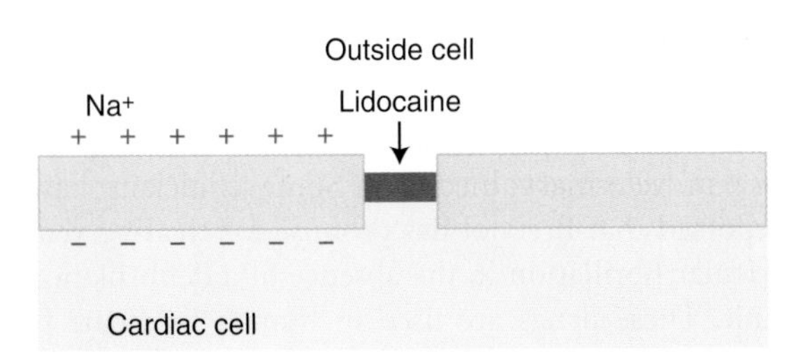

FIGURE 7-7 Effect of lidocaine on sodium channels. Lidocaine blocks sodium channels and reduces the automaticity of cardiac cells.

(Figure 7-7). They are used to treat ventricular arrhythmias, but they have not been approved for this use by the U.S. Food and Drug Administration (FDA).

Lidocaine

Lidocaine is a local anesthetic and antiarrhythmic. It is prepared only in injectable form and is administered intravenously. It is used frequently in emergency medicine and acute care.

Clinical Uses

Lidocaine is primarily used for the control of PVCs and for the treatment of ventricular tachycardia.

Dosage Forms

- Various veterinary brand name forms are available in 1% and 2% solutions.

Adverse Side Effects

These are rare but may include drowsiness, depression, ataxia, and muscle tremors. Cats are potentially sensitive to the central nervous system effects of lidocaine. These should be monitored carefully when a patient is receiving this drug.

> **TECHNICIAN NOTES** When administering lidocaine for an arrhythmia, make certain that it is lidocaine without epinephrine. Epinephrine (a catecholamine) predisposes the heart to arrhythmia.

Tocainide and Mexiletine

Tocainide and mexiletine are other class IB agents that may be given orally.

Class IC

Class IC agents are seldom used in veterinary medicine.

Class II

Class II antiarrhythmics are the beta-adrenergic blockers. Propranolol was the prototype agent in this class for veterinary therapeutics, although atenolol and other agents are now generally favored. Beta blockers may block only $beta_1$ receptors or only $beta_2$ receptors (selective), or they may block both types (nonselective). See Table 4-1. They also are thought to upregulate or increase adrenergic receptors to improve cardiac efficiency (Hamlin, 2003). These drugs may be used to treat atrial or ventricular arrhythmias, decrease cardiac conduction, reduce cardiac output, and decrease blood pressure.

Propranolol

Propranolol reduces automaticity of cardiac conduction cells by blocking $beta_1$ and $beta_2$ receptor sites. Myocardial oxygen demand is reduced by propranolol. Reducing myocardial oxygen demand reduces the tendency for ischemia, which in turn reduces automaticity (Williams and Baer, 1990). Propranolol reduces heart rate, cardiac output, and blood pressure. It also may improve cardiac performance in animals with hypertrophic cardiomyopathy.

Clinical Uses

In veterinary medicine, propranolol is used to treat hypertrophic cardiomyopathy and various atrial and ventricular arrhythmias. It is used in cats to treat systemic hypertension and hyperthyroidism (Plumb, 2011).

Dosage Forms

- Propranolol HCl tablets, 10, 20, 40, 60, 80, and 90 mg, generic
- Propranolol HCl extended-release capsules, 60, 80, 120, and 160 mg (Inderal LA)
- Propranolol for injection, 1 mg/mL in 1-mL ampules or vials (Inderal)
- Propranolol oral solution, 4, 8, and 80 mg/mL concentrate, generic

Adverse Side Effects
These include bradycardia, hypotension, worsening of heart failure, lethargy, bronchospasm, and depression.

> **TECHNICIAN NOTES**
> - Propranolol is contraindicated in patients with overt heart failure, greater than first-degree heart block, and sinus bradycardia (Plumb, 2011).
> - Do not discontinue therapy abruptly because tachycardia or hypertension may occur.

Atenolol
Atenolol is a selective $beta_1$ blocker (Papich, 2011). Atenolol decreases heart rate, slows cardiac conduction, decreases myocardial oxygen demand, reduces blood pressure, and diminishes cardiac output. Because of its selective $beta_1$ effect, atenolol may be safer to use in animals prone to bronchospasm.

Clinical Uses
Atenolol is used in the treatment of supraventricular tachyarrhythmias, premature ventricular contractions, hypertension, and cardiomyopathy.

Dosage Forms
- Atenolol tablets, 25, 50, and 100 mg (Tenormin)
- Atenolol injection, 5 mg/mL (Tenormin)

Adverse Side Effects
Bradycardia, lethargy and depression, hypotension, syncope, or heart failure is most commonly reported in older animals.

Other Beta Blockers
- Carvedilol (Dilatrend)
- Sotalol (Betapace). Sotalol is nonselective with action similar to propranolol. This drug is replacing quinidine as the antiarrhythmic drug of choice by some clinicians.
- Esmolol (Brevibloc). Selective $beta_1$ blocker for short-term use.
- Metoprolol (Lopressor). Metoprolol is a $beta_1$ blocker otherwise similar to propranolol.
- Pindolol (Betapindol)

Class III
The Class III antiarrhythmics bretylium (Bretylol) and amiodarone (Cordarone) are not in common use in veterinary medicine. Some clinicians have reported that Bretylol has promise for treating ventricular fibrillation in the absence of a defibrillation unit. These drugs are used in human medicine to treat ventricular arrhythmias.

Class IV
Class IV antiarrhythmic drugs work by blocking the channels that permit entry of calcium ions through the cardiac cell membrane. This effect causes depression of the contractile mechanism in myocardial and smooth muscle cells and depresses automaticity and impulse transmission (Williams and Baer, 1990).

Verapamil Hydrochloride
Verapamil is a channel-blocking agent and is available in oral and injectable forms. It has had limited use in veterinary medicine.

Clinical Uses
Verapamil is used to treat supraventricular tachycardia, atrial flutter, and atrial fibrillation.

Dosage Forms
Human label products are used.
- Verapamil HCl tablets, 40, 80, and 120 mg (Calan)
- Verapamil HCl sustained-release tablets, 120, 180, 240, and 360 mg (Calan SR, Isoptin SR)
- Verapamil HCl for injection, 5 mg/2 mL in ampules, vials, and syringes—generic

Adverse Side Effects
These include hypotension, bradycardia, tachycardia, pulmonary edema, and worsening of CHF.

Diltiazem
Diltiazem is a channel-blocking agent that is similar in action to verapamil.

Clinical Uses
Diltiazem is used for supraventricular tachyarrhythmias in dogs and cats and for hypertrophic cardiomyopathy in cats.

Dosage Forms

- Diltiazem tablets, 30, 60, 90, and 120 mg (Cardizem)
- Diltiazem oral capsules extended/sustained release, 60, 90, 120, 180, 240, 300, 360, and 420 mg (Cardizem LA, Cardizem CD, Dilacor XR)

Other Class IV Antiarrhythmics

Other channel blockers include nifedipine (Adalat) and amlodipine (Norvasc). These agents are used primarily for the treatment of hypertension rather than as antiarrhythmics.

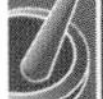

VASODILATOR DRUGS

When heart failure occurs, cardiac output is reduced, which results in hypotension and poor perfusion of tissue. As a reaction to this poor perfusion of tissue, the body activates compensatory mechanisms to increase blood pressure and improve blood supply to tissues. The first compensatory activity is stimulation of the sympathetic nervous system to increase the heart rate and to cause constriction of small arteries, which in turn raises blood pressure. Next, the renin–angiotensin–aldosterone system (RAAS) is activated by the release of renin from poorly perfused kidneys (Figure 7-8). Renin causes angiotensinogen to be converted to angiotensin I. Angiotensin I then is converted by angiotensin-converting enzyme (ACE) to angiotensin II. Angiotensin II causes further vasoconstriction and stimulates the adrenal glands to release aldosterone. Aldosterone acts on the kidney tubules to cause reabsorption of sodium ions and osmotic retention of water. The water that is retained helps to expand the circulating blood volume to improve tissue perfusion.

In the short term, these compensatory mechanisms are beneficial. In the long term, however, they become harmful because the heart must work harder to pump blood through vessels constricted by sympathetic nervous stimulation and by the effects of angiotensin II (increased afterload). The ever-increasing blood volume (increased preload) caused by aldosterone release and water retention also necessitates more strenuous activity by the heart, which in a weakened state initiates the preceding chain of events.

Vasodilator drugs act by dilating arteries (arteriolar dilator), veins (venodilator), or both (combined vasodilator). Dilatory activity may be brought about by direct action on vessel smooth muscle, through blockage of sympathetic stimulation, or by preventing conversion of angiotensin I to angiotensin II. Dilation of constricted arteries tends to decrease the afterload and improve cardiac output. The

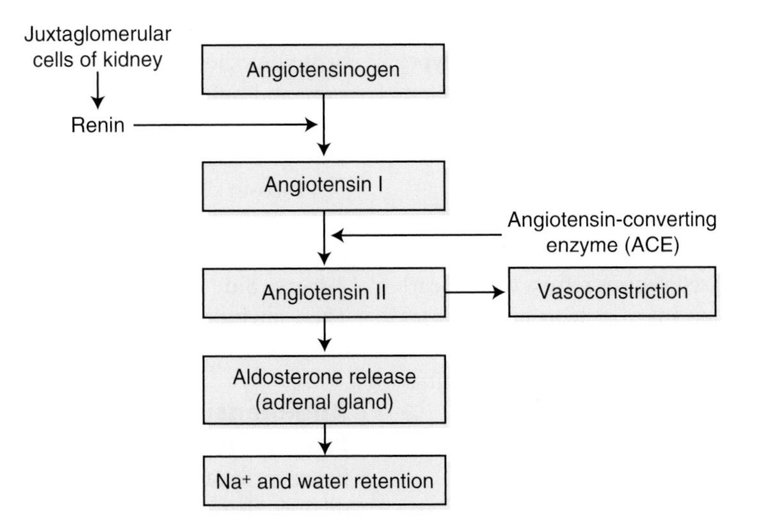

FIGURE 7-8 The renin–angiotensin–aldosterone system (RAAS).

preload is also reduced because of pooling of blood in dilated veins.

Many forms of CHF are improved by the use of vasodilators, which can be used in conjunction with other heart medications.

Hydralazine

Hydralazine is primarily an arteriolar dilator. It acts directly on smooth muscle in the arterial wall by interfering with calcium movement and inhibiting the contractile state (Plumb, 2011). The net result is that peripheral resistance is reduced and cardiac output is often greatly improved in animals with CHF. Some clinicians recommend that hydralazine be used with a diuretic because it may activate the renin–angiotensin system and cause water retention (Bill, 1994).

Clinical Uses

Hydralazine is used for afterload reduction associated with CHF, especially CHF caused by mitral valve insufficiency.

Dosage Forms

Human forms are used.

- Hydralazine HCl tablets, 10, 25, 50, and 100 mg (Apresoline)
- Hydralazine for injection, 20 mg/mL in ampules or vials—generic

Adverse Side Effects

Adverse side effects in small animals include hypotension, vomiting, diarrhea, sodium and water retention, and tachycardia.

Nitroglycerin Ointment

Nitroglycerin is primarily a venodilator that reduces preload as the result of pooling of blood in peripheral vessels and decreased venous return to the heart. Some arteriolar dilation may occur at higher doses. Nitroglycerin is applied topically in hairless areas of small animal patients. The medical vehicle of nitroglycerin causes it not to be explosive.

Clinical Uses

In small animal medicine, nitroglycerin is used as a vasodilator to improve cardiac output and reduce associated pulmonary edema. In equine medicine, nitroglycerin is used as a leg sweat to reduce swelling and to treat laminitis.

Dosage Forms

- Nitroglycerin topical ointment, 2% in 20-g, 30-g, and 60-g tubes (Nitro-Bid, Minitran)—human label

Adverse Side Effects

Adverse side effects are minimal and may include rashes at the application site and hypotension.

TECHNICIAN NOTES

- Gloves should be worn when nitroglycerin is applied.
- Rotate application sites.
- Do not pet animals at application sites.
- The dose is measured in inches by application of a strip of ointment to measuring paper that is supplied with the product.
- The veterinarian should be contacted if a rash appears at the application site.

Prazosin

Prazosin is a combined vasodilator. It reduces blood pressure and peripheral vasoconstriction by blocking alpha$_1$-adrenergic receptor sites. Prazosin apparently does not activate the renin–angiotensin system.

Clinical Uses

Prazosin is used for adjunctive treatment of CHF, dilated cardiomyopathy in dogs, systemic hypertension, and pulmonary hypertension.

Dosage Forms

- Prazosin capsules, 1, 2, and 5 mg (Minipress)—human label.

Adverse Side Effects

These include hypotension, syncope, vomiting, and diarrhea.

Angiotensin-Converting Enzyme Inhibitors

Benazepril, captopril, and enalapril are potent vasodilators that exert their effects on blood vessels by preventing formation of the potent vasoconstrictor angiotensin II. They prevent the conversion of angiotensin I to angiotensin II by inhibiting ACE (Figure 7-8). They are combined vasodilators that produce mild preload and significant afterload reduction. ACE inhibitors also influence several other mediators associated with cardiac remodeling (Boothe, 2012).The drugs in this category are called ACE inhibitors.

Clinical Uses

ACE inhibitors act as vasodilators and may be used in the treatment of Stage B, C, and D heart failure (see Table 7-1). In cats, benazepril and enalapril can also be used to treat hypertension associated with chronic renal failure or hypertrophic cardiomyopathy.

Dosage Forms

- Enalapril tablets, 1, 2.5, 5, 10, and 20 mg (Enacard)—veterinary label
- Enalapril tablets, 2.5, 5, 10, and 20 mg tablets (Vasotec tablets)—human label
- Benazepril, tablets, 5, 10, 20, and 40 mg (Lotensin)—human label
- Captopril, tablets, 12.5, 25, 50, and 100 mg (Capoten)—human label
- Lisinopril (Prinivil)
- Ramipril (Altace)

Adverse Side Effects

These include hypotension, azotemia, vomiting, diarrhea, hyperkalemia, and others. The safety of enalapril in breeding dogs has not been established.

> **TECHNICIAN NOTES**
>
> - Care should be taken when captopril or enalapril is administered with other vasodilators and certain diuretics because of potential hypotension.
> - Concurrent use of nonsteroidal antiinflammatory drugs may reduce the effectiveness of captopril.
> - Captopril may cause a false-positive urine acetone finding.

Other Vasodilators

- Isosorbide (Isordil)
- Isoxsuprine (Vasodilan)
- Nitroprusside (Nitropress); intravenous injection for acute, severe hypertension
- Sildenafil (Viagra); may have use in the treatment of pulmonary hypertension in small animals
- Tadalafil (Cialis); may be useful in treating pulmonary hypertension in dogs

DIURETICS

Diuretics have been some of the most commonly used drugs in the treatment of heart failure because of their ability to promote the reduction of preload through diuresis. Diuretics reduce the harmful effects of CHF (i.e., pulmonary edema, ascites, and increased cardiac work) by reducing plasma volume through various mechanisms.

Many different diuretics are available, and most work by inhibiting reabsorption of sodium and water in the loop of Henle or the distal tubules. If sodium ions remain in the tubules, they exert an increased osmotic "pull" on water molecules to cause them to remain in the tubules and be excreted as urine. The diuretics used most in veterinary medicine include furosemide, the thiazides, and spironolactone.

Furosemide

Furosemide is very powerful and is the most important and efficacious diuretic for removing edema from animals with heart failure (Hamlin, 2003). Furosemide may be administered intravenously, intramuscularly, subcutaneously, or orally and works rapidly to reduce pulmonary edema and other signs of CHF. It causes diuresis by reducing reabsorption of sodium and other electrolytes in the kidney tubules. Because much of the reabsorption occurs in the loop of Henle, furosemide is sometimes called a *loop diuretic.*

Clinical Uses

Furosemide is used for diuretic therapy (in CHF and other conditions) in all species.

Dosage Forms

Injectable and oral (solution, tablet, and bolus) human-label products are used.

- Furosemide, 12.5-mg and 50-mg tablets and 5% injection (Lasix), human label
- Furosemide tablets, 12.5 and 50 mg and 5% injection (Salix), veterinary label
- Furosemide tablets and injection, generic

Adverse Side Effects

These include low blood potassium (hypokalemia), dehydration, low blood sodium (hyponatremia), ototoxicity (cats), weakness, and shock.

> *TECHNICIAN NOTES*
> - Furosemide should be administered carefully to animals that are dehydrated or in shock.
> - Furosemide should be used at the lowest effective dose to prevent hypokalemia, cardiorenal syndrome, and other potential adverse effects.
> - Animals who are receiving diuretics such as furosemide should always have free access to water.
> - Administer the dose at convenient times for the client because urination follows within 20 to 30 minutes.

Thiazides

Thiazide diuretics such as chlorothiazide (Diuril) act on the loop of Henle and distal tubules to inhibit reabsorption of sodium. Thiazides are seldom used in veterinary medicine.

Spironolactone

Spironolactone is a potassium-sparing diuretic (it does not normally cause hypokalemia) and an antagonist of aldosterone. By inhibiting aldosterone, it reduces the amount of sodium reabsorbed from the kidney tubules. Spironolactone (Aldactone) usually is not used alone but is combined with a loop diuretic or a thiazide (Plumb, 2011). Similar to the thiazides, it has limited use in veterinary medicine.

DIETARY MANAGEMENT OF HEART DISEASE

Dietary management is an important part of the overall treatment of patients with heart disease. Dietary measures often are instituted early in the pathogenesis of heart disease (before clinical signs are observed or drug therapy is begun). Two of the primary goals of dietary management of heart disease are sodium restriction and maintenance of good body weight and condition (reduction of obesity or cachexia). Specific nutrient deficiencies (taurine or carnitine), concurrent disease (chronic renal failure), and electrolyte disorders also may have to be addressed (Roudebush et al, 2000).

Sodium restriction has long been recognized as an important part of the management of CHF. As was previously mentioned, increased sodium levels in the body lead to water retention, increased plasma volume, and exacerbation of the clinical signs of heart failure. The primary source of sodium is food. However, water and treats also must be considered when dietary intake is limited. Prescription diets provide sodium-restricted nutrition for dogs and cats. These diets may also be restricted in chloride and phosphorus. They may have added taurine and/or carnitine, B-complex vitamins, and normal or added levels of potassium. Sometimes it is difficult to get an animal to accept a sodium-reduced diet because of palatability issues. These foods may be made more palatable by adding flavor enhancers or warming the food.

Because heart failure may impair other internal organs, such as the kidneys, gastrointestinal tract, and liver, cardiac diets should be highly digestible and easily metabolized. They are balanced with adequate (but not excessive) levels of high-biologic-value protein to address potential renal failure. The energy level may need to decrease or increase on the basis of individual animal type and the cardiac condition of the animal. Improvements in cachexia in dogs with congestive failure have been seen with dietary supplementation of fish oils, which are high in omega-3 fatty acids (Ware, 2002).

> *TECHNICIAN NOTES* Clients should be instructed not to supplement their pet's diet with treats, human foods, or vitamin/mineral supplements when the animal is receiving a prescription sodium-restricted diet.

ANCILLARY TREATMENT OF HEART FAILURE

Various ancillary drugs and procedures are used in the treatment of heart failure. The following section provides a partial list of these therapies.

Bronchodilators

Bronchodilators such as aminophylline and theophylline are sometimes used in the treatment of heart failure. These agents increase the size of lung passageways to allow more efficient oxygenation of blood, to exert a mild positive inotropic effect on heart muscle, and to obtain a mild diuretic effect.

Oxygen Therapy

Oxygen therapy can be crucial in treating animals in the advanced stages of CHF. Animals with pulmonary edema benefit greatly from the administration of 40% to 50% oxygen via cage, mask, or nasal cannula.

Sedation

Animals with pulmonary edema caused by heart failure often experience a great deal of anxiety because of the dyspnea that they encounter. This anxiety often leads to hyperventilation and even greater oxygen demand and anxiety. To break the cycle and calm the animal, sedative drugs are often administered. The clinician may choose morphine, meperidine, diazepam, or other drugs.

Aspirin

Aspirin is known for its ability to reduce pain and inflammation, fever, and platelet aggregation. It is sometimes used in heart disease when clot formation may be a potential problem. It is used by some veterinarians to reduce the tendency for clot formation in heartworm treatment and for the same purpose in congestive cardiomyopathy in cats.

Thoracocentesis and Abdominocentesis

When heart failure is accompanied by excessive fluid (effusion) in the thoracic cavity, drawing fluid from the cavity may be lifesaving. Removal of ascitic fluid is controversial but may relieve pressure on the diaphragm and improve ventilation.

REVIEW QUESTIONS

1. Why is the heart considered to be two pumps functionally? ____________
2. Cardiac cells are connected by intercalated disks and a fusion of cell membranes to form a ____________.
3. Depolarization of cardiac cells is characterized by a rapid influx of ____________ ions, a slower influx of ____________ ions, and the outflow of ____________ ions.
4. A relatively long ____________ is important to cardiac cells to prevent a constant state of contraction from recycling impulses.
5. Define chronotropic and inotropic effects in relation to the heart. ____________
6. Define preload and afterload in relation to the pumping mechanism of the heart.
____
7. List the four basic compensatory mechanisms of the cardiovascular system.
____
8. List five objectives of treatment for heart failure. ____________
9. List four beneficial effects and one potential toxic effect of the use of the cardiac glycosides.
____
10. Catecholamines such as epinephrine are used in veterinary cardiology primarily for
____________.
11. List five factors that may predispose the heart to arrhythmias.
____
12. List six categories of antiarrhythmic drugs and give an example of each.
____
13. List four vasodilator drugs and classify each as arteriolar dilator, venodilator, or mixed.
____
14. Why is Lasix sometimes called a loop diuretic?
____
15. The use of many diuretics can lead to a dangerous loss of what electrolyte?
____
16. List five ancillary methods of treatment for cardiovascular disease.
____

17. ______________________ is characterized by the rapid influx of sodium ions into the cell through channels, the slower influx of calcium ions, and the outflow of potassium ions.
18. The amount of blood that the heart is capable of pumping per minute is called ______________________.
19. ______________________ results when the pumping ability of the heart is impaired to the extent that sodium and water are retained in an effort to compensate for inadequate cardiac output.
20. ACE causes the conversion of ______________________ to ______________________.
21. Nitroglycerin is supplied as an ointment. List the precautions that should be taken when applying.

    ____
22. What diuretic is used most commonly in the treatment of heart failure?

    ____
23. What is hypokalemia?

    ____
24. What are the primary goals of the dietary management of heart disease?

    ____
25. List three effects of administration of catecholamines.
    1. ______________________
    2. ______________________
    3. ______________________
26. The heart is a _____-chambered pump that is responsible for moving blood through the vascular system.
    a. two
    b. four
    c. three
    d. five
27. ______ is a faster-than-normal heart rate.
    a. Bradycardia
    b. Arrhythmia
    c. Tachycardia
    d. Automaticity
28. When situations cause spontaneous depolarization of cardiac muscle or abnormalities of the conduction system, __________ may occur.
    a. bradycardia
    b. arrhythmia
    c. tachycardia
    d. automaticity
29. Which of the following is not a way by which the cardiovascular system may increase its output during times of need, such as during athletic performance or to compensate for cardiac disease?
    a. Decreasing heart rate to such an extent that the myocardium is protected from damage caused by the increased workload
    b. Increasing the stroke volume
    c. Increasing the efficiency of the heart muscle
    d. Physiologic heart enlargement; the heart is composed of muscle that responds to work by increasing its size and becoming stronger
30. Congestive heart failure (CHF) results when the pumping ability of the heart is impaired to the extent that Na and H_2O are retained in an effort to compensate for inadequate cardiac output. It is associated with all of the following, except _____.
    a. exercise intolerance
    b. pulmonary edema
    c. ascites
    d. diaphragmatic hernia
31. Digitalis is a (an) ________________. It is obtained from the dried leaves of the plant *Digitalis purpurea.*
    a. catecholamine drug
    b. bipyridine derivative
    c. cardiac glycoside
    d. antiarrhythmic drug
32. Quinidine is an alkaloid that is obtained from cinchona plants or is prepared from quinine. It is used to treat ventricular arrhythmias, ventricular tachycardia, and atrial fibrillation. Quinidine doses must be ______ in patients who are being treated concurrently with digoxin.
    a. decreased
    b. increased

33. Gloves do not have to be worn when applying nitroglycerin.
 a. True
 b. False

34. Concurrent use of nonsteroidal antiinflammatory drugs may ____ the effectiveness of captopril.
 a. increase
 b. decrease

35. Furosemide may cause _____ in patients.
 a. hypoadrenocorticism
 b. hypokalemia
 c. hypocalcemia
 d. hypothyroidism

36. A 22-lb dog with moderate heart failure will be treated with pimobendan at a dosage of 0.5 mg/kg for 2 weeks. The tablets to be used are 5 mg. How many will you dispense?
____

37. A 12-lb cat with hypertension due to chronic renal failure will be treated with benazepril tablets (5 mg) at a dosage of 0.5 mg/kg. How many tablets will be given in each dose?
____

38. A 50-lb dog with moderate heart failure will be treated with enalapril 0.5 mg/kg twice a day for 14 days and then reevaluated. Enacard tablets (10 mg) are available. How many will you dispense? ______________________________

39. A 10-lb dog with advanced heart failure will be treated with furosemide at 8 mg/kg IV. Salix injection (50 mg/mL) will be used. How much will you draw up? ______________________________

40. A hyperthyroid, hypertensive 8-lb cat will be treated with atenolol at 7 mg/kg, once a day for 3 weeks. Tenormin tablets (25 mg) will be dispensed. How many will you dispense?
____

REFERENCES

Bill R: Drugs affecting the cardiovascular system. In Barragry TB, editor: Cardiac disease: veterinary drug therapy, Philadelphia, 1994, Lea and Febiger.

Boothe DM: Therapy of cardiovascular diseases: small animal clinical pharmacology and therapeutics, Philadelphia, 2012, WB Saunders.

DeFrancesco T: Can we delay progression of heart disease? in Proceedings. Music City Vet Conf, Murfreesboro, Tenn, 2013.

Ettinger S: Therapy of heart failure. In Ettinger S, editor: Textbook of veterinary internal medicine, ed 5, Philadelphia, 2000, WB Saunders.

Ganong W: Origin of the heartbeat and the electrical activity of the heart. In Ganong W, editor: Review of medical physiology, ed 21, New York, 2003, McGraw-Hill.

Hamlin RL: Cardiovascular system, introduction, in Proceedings. Music City Vet Conf, Nashville, Tenn, 2003.

Papich MG: Handbook of veterinary drugs, ed 3, St. Louis, 2011, Saunders.

Plumb DC: Veterinary drug handbook, ed 7, Ames, Iowa, 2011, Wiley-Blackwell.

Roudebush P, Keene BW, Mizelle HL: Cardiovascular disease. In Hand MS, Thatcher CD, Remillard RL, et al, editors: Small animal clinical nutrition, ed 4, Topeka, Kan, 2000, Mark Morris Institute.

Spinelli JS, Enos LR: Drugs for treatment of cardiovascular disorders. In Spinelli JS, Enos LR, editors: Drugs in veterinary practice, St. Louis, 1978, Mosby.

Upson DW: Cardiovascular system. In Upson DW, editor: Handbook of clinical veterinary pharmacology, ed 3, Manhattan, Kan, 1988, Dan Upson Enterprises.

Ware WA: Problems in chronic heart failure management, in Proceedings. Am Vet Med Assoc Annu Conf, Nashville, Tenn, 2002.

Williams BR, Baer C: Antiarrhythmic agents. In Williams BR, Baer C, editors: Essentials of clinical pharmacology in nursing, Springhouse, Pa, 1990, Springhouse Publishing Co.

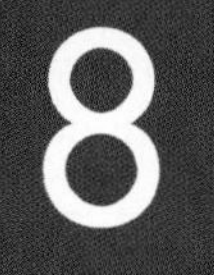

CHAPTER 8

Drugs Used in Gastrointestinal System Disorders

KEY TERMS

Adsorbent
Anticholinergic
Chemoreceptor trigger zone
Cholinergic
Dentifrice
Emesis
Hematemesis
Melena
Motilin
Parietal cell
Peristalsis
Regurgitation
Segmentation
Vomiting center

OUTLINE

Introduction
Anatomy and Physiology
Regulation of the Gastrointestinal System
Vomiting
EMETICS
- Centrally Acting Emetics
- Locally Acting Emetics

ANTIEMETICS
- Phenothiazine Derivatives
- Procainamide Derivatives: Metoclopramide
- Antihistamines (H_1 Blockers)
- Serotonin Receptor (5-HT3) Antagonists
- NK-1 Receptor Antagonists

ANTIULCER MEDICATIONS
- H_2 Receptor Antagonists
- Proton Pump Inhibitors
- Antacids
- Gastromucosal Protectants
- Prostaglandin E1 Analogues

Diarrhea
ANTIDIARRHEAL MEDICATIONS
- Narcotic Analgesics
- Anticholinergics/Antispasmodics
- Protectants/Adsorbents

LAXATIVES
- Saline/Hyperosmotic Agents
- Bulk-Producing Agents
- Lubricants
- Surfactants/Stool Softeners
- Irritants

GASTROINTESTINAL PROKINETICS/STIMULANTS
- Dopaminergic Antagonists
- Serotonergic Drugs
- Motilin-Like Drugs
- Direct Cholinergics
- Acetylcholinesterase Inhibitors

DIGESTIVE ENZYMES
MISCELLANEOUS GASTROINTESTINAL DRUGS
- Antibiotics
- Antiinflammatory Agents
- Antifoaming Agents
- Weight-Loss Products
- Probiotics
- Appetite Stimulants

ORAL PRODUCTS
- Dentifrice and Cleansing Products
- Fluoride Products
- Perioceutic Agents
- Tissue Regeneration Agents
- Polishing Paste
- Disclosing Solution

LEARNING OBJECTIVES

After studying this chapter, you should be able to

1. Exhibit a basic understanding of the anatomy and physiology of the gastrointestinal (GI) system.
2. Describe the various mechanisms of control of the GI system.
3. Explain the difference between vomiting and diarrhea.
4. Exhibit a working knowledge of drugs that induce vomiting and those that inhibit it.
5. List and describe antiulcer medications used in veterinary medicine.
6. Explain the pathophysiology of diarrhea and list the medications used to control this condition.
7. List the different categories of laxatives and explain their respective mechanisms of action.
8. List the two basic categories of GI prokinetics and stimulants.
9. Explain why digestive enzymes are used.
10. Discuss the use of antibiotics and antiinflammatory agents in GI disease.
11. List the categories of oral products and give an example from each category.

INTRODUCTION

Problems of the gastrointestinal (GI) system are common reasons for visits to a veterinary practice. These problems include **regurgitation,** vomiting, diarrhea, weight loss, colic, bloating, flatulence, abnormal stools, and constipation. Because veterinary technicians are expected to answer clients' questions about the GI tract, administer therapeutic GI medications, and monitor the response to GI medications, they must be knowledgeable about this system. They should have a basic knowledge of GI anatomy, physiology, pathophysiology, therapeutic principles, and medications.

ANATOMY AND PHYSIOLOGY

Anatomic and physiologic differences between the GI systems of different animal species are greater than for any other organ system. Despite these differences, the functions are basically the same in each species: (1) intake of food and fluid into the body, (2) absorption of nutrients and fluid, and (3) excretion of waste products. A discussion of the anatomy and physiology of the GI tract with an emphasis on similarities and differences between species follows.

The basic structures of the GI tract include (depending on the species) the mouth, teeth, tongue, salivary glands, esophagus, outpocketings of the esophagus (i.e., crop, reticulum, rumen, and omasum), stomach, liver, pancreas, duodenum, jejunum, ileum, cecum, colon, rectum, and anus.

Carnivorous or omnivorous species (e.g., cats, dogs, and primates) often are described as monogastric or simple-stomach animals because they have no outpocketings or forestomachs arising from the basic configuration (Figure 8-1). The function of the stomach in these monogastric animals is primarily to store ingested material and to begin some enzymatic breakdown of protein. The salivary glands begin enzymatic digestion by producing enzymes that break down starch into simpler carbohydrates. Pancreatic enzymes delivered to the duodenum break down fats, carbohydrates, and proteins, and sodium

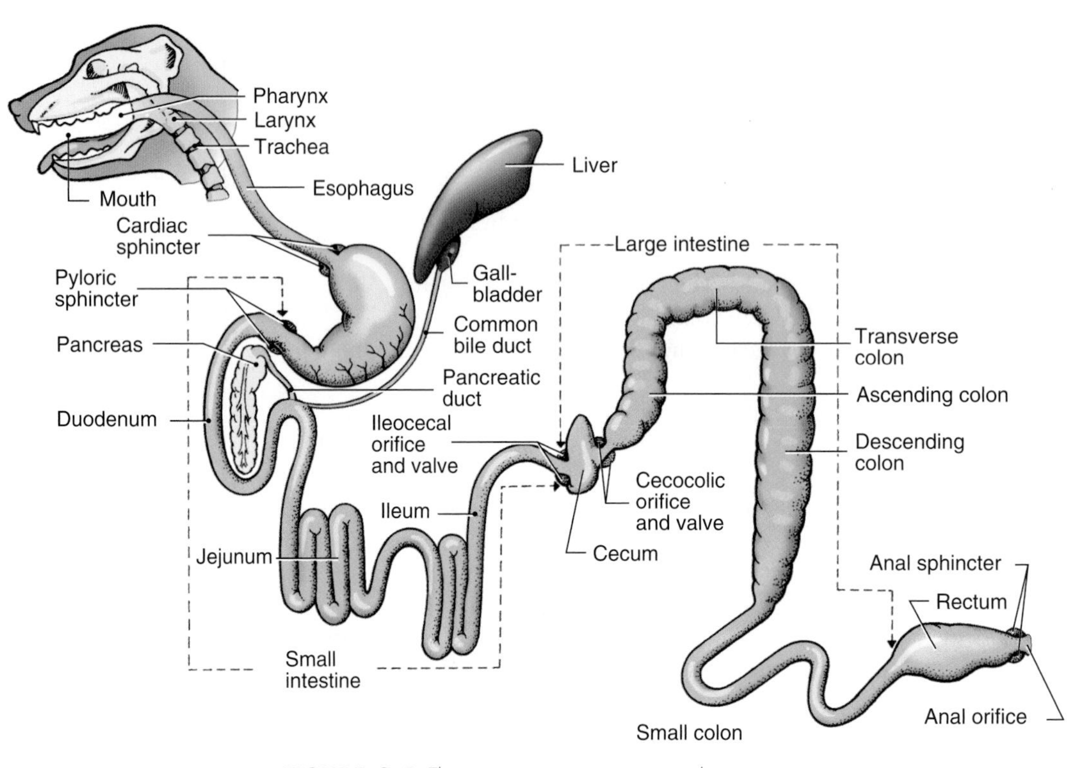

FIGURE 8-1 The monogastric gastrointestinal system.

bicarbonate from the pancreas neutralizes hydrochloric acid from the stomach. Bile salts, produced in the liver and delivered to the duodenum, aid in digestion by emulsifying fats. Bile is stored in the gallbladder, which is absent in some animals (e.g., horses and rats). Digestion and its control mechanisms are complex, and students should consult an appropriate text for further information.

Ruminant animals are herbivorous and have a GI system characterized by three forestomachs, the reticulum, rumen, omasum, and a "true" stomach—the abomasum (Figure 8-2). The reticulum receives ingested material and passes it to the rumen, where it is mixed and acted on by microorganisms to digest cellulose and other coarse plant material (roughage). Some refer to the rumen as a "fermentation vat," where microorganisms break down coarse feeds into forms that can be used by the simple stomach portion of the GI system in ruminants. Partially digested material (cud) in the rumen is regurgitated and remasticated to further facilitate digestion. In an immature ruminant, an esophageal groove allows milk to bypass the rumen and flow directly into the abomasum, and the rumen gains full function only after several months.

Equines, rabbits, and some rodents are chiefly herbivorous animals that have a monogastric GI configuration. They possess, however, a large cecum, which is capable of limited roughage digestion (hindgut fermentation) (Figure 8-3).

Birds have an outpocketing of the esophagus called the *crop,* which is used for food storage. They also have a ventriculus, or gizzard, which serves to grind coarse food material (Figure 8-4).

The small intestine comprises three sections: the duodenum, which has a sharp bend and in which the pancreas is located; the long and highly coiled jejunum; and the short ileum, which connects to the large intestine. In the small intestine, contents passing from the stomach are mixed with intestinal

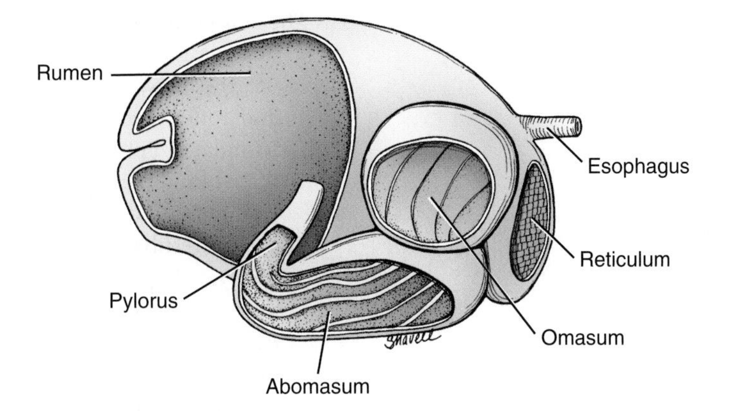

FIGURE 8-2 Compartments of the ruminant forestomach.

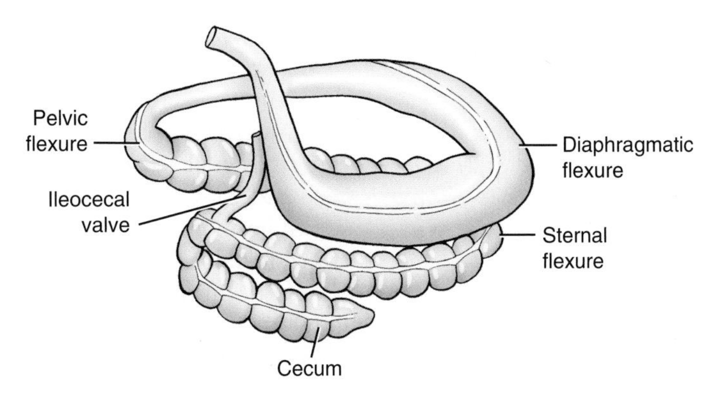

FIGURE 8-3 The large intestine of a horse.

secretions, pancreatic juice, and bile. The digestive process that began in the mouth and stomach is completed in the small intestine. Products of this process are absorbed together with most of the vitamins and a great deal of fluid. Villi and microvilli protrude from the mucosal surface into the lumen of the small intestine and greatly enhance the absorptive process.

Movements of the small intestine mix the intestinal contents, called *chyme,* and move them toward the large intestine. Normal intestinal motility includes two different patterns—peristalsis and segmentation (Figure 8-5). **Peristalsis** is a wave of contractions that propels contents along the digestive tract. **Segmentation** is a periodic, repeating pattern of intestinal constrictions that serves to mix and churn the contents.

The colon has a considerably larger diameter than the small intestine. The colon is connected to the ileum and the cecum through the ileocecocolic valve. The surface of the colon may exhibit one or more longitudinal bands (depending on the species) called *teniae.* The wall of the colon may also form outpocketings, called *haustra.* The colon of monogastric animals has an ascending portion, a transverse portion, and a descending portion that leads into the rectum. Functions of the colon include absorption of water, synthesis of certain vitamins, and storage of waste material.

Movements of the colon include peristalsis and segmentation (as in the small intestine), as well as a third type called *mass action contraction* (Ganong, 2003). Mass action contraction is a result of simultaneous contraction of smooth muscle over a large area and serves to move fecal material from one portion of the colon to another and from the colon into the rectum.

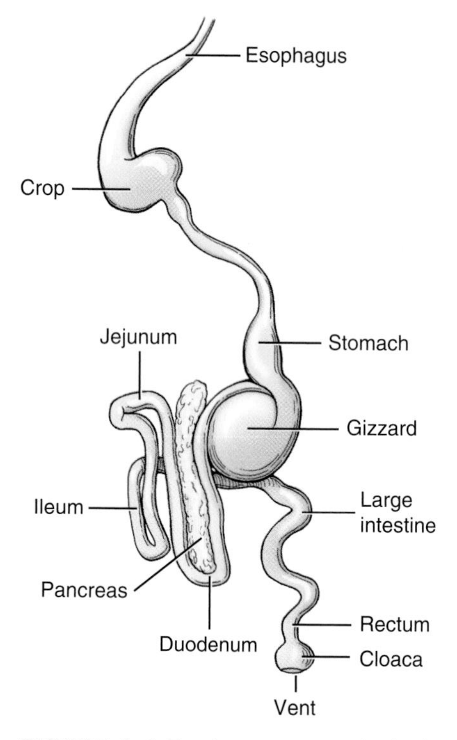

FIGURE 8-4 The digestive system of a bird.

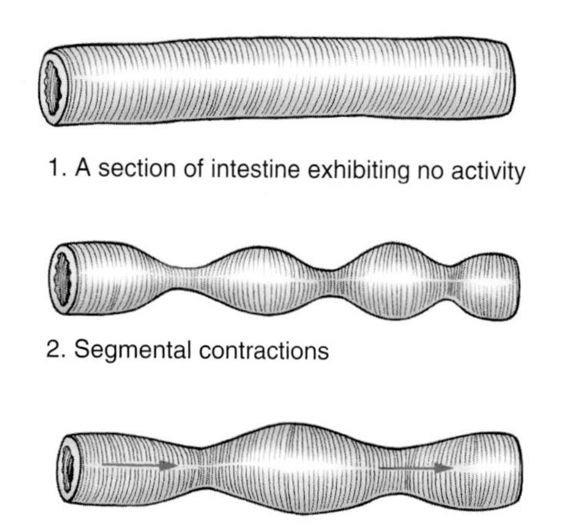

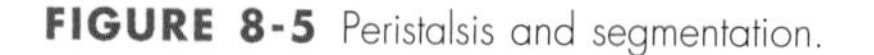

FIGURE 8-5 Peristalsis and segmentation.

REGULATION OF THE GASTROINTESTINAL SYSTEM

Regulation of GI system activity is complex but can be said to be under the influence of the following three basic control systems:

1. The autonomic nervous system (ANS).
   - Stimulation of the parasympathetic portion of the ANS increases intestinal motility and tone, increases intestinal secretions, and stimulates relaxation of sphincters. Drugs that mimic parasympathetic stimulation (i.e., cholinergic or parasympathomimetic) cause similar results. Anticholinergic, or parasympatholytic, drugs inhibit these ANS actions.
   - Stimulation of the sympathetic branch of the ANS decreases intestinal motility and tone, decreases intestinal secretions, and inhibits sphincters.
   - Stimulation of various intrinsic receptors in the GI tract, such as the myenteric plexus (stretch receptor), also may increase peristaltic activity. Some physiologists consider the intrinsic receptors (myenteric plexus and Meissner's plexus) to be a third portion of the ANS called the *enteric nervous system* (Ganong, 2003).
2. GI hormones such as gastrin, secretin, and cholecystokinin, when released from intestinal cells, exert control over many functions such as gastric secretion, emptying of the gallbladder, and gastric emptying.
3. Substances such as histamine, serotonin, and prostaglandin are released from specialized cells of the GI tract. Histamine attaches to H_2 receptors in gastric parietal cells to cause increased release of hydrochloric acid in the stomach. The influences of serotonin and prostaglandin are not as well defined.

Another factor that can have a major influence on GI activity is the presence of bacterial endotoxins. Endotoxins are components of the bacterial cell wall of certain bacteria (often gram-negative bacteria) that may increase the permeability of intestinal blood vessels and cause increased fluid loss and fever.

VOMITING

Vomiting is forceful ejection of the contents of the stomach, and sometimes the contents of the proximal small intestine, through the mouth. Vomiting is initiated by activation of the vomiting (emetic) center in the medulla of the brain. The **vomiting**

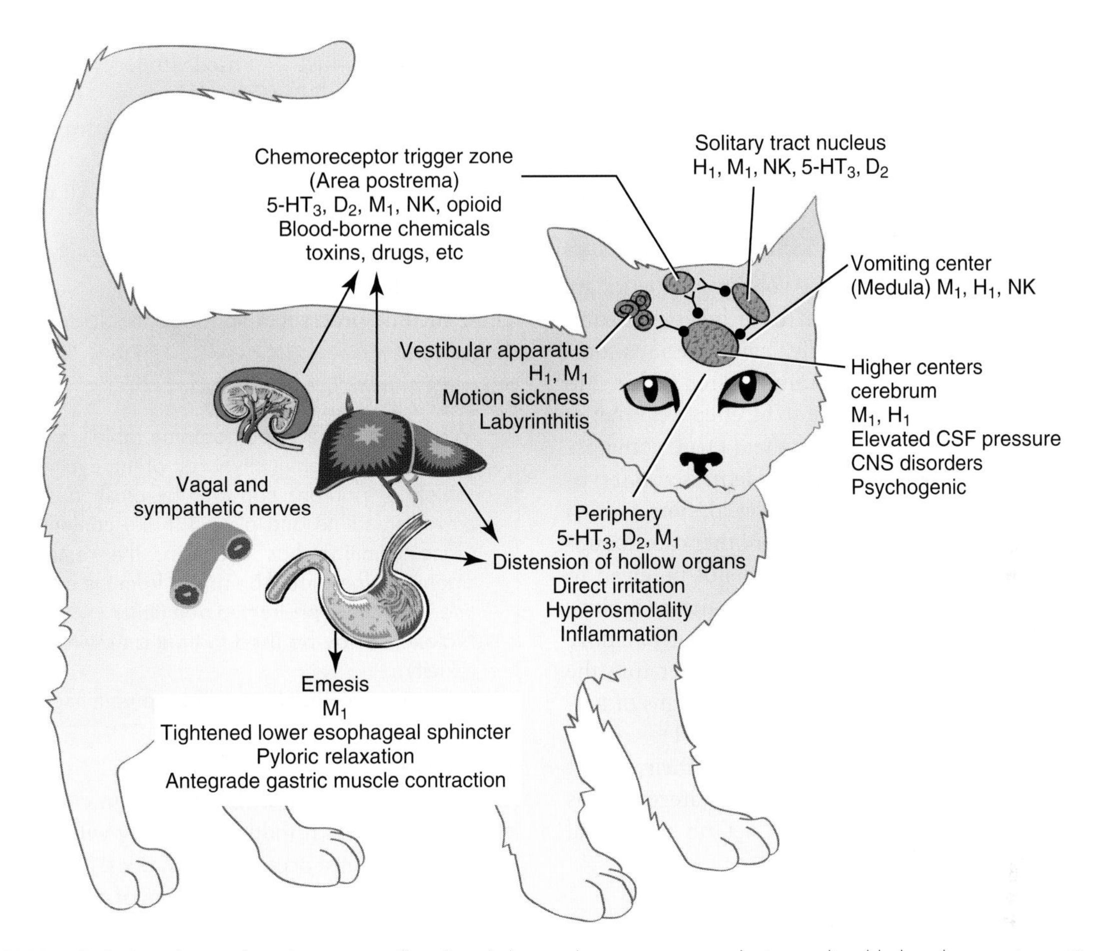

FIGURE 8-6 Sites that mediate the emetic reflex. Stimuli that mediate emesis at each site are listed below the neurotransmitter: *H_1*, histamine; *D_2*, dopaminergic; *5-HT_3*, serotonergic; *NK*, neurokinin; *M_1*, muscarinic (acetylcholine). (From Boothe DM: Gastrointestinal pharmacology. In Small animal clinical pharmacology and therapeutics, Philadelphia, 2012, WB Saunders, Figure 19-2.)

center is connected by nerve pathways to the **chemoreceptor trigger zone (CRTZ),** the cerebral cortex, and peripheral receptors in the pharynx, GI tract, urinary system, and heart. Impulses from any of these areas activate the vomiting reflex; this requires a coordinated effort of the GI, musculoskeletal, respiratory, and nervous systems. Impulses may be generated by (1) pain, excitement, or fear (cortex); (2) disturbances of the inner ear (CRTZ); (3) drugs such as apomorphine and digoxin (CRTZ); (4) metabolic conditions such as uremia, ketonemia, or endotoxemia (CRTZ); and (5) irritation of peripheral receptors.

Multiple neurotransmitters are involved in the vomiting reflexes. Some of those include histamine (H_1), dopaminergic (D_2), serotonergic (5-HT_3), neurokinin (NK), acetylcholine (muscarinic, M_1), substance P, and other neurotransmitters. Agents that prevent **emesis** (antiemetics) exert their effects by blocking one or more of these neurotransmitters (Figure 8-6).

Occasional vomiting by a dog or cat is considered normal. However, persistent vomiting is not normal. Horses and rats do not normally vomit. Persistent vomiting can cause serious problems such as resultant dehydration, electrolyte disturbances, and acid–base imbalances. Sizable quantities of sodium, potassium, and chloride are lost in vomit. However, potassium loss is usually the most significant abnormality.

EMETICS

Emetics are drugs that induce vomiting. Emetics are administered to animals that have ingested toxins, but they must be used carefully to avoid serious complications. Emetics must be administered within 2 to 4 hours of the toxic ingestion to be effective. Emetics should not be used in animals that (1) are comatose or are having a seizure; (2) have depressed pharyngeal reflexes; (3) are in shock or have dyspnea; or (4) have ingested strong acid, alkali, or other caustic substances. Obviously, emetics should not be given to animals that do not normally vomit, such as rabbits, some rodents, and horses. Emetics usually remove about 80% of the stomach contents. Therefore the animal should be closely monitored for signs of toxicity after induced vomiting (Plumb, 2011).

Emetics are classified according to their site of action. Those acting on the CRTZ are categorized as centrally acting, and those that act on peripheral receptors are locally acting.

Centrally Acting Emetics

Apomorphine

Apomorphine is a morphine derivative that stimulates dopamine receptors in the CRTZ, which then activates the vomiting center. This drug is poorly absorbed after oral administration and is therefore usually administered topically in the conjunctival sac or parenterally. Vomiting follows rapidly after intravenous administration, 5 to 10 minutes after intramuscular injection, and variably (10 to 20 minutes) after conjunctival administration.

Clinical Uses

Apomorphine is used primarily for induction of vomiting in dogs. It is considered by many to be the emetic of choice for dogs. Its use in cats is controversial and possibly is contraindicated. Xylazine, which is safer than apomorphine, is effective as an emetic in most cats.

Dosage Forms

Apomorphine must be used under professional supervision.

- Apomorphine HCl soluble tablets, from compounding pharmacies
- Apomorphine injection (Apokyn), 10 mg/mL, human label

Adverse Side Effects

These include protracted vomiting, restlessness, and depression.

> *TECHNICIAN NOTES*
> - Whole or divided apomorphine tablets may be placed in the conjunctival sac of the eye. These tablets or portions can also be crushed or dissolved in saline and placed in the conjunctiva. Once vomiting has occurred, the remaining apomorphine should be rinsed from the conjunctiva to prevent protracted vomiting.
> - Naloxone may be used to treat an overdose or toxicity.
> - Intravenous cefazolin may cause vomiting.

Xylazine

Although xylazine is not classified as an emetic, the label indicates that it induces vomiting within 3 to 5 minutes in cats and occasionally in dogs. Some clinicians consider xylazine to be the agent of choice for inducing vomiting in cats. Normal precautions should be followed regarding administration of this product.

Locally Acting Emetics

Hydrogen peroxide is the primary agent. Other locally acting emetics that have been used with various degrees of effectiveness include mustard and water, syrup of ipecac, and warm salt water.

Hydrogen Peroxide

A 3% solution of hydrogen peroxide can be used orally to induce vomiting. Vomiting is induced by a direct irritant effect on the oropharynx and stomach lining. Dogs and cats usually vomit within 5 to 10 minutes after administration of the hydrogen peroxide. The dosage is 1 teaspoon (5 mL) per 5 pounds of body weight not to exceed 45 mL, and this dose can be repeated once if not successful on the first attempt (Plumb, 2011).

Clinical Uses
Hydrogen peroxide is used for the induction of vomiting in dogs, cats, pigs, and ferrets.

Dosage Form
- Hydrogen peroxide 3% solution

Adverse Side Effects
There are few adverse side effects, but they could include aspiration pneumonia or gastric ulceration.

> **TECHNICIAN NOTES**
> - Ipecac should be administered with caution to animals with an existing heart condition. It is a cardiotoxic drug when given in high doses.
> - Extract of ipecac should never be substituted for syrup of ipecac because it is several times more potent than the syrup.

ANTIEMETICS

Antiemetics are drugs that are used to prevent or control vomiting. The use of antiemetics is a form of symptomatic treatment because these drugs do not necessarily correct the underlying cause of the vomiting. Many cases of vomiting in small animals are self-limiting or can be controlled by withholding food and water for 24 to 48 hours. Other cases are more difficult to control and necessitate the use of antiemetic agents and careful attention to determining the underlying cause. Antiemetics usually are given parenterally because vomiting precludes use of the oral route.

Phenothiazine Derivatives
Phenothiazine-derivative antiemetics act centrally by blocking dopamine receptors in the CRTZ and possibly by direct inhibition of the vomiting center. These agents are in widespread use. They are very useful in preventing motion sickness in dogs and cats but may be less effective against irritant emetics (Upson, 1988). Common side effects include hypotension and sedation.

Chlorpromazine
Chlorpromazine is a phenothiazine-derivative tranquilizer that has little popularity as a tranquilizer in veterinary medicine and is more often used as an antiemetic.

Clinical Uses
Chlorpromazine is used as an antiemetic in dogs and cats. It is more effective in dogs than in cats.

Dosage Forms
- Chlorpromazine tablets (Thorazine), various sizes
- Chlorpromazine extended-release capsules (Thorazine Spansule), various sizes
- Chlorpromazine oral solution (Thorazine), 2 mg/mL, 30 mg/mL, and 100 mg/mL
- Rectal suppositories (Thorazine), 25 mg and 100 mg
- Chlorpromazine injection (Thorazine), 25 mg/mL in ampules and vials

Adverse Side Effects
These are primarily limited to sedation, ataxia, and hypotension.

> **TECHNICIAN NOTES**
> - Chlorpromazine is incompatible when mixed with several other injectable agents. Check the label before administering.
> - Chlorpromazine may interact adversely when given concurrently with several other drugs. Read the label before administering to determine whether the combination is compatible.

Prochlorperazine
Prochlorperazine is a phenothiazine derivative agent with moderate sedative effects and strong antiemetic effects. The approved form of this drug is a combination product that contains an **anticholinergic** agent (Darbazine). Prochlorperazine is available singly as Compazine (human label).

Clinical Uses
These include control of vomiting (prochlorperazine alone) in dogs and cats and treatment of vomiting, gastroenteritis, diarrhea, spastic colitis, and motion sickness (combination product).

Dosage Forms
- Prochlorperazine—injection, oral syrup, sustained-release capsules, and suppositories (Compazine)

- Prochlorperazine/isopropamide—injectable and capsule (Darbazine)

Adverse Side Effects

These are similar to those of chlorpromazine but may also include dry mucous membranes, dilated pupils, and urinary retention caused by the effects of the anticholinergic in the combination product.

Procainamide Derivatives: Metoclopramide

Metoclopramide is a derivative of procainamide and has central and peripheral antiemetic activities. Centrally, it blocks dopamine receptors in the CRTZ, whereas peripherally, it increases gastric contraction, speeds gastric emptying, and strengthens cardiac sphincter tone. Metoclopramide has a limited influence on GI secretions. This drug has a short half-life and may have to be administered often or in a continuous drip in severe cases of vomiting (Plumb, 2011).

Clinical Uses

Metoclopramide is used as an antiemetic for parvoviral enteritis, uremic vomiting, and vomiting associated with chemotherapy. It is also used to treat gastric motility disorders

Dosage Forms

- Metoclopramide HCl tablets (Reglan), 5 and 10 mg
- Metoclopramide HCl oral solution (Reglan), 1 mg/mL in containers of various sizes
- Metoclopramide HCl injection (Reglan), 5 mg/mL

Adverse Side Effects

The most common side effects in horses, dogs, and cats are behavioral or other disorders associated with the central nervous system (CNS). Constipation also may occur.

> *TECHNICIAN NOTES*
>
> - Reglan is contraindicated if GI obstruction is suspected.
> - Atropine and the opioid analgesics may antagonize the actions of metoclopramide.

Antihistamines (H_1 Blockers)

Antihistamines are most effective as antiemetics in dogs and cats when vomiting is a result of motion sickness or inner ear abnormalities. Antihistamines inhibit vomiting at the level of the CRTZ through H_1 blockade. All antihistamines may cause sedation.

Dosage Forms

- Trimethobenzamide HCl (Tigan). Trimethobenzamide is an antiemetic for use in dogs only.
- Dimenhydrinate (Dramamine). Dimenhydrinate is an antihistamine labeled for treatment of motion sickness in dogs and cats. It is available in tablet, liquid, and injectable forms.
- Diphenhydramine (Benadryl). Diphenhydramine is used in veterinary medicine as an antiemetic and for the treatment of motion sickness, pruritus, and allergic reactions. It is available in tablet, capsule, oral elixir, and injectable forms.
- Meclizine (Antivert). Meclizine is used mainly in small animals for the treatment of motion sickness.
- Promethazine (Phenergan)

Serotonin Receptor (5-HT3) Antagonists

Serotonin receptors are found on vagal nerve terminals and in the CRTZ (Plumb, 2011). Blockade of these 5-HT3 receptors causes antiemetic activity.

Dosage Forms

- Ondansetron (Zofran). Zofran is used mainly as an antiemetic during chemotherapy and is noted for its special effectiveness during this application.
- Dolasetron (Anzemet)
- Granisetron (Kytril)

NK-1 Receptor Antagonists

NK-1 antagonists block the binding of substance P (a neurotransmitter involved in vomiting) to NK-1 receptors in the CRTZ.

Clinical Uses

Uses include the prevention and treatment of vomiting in dogs resulting from motion sickness or other causes.

Dosage Forms

- Maropitant citrate (Cerenia) tablets in 16, 24, 60, or 160 mg; injection, 10 mg/mL. Labeled for use in dogs but has been used effectively off-label in cats.

Adverse Side Effects

Side effects noted in a field study included diarrhea, bloody stool, anorexia, endotoxic shock, and otitis.

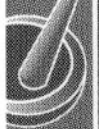

ANTIULCER MEDICATIONS

Gastric ulcers may occur in animals for various reasons, including stress, metabolic disease, gastric hyperacidity, and drug therapy (e.g., corticosteroids or nonsteroidal antiinflammatory agents) (Hall, 2001). Anorexia, **hematemesis,** pain, and **melena** are common signs of gastric ulcer. Most cases of gastric ulceration involve increased gastric acid production and require treatment of the underlying cause and symptomatic therapy. Five classes of drugs are most commonly used to treat gastric ulcers: (1) H_2 receptor antagonists, (2) proton pump inhibitors, (3) antacids, (4) gastromucosal protectants, and (5) prostaglandin E1 analogues.

H_2 Receptor Antagonists

One of the primary stimuli for secretion of hydrochloric acid by gastric **parietal cells** is activation of H_2 receptors by histamine. By blocking H_2 receptors, H_2 receptor antagonists reduce the release of hydrochloric acid, thus decreasing irritation of the eroded mucosa and promoting healing (Figure 8-7). H_2 blockers in current use include cimetidine, ranitidine, famotidine, and nizatidine. These are all available as over-the-counter products.

Cimetidine

Cimetidine competitively inhibits histamine at H_2 receptors of gastric parietal cells, thereby reducing hydrochloric acid secretion by these cells. Cimetidine, the least potent of the H_2 receptors, must be given 3 to 4 times daily to be effective (DeNovo, 2002).

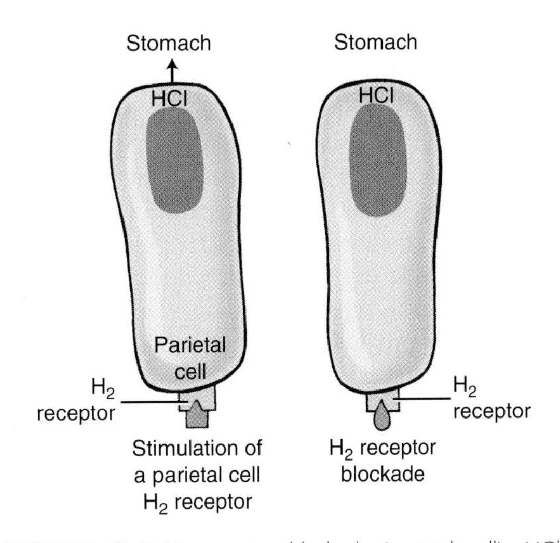

FIGURE 8-7 H_2 receptor blockade (parietal cell). *HCl,* Hydrochloric acid.

Clinical Uses

Cimetidine is used for the treatment or prevention of gastric, abomasal, or duodenal ulcers; hypersecretory conditions of the stomach; esophagitis; gastric reflux; and experimentally as an immunomodulator.

Dosage Forms

Products approved for use in humans are also used in animals.

- Cimetidine tablets (Tagamet), 100, 200, 300, 400, and 800 mg
- Cimetidine oral solution (Tagamet), 60 mg/mL
- Cimetidine HCl for injection (Tagamet)

Adverse Side Effects

These are rare in animals; however, cimetidine does inhibit microsomal enzymes in the liver and thus may alter the rate of metabolism of other drugs.

TECHNICIAN NOTES

- Because of its inhibition of liver microsomal enzymes, cimetidine may prolong the effects of drugs that are highly metabolized by the liver (e.g., lidocaine, propranolol, metronidazole, diazepam, and others). References should be checked before cimetidine is used in combination with other drugs.
- If cimetidine is used with antacids, metoclopramide, digoxin, sucralfate, or ketoconazole, doses should be separated by at least 2 hours.

Ranitidine

Ranitidine is also an H_2 receptor antagonist that competitively inhibits histamine at parietal cell receptors and reduces hydrochloric acid secretion. Ranitidine has little effect on hepatic microenzymes and is unlikely to cause drug interactions. Ranitidine is the H_2 receptor antagonist preferred by many clinicians because of its greater potency (five times that of cimetidine) and greater duration of action. Ranitidine also has prokinetic activity in that it promotes gastric emptying (DeNovo, 2002).

Clinical Uses

Clinical uses are identical to those of cimetidine.

Dosage Forms

- Ranitidine HCl tablets (Zantac), 75, 150, and 300 mg
- Ranitidine HCl oral syrup (Zantac), 15 mg/mL
- Ranitidine injection (Zantac), 25 mg/mL

Adverse Side Effects

Adverse side effects are rare in animals.

> TECHNICIAN NOTES A practical advantage of ranitidine over cimetidine is its reduced frequency of dosing (twice a day rather than three or four times daily).

Famotidine

Famotidine is an H_2 receptor antagonist that is considerably more potent than cimetidine. It is administered once a day and may have fewer drug interactions than cimetidine or ranitidine.

Clinical Uses

Clinical uses are similar to those of cimetidine and ranitidine.

Dosage Forms

- Famotidine film-coated tablets (Pepcid or Pepcid AC), 10, 20, and 40 mg
- Famotidine oral powder (Pepcid)
- Famotidine injection (Pepcid IV)

Adverse Side Effects

Because of limited use, side effects have not been determined.

Nizatidine

Nizatidine is an H_2 receptor antagonist that also has prokinetic activity, similar to ranitidine.

Clinical Uses

Even though nizatidine is an H_2 receptor blocker, it is used primarily in small animal medicine as a prokinetic agent for the treatment of constipation and delayed gastric emptying (Plumb, 2011).

Dosage Forms

- Nizatidine (Axid) tablets
- Nizatidine (Axid) capsules

Proton Pump Inhibitors

These agents bind irreversibly at the secretory surface of the parietal cell to the enzyme Na-K-ATPase. This enzyme is responsible for "pumping" hydrogen ions into the stomach against a concentration gradient. When bound in this way, the enzyme is inactivated and the cell is unable to secrete acid until a new enzyme is synthesized.

Clinical Uses

These agents are used to treat gastric or duodenal ulcers and esophagitis and may be useful in treating parietal hypersecretion associated with gastrinoma and mastocytosis (DeNovo, 2002). Omeprazole has a veterinary-approved label for the treatment and prevention of recurrence of gastric ulcers in horses and foals (Foushee, 2000).

Dosage Forms

- Omeprazole oral sustained-release capsules (Prilosec), 10 and 20 mg
- Omeprazole (Losec) (Canada)
- Omeprazole Oral Paste
- GastroGard (equine product)
- Lansoprazole (Prevacid)
- Pantoprazole (Pantoloc), oral or IV
- Rabeprazole (AcipHex)

Adverse Side Effects

These include constipation, sedation, ileus, pancreatitis, and CNS effects.

Antacids

Antacids used in veterinary medicine are (relatively) nonabsorbable salts of aluminium, calcium, or magnesium. Antacids are used to decrease hydrochloric acid levels in the stomach as an aid in the treatment of gastric ulcers. In ruminants, antacids such as magnesium hydroxide are used to treat rumen acidosis (rumen overload syndrome) and are used as a laxative. Antacids also may be used in patients with renal failure to bind with (chelate) intestinal phosphorus and reduce hyperphosphatemia.

Clinical Uses

These include treatment of gastric ulcer, gastritis, esophagitis, and hyperphosphatemia in small animals. In ruminants, they are used to treat rumen overload.

Dosage Forms

- Human label
  - Aluminum/magnesium hydroxide (Maalox, Mylanta)
  - Aluminum carbonate (Basaljel)
  - Aluminum hydroxide (Amphojel)
  - Magnesium hydroxide (milk of magnesia)
- Veterinary label
  - magnesium hydroxide (Magnalax)

Adverse Side Effects

Adverse side effects in monogastric animals include constipation (with aluminium- and calcium-containing products) and diarrhea (with magnesium-containing products).

TECHNICIAN NOTES

- Generally, do not give oral antacids within 1 to 2 hours of other oral medications because of their ability to decrease the absorption of drugs such as tetracycline, cimetidine, ranitidine, digoxin, captopril, corticosteroids, and ketoconazole.
- Magnesium-containing antacids are contraindicated in animals with renal disease.

Gastromucosal Protectants

Sucralfate is the only gastromucosal protectant in common use in veterinary medicine. This drug is a disaccharide that, when administered orally, forms a pastelike substance in the stomach that binds to the surfaces of gastric ulcers. This pastelike material forms a barrier over the ulcer to protect it from further damage and to promote healing. Because sucralfate binds better to ulcers in an acidic environment, it should be administered 30 minutes to 1 hour before H_2 receptor antagonists are given. It also may reduce the availability of some other drugs.

Clinical Uses

Sucralfate is used in the treatment of oral, esophageal, gastric, and duodenal ulcers.

Dosage Form

- Sucralfate (Carafate), 1-g tablets

Adverse Side Effects

These usually are limited to constipation. However, drug interactions may be notable.

TECHNICIAN NOTES

- Sucralfate should be given 2 hours before cimetidine, tetracycline, phenytoin, fluoroquinolones, or digoxin is administered.
- Sucralfate should be given a half hour before H_2 receptor antagonists or antacids are given because it requires an acid environment to be effective.

Prostaglandin E1 Analogues

Misoprostol is a prostaglandin E1 analogue that directly inhibits the parietal cell from secreting hydrogen ions into the stomach. It also protects the gastric mucosa by increasing the production of mucus and bicarbonate.

Clinical Uses

Prostaglandin E1 analogues are used primarily to prevent or treat gastric ulcers associated with the use of nonsteroidal antiinflammatory drugs (NSAIDs).

Dosage Form

- Misoprostol oral tablets (Cytotec), 100 and 200 g

Adverse Side Effects

Side effects include diarrhea, vomiting, flatulence, and abdominal pain.

TECHNICIAN NOTES Misoprostol causes abortion and should not be used in pregnant animals.

DIARRHEA

Diarrhea is the passage of loose or liquid stools, often with increased frequency. Diarrhea can result from primary disease of the intestinal tract or may accompany non-GI disease. Explanation of the pathophysiology of diarrhea is beyond the scope of this text. However, categories of mechanisms described in veterinary references include hypersecretion, increased permeability, osmotic overload, and altered intestinal motility. Parasitism is a common cause of diarrhea in all domestic animal species; it results in diarrhea through a combination of previously described mechanisms. Parasitism always should be ruled out when a diagnosis is determined.

Increased secretion of fluid from the intestine may result from the actions of bacterial endotoxins from microorganisms such as *Escherichia coli, Clostridium perfringens, Clostridium difficile, Campylobacter jejuni,* and *Helicobacter.* Intestinal epithelium damaged by viruses or other organisms may lose fluid as the result of increased permeability. Osmotic overload may occur because of poorly digestible foods, a rapid change in diet, or maldigestion or malabsorption. Although diarrhea has often been associated with hypermotility of the GI tract, the current belief is that most patients with diarrhea actually have hypomotility.

Decreased segmental contractions (hypomotility) increase the diameter of the lumen and allow rapid passage of contents, resulting in diarrhea. Normal segmental constrictions narrow the diameter of the intestinal lumen and actually slow the passage of contents. Diarrhea, if not controlled, can result in substantial fluid and electrolyte (i.e., sodium, chloride, potassium, and bicarbonate) losses. Dehydration, acidosis, weakness, and anorexia may follow.

Acute diarrhea, similar to acute vomiting, in dogs and cats often responds to dietary management and conservative treatment. In cases that do not respond to conservative management, symptomatic and specific treatments are essential.

ANTIDIARRHEAL MEDICATIONS

Narcotic Analgesics

Narcotic analgesics (opiates) are effective agents in the control of diarrhea because of their ability to (1) increase segmental contractions, (2) decrease intestinal secretions, and (3) enhance intestinal absorption. Many clinicians consider opiates to be the drugs of choice for the control of diarrhea in dogs. They also are used for the treatment of diarrhea in calves, but their use in cats and horses is controversial because of their tendency to cause CNS stimulation. Narcotic agents are sometimes prepared as combination products with other classes of antidiarrheals.

Clinical Uses

The opiates are used in GI therapy for the control of diarrhea.

Dosage Forms

- Diphenoxylate (Lomotil). Diphenoxylate is a synthetic narcotic agent (Class V) that is structurally similar to meperidine. Atropine sulfate is added to commercial preparations to discourage substance abuse.
- Loperamide (Imodium). Loperamide is a synthetic narcotic that is available in a nonprescription preparation. Loperamide poorly penetrates the CNS in cats and is acceptable in this species (Willard, 1998).
- Paregoric/kaolin/pectin (Parepectolin)

Adverse Side Effects

Adverse side effects of all the opiates include constipation, ileus, sedation, and CNS excitement (cats and horses).

Anticholinergics/Antispasmodics

Anticholinergics and antispasmodics have been widely used in veterinary medicine for the treatment of diarrhea. Because hypomotility rather than hypermotility is now considered to be associated with most cases of diarrhea, anticholinergics and antispasmodics should be used with caution for the treatment of diarrhea. A few commercial antidiarrheal preparations contain an anticholinergic plus a CNS depressant.

Clinical Uses

Anticholinergics/antispasmodics are used for the treatment of diarrhea.

Dosage Forms

- Aminopentamide (Centrine)
- N-butylscopolammonium bromide (Buscopen)
- Hyoscyamine (Levsin)
- Propantheline (Pro-Banthine)
- Clidinium/chlordiazepoxide (Librax)
- Hyoscyamine/phenobarbital (Donnatal)

Adverse Side Effects

Adverse side effects are addressed in the section on antiemetics.

Protectants/Adsorbents

Products in this category may have protectant or **adsorbent** qualities in the GI tract. The coating action of these drugs protects inflamed mucosa from further irritation. Their adsorbent activity binds bacteria or their toxins to protect against the harmful effects of these organisms. Kaolin and pectin are two ingredients often used in protectant compounds. The ability of protectants to control diarrhea has been questioned by some clinicians.

Bismuth subsalicylate is a compound found in products such as Corrective Suspension and Pepto-Bismol. Bismuth subsalicylate is converted to bismuth carbonate and salicylate in the small intestine. The bismuth has a coating and antibacterial effect, and the salicylate (an aspirin-like compound) has an antiinflammatory effect and reduces secretion by inhibiting prostaglandins (Boothe, 2012).

Activated charcoal is an adsorbent that is used primarily to treat poisoning.

Clinical Uses

These agents are used to control diarrhea and act as adsorbents.

Dosage Forms

- Bismuth subsalicylate
  - Corrective Suspension (veterinary approved)
  - Pepto-Bismol (human label)
- Kaolin/pectin
  - Kaopectolin
  - Kaolin Pectin Plus
  - Kao-Pect
- Activated charcoal
  - ToxiBan Suspension and Granules
  - CharcoAid

Adverse Side Effects

Adverse side effects are rare and usually are limited to constipation.

> *TECHNICIAN NOTES*
> - Bismuth subsalicylate compounds should be used with caution in cats because of the conversion to aspirin.
> - Bismuth may appear opaque on radiographs.
> - Administration of bismuth subsalicylate can result in black stools that resemble melena.

LAXATIVES

Laxatives are substances that loosen bowel contents and encourage their evacuation. Laxatives with a strong or harsh effect are called cathartics, or purgatives. Categories of laxatives include saline/hyperosmotic agents, bulk-producing agents, lubricants, surfactants/stool softeners, irritants, and miscellaneous agents.

Saline/Hyperosmotic Agents

Saline or hyperosmotic laxatives contain magnesium or phosphate anions that are very poorly absorbed from the GI tract. It generally is believed that these anions hold water in the tract osmotically. Increased water in the GI tract then softens the stool and stimulates stretch receptors in the gut wall to enhance peristalsis.

Clinical Uses

These agents are used for the relief of constipation.

Dosage Forms
Dosage forms include suspensions, crystals, powders, and boluses.
- Lactulose (Cephulac, Constulose, or Enulose). Lactulose also reduces blood ammonia levels in some hepatic diseases.
- Magnesium hydroxide
  - Milk of Magnesia is a suspension for use in dogs and cats.
  - Carmilax Powder and Bolets is for use in cattle (laxative/antacid).
  - Magnalax Bolus and Powder is for use in cattle.
  - Polyox II Bolus is for use in cattle.
- Magnesium sulfate
  - Epsom salts has been used in horses and birds.

Adverse Side Effects
These are rare but may include cramping or nausea. Overdose or overuse may result in dehydration or electrolyte imbalances.

Bulk-Producing Agents
Bulk-producing agents are often indigestible plant materials (e.g., cellulose or hemicellulose) that act by absorbing water and swelling to increase the bulk of intestinal contents, thereby stimulating peristalsis.

Clinical Uses
Bulk-producing agents are used for relief of constipation and for relief of some types of impaction (sand primarily) in horses.

Dosage Forms
Dosage forms primarily consist of psyllium preparations. Psyllium is obtained from the ripe seed of a species of *Plantago* (Plumb, 2011).
- Metamucil
- Equine Enteric Colloid
- Equi-Phar Sweet Psyllium
- SandClear
- Bran—a bulk-producing agent often used for horses (bran mash)
- Vetasyl Fiber Tablets for Cats

Adverse Side Effects
Adverse side effects are rare.

Lubricants
Lubricants are typically oils or other hydrocarbon derivatives (petrolatum) that soften the fecal mass and make it easier to move through the GI tract.

Clinical Uses
These include treatment of constipation and fecal impaction.

Dosage Forms
Dosage forms include liquids (mineral oil) and a jellylike mass (petrolatum).
- Mineral oil. Mineral oil is used in horses for the treatment of constipation, colic, and impaction. This substance is also used as a laxative in other species. Heavy mineral oil is preferred over light mineral oil.
- Petrolatum. This is a jellylike mass that is insoluble in water and is only slightly soluble in alcohol. Petrolatum is the principal ingredient in many of the oral laxatives for hairball treatment in cats.
  - Laxatone
  - Felilax
  - Cat Lax

Adverse Side Effects
These are minimal when used appropriately.

> **TECHNICIAN NOTES** When mineral oil is administered orally to a patient, care should be taken to avoid aspiration. Mineral oil is very bland and may not readily stimulate a swallowing reflex.

Surfactants/Stool Softeners
Surfactants reduce surface tension and allow water to penetrate GI contents, thus softening the stool. They also may increase intestinal secretions.

Clinical Uses
Clinical uses include the treatment of hard, dry feces in small animals; impaction in horses; and occasionally digestive upset in cattle.

Dosage Forms
These products are available in liquid, syrup, capsule, tablet, and enema forms. Docusate sodium, also

called dioctyl sodium sulfosuccinate, is the main ingredient.

- Disposable Enema
- Enema SA
- Pet-Enema
- Docusate Sodium Enema, 5% solution water miscible solution in 1-gallon containers
- Docusate sodium oral liquid (Veterinary Surfactant) 5% in gallons

Adverse Side Effects

Adverse side effects are rare.

TECHNICIAN NOTES

- Docusate sodium given with mineral oil may result in some absorption of mineral oil.
- Phosphate enemas (human label) should not be used in cats or puppies because of the potential for causing electrolyte imbalances.

Irritants

Irritants act by irritating the gut wall, causing stimulation of GI smooth muscle and increased peristalsis. These drugs are seldom used in veterinary medicine. This category includes several agents that are sometimes used in the treatment of constipation in humans.

- Bisacodyl (Dulcolax)
- Castor oil

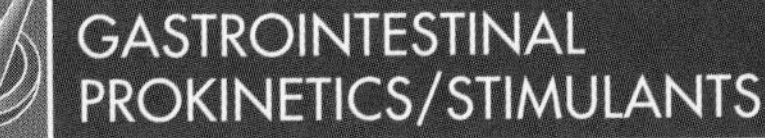

GASTROINTESTINAL PROKINETICS/STIMULANTS

Prokinetic/stimulant drugs increase the motility of a part or parts of the gastrointestinal tract and by doing this enhance the transit of material through the tract. Several classes of drugs, including dopaminergic antagonists, serotonergic drugs, **motilin**-like drugs, direct **cholinergics,** and acetylcholinesterase inhibitors, have the ability to enhance gastrointestinal motility. As was previously noted, some H_2 receptor antagonists exhibit prokinetic activity (see ranitidine earlier).

Dopaminergic Antagonists

Dopaminergic antagonists used as prokinetics in veterinary medicine include metoclopramide and domperidone (Hall and Washabau, 1997). These agents stimulate motility of the gastroesophageal sphincter, stomach, and small intestine. Domperidone has had limited use as a prokinetic in the United States but is approved in Europe for the treatment of nausea, vomiting, and gastric reflux in humans (Parker, 2001).

Clinical Uses

Metoclopramide is used for treatment of gastroesophageal reflux and delayed gastric emptying, for stimulation of the gastrointestinal tract in foals, and for gastrointestinal motility disorders in dogs and cats. Metoclopramide has been shown to enhance gastric emptying. The use of metoclopramide as an antiemetic is discussed in a previous section.

Dosage Forms

- Metoclopramide (Reglan) tablets, syrup, and injection
- Domperidone (Motilium, Equidone). Domperidone may have use in regulating gastrointestinal motility in horses, cats, and dogs.

Adverse Side Effects

Side effects include behavioral changes in dogs, cats, and adult horses. Cats have shown frenzied behavior (Plumb, 2011), and adult horses have exhibited alternating periods of sedation and excitement.

Serotonergic Drugs

Cisapride is the serotonergic prokinetic that is used in veterinary medicine. Cisapride stimulates motility of the proximal and distal gastrointestinal tract, including the gastroesophageal sphincter, stomach, small intestine, and colon (Boothe, 2012). Cisapride is not effective as an antiemetic but may be better than metoclopramide in treating some motility disorders and in promoting gastric emptying of solid material.

Clinical Uses

Uses include the treatment of constipation (along with dietary and/or surgical considerations) in cats and gastroesophageal reflux and gastrointestinal stasis in dogs, cats, and horses.

Dosage Form

- Cisapride. This drug has been removed from the human market but may be available from compounding pharmacies.

Adverse Side Effects

Side effects may include diarrhea and abdominal pain.

Motilin-Like Drugs

Erythromycin has been used by veterinarians to treat bacterial and mycoplasmal infections for many years. This drug has been shown to stimulate gastrointestinal motility by mimicking the effect of the hormone motilin (Hall and Washabau, 2000). Erythromycin stimulates motility in the esophageal sphincter, stomach, and small intestine at microbially ineffective doses.

Clinical Uses

Uses may include increasing lower esophageal sphincter pressure, accelerating gastric emptying, and facilitating intestinal transit time.

Dosage Form

- Erythromycin (Erythro)

Adverse Side Effects

Side effects may include anorexia, vomiting, diarrhea, and abdominal pain.

Direct Cholinergics

Clinical Uses

These include postoperative treatment of ileus—or retention of flatus or feces—and equine colic (without obstruction).

Dosage Forms

- Dexpanthenol (D-Panthenol Injectable, D-Panthenol Injection)—veterinary label
- Dexpanthenol (Ilopan injection)—human label

Adverse Side Effects

Adverse side effects are rare but may include cramping and diarrhea.

TECHNICIAN NOTES Dexpanthenol should not be used within 12 hours of the use of neostigmine, parasympathomimetic agents, or succinylcholine.

Acetylcholinesterase Inhibitors

These drugs increase the amount of acetylcholine available to bind smooth muscle receptors.

Clinical Uses

These agents are used to treat rumen atony, to enhance gastric emptying (ranitidine), to stimulate peristalsis, to empty the bladder of large animals, and to aid in the diagnosis of myasthenia gravis (neostigmine) in dogs. They also may be used to treat curare overdose.

Dosage Forms

- Neostigmine methylsulfate (Stiglyn injection)
- Ranitidine (Zantac)

Adverse Side Effects

Adverse side effects are cholinergic and may include nausea, vomiting, diarrhea, drooling, sweating, lacrimation, bradycardia, and various others.

TECHNICIAN NOTES Ranitidine and nizatidine, H_2 receptor antagonists, increase acetylcholine by inhibiting acetylcholinesterase. The increase in acetylcholine stimulates smooth muscle in the stomach and promotes gastric emptying to reduce vomiting in patients with gastritis and related disorders.

DIGESTIVE ENZYMES

Pancrelipase is a product that contains pancreatic enzymes that aid in the digestion of fats, proteins, and carbohydrates. The powder that contains the enzymes is mixed with the animal's food, which is allowed to stand for 15 to 20 minutes before feeding.

Clinical Uses

This product is used to treat pancreatic exocrine insufficiency.

Dosage Forms
- Pancrelipase (Viokase-V powder, Pancrezyme powder, Epizyme, Panakare)

Adverse Side Effects
Adverse side effects of high doses include cramping, nausea, and diarrhea.

> TECHNICIAN NOTES
> - Powder spilled onto the skin should be washed off to prevent irritation.
> - Inhaled powder can cause nasal irritation or can precipitate an asthma attack.

MISCELLANEOUS GASTROINTESTINAL DRUGS

Antibiotics
Antibiotics are not routinely used in the treatment of GI tract disease in small animals because these agents may destroy normal inhabitants of the GI tract and allow pathogenic bacteria (e.g., *Salmonella* species, *C. jejuni, C. perfringens, C. difficile, Helicobacter,* and others) to grow on the mucosal surface. Bloody diarrhea or signs of sepsis may indicate the need for antibiotic therapy. Antibiotics that are often used for treating bacterial overgrowth and other GI conditions include metronidazole, amoxicillin, clavamox, and tylosin.

Metronidazole
Metronidazole is a synthetic antibacterial and antiprotozoal agent. This drug is prohibited from use in food-producing animals.

Clinical Uses
Metronidazole is used for treatment of giardiasis, trichomoniasis, balantidiasis, plasmacytic/lymphocytic enteritis, ulcerative colitis, hepatic encephalopathy, and anaerobic infection in dogs. It is also used to treat giardiasis and anaerobic infections in cats and anaerobic infections in horses.

Dosage Form
- Metronidazole (Flagyl tablets, Flagyl capsules, Metronidazole Injection)

Adverse Side Effects
These include anorexia, hepatotoxicity, neutropenia, vomiting, and diarrhea.

> TECHNICIAN NOTES
> - Metronidazole should not be given to debilitated, pregnant, or nursing animals.
> - Metronidazole is prohibited by the FDA for use in food animals.
> - Tylosin is a macrolide antibiotic that is sometimes used to treat chronic colitis in animals.

Antiinflammatory Agents
Antiinflammatory agents are used in the treatment of idiopathic inflammatory bowel disease in animals. Increased numbers of lymphocytes, macrophages, plasma cells, or eosinophils in the intestinal wall characterize these diseases. Treatment often involves the use of hypoallergenic diets and antiinflammatory agents.

Dosage Forms
Antiinflammatory agents used in the treatment of inflammatory bowel disease include prednisone, azathioprine, sulfasalazine, and olsalazine.
- Prednisone/prednisolone—Many generic and trade name products are available.
- Azathioprine (Imuran)—A purine antagonist antimetabolite that may be used in the treatment of inflammatory bowel disease because of its immunosuppressive effects.
- Sulfasalazine (Azulfidine)—A drug that is converted by intestinal bacteria to a sulfa drug (sulfapyridine) and aspirin (salicylic acid). Aspirin is the active component that has an antiinflammatory effect and is useful in many cases of colitis in dogs and cats. It should be used with care in cats because of their poor ability to metabolize aspirin.
- Olsalazine (Dipentum)—Olsalazine is used for the treatment of dogs with chronic colitis that cannot tolerate sulfasalazine or respond poorly to the product.

Antifoaming Agents
Antifoaming agents are used to treat frothy bloat in ruminants. In this condition, gas bubbles form and become trapped in the rumen fluid as a result of

consumption of wheat pasture or legumes, such as alfalfa or clover. The trapped bubbles cause a form of bloat that cannot be relieved by usual means.

Antifoaming agents act as surfactants (reduce surface tension) and cause bubbles to break down so that gas can be relieved by eructation or by the stomach tube. These products are given orally.

Clinical Uses

Antifoaming agents are used for the treatment of frothy bloat in ruminants.

Dosage Forms

- Bloat Guard
- Bloat Treatment
- Bloat-Pac
- Therabloat

Adverse Side Effects

These are rare if the products are given as directed.

Weight-Loss Products

Dirlotapide

Dirlotapide is a selective microsomal triglyceride transfer protein inhibitor that blocks the assembly and release of lipoprotein particles into the bloodstream in dogs.

Clinical Uses

Dirlotapide is indicated for the management of obesity in dogs.

Dosage Form

- Slentrol solution containing 5 mg/mL for oral administration

Adverse Side Effects

Side effects include vomiting, diarrhea, lethargy, anorexia, constipation, and dehydration.

Probiotics

In healthy animals a balance exists between beneficial and harmful bacteria in the GI tract. Beneficial bacteria contribute to the maintenance or restoration of good health by modulating the immune system, competitively inhibiting enteropathogens, processing nutrients, and producing vitamins and fatty acids. Probiotics are beneficial live microbes that are administered orally to animals to support intestinal and overall health. Commercial probiotic products typically contain strains of *Lactobacillus* species, *Bifidobacterium* species, and *Enterococcus* species. The number of microbes, bacteria, or yeast in a commercial product is usually quantified on the label and in promotional literature as colony-forming units (CFUs). One billion to ten billion CFUs per day is a recommended dose (Loes, 2012). The composition of the microbe mixture and the number of microbes are both likely to be important in the effectiveness of the product (Tams, 2012).

Prebiotics are nondigestable food ingredients that are beneficial to the bacterial population. Synbiotics contain both prebiotics and probiotics.

Clinical Uses

Probiotics are used to treat stress-related GI upset, antibiotic-associated diarrhea, diarrhea associated with dietary change, inflammatory bowel disease, gingival disease, and some conditions associated with other body systems.

Dosage Forms

- FortiFlora
- Proviable KP
- Proviable DC
- Proviable EQ
- Proflora
- Probios
- Bactaquin
- Culturelle
- Numerous others

Appetite Stimulants

Stimulating an animal to eat can be an important component of a therapy regimen. Proper nutrition is essential for optimal functioning of the immune system as well as for proper organ function. Cats who do not eat adequately for a period of time may develop a “fatty liver” syndrome that can be life threatening. The following is a partial list of appetite stimulants:

- Diazepam—medication that produces a transient appetite stimulation when given intravenously
- Oxazepam (Serax)—used in dogs and cats

- Cyproheptadine—antihistamine used as an appetite stimulant primarily in cats
- Mirtazapine (Remeron)—used in dogs and cats

ORAL PRODUCTS

An increased emphasis on dentistry in veterinary practice in recent years has fueled a demand for products that promote and maintain oral health. Many of these products help to remove food particles and plaque and assist in the maintenance of pleasant-smelling breath. Some are labeled as a **dentifrice,** and others may be applied as an oral rinse or with a toothbrush. They are prepared as solutions, gels, and premoistened gauze sponges. Various flavors are available, as are products with fluoride. These products should not be considered a substitute for veterinary dental treatment. Clients should be advised to look for products with the Veterinary Oral Health Council (www.vohc.org) seal when purchasing dental hygiene products.

Other oral products include grit impregnated in paste for polishing teeth and smoothing rough surfaces left by scaling, as well as disclosing solution used to help identify plaque.

Dentifrice and Cleansing Products

- C.E.T. Enzymatic Toothpaste
- Nolvadent oral cleansing solution—active ingredient: chlorhexidine acetate; also contains a peppermint flavor; may be used with a toothbrush or as a rinse
- OraVet Plaque Prevention Gel
- OraVet Barrier Sealant
- C.E.T. Oral Hygiene Rinse
- C.E.T. HEXtra Premium Chews for Dogs
- Friskies Chew eez Beefhide treats
- C.E.T. Oral Hygiene Chews for Cats
- Hills t/d Diets
- Friskies Feline Dental Diet
- C.E.T. Dental Reward
- Purina Veterinary Diet
- Eukanuba Adult Maintenance Diet
- Canine Greenies
- Healthy Mouth Water Additive
- C.E.T. Oral Tatar Control Toothpaste
- CHX Rinse
- Sanos Dental Sealant
- Petsmile Toothpaste

Fluoride Products

- SF04 Stannous Fluoride Gel
- C.E.T. Flurafoam

Perioceutic Agents

Doxirobe

Doxirobe is placed in the periodontal pocket after dental cleansing with the use of a cannula. Upon contact with the aqueous environment, the product coagulates and releases doxycycline for several weeks.

Tissue Regeneration Agents

- Consil Dental—a substance used to promote the regeneration of bone lost as the result of periodontal disease or tooth extraction
- Enamel matrix protein (Emdogain)—a substance derived from fetal pig teeth that may be used to promote periodontal ligament growth and proliferation

Polishing Paste

Polishing paste is used as a part of the dental prophylaxis to remove irregularities on the tooth surface which may promote the accumulation of plaque.

- C.E.T. prophypaste
- Human products

Disclosing Solution

Disclosing solution contains a dye that stains plaque a bright color allowing it to be visualized and removed.

- Duo 128 Disclosing Solution

REVIEW QUESTIONS

1. List three general functions of the GI tract.

   ____
2. List three examples of monogastric animals.

   ____
3. What is the GI configuration of ruminant animals? ______________________
4. What is the difference between vomiting and regurgitation? ______________________
5. Ruminants are animals that use ______________________ to digest coarse plant material.
6. What are the three basic control mechanisms of the GI tract? ______________________
7. What is the significance of the presence of bacterial endotoxins in the GI tract?

   ____
8. The CRTZ stimulates vomiting when activated by ______________________.
9. List two examples of centrally acting emetics and two examples of peripherally acting emetics. ______________________
10. Drugs that inhibit vomiting are called ______________________.
11. H_2 receptor antagonists promote the healing of GI ulcers by ______________________.
12. List two H_2 receptor antagonists.

    ____
13. What are the two types of intestinal motility patterns? ______________________
14. Acute vomiting and diarrhea in dogs and cats often respond to conservative management such as ______________________.
15. List two species that do not vomit.

    ____
16. What is the mechanism of action of saline/hyperosmotic laxatives?

    ____
17. What is the active ingredient of Metamucil?

    ____
18. Direct cholinergic drugs stimulate the GI tract by what mechanism?

    ____
19. A synthetic antibiotic/antiinflammatory agent used to treat giardiasis and anaerobic bacterial infection in animals is called

    ______________________.
20. List four products used as dentifrice/oral cleansing agents. ______________________
21. What is the difference between peristalsis and segmentation? ______________________
22. Stimulation of the parasympathetic portion of the ANS decreases intestinal motility.
    a. True
    b. False
23. About what percent of the stomach's contents do emetics usually remove?

    ____
24. How does sucralfate work to treat/prevent gastric ulcers?

    ____
25. Bismuth subsalicylate compounds should be used with caution in what species?

    ____
26. All the following are basic functions of the GI system, except __________.
    a. intake of food and fluid into the body
    b. absorption of nutrients and fluid
    c. excretion of waste products
    d. excretion of urine
27. Which of the following species has no gallbladder?
    a. Canines
    b. Equines
    c. Felines
    d. Bovines
28. Ruminants remasticate food to facilitate the digestion process.
    a. True
    b. False
29. The crop in birds is used for ______.
    a. a stomach
    b. food storage
    c. feces storage
    d. a place where food goes to mix with hydrochloric acid to aid in the breakdown of foodstuffs
30. All of the following are parts of the small intestine, except the __________.
    a. ilium
    b. duodenum
    c. jejunum
    d. ileum

31. _______ is an emetic.
    a. Tigan
    b. Meclizine
    c. Promethazine
    d. Apomorphine
32. Cimetidine is ________.
    a. a proton pump inhibitor
    b. an antacid
    c. a gastromucosal protectant
    d. an H_2 receptor antagonist
33. ________ are substances that loosen bowel contents and encourage their evacuation.
    a. Protectants
    b. Adsorbents
    c. Antispasmodics
    d. Laxatives
34. Mg sulfate is found in _______.
    a. Magnalax boluses
    b. Fleet Enemas
    c. Epsom salts
    d. milk of magnesia
35. Viokase-V powder is _______.
    a. an anticholinergic substance
    b. a digestive enzyme
    c. approved for use in dogs and cats
    d. both b and c
36. A 20-lb puppy will be given a continuous IV infusion of metoclopramide over 24 hours for vomiting. The dosage is 2 mg/kg and the Reglan solution contains 5 mg/mL. How many milliliters of Reglan will you draw up to add to the IV fluids? ____________________
37. A 30-lb dog will be treated with Cerenia for vomiting associated with pancreatitis. The Cerenia solution contains 1 mg/mL. How much will you draw up? ____________________
38. A 1200-lb horse will be treated with omeprazole for gastric ulcers at 4 mg/kg once daily for 2 weeks. GastroGard oral paste is available in syringes containing 2.28 g. How many syringes will you dispense?

    ____
39. A 12-lb cat with anorexia due to chronic renal failure will be treated with cyproheptadine at a dosage of 0.35 mg/kg. Cyproheptadine tablets (4 mg/mL) will be used twice a day for 1 week. How many tablets will you dispense?

    ____
40. A 15-lb cat will be treated with prednisolone at 0.55 mg/kg once a day for inflammatory bowel disease (IBD). Prednisolone tablets (2.5 mg) will be used. How tablets many will you give each day? ____________________

REFERENCES

Boothe DM: Gastrointestinal pharmacology. In Small animal clinical pharmacology and therapeutics, Philadelphia, 2012, WB Saunders.

DeNovo RC: Chronic vomiting in the cat and dog. In Proceedings. Annu Meet Am Vet Med Assoc, Nashville, Tenn, 2002.

Foushee LL: Omeprazole, Compend Contin Educ Pract Vet 22(8):746–749, 2000.

Ganong W: Regulation of gastrointestinal function. In Ganong W, editor: Review of medical physiology, ed 21, New York, 2003, McGraw-Hill.

Hall JA: Diseases of the stomach. In Ettinger SJ, editor: Pocket companion to textbook of veterinary internal medicine, Philadelphia, 2001, WB Saunders.

Hall JA, Washabau RJ: Gastrointestinal prokinetic therapy: dopaminergic antagonist drugs, Compend Contin Educ Pract Vet 19(2):214–219, 1997.

Hall JA, Washabau RJ: Gastrointestinal prokinetic agents. In Kirk's current veterinary therapy XIII: small animal practice, Philadelphia, 2000, WB Saunders.

Loes N: Probiotics: healthy from the inside out. In Proceedings. Annu Meet Tennessee Vet Med Assoc, Nashville, Tenn, 2012.

Parker AR: Domperidone, Compend Contin Educ Pract Vet 23(10):906–908, 2001.

Plumb DC: Veterinary drug handbook, ed 7, Ames, Iowa, 2011, Wiley-Blackwell.

Tams TR: Gastrointestinal medicine—diarrhea. In Proceedings. Annu Meet Tennessee Vet Med Assoc, Nashville, Tenn, 2012.

Upson DW: Gastrointestinal system. In Upson DW, editor: Handbook of clinical veterinary pharmacology, ed 3, Manhattan, Kan, 1988, Dan Upson Enterprises.

Willard MD: Gastrointestinal drugs. In Boothe DM, editor: The veterinary clinics of North America, small animal practice, Philadelphia, 1998, WB Saunders.

CHAPTER

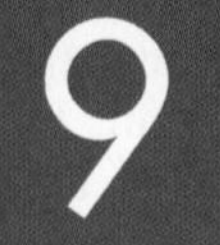

Drugs Used in Hormonal, Endocrine, and Reproductive Disorders

KEY TERMS

Anabolism
Analogue
Cushing's syndrome
Dystocia
Endometrium
Euthyroid
Feed Efficiency
Feedback
Gonadotropin
Hypophyseal Portal System
Iatrogenic
Involution
Levo Isomer
Myofibril
Nitrogen Balance
Primary Hypothyroidism
Releasing Factor (Releasing Hormone)
Trophic Hormone

OUTLINE

LEARNING OBJECTIVES

After studying this chapter, you should be able to

1. Discuss the control mechanisms (physiology) of the endocrine system.
2. List the endocrine glands.
3. List the reasons why hormones are clinically used.
4. Describe the difference between an endogenous and an exogenous hormone.
5. Describe the location and functions of the pituitary gland.
6. Differentiate between a positive and a negative feedback control mechanism.
7. Describe a neurohormonal reflex.
8. Discuss the uses and classes of gonadotropins, gonadal hormones, progestins, and prostaglandins used in veterinary medicine.
9. Describe the uses and classes of drugs that affect uterine contractility.
10. Define *pheromone* and give an example.
11. Describe the location, function, and hormonal products of the thyroid gland.
12. Describe the hormonal treatment of hypothyroidism and hyperthyroidism.
13. List the two forms of spontaneous Cushing's syndrome.
14. List two or more drugs used to treat Cushing's syndrome.
15. List the endogenous source of insulin and its metabolic effects.
16. List the classes of insulin products and their general characteristics.
17. Describe the method of action of the growth promoters.
18. List the clinical uses for the anabolic steroids.

INTRODUCTION

The traditional definition of the endocrine system states that it is composed of organs (glands) or groups of cells that secrete regulatory substances (hormones) directly into the bloodstream. This definition has now been extended to include regulatory substances that are distributed by diffusion across cell membranes.

The endocrine system and the nervous system constitute the two major control mechanisms of the body. These two control mechanisms are linked together through the complex integrating action of the hypothalamus (Figure 9-1). Coordination of these two systems allows an individual to adapt its reproductive and survival strategies to changes in the environment.

Endocrine glands include the pituitary, adrenals, thyroid, ovaries, testicles, pancreas, and kidneys. These glands produce hormones that are carried to target organs, where they influence the physiologic activity of these structures.

Hormones generally are administered to animals for one of two reasons: (1) to correct a deficiency of that hormone or (2) to obtain a desired effect (e.g., to postpone estrus). Hormones that are administered to an animal are called *exogenous* hormones, whereas those produced naturally in the body are *endogenous* hormones.

ANATOMY AND PHYSIOLOGY

Pituitary Gland

The pituitary gland has been called the master gland of the endocrine system because of the control it exerts over the regulation of this system. It is located at the base of the brain just ventral to the hypothalamus and is connected to the brain by

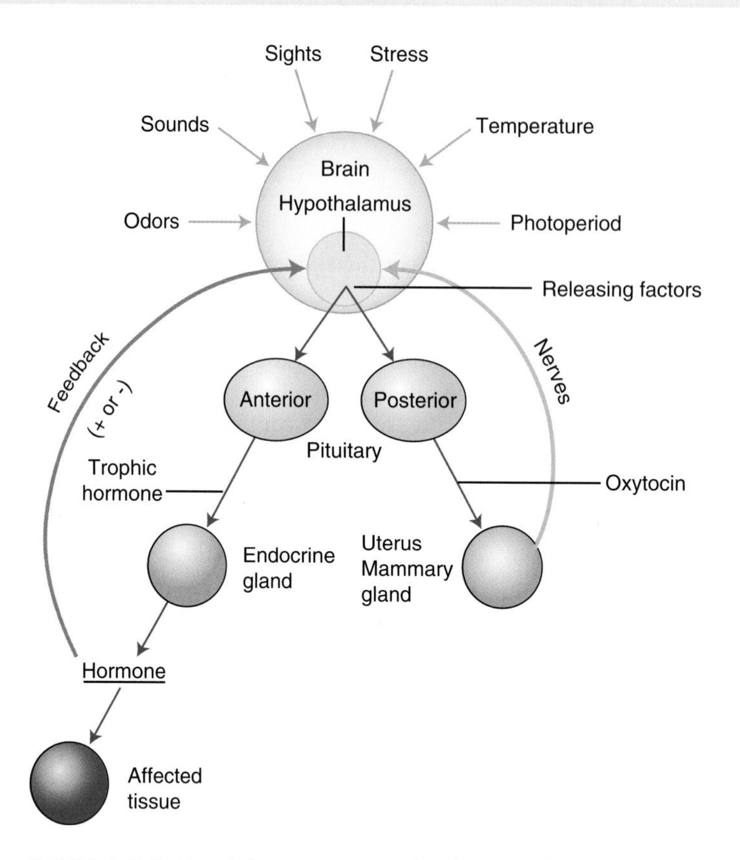

FIGURE 9-1 Hypothalamic integration of endocrine and nervous systems.

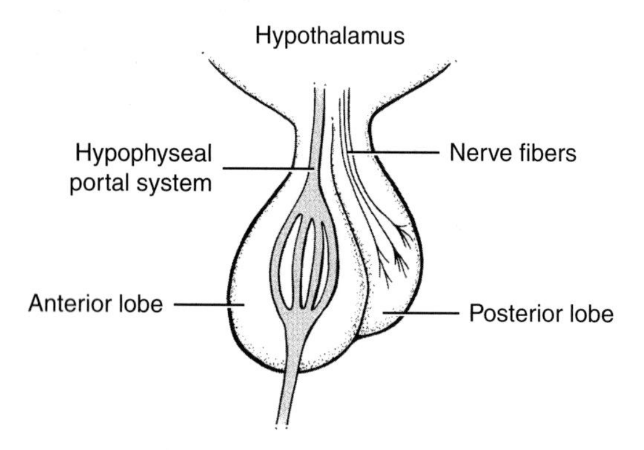

FIGURE 9-2 Lobes of the pituitary gland.

a stalk. It is divided into two main lobes—an anterior lobe (adenohypophysis), which arises from the embryologic pharynx, and a posterior lobe (neurohypophysis), which arises from the brain (Figure 9-2).

The hypothalamus exerts control over the anterior pituitary through the transport of **releasing hormones,** or **factors,** down the **hypophyseal portal system.** In the anterior pituitary, these releasing factors cause the secretion of **trophic hormones** into the circulation. Trophic hormones produced by the anterior pituitary include thyroid-stimulating hormone (TSH), adrenocorticotropic hormone (ACTH), luteinizing hormone (LH), follicle-stimulating hormone (FSH), prolactin (LTH), and growth hormone (GH or somatotropin). These trophic hormones are sometimes called *indirect-acting hormones* because they cause their target organ to produce a second hormone, which in turn influences a second target organ or tissue (Table 9-1). For example, TSH stimulates the thyroid gland to produce triiodothyronine (T_3) and tetraiodothyronine (T_4), which are hormones that in turn influence the metabolic rate of all tissues in the body.

TABLE 9-1 Pituitary Hormones

SOURCE AND NAME	TARGET AND ACTIONS
Anterior Lobe	
Thyroid-stimulating hormone (TSH)	Stimulates the thyroid to produce T_3/T_4
Follicle-stimulating hormone (FSH)	Stimulates ovarian follicle growth (female) and spermatogenesis (male)
Luteinizing hormone (LH)	Stimulates ovulation (female) and testosterone production (male)
Growth hormone (somatotropin)	Accelerates body growth and increases milk production
Adrenocorticotropic hormone (ACTH)	Stimulates production of corticosteroids by adrenal cortex
Posterior Lobe	
Oxytocin	Stimulates uterine contraction and milk letdown
Vasopressin (antidiuretic hormone, ADH)	Stimulates water retention

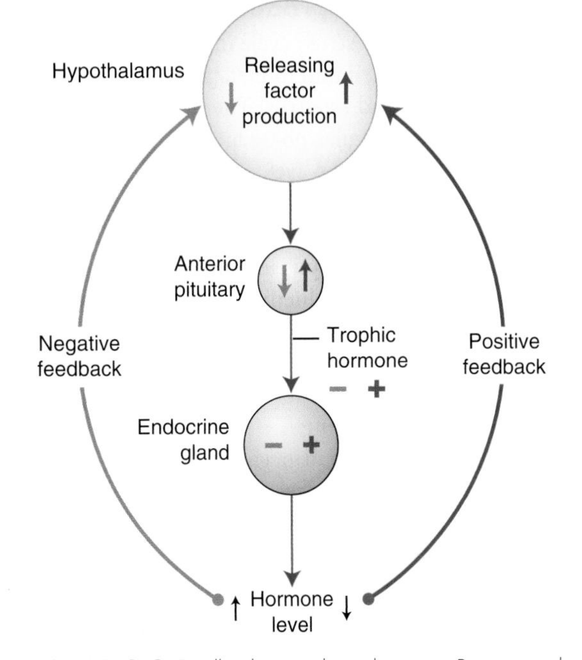

FIGURE 9-3 Feedback control mechanisms. Positive and negative feedback mechanisms control the quantity of a particular hormone.

The two hormones of the posterior pituitary are vasopressin (antidiuretic hormone) and oxytocin. These hormones are produced in the hypothalamus and subsequently travel down nerve fibers to the posterior pituitary, where they are stored for release into the circulation. The hormones of the posterior pituitary are called *direct-acting hormones* because they produce the desired activity (e.g., contraction of the uterus) directly in the target organ.

Control of the Endocrine System

Feedback Mechanism

The nervous system is sensitive to levels of hormones through a mechanism called **feedback.** By this mechanism, the plasma level of a particular hormone controls the activity of the gland that produces it. The feedback may be negative or positive (Figure 9-3).

With negative feedback, high plasma levels of a hormone are sensed by the hypothalamus, which then reduces the amount of the appropriate releasing factor (or hormone). A decreased amount of releasing factor reduces the amount of trophic hormone released from the pituitary, causing less activity in the organ that is producing the hormone in question. The overall effect is to lower the amount of the hormone in the plasma.

In the positive feedback scheme, low levels of a hormone are sensed by the hypothalamus, and release of the appropriate releasing factor increases. Increased amounts of the corresponding trophic hormone are then secreted, causing increased activity in the target organ and a corresponding rise in the plasma levels of the hormone.

Neurohormonal Reflex

The neurohormonal reflex applies to the release of oxytocin by the posterior pituitary. The first step in this reflex can be initiated by (1) stimulation of the udder by a nursing calf or by preparation of the udder for milking, (2) stimulation of the uterus and vagina in parturition, or (3) stimulation of the cerebral cortex by sensory stimuli associated with nursing or milking.

Control of the Reproductive System

The reproductive (estrus) cycle in animals traditionally has been divided into four stages called *proestrus, estrus, diestrus,* and *anestrus.* The cycle also may be divided into a follicular phase and a luteal phase. In the follicular phase, the cycle is under the influence of estrogen produced by a developing follicle, and in the luteal phase, it is under the influence of progesterone made by the corpus luteum.

Control of the reproductive system is coordinated in the hypothalamus, where the gonadotropin-releasing hormone (GnRH) is produced in response to various stimuli (Figure 9-4). These stimuli can include day–night length (photoperiod), pheromones, and positive and negative internal feedback mechanisms. GnRH causes the release of FSH and LH from the anterior pituitary.

FSH causes the growth and maturation of a follicle, which begins to produce increasing amounts of estrogen as it matures. Estrogen causes the changes that occur in proestrus and estrus, including the behavioral characteristics associated with estrus (e.g., standing to be mounted). The follicle also produces inhibin, which—along with estrogen—serves as negative feedback to the hypothalamus to inhibit the release of GnRH.

LH release causes ovulation of the mature follicle and the formation of a corpus luteum in its place. This event signals the beginning of diestrus and the beginning of the luteal phase of the cycle. The corpus luteum produces progesterone, which prepares the uterus for pregnancy. Once pregnancy occurs, the corpus luteum maintains a uterine environment conducive to normal progression of the pregnancy. Progesterone levels in the blood serve as negative feedback to prevent the release of GnRH and the development of new follicles during pregnancy.

When the gestation period nears its end, the fetus begins to produce increasing amounts of ACTH. ACTH causes increased amounts of cortisol to be produced by the adrenal glands. The increased cortisol levels result in increased production of estrogen and prostaglandin by the uterus. These two substances sensitize the uterus to the

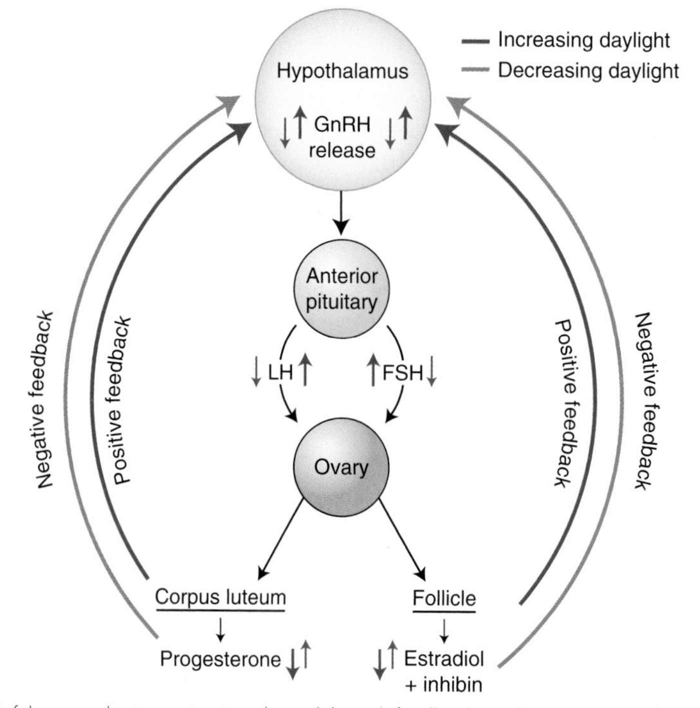

FIGURE 9-4 Control of the reproductive system is achieved through feedback mechanisms responding to increased or decreased levels of estradiol and progesterone in the bloodstream and increasing or decreasing daylight. *FSH,* Follicle-stimulating hormone; *GnRH,* gonadotropin-releasing hormone; *LH,* luteinizing hormone.

contraction-producing effects of oxytocin and allow parturition to begin. Prostaglandin also causes the breakdown (lysis) of the corpus luteum at the end of pregnancy and at the end of diestrus if pregnancy does not occur.

HORMONAL DRUGS ASSOCIATED WITH REPRODUCTION

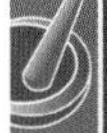

GONADOTROPINS AND GONADAL HORMONES

Products in this category are used in veterinary medicine for various reasons. Some of these include synchronization of estrus, suppression of estrus, induction of estrus, treatment of cystic ovaries, and termination of pregnancy.

Gonadotropins

Gonadotropins are drugs that act similarly to GnRH, LH, or FSH. Gonadotropins cause the release of LH and FSH or cause activity similar to that of LH or FSH. LH may be prepared from the pituitary glands of slaughtered animals, from the urine of pregnant women in the form of human chorionic gonadotropin (hCG), or in pure form through recombinant techniques. FSH may be obtained from pituitary glands (FSH-P), from the serum of pregnant mares (PMS) between the 40th and 140th days of pregnancy, or from recombinant sources. GnRH is prepared synthetically.

FSH that is released endogenously by the anterior pituitary causes growth and maturation of the ovarian follicle in females and spermatogenesis in males. LH, also released by the anterior pituitary, causes ovulation in females and production of testosterone in males.

Gonadorelin

Gonadorelin (GnRH) is produced endogenously by the hypothalamus. Gonadorelin causes the release of FSH and LH by the anterior pituitary.

Clinical Uses

Gonadorelin is used to treat cystic (follicular) ovaries in dairy cattle. It has also been used in cats and horses (with limited success) to induce estrus.

Dosage Forms

- Gonadorelin (Cystorelin) for injection
- Gonadorelin (Factrel) for injection
- Gonadorelin (Fertagyl) for injection
- Deslorelin (SucroMate, Ovuplant); deslorelin is used to induce and time ovulation in mares and may have some potential as a contraceptive agent in dogs.

Adverse Side Effects

These are minimal with the use of this product.

Chorionic Gonadotropin

hCG is a hormone secreted by the uterus and obtained from the urine of pregnant women. It mimics the effects of LH, although it has limited FSH activity. In males, it stimulates the production of male hormones by the testicles and may facilitate descent of the testicles.

Clinical Uses

Chorionic gonadotropin is used to treat cystic ovaries (nymphomania) in dairy cattle. In males, it has been used to treat cryptorchidism and infertility caused by low testosterone levels.

Dosage Forms

- hCG injection (Follutein)
- Combination hCG and PMS (P.G. 600); contains both LH and FSH activity
- hCG injection (Chorulon)
- Chorionic gonadotropin injection (generic)
- Chorionad

Adverse Side Effects

These are limited but may include hypersensitivity reaction and abortion in mares if given before the 35th day of pregnancy.

Follicle-Stimulating Hormone

FSH causes growth and maturation of the ovarian follicle. FSH-P, prepared from the pituitary glands from slaughtered animals, is no longer available. Purified recombinant human FSH may be obtained, but it is expensive. Chorionic gonadotropin is readily available and causes FSH-like activity (and LH activity) and is more likely to be used in reproductive cases.

Clinical Uses

FSH has been used in veterinary medicine to induce superovulation and for out-of-season breeding.

Dosage Form

- FSH (Follitropin alpha), human label

Adverse Side Effects

These include endometrial hyperplasia, superovulation, and follicular cysts.

Estrogens

Estrogens are a group of hormones synthesized by the ovaries and—to a lesser extent—by the testicles, adrenal cortex, and placenta. Estrogens are classified as sex steroids and are synthesized from a cholesterol precursor. Estrogens are necessary for normal growth and development of the female gonads. They cause secondary female characteristics and are responsible for female sex drive. These hormones inhibit ovulation, increase uterine tone, and cause proliferation of the **endometrium.**

Clinical Uses

In cattle, estrogens are used to treat persistent corpus luteum, to expel purulent material from the uterus, to expel retained placentas and mummified fetuses, and to promote weight gain. In dogs, estrogens may be used to control urinary incontinence. In horses, they may be used for induction of estrus in the nonbreeding season.

Dosage Forms

- Estradiol cypionate (ECP) injection
- Estradiol cypionate for injection (Depo-Estradiol), human label
- Estradiol valerate for injection (Delestrogen), human label
- Diethylstilbestrol (DES) compounded capsules and tablets
- Estriol (Incurin), for control of urinary incontinence in spayed dogs
- Implants to promote weight gain (discussed in a later section)

Adverse Side Effects

These include severe anemia, prolonged estrus, genital irritation, and follicular cysts.

> *TECHNICIAN NOTES*
> - Estrogens should not be given during pregnancy.
> - Estrogen administration can cause severe anemia.
> - Synthetic DES has been banned from use in food-producing animals because of its possible link with cervical cancer in women.

Androgens

Androgens are male sex hormones produced in the testicles, the ovaries, and the adrenal cortex. Similar to the other gonadal hormones, they have a steroidal parent molecule. These hormones are necessary for growth and development of the male sex organs. They cause secondary male sex characteristics and produce male libido. The androgens promote tissue **anabolism,** weight gain, and red blood cell formation.

Methyltestosterone, Testosterone Cypionate, Testosterone Enanthate, and Testosterone Propionate

These injectable testosterone products are available under a human label.

Clinical Uses

These androgens are used to treat urinary incontinence in male dogs and to increase libido and fertility in domestic animals (with generally poor results).

Dosage Forms

- Methyltestosterone (Android), human label
- Danazol (Danocrine), synthetic androgen (human label)
- Testosterone cypionate injection (generic)
- Testosterone enanthate (generic)
- Testosterone propionate injection (generic)
- Depo-Testosterone
- Combination products with estradiol as growth-promoting implants

Adverse Side Effects

These are uncommon when the products are used as directed.

> *TECHNICIAN NOTES* Testosterone products are now Class III controlled substances.

Mibolerone

Mibolerone is an androgen used for prevention of estrus in dogs. Mibolerone blocks the release of LH by the pituitary and prevents complete development of the follicle. Ovulation does not occur.

Clinical Uses

This product is used for prevention of estrus in adult female dogs and for treatment of pseudocyesis.

Dosage Forms

- Oral liquid preparation (Cheque Drops)
- Implants to promote weight gain (discussed later)

Adverse Side Effects

Adverse side effects reported in the product insert include premature epiphyseal closure and vaginitis in immature females. In mature females, vulvovaginitis, clitoral hypertrophy, riding behavior, increased body odor, and various other side effects have been reported. It is further reported that side effects usually resolve with discontinuation of therapy.

> TECHNICIAN NOTES Mibolerone should not be used in cats because of a very low margin of safety in this species.

Progestins

Progestins are a group of compounds that are similar in effect to progesterone. Endogenous progestins are produced by the corpus luteum. They cause increased secretions by the endometrium, decreased motility in the uterus, and increased secretory development in the mammary glands. They also inhibit the release of gonadotropins by the pituitary to produce an inactive ovary. In some situations, they can cause elevated blood glucose levels (antiinsulin effect) or serious suppression of the adrenal glands. These hormones are used clinically to suppress estrus and to treat false pregnancy, behavioral disorders, and progestin-responsive dermatitis. The root "gest" often allows name recognition of the progestins.

Megestrol Acetate

Megestrol acetate is a synthetic progestin labeled for use in dogs. It is used, however, in cats for some behavioral and dermatologic conditions.

Clinical Uses

Megestrol acetate is labeled for use in dogs to control estrus, treat false pregnancy, prevent vaginal hyperplasia, treat severe galactorrhea, and control unacceptable male behavior. Megestrol acetate has been used in cats for various dermatologic and behavioral problems and for suppression of estrus.

Dosage Forms

- Megestrol acetate (Ovaban) tablets in bottles or foil strips
- Oral tablet preparation of megestrol acetate (Megace) approved for use in humans

Adverse Side Effects

These can include hyperglycemia, adrenal suppression, endometrial hyperplasia, and increased appetite.

> TECHNICIAN NOTES Clients should be made aware of the potential dangers associated with the use of megestrol acetate and should be asked to report any changes in their pet's health status that occur after initiation of therapy.

Medroxyprogesterone Acetate

Medroxyprogesterone acetate (MPA) is a human label progestin that has been used to treat certain behavioral and dermatologic problems and to suppress estrus in dogs and cats.

Clinical Uses

MPA is used for (1) treatment of behavioral problems, such as aggression, roaming, spraying, or mounting in males, and (2) treatment of certain dermatologic conditions.

Dosage Forms

- MPA for injection (Depo-Provera); human label
- MPA tablets (Provera); human label

Adverse Side Effects

These are potentially numerous and include pyometra, personality changes, depression, lethargy, mammary changes, and increased appetite.

TECHNICIAN NOTES Progestins should be administered with strict adherence to an accepted protocol to minimize side effects such as pyometra.

Altrenogest

Altrenogest is an oral progestin labeled for use in horses and swine. This drug is used to suppress estrus in mares and sexually mature gilts. Mares stop cycling within 3 days of treatment and begin cycling again 4 to 5 days after treatment is stopped. It is also used to manage other reproductive conditions that are listed later.

Clinical Uses

Altrenogest is used to suppress estrus for synchronization, to suppress estrus for long periods, or to maintain pregnancy in mares with low levels of progesterone.

Dosage Form

- Altrenogest in oil oral solution (Regu-Mate) for use in horses
- For use in sexually mature gilts (Matrix); extralabel use is prohibited.

Adverse Side Effects

These have been reported as minimal when altrenogest is used correctly.

TECHNICIAN NOTES Altrenogest can be absorbed through the skin and should be used with great caution by pregnant women or anyone with vascular disorders. Read the label carefully before using.

Norgestomet

Norgestomet is a synthetic progestin that is used in combination with an estrogen (estradiol valerate) for synchronization of estrus in beef cows and nonlactating dairy cows. A treatment consists of one implant and an injection at the time of implantation.

Clinical Uses

Norgestomet is used for synchronization of estrus in cattle.

Dosage Form

- Syncro-Mate-B

Adverse Side Effects

Adverse side effects are not reported in the insert.

Melengestrol Acetate

Melengestrol acetate is a progestin used in implants that promotes weight gain (discussed in a separate section).

PROSTAGLANDINS

Prostaglandins consist of a group of naturally occurring, long-chain fatty acids that mediate various physiologic events in the body. The primary use of prostaglandins in veterinary medicine is for regulation of activity in and treatment of conditions of the female reproductive tract. Of the six classes (A, B, C, D, E, and F), only prostaglandin F_{2alpha} has significant clinical application in the reproductive system.

Prostaglandin F_{2alpha} causes lysis of the corpus luteum, contraction of uterine muscle, and relaxation of the cervix. Lysis of the corpus luteum results in a decline in plasma levels of progesterone and, through the negative feedback mechanism, initiation of a new estrus cycle. Contraction of uterine muscle can facilitate evacuation of uterine contents (pus or a mummified fetus) or produce an abortion.

Bronchoconstriction, increased blood pressure, and smooth muscle contraction have been reported in other species, including humans. For these reasons, pregnant women and asthmatic individuals should handle prostaglandin products with extreme caution; exposure (through injection or skin contact) can cause abortion or an asthma attack.

Name recognition of the prostaglandins is made easier by looking for "prost" in the drug name.

Dinoprost Tromethamine

Dinoprost tromethamine is a salt of the naturally occurring prostaglandin F_{2alpha} and is labeled for use in cattle, horses, and swine. It also has accepted clinical uses in dogs, cats, sheep, and goats. It is effective only in animals with a corpus luteum.

Clinical Uses
Labeled clinical uses include estrus synchronization, treatment of silent estrus, and pyometra in cattle. It is also used for abortion of feedlot and other non-lactating cattle. In swine, dinoprost tromethamine induces parturition. It can be used for controlling the timing of estrus in cycling mares and in anestrous mares that have a corpus luteum. In dogs and cats, dinoprost tromethamine is used to treat pyometra and endometrial hyperplasia and as an abortion-producing agent. In sheep and goats, the uses are similar to those for cattle.

Dosage Forms
- Dinoprost tromethamine for injection (Lutalyse)
- AmTech ProstaMate
- In Synch
- ProstaMate

Adverse Side Effects
These can include sweating (horses), abdominal pain (horses, dogs, cats, and swine), urination/defecation (dogs, cats, and swine), dyspnea and panting (dogs and cats), tachycardia (dogs), and increased vocalization (cats and swine). Most of the side effects are self-limiting and disappear within a short time.

Cloprostenol Sodium
Cloprostenol sodium is an analogue of prostaglandin F_{2alpha} for use in cattle. This product is chemically very similar to dinoprost and fenprostalene and is labeled for uses that are very similar to those of dinoprost and fenprostalene in cattle. The same precautions should be taken when this drug is used as are taken with the other prostaglandins.

Clinical Uses
This drug is used for treatment of luteal cysts and mummified fetuses, termination of pregnancy, and estrus synchronization.

Dosage Forms
- Cloprostenol (Estrumate) for injection
- estroPLAN

Adverse Side Effects
At high doses, adverse side effects may include uneasiness, frothing at the mouth, and milk letdown.

> **TECHNICIAN NOTES**
> - When administering any of the prostaglandinsm do not administer by intravenous injection.
> - Skin that is accidentally exposed during administration should be washed off immediately.
> - Pregnant women and individuals with asthma or bronchial disease should handle this product with great caution.

DRUGS THAT AFFECT UTERINE CONTRACTILITY

Several drugs have the ability to increase the contractility of uterine muscle. Some are used during pregnancy to cause abortion, and others are used at term to induce parturition, to aid in delivery of the fetus or the placenta, and to cause **involution** of the uterus after delivery. Great care should be taken to ensure that the cervix is dilated before these drugs are administered.

One of these drugs, oxytocin, also causes contraction of the myoepithelial cells in the mammary glands to facilitate milk letdown.

Oxytocin
Oxytocin is a polypeptide made in the hypothalamus and stored in the posterior pituitary for release in response to appropriate stimuli from the reproductive tract or mammary glands. This hormone causes stronger uterine contractions by increasing the contractility of uterine **myofibrils.** The uterus must be primed for a period by progesterone and estrogen before oxytocin is effective in stimulating the uterus.

Oxytocin is used clinically to cause more forceful uterine contractions as an aid in delivery of a fetus. It is also used to assist delivery of the placenta, to cause uterine involution, and to reduce bleeding of the uterus after delivery. It should be used only when the cervix is sufficiently dilated and when it can be determined that the fetus can be delivered normally through the pelvic canal.

This hormone is responsible for milk letdown from the mammary glands through its stimulation of myoepithelial cells in the alveolar wall of the glands. It is released endogenously after stimulation of the udder or in response to environmental stimuli, such as the sound of milking machines or other sights, sounds, or smells associated with nursing/milking.

Clinical Uses

Oxytocin is used to augment the force of uterine contractions during delivery, aid in delivery of the placenta, facilitate involution of the uterus (for reduction of bleeding or replacement of a prolapse), induce milk letdown, and assist in the treatment of agalactia in sows.

Dosage Form

- Oxytocin injection; generic form from many sources.

Adverse Side Effects

These are minimal when used according to recommendations.

> **TECHNICIAN NOTES**
> - Oxytocin should be used in **dystocia** only when the reproductive tract has been adequately examined. Inappropriate use can result in uterine torsion or rupture and can lead to death.
> - A single dose of oxytocin lasts approximately 15 minutes.
> - Oxytocin is stored under refrigeration.

Ergot

Ergot is a fungus that grows on rye grass and possibly on some pasture grasses. It causes smooth muscle contraction and can cause intense vasoconstriction. If the vasoconstriction is severe enough, gangrene and sloughing may occur.

Ergonovine maleate has been used in veterinary medicine because it produces uterine contractions similarly to oxytocin; however, it results in very little vasoconstrictive action. This product is not commonly used.

Prostaglandins

Prostaglandins, as mentioned in a previous section, stimulate uterine smooth muscle and can be used to induce parturition or abortion.

Corticosteroids

Corticosteroids comprise a group of hormones produced by the adrenal cortex that are used primarily for their antiinflammatory effect but can cause induction of parturition in the last trimester of pregnancy. This effect occurs because exogenous administration of the drug mimics the natural rise in production of corticosteroids by the fetus as the time for delivery draws near. Induction of parturition or abortion is not a labeled use for the corticosteroids, but they have been applied clinically for this purpose.

MISCELLANEOUS REPRODUCTIVE DRUGS

Bromocriptine

Bromocriptine is a dopamine agonist and prolactin inhibitor that has been used mainly in dogs for pregnancy termination after mismating or for the treatment of pseudopregnancy.

Cabergoline

Cabergoline is an ergot derivative used in dogs and cats for reduction of milk production, for pregnancy termination, and for estrus induction (dogs).

Leuprolide

Leuprolide is a synthetic analogue of GnRH that is used for the treatment of adrenal endocrinopathy in ferrets and for the treatment of inappropriate egg laying in cockatiels.

Melatonin

Melatonin is a naturally occurring hormone that is produced in the pineal gland. In addition to its use in the treatment of alopecia in dogs and sleep disorders in cats and dogs, melatonin has been used to improve early breeding and ovulation in sheep and goats.

Metergoline

Metergoline is a serotonin antagonist that may be used for treating pseudopregnancy in dogs.

Neutersol

Neutersol is a U.S. Food and Drug Administration (FDA)-approved product that contains the amino acid L-arginine and a zinc salt; it is administered directly into the testicles of puppies to cause permanent sterility. However, it reportedly does not eliminate testosterone production and its associated behavioral characteristics. This product is not currently available.

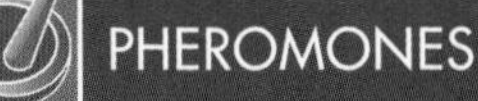

PHEROMONES

Pheromones are odors released by animals that influence the behavior of other animals of the same species. Although pheromones do not fit exactly into the endocrine category, they are considered in this section.

The first pheromone made commercially available was a boar odor aerosol called SOA/Sex. This product is a synthetic version of the natural pheromone that causes the typical boar odor and is used for heat detection in sows and gilts. Label instructions call for spraying the pheromone directly at the nostrils of the sow or gilt for 2 seconds. If the sow or gilt is in heat, she will demonstrate mating reflexes, such as rigid posture, deviations of the tail, and erect ears.

Other products (Feliway, Comfort Zone-Feline) are analogues of the feline facial pheromone. They are labeled for use in stopping or preventing urinary marking by the cat and to comfort the cat in an unknown or stressful environment. Cats deposit facial pheromones by rubbing an object with the side of the face. The manufacturers recommend spraying this product directly onto the places soiled by the cat and also on prominent objects that could be attractive to the cat. The products should be applied daily at a height of 8 inches from the floor until the cat is seen rubbing the area with its head. Pheromones can also be used to familiarize cats with new environments, such as carriers and cages. They may be dispensed over a large area with the use of a plug-in diffuser.

Another pheromone available in the veterinary market is called dog-appeasing hormone (D.A.P. and Comfort Zone-Canine). The manufacturers indicate that this product mimics the appeasement pheromones, which female dogs secrete to comfort and reassure their nursing puppies. Label indications for use include calming dogs during stressful situations, such as thunderstorms, fireworks, visits by strangers, or moving the dog to a new environment. It is available as a spray, collar, or room diffuser.

THYROID HORMONES

The thyroid gland is made up of two lobes (one on each side of the trachea) and is located near the thyroid cartilage of the larynx. Microscopically, the thyroid is composed of follicles that, on stimulation by TSH from the anterior pituitary, produce two metabolically active hormones. The thyroid synthesizes these hormones by first trapping iodide from the blood and then oxidizing the iodide to iodine. The iodine is combined with the amino acid tyrosine to form (through several intermediary steps) T_3 and T_4. T_3 is considered to be the active form at the cellular level. Although both T_3 and T_4 are released from the thyroid gland, some of the T_4 is converted to T_3 after release. T_4, also called *thyroxine,* is found in higher levels than T_3 in **euthyroid** animals.

Thyroid hormones control many events in the body, including metabolic rate, growth and development, body temperature, heart rate, metabolism of nutrients, skin condition, resistance to infection, and others. Two abnormalities of thyroid function that are encountered in veterinary medicine are hypothyroidism and hyperthyroidism.

Hypothyroidism is noted most often in dogs and is characterized by lethargy, cold intolerance, dry haircoat, and bradycardia. Hyperthyroidism is encountered more often in older cats and is accompanied by weight loss, increased appetite, restlessness, hyperexcitability, and tachycardia. Diagnosis of thyroid conditions is made by observing clinical signs and by measuring serum levels of T_3 and T_4 before and after TSH administration.

Goiter is a condition that is caused by inadequate levels of iodide in the diet. Lack of iodide causes the thyroid to be unable to produce T_3 or T_4. The thyroid attempts to increase its output by enlarging, often to a size that can be palpated and visualized. Goiter is almost nonexistent in animals receiving a commercial diet.

DRUGS USED TO TREAT HYPOTHYROIDISM

Treatment of hypothyroidism consists of supplementation of thyroid hormones on a daily basis. Clinical signs usually resolve within a short time of treatment initiation, but lifelong therapy is required.

Thyroid hormones can be extracted from thyroid glands or can be prepared synthetically. Purification of the animal source hormones is difficult and has led to the common use of synthetic products. Synthetic thyroxine (T_4) is considered to be the compound of choice in the treatment of hypothyroidism. T_3 products are recommended only when a poor response to T_4 occurs.

Levothyroxine Sodium (T_4)

Levothyroxine is a synthetic **levo isomer** of T_4. It is the compound of choice for the treatment of hypothyroidism in all species.

Clinical Uses

Levothyroxine is used for the treatment of hypothyroid conditions.

Dosage Forms

- Levothyroxine tablets (Soloxine), approved for dogs
- Levothyroxine chewable tablets (Thyromed), approved for dogs
- Levothyroxine tablets (Thyro-Tabs) for dogs
- Levothyroxine tablets (Thyrozine Tablets) for dogs
- Levothyroxine chewable tablets (NutriVed T-4 Chewables), approved for dogs
- Levothyroxine powder (Thyro-L), approved for horses
- Equine Thyroid Supplement
- Levothyroxine tablets (Synthroid), approved for humans
- Various others

Adverse Side Effects

These are rare when used according to recommendations.

Liothyronine Sodium

Liothyronine sodium (T_3) is a synthetic salt of endogenous T_3. T_3 is not the compound of choice for the treatment of hypothyroidism. It may be useful, however, in cases that do not respond well to T_4.

Clinical Uses

T_3 is used for the treatment of hypothyroidism in cases that respond poorly to T_4.

Dosage Forms

- Triostat, human label
- Cytomel, human label

Adverse Side Effects

These are probably minimal with careful use.

Thyroid-Stimulating Hormone

Thyrotropin alpha is a recombinant TSH. It is used as an aid in the diagnosis of hypothyroidism. The bovine source of TSH is no longer available.

Clinical Uses

In veterinary medicine, thyrotropin is used for diagnosis of **primary hypothyroidism** in the TSH stimulation test.

Dosage Form

- Thyrogen powder for injection

Adverse Side Effects

Allergic reactions may occur in animals sensitive to human protein.

DRUGS USED TO TREAT HYPERTHYROIDISM

Treatment of hyperthyroidism is directed at lowering blood levels of T_3 and T_4. This can be accomplished by destruction or removal of the overproducing thyroid or by blocking of hormone production. The thyroid can be removed surgically or destroyed with radioactive iodine. Drug therapy to block hormone production can be effective but is continuous and is not curative (Boothe, 2012).

The two antithyroid drugs used most often are methimazole and carbimazole. These compounds are used for long-term therapy and for presurgical preparation of patients. Cats with hyperthyroidism are often high surgical risks, primarily because of tachycardia and other potential cardiac abnormalities.

Methimazole

Methimazole is a compound that interferes with incorporation of iodine into the precursor molecules of T_3 and T_4. It does not alter thyroid hormones already released into the bloodstream.

Clinical Uses

Methimazole is used for the treatment of feline hyperthyroidism.

Dosage Form

- Methimazole tablets (Felimazole), approved for cats
- Methimazole tablets (Tapazole), human approved

Adverse Side Effects

These include anorexia, vomiting, and skin eruptions. Kittens should receive a milk replacement after receiving colostrum from mothers given methimazole.

Carbimazole

Carbimazole is a product similar to methimazole that is used in Canada and other countries. Most of this drug is converted to methimazole after administration to the cat. It inhibits the synthesis of thyroid hormones.

Clinical Uses

Carbimazole is used for the treatment of feline hyperthyroidism.

Dosage Forms

- Carbimazole (Carbizole), human label
- Carbimazole (Neo-Mercazole), human label

Adverse Side Effects

Side effects are similar to those of methimazole.

Ipodate

Ipodate is an orally administered, radiopaque, organic iodine compound that is thought to inhibit the conversion of T_4 to T_3.

Clinical Uses

Ipodate may be helpful in the treatment of hyperthyroidism in cats that cannot tolerate methimazole or carbimazole.

Dosage Form

- Ipodate: obtained from compounding pharmacies

Propylthiouracil

Propylthiouracil has been used as an antithyroid drug but is considered dangerous for use in cats because of potential hematologic complications.

Radioactive Iodine

Radioactive iodine (I-131) may be given intravenously to destroy overproductive thyroid tissue. I-131 concentrates in the thyroid, where it remains and destroys thyroid tissue. This method has appeal because it is performed only once and is not especially stressful to patients. However, it must be done at facilities that can handle radioactive materials.

Propranolol

Propranolol (Inderal) may be used preoperatively to treat the tachycardia associated with hyperthyroidism in cats.

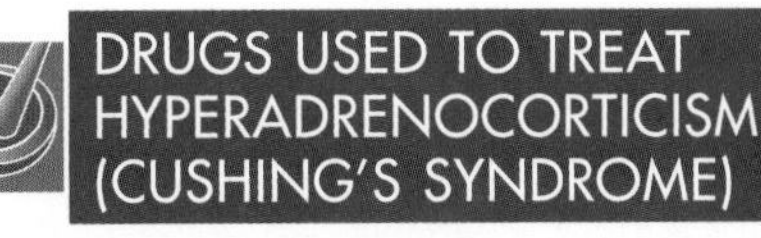

DRUGS USED TO TREAT HYPERADRENOCORTICISM (CUSHING'S SYNDROME)

Hyperadrenocorticism or **Cushing's syndrome** is one of the most commonly diagnosed endocrine disorders in dogs and horses. Cushing's syndrome is usually seen in older dogs and can be spontaneous or **iatrogenic.** The signs associated with this syndrome occur because of an excess of circulating glucocorticoids, especially cortisol. Cortisol (see Chapter 14) is a hormone produced in the cortex of the adrenal gland on stimulation by ACTH from the pituitary. Its function is to help the body respond to stress and to prepare the body for the flight-or-fight response. It does this by mobilizing nutrients, modifying the response to inflammation, raising the blood glucose level, and controlling the amount of water in the body.

There are two forms of spontaneous Cushing's syndrome:

- Pituitary-dependent hyperadrenocorticism (PDH). This is the most common of spontaneous cases and often occurs due to a benign tumor of the pituitary gland. This tumor causes the pituitary to produce large amounts of ACTH, which stimulates the adrenal to make large amounts of cortisol.
- Adrenal-dependent hyperadrenocorticism (ADH). This is a less common form of the spontaneous disease. It occurs due to a tumor of one or both of the adrenal glands and results in the production of a large amount of cortisol independent of ACTH.

Differentiating between these two forms of disease in the dog can be difficult.

In the equine patient, Cushing's syndrome is a disease of older horses that is the result of pituitary pars intermedia dysfunction (PPID), which makes it different from Cushing's syndrome in the dog. Adrenal gland tumors are apparently rare in the horse.

Ketoconazole

Ketoconazole is an antifungal agent that can be used in the treatment of hyperadrenocorticism if other agents like mitotane are not effective.

Dosage Form

- Ketoconazole tablets, human label

Adverse Side Effects

Side effects include vomiting, diarrhea, and anorexia.

Metyrapone

Metyrapone is an agent used to treat cats with hyperadrenocorticism, especially for stabilization of patients before adrenalectomy.

Dosage Form

- Metyrapone (Metopirone), oral capsule, human label

Adverse Side Effects

Metyrapone is relatively well tolerated in cats.

Mitotane

Mitotane is used for the treatment of PDH. This agent is an adrenal cytotoxic agent that inhibits or destroys the cortisol-producing layers of the adrenal gland.

Dosage Form

- Mitotane tablets, Lysodren, human label

Adverse Side Effects

Side effects include lethargy, ataxia, weakness, vomiting, diarrhea, and others. Long-term glucocorticoid and possibly mineralocorticoid replacement therapy may be needed in some patients treated with mitotane.

Selegiline

Selegiline is a monoamine oxidase-B (MAO-B) inhibitor that is used for cognitive dysfunction and PDH in dogs. Its use for Cushing's syndrome is controversial because of disappointing clinical studies (Plumb, 2011).

Dosage Forms

- Selegiline tablets (Anipryl), veterinary label
- Selegiline tablets (Eldepryl), human label

Adverse Side Effects

Side effects may include vomiting, diarrhea, restlessness, salivation, and others.

Trilostane

Trilostane is an adrenal steroid synthesis inhibitor that may be used to treat PDH or hyperadrenocorticism due to adrenal tumors in dogs.

Dosage Form

- Trilostane capsules (Vetoryl)

Adverse Side Effects

Side effects may include loss of appetite, lethargy, weakness, diarrhea, or vomiting.

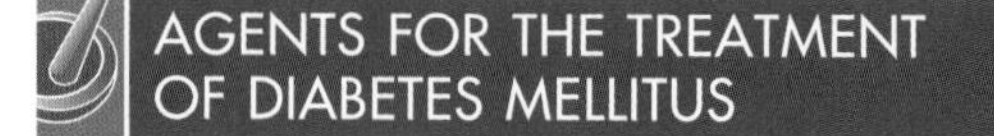

AGENTS FOR THE TREATMENT OF DIABETES MELLITUS

Insulin

The pancreas produces two principal hormones in special cells of the islets of Langerhans: insulin and glucagon. Insulin is produced by beta cells, and glucagon is produced by alpha cells. Insulin causes a decrease in blood glucose levels, and glucagon promotes an increase. Only insulin is used clinically.

Insulin facilitates cellular uptake of glucose and its storage in the form of glycogen and fat. It inhibits the breakdown of fat, protein, and glycogen into forms that may be used as energy sources. Further, it promotes synthesis of protein, fatty acids, and glycogen. In the absence of insulin, the body cannot use glucose and must break down its own fat and protein that can be used for energy.

Diabetes mellitus is a complex disease that results from the inability of the beta cells of the pancreas to produce enough insulin or from altered insulin action within cells. Diabetes mellitus that results from inadequate secretion of insulin is called *type I,* or *insulin-dependent, diabetes mellitus.* This is the most common type of diabetes mellitus in dogs and cats. Diabetes mellitus that results from resistance of tissue to the action of insulin is called *type II,* or *non*insulin-dependent, diabetes mellitus (NIDDM). NIDDM is rare in dogs but is occasionally encountered in cats.

Both forms of diabetes mellitus eventually cause polydipsia, polyuria, polyphagia, and weight loss. Untreated diabetes mellitus proceeds to the condition called *diabetic ketoacidosis,* in which body fat is metabolized as a substitute energy source. Metabolism of body fat results in accumulation of by-products of this process called *ketone bodies,* which promote a metabolic acidosis that can lead to death.

Because blood glucose levels can be increased by corticosteroids, epinephrine, and progesterone, these drugs should be given with caution to diabetic animals. Sudden changes in diet and exercise level should also be avoided because they can alter blood glucose levels and cause an imbalance in the ratio of insulin to glucose.

Insulin is not effective when given orally because the digestive tract breaks down the protein molecule before it can be absorbed. Insulin usually is administered by subcutaneous injection. However, some forms may be given intravenously or intramuscularly.

Sources of insulin have traditionally included beef or pork pancreas and preparations consisting of a purified (pure beef source or pure pork source) form or a combination beef/pork form. The beef/pork form is best suited to the treatment of diabetes mellitus in dogs and cats. Pork insulin is very close in structure to dog and human types of insulin, whereas beef insulin is very similar to cat insulin.

Most human insulin products are now prepared through recombinant DNA or synthetic processes. Only two animal labeled products (ProZinc and Vetsulin) are currently approved for use in the United States. The availability of insulin products is subject to change, and technicians should always consult current information when dealing with products for diabetic patients.

Insulin concentration is measured in units of insulin per milliliter. It is available in concentrations of 40 (U-40), 100 (U-100), and 500 (U-500) U/mL. Most products for human use are U-100 concentrations (U-500 is only used for people who need very high insulin doses). Animal-approved products are U-40. Both animal-approved and human-approved insulin preparations are used in animals.

U-40 syringes should be used with U-40 insulin, and U-100 syringes should be used with U-100 insulin. U-40 syringes have a red top, and U-100 syringes have an orange top (Figure 9-5). U-100 syringes are available in 0.3 mL (30 units), 0.5 mL (50 units), and 1.0 mL (100 units) sizes (Figure 9-6). U-40 syringes are also produced in 0.3 mL (12 units), 0.5 mL (20 units), and 1.0 mL (40 units) sizes. Table 9-2 lists insulin syringe manufacturers.

When U-40 insulin is drawn into a U-40 syringe, each mark on the syringe barrel denotes 1 unit of insulin. A 100-unit, 1 mL syringe may be marked

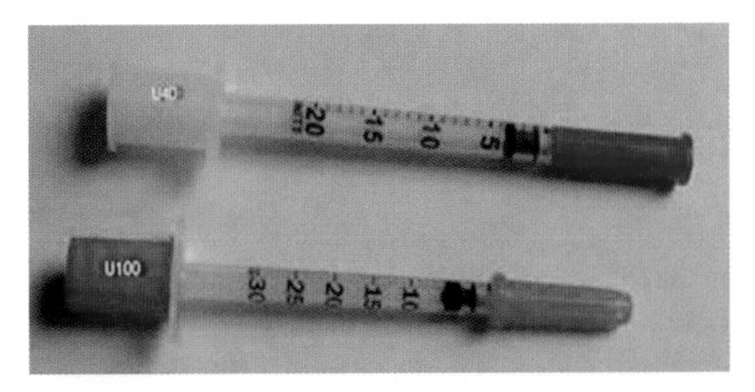

FIGURE 9-5 U-40 syringe (red top) and U-100 syringe (orange top).

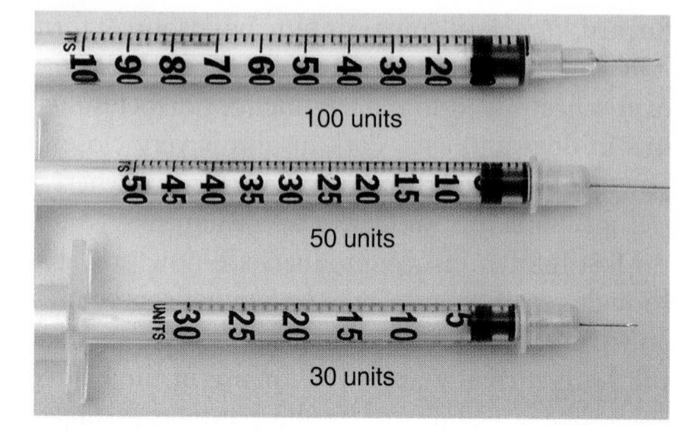

FIGURE 9-6 U-100 insulin syringes: 30 unit, 50 unit, and 100 unit. (From Mulholland J: The nurse, the math, the meds, St. Louis, 2011, Elsevier.)

TABLE 9-2 Insulin Syringe Manufacturers

U-100	U-40
BD (Becton Dickinson)	Ulti Care
Turemo	Ulti Guard
Monoject	MVP
Ulti Med	Vetsulin
Aimsco	BD
ReliOn (Walmart)	
Abbott Laboratories	
Can-Am Care	
Inviro Medical Devices	
Excel International	

TABLE 9-3 Insulin Products Commonly Used in Dogs and Cats

BRAND NAME	GENERIC NAME	SOURCE	DURATION	MANUFACTURER	CONCENTRATION
Humulin R Novolin R	Regular insulin	Human recombinant	Short	Eli Lilly Novo Nordisk	U-100
Humulin N Novolin N	NPH	Human recombinant	Intermediate	Eli Lilly Novo Nordisk	U-100
Vetsulin	Lente	Pork	Intermediate	Merck	U-40
ProZinc	Protamine zinc	Human recombinant	Intermediate	Boehringer Ingelheim	U-40
Lantus	Glargine	Human recombinant	Intermediate to long	Aventis	U-100

in 2-unit increments (e.g., 2, 4, 6, 8) or in 1-unit increments (e.g., 1, 2, 3, 4, 5); care should be taken to note which is being used. Small volume 100-unit (0.3 mL and 0.5 mL) syringes are marked in 1-unit increments.

U-100 syringes can be used to administer U-40 insulin by multiplying the required units of U-40 insulin by 2.5 (Plumb, 2011). A conversion chart is also available at www.medi-vet.com/Insulin_Syringe_Conversion_Chart.aspx

Needles for insulin syringes are either $\frac{1}{2}$ or $\frac{5}{16}$ inches in length and standard gauges are 28, 29, and 31.

Insulin Classifications

Insulin is usually classified according to its duration of action, that is, short acting, intermediate acting, or long acting. Short-acting insulins include regular, lispro, and aspart. Neutral protamine Hagedorn (NPH), protamine zinc insulin (PZI), and Lente are intermediate-acting insulins. Glargine and detemir are long-acting products (Hess, 2006). Two different forms are sometimes combined in the same preparation. See Table 9-3 for a partial listing of insulin products in each category. Because insulin products and classifications tend to change periodically, the technician involved in treating diabetic animals should remain current with the literature on this topic.

The onset of effect and route of administration are other important characteristics of insulin preparations to be considered. For an in-depth discussion of insulin forms and characteristics, other references should be consulted.

Short-Acting Insulin

Regular insulin/lispro/aspart. Regular insulin is a fast-acting insulin that is made from zinc insulin crystals; it is a clear solution that may be administered intravenously, intramuscularly, or subcutaneously. It is used mainly to treat diabetic ketoacidosis until blood glucose levels are reduced and the animal is metabolically stable. At that time, the animal is usually switched to a longer-acting form. Lispro and aspart insulins are not used in dogs and cats at this time.

Clinical Uses
Regular, lispro, and aspart insulin types are used primarily for the treatment of diabetic ketoacidosis.

Dosage Forms
Many products approved for humans are available. Following is a partial listing:
- Humulin R
- Novolin R
- Humalog

Adverse Side Effects
These usually are related to overdose and may include weakness, ataxia, shaking, and seizures.

> **TECHNICIAN NOTES**
> - Although not required by label on the newer products, refrigeration probably enhances storage life. Do not freeze.
> - Do not use regular insulin preparations if discoloration or precipitates are present.

Intermediate-Acting Insulin

NPH/PZI/Lente. NPH insulin is a cloudy suspension of zinc insulin crystals and protamine zinc. Protamine (a fish protein) and zinc prolong the absorption and activity of the product. These insulin types are longer acting than regular insulin. They are commonly used for the control of uncomplicated diabetes in dogs and cats. Lente insulin is similar in activity to NPH insulin but is made without the use of protamine.

Clinical Uses
NPH insulin is used in the treatment of uncomplicated diabetes mellitus.

Dosage Forms
A partial listing follows:
- Humulin N
- Novolin N
- Vetsulin (U-40), approved for use in cats and dogs. This product was withdrawn from the market in 2009 because of concentration issues but was reapproved by the FDA and placed back on the market by the manufacturer in 2013.
- ProZinc (U-40), approved for use in cats

Adverse Side Effects
These are similar to those of regular insulin.

> **TECHNICIAN NOTES**
> - Resuspension, by gently rolling the bottle, is required before the product is withdrawn from the bottle An exception to this rule is Vetsulin whose label reads: "Shake the vial thoroughly until a homogenous, uniformly milky suspension is obtained."
> - Store in the manner of regular insulin. Do not freeze.
> - NPH insulin is usually administered once a day although maintenance doses of insulin in dogs and cats can be highly individualized.

Long-Acting Insulin

Glargine (Lantus) and detemir (Levemir) insulin are long-acting insulins with a human label. Lantus is marketed as a peakless insulin. Care should be taken to avoid confusing Lantus and Levemir with other clear insulins.

Clinical Uses
Glargine is used for the treatment of uncomplicated diabetes mellitus.

Dosage Forms
- Clear, long-acting glargine insulin (Lantus)
- Clear, detemir insulin (Levemir)

Adverse Side Effects
These are similar to those of regular and intermediate-acting insulins.

> **TECHNICIAN NOTES** Humulin L, Humulin U, Iletin II regular pork insulin, and Iletin II NPH pork insulin were discontinued by Eli Lilly in 2005.

Use of Insulin Products

Technicians who are counseling clients about the use of insulin products should take great care to become thoroughly familiar with the products they are using. The onset of action of various insulin products can vary from a few minutes to a few hours. Peak activity time and duration of activity can also vary greatly between products. Exercise levels and eating patterns may influence insulin activity. An overdose of insulin can lead to various degrees of hypoglycemia that produce clinical signs ranging from mild weakness to coma. Clients should be shown how to give subcutaneous injections of insulin, and they should be given written instructions about monitoring the insulin response and making appropriate adjustments. Tips regarding the use of insulin products follow as technician's notes.

One of the issues involved in treating animals with human insulin products is the high cost. To reduce the cost of these products many veterinarians are choosing the ReliOn (Walmart) line of products, which may reduce the cost of some products by half or more (Jordan, 2013).

> *TECHNICIAN NOTES*
>
> - It is usually best to feed the animal 30 minutes before giving the insulin injection.
> - Roll "cloudy" insulins between your palms; do not shake (except Vetsulin).
> - NPH insulin should not be mixed with any Lente insulin.
> - It is the opinion of some people that insulin should be disposed of after 30 days or 100 injections.
> - Injection sites should be rotated (Figure 9-7).
> - Clients should be advised to use insulin syringes only once.
> - Mild to moderate hypoglycemia resulting from an overdose can be treated by feeding the animal or administering corn (Karo) syrup.

Oral Hypoglycemic Agents

Oral hypoglycemic agents such as the sulfonylureas are extensively used in human diabetic patients to control type II diabetes mellitus (NIDDM). They have little apparent effectiveness in diabetic dogs but may be useful in some cats with type II diabetes.

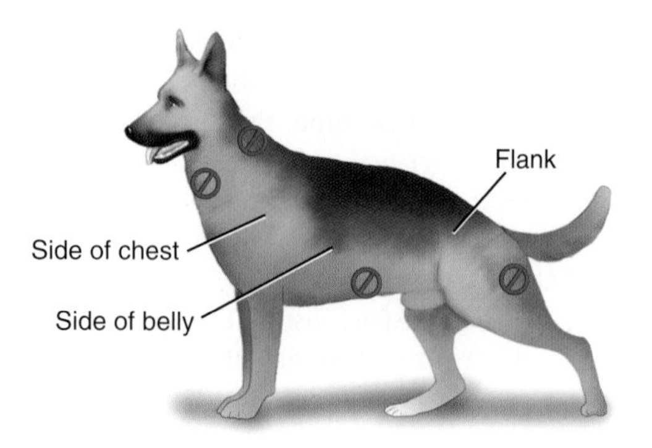

FIGURE 9-7 Insulin injection sites include the side of the chest, belly or at the flank. The red circle indicate an area where injections should not be made. (From Civco T: Diabetic treatment & management protocols, 2010 [website]. http://abbottanimalhealthce.com. Accessed March, 28, 2013.)

Drugs in this category include glipizide (Glucotrol) and metformin (Glucophage XR).

HYPERGLYCEMIC AGENTS

Several drugs such as corticosteroids, epinephrine, and progesterone incidentally elevate blood glucose levels. Two products that are marketed for this purpose, however, are diazoxide (Proglycem) and octreotide (Sandostatin). These are used to treat the low blood glucose levels associated with hypersecretion of insulin that occurs in tumors of the beta cells of the pancreas (insulinoma) in dogs and ferrets (Plumb, 2011). These products act by inhibiting the release of insulin from beta cells of the pancreas.

HORMONES THAT ACT AS GROWTH PROMOTERS

SEX STEROIDS, SYNTHETIC STEROID ANALOGUES, AND NONSTEROIDAL ANALOGUES

The factors that control growth, **feed efficiency,** and carcass composition in animals involve a complex interrelationship between genetic, metabolic, and hormonal mechanisms that are not always totally understood. It is possible, however, to increase growth (weight gain) in ruminants by administering sex steroid hormones (estrogen, testosterone, or progesterone), synthetic steroid hormone analogues (trenbolone), or certain nonsteroidal hormone analogs (zeranol).

The primary sex steroid used to promote weight gain is estrogen (estradiol). The mechanisms by which estradiol promotes weight gain include (1) increased water retention, (2) increased protein synthesis, (3) increased fat deposition, and (4) possible increased release of growth hormone (bovine somatotropin).

Testosterone is used as an adjunct to estradiol in some growth-promotion products because it is an anabolic agent in itself and because a second component in the compound slows down the release of estradiol and prolongs its effective life span.

Progesterone is also added to growth promoters to slow the release of estradiol. It apparently has little anabolic effect of its own.

Trenbolone is a synthetic anabolic agent that improves feed efficiency and promotes weight gain in steers. It is used as the sole agent in some growth-promoting preparations.

Zeranol is an analogue of a naturally occurring plant estrogen that increases feed efficiency, protein synthesis, and growth rate.

All of the growth-promoting products for use in cattle and sheep are prepared as compressed pellets that are implanted in the subcutaneous tissue of the dorsal, middle third of the ear (Figure 9-8). These pellets are designed for use with corresponding needle devices and should be implanted with close adherence to product instructions (failure to do so is a violation of federal law in some cases).

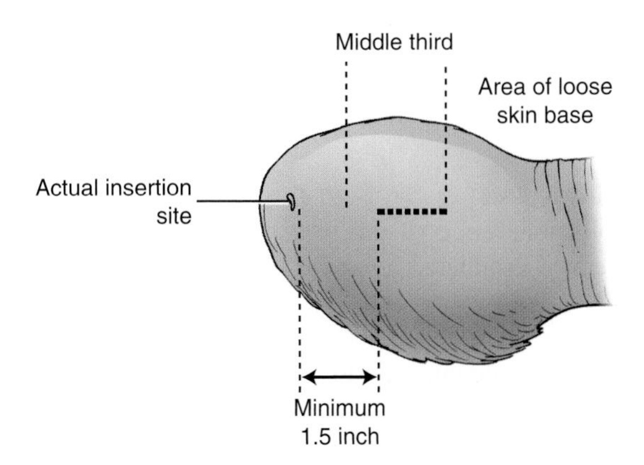

FIGURE 9-8 Implantation site for growth-promoting pellets (posterior view of the ear).

The growth-promotion products are considered here as a group, and minimal information is provided about each product.

Clinical Uses

These drugs are used to promote feed efficiency and weight gain in calves, steers, heifers, or sheep (depending on the product).

Dosage Forms

- Estradiol/progesterone implant for use in calves older than 45 days (Synovex C)
- Estradiol/testosterone implant for use in heifers (Synovex H)
- Estradiol/testosterone implant for use in steers (Synovex S)
- Estradiol implant for use in steers (Compudose)
- Estradiol/testosterone implant for use in heifers (Implus-H)
- Trenbolone implant for use in feedlot heifers (Finaplix-H)
- Trenbolone and estradiol implant for use in feedlot steers (Revalor-S)
- Zeranol implant for use in growing cattle, feedlot heifers, feedlot steers, and suckling and weaned calves (Ralgro beef cattle implant)

Adverse Side Effects

These may include mounting, elevated tail heads, rectal prolapse, and udder development.

TECHNICIAN NOTES

- Most growth-promoting implants should not be given to animals intended for breeding purposes or to dairy cattle.
- Product insert instructions should be read and followed carefully.

GROWTH HORMONE: BOVINE SOMATOTROPIN, BOVINE GROWTH HORMONE

Growth hormone, also called *somatotropin,* is a hormone produced by the anterior pituitary. Its function before the onset of puberty is to stimulate growth. It is released throughout life to promote anabolic activity (e.g., to increase protein synthesis). It has been shown to increase growth rate and feed efficiency in farm animals. Many of the growth-promoting agents listed in the previous section may work by stimulating the release of somatotropin. Somatotropin is also a potent stimulator of milk production. Claims of a 20% boost in milk production in dairy cows have been made after administration of somatotropin.

The FDA approved a recombinant (genetically engineered) bovine somatotropin (BST) for commercial production in 1993. This product, Posilac, was manufactured originally by Monsanto and was later acquired by Elanco. Its market availability has sparked intense debate among certain groups. Some dairy producers have opposed its use because of their fear that increased production would drive milk prices down and reduce their overall income. Other groups have resisted the use of BST because of their concerns about residues of the hormone in milk products, even though the FDA has stated that milk from cows receiving BST is completely safe. People who advocate the use of "organic" food products may oppose the use of this product.

ANABOLIC STEROIDS

Anabolic steroids are steroids that produce a tissue-building (anabolic) effect. Testosterone is a naturally occurring anabolic steroid that produces masculinization in addition to its anabolic effects. Synthetic anabolic steroids are designed to prevent most masculinizing effects.

Anabolic steroid administration causes positive **nitrogen balance** and reverses processes that break down tissue. An increase in appetite, weight gain, improved overall condition, and recovery are promoted. These products are labeled for clinical use in dogs, cats, and horses for anorexia, weight loss, and debilitation. In working animals, they may be used in cases of overwork or overtraining. Anabolic steroids also promote red blood cell formation and are used to treat some forms of anemia. The product insert for a commonly used anabolic steroid states that "anabolic therapy is intended primarily as an adjunct to other specific and supportive therapy, including nutritional therapy."

Because of the potential for abuse by bodybuilders and other athletes, the FDA has now classified anabolic steroids as Class III controlled substances.

Stanozolol

Stanozolol is an anabolic steroid that has been found to have an unusual pattern of biologic activity in that its anabolic effect far outweighs its weak androgenic influence.

Clinical Uses

Stanozolol is used for the treatment of anorexia, debilitation, weight loss, overwork, and anemia.

Dosage Forms

- Stanozolol sterile suspension for injection in dogs, cats, and horses (Winstrol-V)
- Stanozolol tablets for use in dogs and cats (Winstrol-V)

Adverse Side Effects

These may include mild androgenic effects after prolonged use or overdose.

> *TECHNICIAN NOTES*
> - Winstrol-V should not be used in pregnant dogs, mares, or stallions.
> - Winstrol-V should not be given to horses intended for food uses.

Boldenone Undecylenate

Boldenone undecylenate is a steroid ester that possesses marked anabolic activity and a minimal amount of androgenic activity. It is labeled for use in horses.

Clinical Uses

Boldenone undecylenate acts as an aid in the treatment of debilitated horses.

Dosage Form

- Boldenone injection for horses (Equipoise)

Adverse Side Effects

These include androgenic effects such as overaggressiveness.

TECHNICIAN NOTES

- Boldenone should not be used in horses intended as food.
- Boldenone should not be used in stallions or in pregnant mares.

Nandrolone Decanoate

Nandrolone decanoate is an injectable anabolic steroid that was previously sold under the human label Deca-Durabolin. It is no longer commercially produced but may be available from compounding pharmacies. It exhibits activity similar to that of the other anabolic agents.

REVIEW QUESTIONS

1. Describe the relationship between hormonal releasing factors, trophic hormones, and the hormones produced by specific tissues or glands.
   ____
2. List the major endocrine glands.
   ____
3. What are the reasons for using hormonal therapy in veterinary medicine?
   ____
4. Endogenous hormones are those that are produced ______________________, whereas exogenous hormones come from ______________________ sources.
5. Where is the pituitary gland located, and what is its function?
   ____
6. Describe the difference between a negative and a positive feedback control mechanism in the endocrine system.
   ____
7. The release of oxytocin by the posterior pituitary is controlled through the ______________________ mechanism.
8. GnRH is classified as a/an ______________________.
9. Hormonal products with "gest" in their name are classified as ______________________.
10. List three potential uses of the prostaglandins in veterinary medicine.
    ____
11. Human skin contact or injection with prostaglandins can be a serious health risk to ______________________ women and individuals with ______________________.
12. Before oxytocin can exert its effects on the uterus, the uterus must first be primed by ______________________ and ______________________.
13. What precautions should be taken before oxytocin is administered?
    ____
14. What two active hormones are produced by the thyroid gland? ______________________
15. List two drugs used in the treatment of hypothyroidism. ______________________
16. List the three major classes of insulin.
    ____
17. Which form of insulin is used in the treatment of diabetic ketoacidosis?
    ____
18. Which form(s) of insulin must be resuspended before administration?
    ____
19. What are some signs of insulin overdose?
    ____
20. Growth promoters generally should not be used in animals intended for ______________________.
21. Why are anabolic steroids classified as controlled substances?
    ____
22. Which insulin product should be shaken thoroughly prior to use? ______________
23. What precautions should be taken by pregnant women when Regu-Mate is administered?
    ____
24. Why was synthetic DES banned from use in food-producing animals?
    ____

25. Prostaglandin causes lysis of the ________________________________ at the end of pregnancy or at the end of diestrus if pregnancy does not occur.
26. Endometrium lines the ________________.
   a. kidney
   b. stomach
   c. intestines
   d. uterus
27. A ________________ hormone is one that results in the production of a second hormone within a target gland.
   a. gonadotropin
   b. euthyroid
   c. trophic
   d. myofibril
28. GnRH is produced in the ________________.
   a. pancreas
   b. thymus
   c. thyroid gland
   d. hypothalamus
29. All the following drugs are gonadotropins, except ________________.
   a. estradiol cypionate
   b. Cystorelin
   c. Factrel
   d. Fertagyl
30. Androgens are female sex hormones produced in the ovaries, adrenal cortex, and testicles.
   a. True
   b. False
31. Prostaglandins are a group of naturally occurring, long-chain fatty acids that mediate various physiologic events in the body.
   a. True
   b. False
32. ________________ causes uterine contractions.
   a. Regu-Mate
   b. Bovilene
   c. Oxytocin
   d. Cystorelin
33. Corticosteroids are produced by the ________________.
   a. thyroid gland
   b. adrenal cortex
   c. kidneys
   d. hypothalamus
34. Pheromones are ________________ released by an animal that influence the behavior of other animals of the same species.
   a. hormones
   b. gonadotropins
   c. steroids
   d. odors
35. Levothyroxine is used in the treatment of ________________ in all species.
   a. hypoglycemia
   b. hypothyroidism
   c. hypokalemia
   d. hypocalcemia
36. Cushing's syndrome is caused by an excess of circulating ________________.
   a. cortisol
   b. T_3
   c. estrogen
   d. insulin
37. Pituitary-dependent hyperadrenocorticism in dogs may be treated with ________________.
   a. Lysodren
   b. Vetoryl
   c. Captopril
   d. both a and b
38. U-40 syringes have a/an ________________ top.
   a. green
   b. purple
   c. orange
   d. red
39. Insulin should be frozen to prolong its effectiveness.
   a. True
   b. False
40. Two veterinary-approved insulin products include ________________.
   a. Vetsulin
   b. Glargine
   c. ProZinc
   d. both a and c

41. A 1200-lb Holstein cow will be treated for an ovarian cyst with 100 mcg of Cystorelin. Cystorelin contains 50 mcg/mL. How much of the product will you draw up?

____

42. A 1100-lb mare will be given altrenogest at 0.044 mg/kg daily to maintain pregnancy. The concentration of altrenogest (Regu-Mate) is 0.22%. What quantity will you give daily?

____

43. A 50-lb Golden Retriever with hypothyroidism will be treated with Soloxine at 0.02 mg/kg twice a day. Soloxine tablets (0. 5 mg) will be used. How many tablets will you give with each dose? ______________________

44. A 13-lb diabetic cat with a blood glucose of 450 mg/dL will be treated with ProZinc (U-40) at a dosage of 0.5 U/kg twice a day. How many units will you give with each dose? ______________________

45. A 20-lb poodle with pituitary-dependent hyperadrenocorticism will be treated with trilostane (Vetoryl) at a dosage of 3 mg/lb once a day for 2 weeks. How many 60-mg capsules will you dispense?

____

46. An 8-lb cat with hyperthyroidism will be treated with methimazole at 2.5 mg twice a day for 3 weeks. Felimazole tablets (2.5 mg) will be used. How many will you dispense?

____

REFERENCES

Boothe DM: Drug therapy for endocrinopathies. In Boothe DM, editor: Small animal clinical pharmacology, Philadelphia, 2012, WB Saunders.

Hess RS: New and old insulin products. In Proceedings. Intl Vet Emerg Crit Care Symp (IVECCS), San Antonio, Tex, September 17-21, 2006.

Jordan DG: Trends in veterinary therapeutics. In Proceedings. Music City Vet Conf, Murfreesboro, Tenn, 2013.

Plumb DC: Veterinary drug handbook, ed 7, Ames, Iowa, 2011, Wiley-Blackwell.

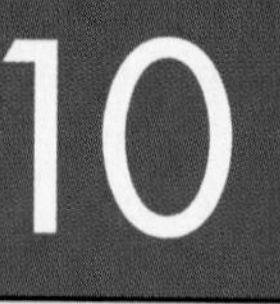

CHAPTER 10

Drugs Used in Ophthalmic and Otic Disorders

KEY TERMS

Blepharospasm
Cerumen
Conjunctivitis
Cycloplegia
Distichia (distichiasis)
Ectropion
Entropion
Glaucoma
Horner's syndrome
Hyphema
Intracameral injection
Keratitis
MRSA
Mydriasis
Open-angle glaucoma
Otoacariasis
Uvea
Uveitis

OUTLINE

Introduction

Diagnostic Agents
- Fluorescein Sodium
- Lissamine Green
- Phenol Red Thread
- Rose Bengal
- Schirmer Tear Test

Ocular Anesthetics
- Proparacaine HCl
- Tetracaine HCl
- Benoxinate

Parasympathomimetics
- Carbachol
- Pilocarpine HCl
- Demecarium Bromide

Sympathomimetics
- Apraclonidine
- Brimonidine
- Epinephrine

Beta-Adrenergic Antagonists
- Timolol

Carbonic Anyhydrase Inhibitors
- Brinzolamide HCl
- Dorzolamide HCl

Prostaglandins
- Latanoprost
- Bimatoprost
- Travoprost
- Unoprostone Isopropyl

Osmotic Agents for the Treatment of Glaucoma

Mydriatic Cycloplegic Vasoconstrictors
- Cyclopentolate
- Phenylephrine HCl
- Atropine Sulfate
- Tropicamide

Antiinflammatory/Analgesic Ophthalmic Agents
- Cromolyn Sodium
- Lodoxamide Tromethamine
- Olopatadine HCl

Nonsteroidal Anatiinflammatory Agents

Steroidal Antiinflammatory Agents
- Prednisolone
- Dexamethasone
- Betamethasone
- Fluorometholone
- Loteprednol
- Rimexolone

Ophthalmic Analgesics
- Morphine Sulfate

Antimicrobial Ophthalmic Therapy
- Amikacin Sulfate
- Neomycin Sulfate
- Gentamicin Sulfate
- Tobramycin Sulfate
- Ocular Fluoroquinolones

Miscellaneous Ocular Antibiotics
- Chloramphenicol
- Polymyxin B
- Sulfacetamide
- Vancomycin

Ocular Antifungals
- Amphotericin B
- Natamycin
- Povidone Iodine
- Silver Sulfadiazine
- Itraconazole

Ocular Antivirals
- Trifluridine
- Idoxuridine
- Interferon Alpha

- Acyclovir, Valacyclovir, Famciclovir, Ganciclovir, Cidofovir, and Penciclovir

Drugs for Keratoconjunctivitis Sicca
- Cyclosporine
- Tacrolimus
- Pimecrolimus

Ocular Lubricants/Artificial Tear Products
- Artificial Tears
- Ophthalmic Irrigants

Anticollagenase Agents
- Acetylcysteine
- Edetate Disodium

Otic Drugs
- Ceruminolytic Agents
- Cleaning/Drying Agents
- Antiseptic Agents
- Antibiotic Potentiating Agents
- Corticosteroid Preparations
- Antibacterials
- Antifungals
- Corticosteroid Plus Antimicrobial Preparations
- Antiparasitic Preparations

LEARNING OBJECTIVES

After studying this chapter, you should be able to

1. Describe the clinical indications for common ophthalmic and otic agents.
2. Describe the products used to diagnose ocular problems.
3. Identify the different classes of ophthalmic and otic agents.
4. Identify the possible adverse reactions and contraindications of many commonly used agents.

INTRODUCTION

The sense of smell is highly developed in animals, but the sense of sight also plays an important role in an animal's health and well-being. Cats rely on excellent eyesight because they are animals of prey. This prey trait can provide cat owners with much laughter as a string or a feather toy is pulled around the house. Horses rely on good eyesight to perform their best in equestrian events. Police dogs, hunting dogs, seeing-eye dogs, and herd dogs rely on their eyesight to interpret hand signals when working in the field.

An ophthalmic examination includes the use of diagnostic agents to determine any ocular problems that may be present in the patient. Additionally, an examination of the ocular features (eyelids, eyelashes, sclera, cornea, third eyelid [i.e., nictitating membrane]), pupil, anterior chamber, iris, and lens), all of which can be seen without highly specialized equipment (McCurnin, 2006), are also important to evaluate. Some dog breeds (shar-pei, cocker spaniels, English bulldogs, and others) are genetically predisposed to conditions that may require cosmetic surgery to correct faults. Three of these conditions are known as **entropion, ectropion,** and **distichiasis.**

Topical administration of eye drops or ointment is the most common method of treatment involving disorders of the eye. It is the veterinary technician's duty to educate the client by demonstrating the proper way to administer eye medication. Products for ocular treatment are usually available as solutions or ointments. Drug penetration is one factor that veterinarians must consider when choosing a topical ophthalmic agent. Topical agents are more readily absorbed into the anterior chamber than the posterior chamber. For this reason, these agents have limited use in posterior eye disorders. Systemic

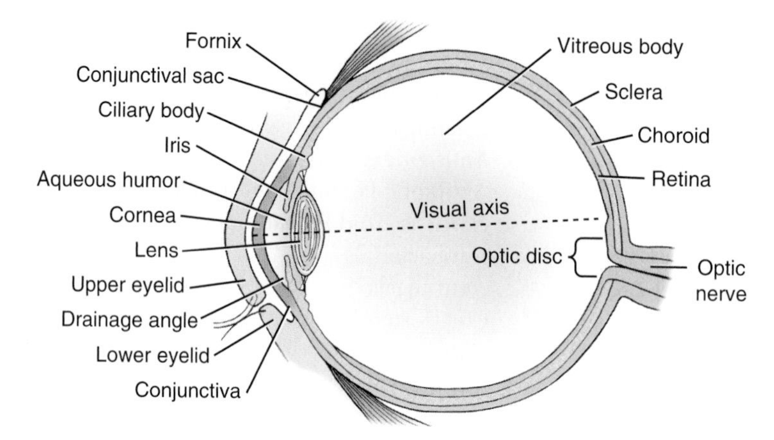

FIGURE 10-1 Internal structures of the eyeball.

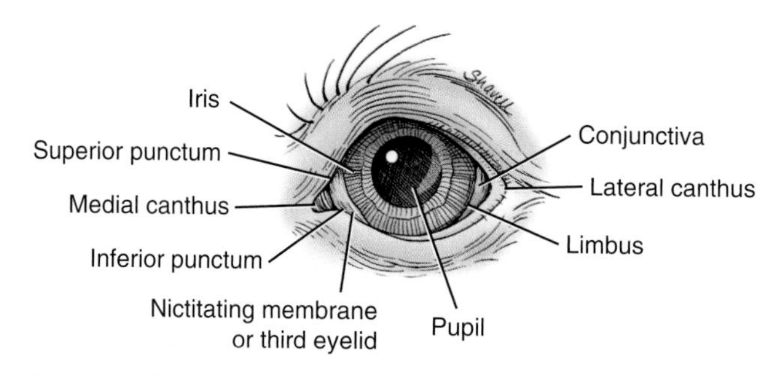

FIGURE 10-2 External structures of the eye.

agents may be more effective. Lipid-soluble agents readily penetrate the corneal epithelium and endothelium layers. Water-soluble agents readily penetrate the corneal stroma layer (Figures 10-1 and 10-2). Most topical ophthalmic medications require several applications per day because the eye continuously secretes tears that wash away the medication. Ointments tend to necessitate less frequent applications than drops. However, ointments may blur an animal's vision for a short period after application. Recently, some clinicians believe that ophthalmic drops may be more effective than ointments.

Client education is invaluable for proper treatment of an eye disorder. It is important that clients understand that the applicator tip of the drug's container should not touch the eye's surface or the conjunctiva because bacteria from the patient's eye may contaminate the remaining drug contents inside the container. This is also important to remember when veterinary personnel are treating several patients in a veterinary hospital with the same drug container.

Clients placing telephone calls to the veterinary hospital to discuss a potential eye problem in a companion animal should be made to realize that these situations may be considered an emergency. Unfortunately, some clients tend to let an ocular problem progress to severe stages before treatment is sought. Veterinary technicians should remind clients that animals have only two eyes and the importance of vision should not be minimized.

DIAGNOSTIC AGENTS

The use of diagnostic agents to determine what problems may exist with the eyes is an important part of the ophthalmic examination. Some diagnostic agents should be used before others so that results are not misinterpreted.

TECHNICIAN NOTES The Schirmer tear test is one of the first diagnostic procedures to be employed so that tear evaluation is calculated correctly.

TECHNICIAN NOTES If a bacterial culture is indicated, the culture should be obtained before cleaning the eye or administering other ophthalmic drugs. Therefore, an eye examination should be carried out in a methodical manner in order for a proper diagnosis to be made.

Fluorescein Sodium

Clinical Uses

Fluorescein stain is commonly used to stain the patient's cornea in cases in which a corneal ulcer is suspected. The stain fluoresces, and if a corneal ulcer is present it can be observed with the use of a cobalt blue filter and a light source. The corneal epithelium will not stain because the corneal stroma, which is a lipid membrane, repels the stain. Fluorescein stain is also used to diagnose patency of the nasolacrimal outflow duct.

Dosage Forms

Fluorescein stain is manufactured on paper strips.

- Ful-Glo
- Fluor-I-Strip
- Bio-Glo

TECHNICIAN NOTES

- Do not allow the fluorescein strip to touch the cornea because this could potentially produce a paper cut on the cornea.
- Obtain a sterile 6-mL syringe and place the fluorescein strip into the syringe barrel. Fill the syringe with sterile water and replace the plunger. Invert the syringe several times until the water turns yellow. Simply administer this solution into the eye for the staining procedure.
- Horses have strong palpebral muscles. If stain is to be used in this species, it may be necessary to have another person keep the eyelids spread apart while the stain is introduced into the eye.
- Fluorescein stains the hair if allowed to drain on the face. Use cotton to wipe away excess fluorescein stain because it is softer than a paper towel.
- Use care to prevent the stain from causing temporary staining of the patient's fur, as this may make some owners unhappy (especially on white-coated breeds that have just been groomed).

Lissamine Green

Clinical Uses

Lissamine green is used to diagnose corneal damage and to quantify tear production. This product does not sting like Rose Bengal, but interpretation requires more experience. Fluorescein stain is a more reliable indicator of corneal damage.

Dosage Form

- Manufactured on paper strips

Adverse Side Effects

Side effects are uncommon.

Phenol Red Thread

Clinical Uses

This product is used to evaluate tear production. Phenol red thread is a new accurate way to measure tear production as compared with the Schirmer tear test.

Dosage Form

- A long (75-mm) yellow-colored thread impregnated with phenol red, which is a sensitive pH indicator (Zone-Quick Diagnostic Threads)

Adverse Side Effects

Side effects are uncommon.

Rose Bengal

Clinical Uses

Rose bengal is used most commonly to detect the presence of viral **keratitis** in felines. It can also be used to evaluate corneal epithelium that may be damaged due to keratoconjunctivitis sicca (KCS).

Dosage Forms

- Manufactured by Akorn as a solution or an impregnated strip (Rosets)

Adverse Side Effects
This product may be toxic to the cornea and should be thoroughly flushed from the eye to prevent irritation. Hypersensitivity reactions may occur. It may also stain clothing.

Schirmer Tear Test
Clinical Uses
It is used clinically to measure tear production.

Dosage Forms
Paper strips inserted near the lateral canthus of the eye and adjacent to the conjunctiva
- Schirmer Tear Test
- Clement Clarke Schirmer Tear Test Strips—human label

Adverse Side Effects
These are uncommon.

OCULAR ANESTHETICS

Ocular anesthetics are used during tonometry or for relief of corneal pain during performance of an ocular examination.

Proparacaine HCl
Clinical Uses
Proparacaine HCl is a topical anesthetic used for a variety of ophthalmic procedures. Proparacaine should be protected from light and should be refrigerated.

Dosage Forms
Drops placed in the eye
- Ophthaine
- Ophthetic
- Alcaine
- AK-Taine

Adverse Side Effects
Side effects are uncommon.

Tetracaine HCl
Clinical Uses
Tetracaine HCl is used to produce local anesthesia of short duration for ophthalmic procedures.

Dosage Forms
Drops placed in the eye
- Ocu-Caine
- Spectro-Caine

Adverse Side Effects
Tetracaine may be more irritating than proparacaine; it is only sometimes used in veterinary medicine. Prolonged use may cause delayed wound healing and corneal ulcers and may retard the blink reflex. Repeated use may cause development of tolerance to the drug.

Benoxinate
Benoxinate is supplied as drops for topical anesthesia of the eye. This drug is a human product and has not been evaluated for use in veterinary medicine.

PARASYMPATHOMIMETICS

These are also known as *miotics.* Parasympathomimetics are used to induce contraction of the intraocular smooth muscle (miosis), which helps to reduce intraocular pressure (IOP).

Carbachol
Clinical Uses
Carbachol may be used to cause miosis in the treatment of glaucoma. Veterinary ophthalmologists may also use it at the conclusion of cataract removal to prevent cases of postoperative increased IOP.

Dosage Forms
Intracameral injection
- Carbastat
- Miostat Intraocular
- Isopto Carbachol
- Carboptic

Adverse Side Effects
In humans, the following have been reported: headaches, muscle spasms of accommodation, retinal detachment, and iritis (postoperatively).

Pilocarpine HCl

Clinical Uses

Pilocarpine is a cholinergic agonist (miotic) that is sometimes used in the treatment of canine primary glaucoma. It may be used orally as a primary treatment of neurogenic KCS in dogs because this condition does not respond to cyclosporine or tacrolimus (Plumb, 2011).

Dosage Forms

Various solutions and gels

- Isopto Carpine
- Ocu-Carpine
- Piloptic
- Pilostat

Adverse Side Effects

In humans, pilocarpine may cause local irritation, miosis, decreased visual ability, inflammation of the **uveal** tract (especially with repeated doses), and **hyphema**. This drug should not be used in secondary glaucoma cases. With repeated use, it may cause vomiting, diarrhea, increased salivation, bronchiolar spasm, and pulmonary edema.

Demecarium Bromide

Clinical Uses

Used to reduce IOPs for up to 48 hours in dogs. Causes miosis. Generally, this drug is used to manage potential glaucoma in the eye opposite from which a diagnosis of an acute congestive crisis of primary glaucoma is made.

Dosage Form

- Ophthalmic drops (Humorsol)

Adverse Side Effects

Do not use in pregnant animals. Use with caution when other cholinesterase inhibitors are used. May cause ciliary muscle spasm, headache, blurred vision, local inflammation, vomiting, diarrhea, increased salivation, and cardiac effect especially when used in high doses in small breed dogs.

SYMPATHOMIMETICS

These are also known as *alpha$_2$-agonists.* Sympathomimetic drugs decrease IOP. Long-term use may result in an increase in uveoscleral outflow.

Apraclonidine

Clinical Uses

Apraclonidine is used to reduce aqueous humor formation. Effects are usually noted 3 to 5 hours after a single dose.

Dosage Forms

- Ophthalmic solution (Iopidine)

TECHNICIAN NOTES Do not use apraclonidine in cats.

Brimonidine

Clinical Uses

Brimonidine has a longer duration of action than does apraclonidine. It reduces aqueous humor formation and increases uveoscleral outflow.

Dosage Forms

Ophthalmic solution

- Alphagan P
- Combigan

Adverse Side Effects

Animals seem to better tolerate side effects from brimonidine than from apraclonidine. In humans, allergic **conjunctivitis**, eye itching, oral dryness, and visual disturbance have been noted.

Epinephrine

Clinical Uses

Epinephrine is used clinically as an **intracameral injection** to cause **mydriasis** and to prevent bleeding after intraocular surgical procedures.

Dosage Forms

Topical ophthalmic solution

- Epifrin
- Glaucon
- Eppy/N
- Epinal

Adverse Side Effects

These include possible eye irritation at administration.

BETA-ADRENERGIC ANTAGONISTS

These drugs aid in reducing IOP.

Timolol

Clinical Uses

Timolol is primarily used to prevent glaucoma from developing in the contralateral eye of a dog that has primary glaucoma in one eye. The drug reduces IOP.

Dosage Forms

Ophthalmic solution; no veterinary product is available

- Timoptic—human label
- Istalol—human label

Adverse Side Effects

These include miosis in dogs and cats to a slight degree.

> *TECHNICIAN NOTES* Caution should be used if timolol is prescribed for cats with asthma.

CARBONIC ANYHYDRASE INHIBITORS

These drugs are most useful in treating primary **open-angle glaucoma** and secondary glaucoma in humans.

Brinzolamide HCl

Clinical Uses

Brinzolamide reduces aqueous humor production.

Dosage Forms

- Ophthalmic topical solution (Azopt)

Adverse Side Effects

Because cats seem to be quite sensitive to dorzolamide, brinzolamide can sometimes be used.

Dorzolamide HCl

Clinical Uses

This drug is often used in the contralateral eye of a dog with primary glaucoma to prevent development of bilateral disease. It is also used for secondary glaucoma in dogs and cats because it does not affect pupil size.

Dosage Forms

Ophthalmic topical solution

- Trusopt
- Cosopt

Adverse Side Effects

These may include a stinging sensation in cats. Hypersensitivity may also occur.

PROSTAGLANDINS

These drugs act on prostanoid receptors to lower IOP.

Latanoprost

Clinical Uses

Latanoprost reduces IOP, especially in canine primary glaucoma cases; results are even better when this drug is combined with carbonic anhydrase inhibitors.

Dosage Form

- Latanoprost ophthalmic solution (Xalatan)

Adverse Side Effects

Topical irritation and hyperemia of the conjunctiva may be noted. Various other effects may also occur.

> *TECHNICIAN NOTES*
> - Do not use latanoprost in cats or horses because of adverse side effects.
> - Refrigerate until use; store at room temperature for 6 weeks after opening.

Bimatoprost

Dosage Forms

Ophthalmic drops

- Lumigan
- Latisse

Travoprost

Dosage Form

- Travatan

Unoprostone Isopropyl

Clinical Uses

Clinical uses of unoprostone isopropyl include lowering IOP in dogs. None of the three previously mentioned drugs work very well in cats to reduce IOP.

Dosage Forms

- Not currently available in the United States; may be obtained through importation or through the services of a qualified pharmacy

Adverse Side Effects

It may cause hyperemia of the conjunctiva.

OSMOTIC AGENTS FOR THE TREATMENT OF GLAUCOMA

Osmotic agents increase osmotic pressure of plasma and create a concentration gradient that will draw fluid out of the intraocular environment. These agents are systemically administered with concurrent water deprivation (4 to 6 hours) and are indicated only for acute episodes of **glaucoma** not maintenance (Plumb, 2011).

MYDRIATIC CYCLOPLEGIC VASOCONSTRICTORS

Cyclopentolate

Clinical Uses

This drug is an anticholinergic agent that causes the sphincter of the iris and ciliary muscles to relax. This drug is mainly used to induce mydriasis and **cycloplegia** for diagnostic purposes.

Dosage Forms

Ophthalmic solution

- AK-Pentolate
- Cyclogyl

> *TECHNICIAN NOTES* Cyclopentolate increases IOP and should never be used in animals with glaucoma.

Phenylephrine HCl

Clinical Uses

Phenylephrine is a direct acting, $alpha_1$-agonist vasoconstrictor drug that is commonly used in veterinary medicine to induce mydriasis before cataract removal. This drug can also be used to control bleeding for minor surface procedures. On administration, phenylephrine HCl lasts approximately 2 to 18 hours. It can be used in the treatment of **Horner's syndrome.**

Dosage Form

- Ophthalmic solution (Neo-Synephrine)

Adverse Side Effects

Local irritation may occur. In cats and rabbits, stromal clouding may occur if the corneal epithelium is damaged.

Atropine Sulfate

Clinical Uses

Atropine controls pain caused by corneal and/or uveal disease. It may be used to dilate the pupil for an ophthalmic examination or before ophthalmic surgery.

Dosage Forms

- Manufactured as an ophthalmic solution or ophthalmic ointment (Atrophate)

Adverse Side Effects

This drug causes mydriasis and accommodation paralysis. Hypersalivation may occur in cats when atropine drops are administered. Atropine can cause a decrease in tear production in small animals. In horses, repeated treatment with atropine may cause colic, although this is rare.

> *TECHNICIAN NOTES*
> - In the dog, dilation may persist for up to 120 hours.
>
> Dogs and cats should be placed in darkened quarters until the pupil is at its normal size.
> - Ointments or drops may be used in dogs.
> - Atropine is very long lasting when used in horses, and dilation may last for days to weeks.
> - Do not use in patients with primary glaucoma.
> - Atropine ointment should be used in cats to prevent hypersalivation caused by the bitter taste of atropine drops.

Tropicamide

Clinical Uses

This drug causes mydriasis more than cycloplegic activity of the eye. Tropicamide has a more rapid onset of action and a shorter duration of action than atropine. This drug's effects make it useful for funduscopic examinations. In dogs, IOP does not seem to be affected by the action of tropicamide.

Dosage Forms

Ophthalmic solution

- Mydriacyl
- Opticyl
- Tropicacyl

Adverse Side Effects

Side effects include less effective pain control than atropine; hypersalivation, especially in cats; stinging of the eye on administration; and acute congestive glaucoma in some patients.

ANTIINFLAMMATORY/ANALGESIC OPHTHALMIC AGENTS

Cromolyn Sodium

Clinical Uses

Cromolyn sodium is a mast cell stabilizing agent. This drug blocks the release of histamine from mast cells after antigen recognition. This drug is particularly useful in treating patients with allergic conjunctivitis and may help alleviate seasonal allergies affecting the eyes.

Dosage Form

- Ophthalmic solution (Crolom)

Adverse Side Effects

In humans, a stinging sensation has been reported at administration.

Lodoxamide Tromethamine

Clinical Uses

This drug is used for treating allergies of the eyes. It may be used in horses and small animal patients.

Dosage Form

- Ophthalmic product (Alomide)

Adverse Side Effects

Lodoxamide may produce a stinging sensation on administration of the drug.

Olopatadine HCl

Clinical Uses

This drug is used to stop the symptoms of ocular allergies.

Dosage Form

- Ophthalmic solution (Patanol)

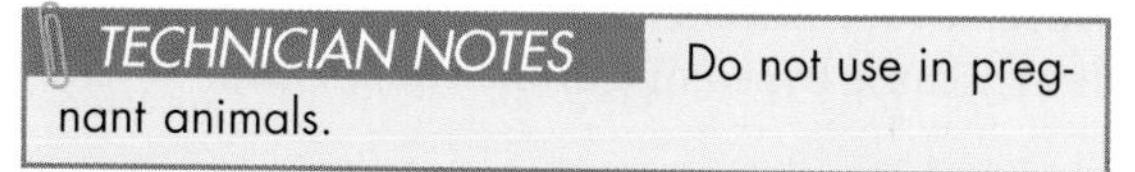

TECHNICIAN NOTES Do not use in pregnant animals.

NONSTEROIDAL ANATIINFLAMMATORY AGENTS

Nonsteroidal antiinflammatory drugs (NSAIDs) are used in veterinary medicine to control inflammation and to provide pain relief. They may be used postoperatively to help the cornea to heal. Additionally, they may also be used to treat allergic conjunctivitis.

Clinical Uses

Bromfenac is used after cataract removal to minimize inflammation. Diclofenac sodium is used for the treatment of **uveitis**. Diclofenac is the drug of choice in diabetic patients whose insulin regulation could be altered by the systemic uptake of topical corticosteroids (Plumb, 2011). Flurbiprofen sodium may be useful in the management of uveal inflammation, especially if topical steroids are also used. Ketorolac tromethamine is most commonly used to control surgical or nonsurgical uveitis, especially in cases with corneal bacterial infection or ulceration. Nepafenac is used in veterinary medicine to control the pain and inflammation that accompanies cataract surgery. Suprofen may be useful in the management of uveal inflammation.

Dosage Forms

Ophthalmic solution

- Bromfenac (Xibrom)
- Diclofenac sodium (Voltaren)
- Flurbiprofen sodium (Ocufen)
- Ketorolac tromethamine (Acular)

- Nepafenac (Nevanac)
- Suprofen (Profenal)

Adverse Side Effects

Bromfenac is not to be used in patients with known hypersensitivity to any ingredient found in bromfenac. Do not use flurbiprofen in patients with infected corneal ulcers because this drug can be as immunosuppressive as topical corticosteroids. Nepafenac may cause bleeding of ocular tissues. All topical NSAIDs may slow healing time. Other adverse reactions also exist.

STEROIDAL ANTIINFLAMMATORY AGENTS

This group of drugs is used to treat diseases of the eye that may include the conjunctiva, the sclera, the cornea, and the anterior chamber. For maximum results from these agents, the frequency of administration should be increased instead of increasing the drug's concentration. Some side effects may occur when steroidal antiinflammatory agents are used. These are more common in humans than in animals but may include the development of cataracts, increased IOP, infection, decreased wound healing, mydriasis, and calcific keratopathy. These drugs should not be used to treat conjunctivitis in cats.

Prednisolone

Clinical Uses

This drug is typically used in the treatment of anterior uveitis.

Dosage Forms

Suspension drops

- Pred Mild
- Econopred
- Econopred Plus
- Pred Forte
- Mydrapred

Adverse Side Effects

These are uncommon.

Dexamethasone

Clinical Uses

This drug is used for antiinflammatory purposes.

Dosage Forms

Manufactured as an ophthalmic solution and ophthalmic ointment.

Betamethasone

Clinical Uses

Antimicrobial-steroid combination.

Dosage Form

- Ophthalmic drops (Gentocin Durafilm)

TECHNICIAN NOTES

- Never use this product if corneal ulceration or abrasion is suspected.
- Do not use to treat herpes keratitis in cats.

Fluorometholone

Clinical Uses

This drug is used for antiinflammatory purposes.

Dosage Forms

Manufactured as an ophthalmic ointment and ophthalmic suspension

- FML S.O.P.
- FML Forte
- FML
- Flarex

Adverse Side Effects

High concentrations of this drug may raise IOP.

Loteprednol

Clinical Uses

Loteprednol is used for antiinflammatory purposes. It is not apt to raise IOP.

Dosage Forms

Ophthalmic suspension

- Lotemax
- Alrex

Rimexolone

Dosage Form

- Ophthalmic suspension (Vexol)

OPHTHALMIC ANALGESICS

These agents are for eye pain relief.

Morphine Sulfate

Clinical Use

Morphine sulfate is used for corneal ulcer pain relief and may also be used to lessen **blepharospasms.** Morphine sulfate is a Class II controlled substance.

Dosage Forms

- No veterinary- or human-label products available
- May be compounded as a 1% solution

ANTIMICROBIAL OPHTHALMIC THERAPY

Antimicrobials aid in the treatment and management of ocular disease.

Amikacin Sulfate

Clinical Uses

This drug is useful in the treatment of corneal infections, as well as in treating endophthalmitis. It does not cause retinal toxic effects.

Dosage Forms

- Not available as a veterinary- or human-label drug
- Must be compounded into a topical preparation at 8 mg/mL (Plumb, 2011)

Neomycin Sulfate

Clinical Uses

This drug is useful in treating superficial corneal ulcers or infections of the ocular surface.

Dosage Forms

This drug is manufactured as an ophthalmic ointment or ophthalmic solution. Most are a combination of bacitracin/neomycin/polymyxin B.

- Mycitracin
- Neobacimyx
- TriOptic
- Vetropolycin
- Optiprime

Adverse Side Effects

The neomycin in this product may cause contact sensitivity and should not be used in patients with a history of this problem.

Gentamicin Sulfate

Clinical Use

This drug is most commonly used for keratitis caused by *Pseudomonas aeruginosa.*

Dosage Forms

- Ophthalmic ointment and ophthalmic solution available (Gentocin)

Tobramycin Sulfate

Clinical Uses

This is an antimicrobial product.

Dosage Forms

Manufactured as an ophthalmic ointment and ophthalmic solution

- No veterinary-label products available
- Tobrex—human label

Adverse Side Effects

Systemic use of this drug is not beneficial in ocular infections.

Ocular Fluoroquinolones

Clinical Uses

These drugs are used for bactericidal purposes. Fluoroquinolones are commonly used against gram-negative corneal infections that have established themselves in the eye.

Dosage Forms

- Ciprofloxacin (Ciloxan)
- Gatifloxacin (Zymar)
- Levofloxacin (Quixin)
- Norfloxacin (Chibroxin)
- Ofloxacin (Ocuflox)

Adverse Side Effects

These drugs should not be used prophylactically before or after surgery. They may cause retinal neurotoxicity in cats if administered systemically. These drugs may cause crusting around the superficial part of corneal defects, conjunctival hyperemia, bad taste in the mouth, foreign body itching sensation, photophobia, edema of the eyelid(s), keratitis, and nausea. Some allergic reactions have been reported.

MISCELLANEOUS OCULAR ANTIBIOTICS

Chloramphenicol

Clinical Uses

This is a broad-spectrum antibiotic that is able to cross the corneal barrier and gain entrance into the anterior chamber. (Very few infections, however, happen in the anterior chamber.) Generally speaking, *Staphylococcus* spp. and *Streptococcus* spp. are destroyed by chloramphenicol, but *Pseudomonas* spp. are resistant to it.

Dosage Forms

- Chloromycetin
- Chloroptic

Polymyxin B

Clinical Uses

This drug is a surface detergent (cationic). Its efficacy is against gram-negative organisms and can be combined with other antimicrobials with gram-positive activity.

Dosage Form

- Terramycin Ophthalmic Ointment

Sulfacetamide

Clinical Uses

This drug is useful in the treatment of conjunctivitis and superficial eye infections.

Dosage Forms

No veterinary products are available.

- Sulf-10—human label
- AK-Sulf—human label
- Bleph-10—human label

Adverse Side Effects

Side effects include GI disturbances, allergies, renal damage, and damage to lacrimal acinar cells. This drug is contraindicated in patients with hypersensitivity problems or in patients with blood dyscrasias.

> *TECHNICIAN NOTES* Warn owners who may be allergic to sulfa.

Vancomycin

Clinical Uses

This drug is used in rabbits to treat methicillin-resistant *Staphylococcus aureus* **(MRSA).**

Dosage Forms

- Must be compounded

> *TECHNICIAN NOTES* This should be the last drug of choice because it has a high potential for ototoxicity (leading to deafness) and nephrotoxicity that can lead to death.

OCULAR ANTIFUNGALS

Aspergillus is a common pathogen causing fungal keratitis in horses. These drugs are used to treat fungal infections in animals.

Amphotericin B

Clinical Uses

This is a broad-spectrum antifungal agent (derived from *Streptomyces nodosus*) used to treat equine fungal keratitis.

Dosage Forms

- No veterinary-label products
- Must be prepared by reconstituting commercially available amphotericin B with sterile water

> *TECHNICIAN NOTES* Do not reconstitute amphotericin B with sodium chloride because it may cause degradation of the drug. Only reconstitute with sterile water.

Natamycin

Clinical Uses

This drug is used to treat fungal keratitis.

Dosage Form

- Ophthalmic suspension (Natacyn)

Adverse Side Effects

Natamycin may cause worsening of corneal edema.

Povidone Iodine

Clinical Uses

This drug can be used for chemical débridement of loose epithelium in canine ulcers.

Dosage Forms

- Must be compounded and diluted from commercially available povidone iodine 10% solutions

Adverse Side Effects

These solutions need to be lavaged from the eye after no more than 5 minutes to prevent corneal epithelial damage.

Silver Sulfadiazine

Dosage Forms

- Ophthalmic aqueous cream base sometimes dispensed aseptically in single-use tuberculin syringes for application to the conjunctival sac
- Silvadene
- Flint SSD

Adverse Side Effects

This product is not labeled for use in the eye. The drug insert specifically states, "not to be used in the eyes" (Plumb, 2011). Therefore, liability for use in the eyes rests solely with the prescribing doctor.

Itraconazole

Clinical Uses

This is a broad-spectrum antifungal agent. Itraconazole is insoluble in water and must be diluted in dimethyl sulfoxide (DMSO) in order to form a solution for instillation into the eyes. This drug may be used in horses to treat fungal keratitis.

Dosage Forms

- Must be compounded by a reputable pharmacy

Adverse Side Effects

Personnel treating horses with this drug should wear gloves to avoid having their skin absorb the DMSO.

OCULAR ANTIVIRALS

These drugs are most commonly used to treat feline ocular herpes virus infections.

Trifluridine

Clinical Uses

This drug is used to treat feline herpes virus infections of the eye. This agent may also be used to treat superficial punctate keratitis in equines, which is thought to occur due to equine herpes virus (EHV-2), which may cause problems with the cornea.

Dosage Forms

Ophthalmic solution

- Trifluorothymidine (Viroptic)

Adverse Side Effects

Trifluridine must be administered quite frequently to obtain acceptable results. If cats do not respond well within a 3-week period, they are not likely to respond to this drug at all. Therefore, use should be discontinued. The conjunctiva and eyelid margins may be irritated in cats during therapy with this drug.

Idoxuridine

Clinical Uses

This drug may be used to treat herpes virus infections of the eye in cats.

Dosage Forms

- No veterinary products exist
- Must be compounded by a qualified pharmacy for ophthalmic ointment to be created

Interferon Alpha

Clinical Uses

This drug is used to treat feline herpes viral keratitis.

Dosage Form

- Intron-A—human label

Acyclovir, Valacyclovir, Famciclovir, Ganciclovir, Cidofovir, and Penciclovir

These drugs are used in the treatment of feline herpes ocular virus. Cats are sensitive to acyclovir and valacyclovir; these drugs may cause fatal myeloid dysplasia in the species. Famciclovir should be used in cats with extreme caution because the pharmacokinetics of this drug are extremely complex (Plumb, 2011).

DRUGS FOR KERATOCONJUNCTIVITIS SICCA

KCS is a common disorder in dogs, and it is believed from recent research that the disease may be due to an immune-mediated disease process.

Cyclosporine

Clinical Uses

Cyclosporine is used in the treatment of KCS. Reported success rates with this drug in stopping the signs of KCS are 75% to 80%. Cyclosporine is also used in the treatment of pannus.

Dosage Forms

Ophthalmic ointment

- Optimmune
- Restasis—human label

Adverse Side Effects

Patients are usually given this drug for life to keep KCS symptoms under control. If the therapy is stopped, the clinical signs often return.

Tacrolimus

Clinical Uses

Tacrolimus was originally studied at the University of Tennessee College of Veterinary Medicine. Investigators there found this drug to be as equally effective as cyclosporine and effective for cyclosporine-resistant cases of KCS.

Dosage Form

- Must be compounded by a qualified compounding pharmacy

Pimecrolimus

This drug is also used in dogs with KCS.

OCULAR LUBRICANTS/ARTIFICIAL TEAR PRODUCTS

These agents are used as a lubricant for dry eyes, to relieve eye irritation, and are also used during anesthetic periods when the patient's eyes remain open and tear production is reduced.

Artificial Tears

- Adsorbotear
- Comfort Tears
- GenTeal
- Isopto-Tears
- Tears Naturale
- Lacril
- Various others

Ophthalmic Irrigants

The main purpose of these agents is to maintain the shape of the anterior chamber during cataract surgery.

ANTICOLLAGENASE AGENTS

These agents are used to stop the melting effect of collagenases and proteases on the cornea.

Acetylcysteine

Dosage Form

- No veterinary product is available
- Mucomyst—human label

Edetate Disodium

Clinical Uses

This drug is used to stop the melting effect of collagenases and proteases on the cornea but are not useful for melting caused by infectious agents.

Dosage Form

- No veterinary product is available

OTIC DRUGS

When a client obtains a new puppy, the veterinary technician should demonstrate the proper way to clean the pup's ears. Performance of the ear cleaning process at an early age will allow the puppy to submit more readily to the task as an adult dog. Unfortunately, those breeds with pendulous ears may tend to have otic problems. Long ear flaps (i.e., pinnae) tend to keep air from circulating into the external ear canal; consequently, the ear canal remains moist, which creates a perfect environment for yeast formation. Yeast is not the only problem that veterinarians encounter in dogs and cats. External parasites such as *Otodectes cynotis* (i.e., ear mites) can cause extreme discomfort in animals that are infested by these creatures. Patients whose ears remain untreated often experience aural hematomas caused by extreme shaking of the head and scratching of the ears. (Hendrix. 1998)

Generally, ear problems are treated with topical medications. Sometimes, ear infections also must be treated with systemic medications. Topical preparations used to treat ear infections are often a combination of different types of drugs, such as antibacterial, antifungal, antipruritic, and antiinflammatory agents. Still other preparations are cleansers, drying agents, and parasiticides.

> **TECHNICIAN NOTES** When a ruptured eardrum is suspected or confirmed, oil-based or irritating external ear preparations (e.g., chlorhexidine) and aminoglycosides should be avoided (Figure 10-3).

Ceruminolytic Agents

Clinical Uses

These products emulsify **cerumen** and purulent exudate. They work by providing a surfactant, detergent, and bubbling action. Do not use these products in patients with ruptured ear drum(s).

Dosage Forms

- ADL Foaming Ear Cleanser
- Cerumene
- CleaRx Ear Cleaning Solution
- Corium-20
- KlearOtic Ear Cleanser
- Douxo Micellar Solution
- Ear Cleansing Solution
- Earoxide Ear Cleanser
- OtiFoam

Cleaning/Drying Agents

Clinical Uses

These products are used after cleaning of the ears has occurred. These agents can be used as maintenance agents to prevent ear infections after swimming or bathing.

Dosage Forms

- ADL Ear Flushing Drying Lotion
- AloCetic Ear Rinse

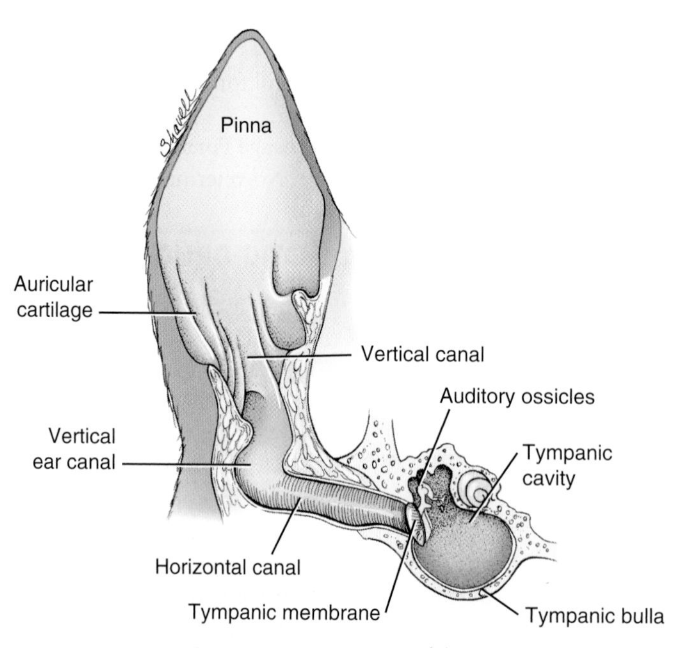

FIGURE 10-3 Structures of the ear.

- CleaRx Ear Drying Solution
- Corium-20
- Domeboro Otic—human product
- Ear Cleansing Solution
- Epi-Otic cleanser with Spherulites
- Epi-Otic Advanced
- Euclens Otic Cleanser
- Gent-L-Clens
- MalAcetic Otic
- OtiCalm
- Oti-Clens
- Oti-Soothe with aloe vera
- Oti-Soothe with cucumber melon
- OtiRinse solution
- OtoCetic solution

Antiseptic Agents

Clinical Uses

These products are commonly used with other products to help heal ear infections. Chlorhexidine-containing products should be used carefully in animals with ruptured tympanic membranes.

Dosage Forms

- Acetic Acid 2% in Aqueous Aluminum Acetate Otic Solution
- MalAcetic Otic
- MalAcetic Ultra Otic
- Mal-A-Ket Plus TrizEDTA Flush
- OtoCetic Solution

Antibiotic Potentiating Agents

Clinical Uses

Tromethamine-ethylenediaminetetraacetic acid (tris-EDTA) has antimicrobial and antibiotic potentiating activity. It is nonototoxic and safe to use in the middle ear. These products work better when used 15 to 30 minutes before a topical antibiotic.

Dosage Forms

- KetoTRIS Flush
- Mal-A-Ket Plus TrizEDTA Flush
- TrizEDTA Aqueous or Crystals
- TrizULTRA + Keto
- TrizChlor
- T8 Keto Flush
- T8 Solution Ear Rinse

Corticosteroid Preparations

Clinical Uses

These products are used in cases of acute or chronic otitis. They help to reduce the buildup of sebaceous and apocrine gland secretion.

Dosage Forms

- CleaRx Drying Solution
- Cort/Astrin Solution
- MalAcetic Ultra Otic
- Synotic Otic Solution

Antibacterials

Clinical Uses

Many antibacterials used in the ears are designed to treat infections caused by *Staphylococcus* spp. or *Pseudomonas* spp. Very few products contain an antibiotic to treat bacterial otitis; therefore the veterinarian may resort to using ophthalmic products or injectable antibiotics directly into the ear canal to treat such infections.

Dosage Forms

- Baytril Otic
- Gentamicin Ophthalmic Solution
- Tobrex Ophthalmic Solution

Antifungals

Clinical Uses

These are mainly used to treat *Malassezia* otitis and sometimes otic candidiasis.

Dosage Forms

- ClotrimaTop Solution
- Clotrimazole Solution
- Lotrimin Solution
- MicaVed Lotion
- Micazole Lotion
- Miconosol Lotion
- Priconazole Lotion

Corticosteroid Plus Antimicrobial Preparations

Clinical Uses

These products are used in cases of acute and chronic otitis. They help reduce inflammation, decrease edema, tissue hyperplasia, pain, and pruritis, and to help eliminate any infectious organisms that may be present.

Dosage Forms

- Antibiotic Ear Solution
- Cortisporin Otic Suspension
- Cortomycin
- Oti-Sone Otic Suspension
- PediOtic Suspension
- Betagen Otic Solution
- GenOne Otic Solution
- Gentaotic
- GentaVed Otic Solution
- Topagen Ointment
- Animax Ointment
- Derma Vet Ointment
- Dermalog Ointment
- Dermalone Ointment
- Quadritop Ointment
- Panalog Ointment
- MoMetaMax Otic Suspension

Antiparasitic Preparations

Clinical Uses

The following preparations are designed for use inside the ears to stop **otoacariasis**. Because *O. cynotis* are known to live outside the ears and can reinfest the ears, products such as selamectin or fipronil are preferred (Plumb, 2011).

Dosage Forms

- Acarexx Otic Suspension
- Adams Pene-Mite
- Cerumite 3x
- Cooper's Best Ear Mite Lotion
- Ear Mite Solution
- Ear Miticide
- EarMed Mite Lotion
- Eradimite
- MilbeMite Otic
- Mita-Clear Lotion
- Otomite Plus
- Performer Ear Mite Killer
- QuadraClear Ear Drops

REVIEW QUESTIONS

1. Mydriatic agents are used to __________________ the pupils.
2. Atropine is contraindicated in __________________ and __________________.
3. Miotic agents produce __________________ __________________ constriction.
4. Why are ophthalmic stains used? __________ __________________
5. ______ stain is the most commonly used dye for the detection of corneal epithelial defects.
6. Patients with ear mites, whose ears are left untreated, often experience ______________ hematomas caused by excessive shaking of the head.
7. What type of administration is the most common method of treating disorders of the eye? __________________
8. Why do most topical ophthalmic medications require several applications per day? __________________
9. What is Ophthaine used for? __________________
10. The appearance of fluorescein stain at the nostril opening is an abnormal finding when a fluorescein stain test is performed.
    a. True
    b. False
11. The nictitating membrane is also known as __________________.
    a. sclera
    b. cornea
    c. third eyelid
    d. ciliary body
12. Mydriatic agents are used to ______________ the pupils.
    a. dilate
    b. constrict
    c. hydrate
    d. teach

13. Atropine ophthalmic agents are used to produce __________________.
a. miosis
b. mydriasis

14. Epinephrine is contraindicated in _________-angle glaucoma.
a. closed
b. open

15. Mannitol is a loop diuretic.
a. True
b. False

16. The local anesthesia provided by proparacaine HCl usually lasts ___ to ___ minutes.
a. 5; 10
b. 30; 60
c. 60; 90
d. 90; 120

17. Fluorescein stain is used commonly to diagnose _____________.
a. glaucoma
b. corneal ulcers
c. entropion
d. ectropion

18. _______________ have very strong palpebral muscles, and it may be necessary to have another person assist when one is applying ophthalmic drugs.
a. Canines
b. Felines
c. Equines
d. Caprines

19. It is acceptable to use corticosteroid-type ointments in patients with corneal ulcers.
a. True
b. False

20. __________________ has been developed for the treatment of *Otodectes* spp.
a. Chloramphenicol
b. Enrofloxacin
c. Optimmune
d. Acarexx

21. How many milligrams of tropicamide are in a 0.5% solution?
a. 50 mg
b. 500 mg
c. 5 mg
d. 0.5 mg

22. If the veterinarian prescribes amphotericin B in a 0.15% solution for ocular administration at a rate of 0.2 mL in the eye every 4 hours for 14 days, how much solution should be prepared for the patient?
a. 8.4 mL
b. 4.2 mL
c. 16.8 mL
d. 32.16 mL

23. If proparacaine anesthetizes the cornea for 8 minutes at the usual dose of two drops, how many drops will need to be administered if an ophthalmic procedure takes half an hour?
a. 7.5 drops
b. 5.5 drops
c. 9.5 drops
d. 12.5 drops

24. A veterinary ophthalmologist must perform fluorescein staining on 21 dogs in a 1-week period. How many fluorescein strips need to be on hand to accomplish this task for a month?
a. 64 strips
b. 66 strips
c. 94 strips
d. 84 strips

REFERENCES

Hendrix CM, Robinson E, editors: Diagnostic veterinary parasitology, ed 2, St. Louis, 1998, Mosby.

McCurnin DM, Bassert JM, editors: Clinical textbook for veterinary technicians, ed 6, Philadelphia, 2006, WB Saunders.

Plumb DC: Veterinary drug handbook, ed 7, Ames, Iowa, 2011, Wiley-Blackwell.

CHAPTER

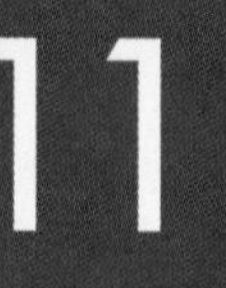

Drugs Used in Skin Disorders

KEY TERMS

Antiseptic
Astringent
Collagen
Comedo (pl. comedones)
Dermatitis
Dermatophyte
Dermatophytosis
Erythema
Fatty acid
Furuncle (furunculosis)
Granulation tissue
Integumentary system
Keratolytic
Keratoplastic
Pruritus
Pseudomembranous colitis
Pyoderma
Seborrhea
Seborrhea oleosa
Seborrhea sicca

OUTLINE

Introduction
Anatomy and Physiology
Wound Healing
TOPICAL ANTIPRURITICS AND ANTIINFLAMMATORIES
- Noncorticosteroids
- Topical Corticosteroids

TOPICAL ANTIMICROBIALS
- Benzoyl Peroxide
- Topical Clindamycin
- Topical Gentamicin Sulfate
- Mupirocin (Pseudomonic Acid A)
- Topical Nitrofurazone
- Silver Sulfadiazine (SSD)

ANTISEPTICS
- Acetic Acid/Boric Acid
- Chlorhexidine
- Chloroxylenol (PCMX)
- Topical Enzymes
- Ethyl Lactate

ANTIFUNGALS
- Enilconazole
- Topical Ketoconazole
- Lime Sulfur
- Topical Miconazole
- Nystatin
- Selenium Sulfide
- Topical Terbinafine HCl
- Salicylic Acid
- Precipitated Sulfur
- Coal Tar

TOPICAL RETINOIDS
- Tretinoin

TOPICAL ANTIPARASITIC AGENTS
- Amitraz
- Crotamiton
- Deltamethrin
- Dinotefuran Plus Pyriproxyfen (Plus Permethrin)
- Fipronil or Fipronil/(S)-Methoprene
- Imidacloprid, Imidacloprid With Permethrin, and Imidacloprid With Moxidectin
- (S)-Methoprene Combinations
- Permethrin
- Topical Pyrethrins and Pyrethrin Combinations
- Topical Pyriproxyfen and Pyriproxyfen Combinations
- Spinetoram

LEARNING OBJECTIVES

After studying this chapter, you should be able to

1. Exhibit a basic understanding of the anatomy and physiology of the skin.
2. List the common ingredients of topical antiseborrheics.
3. Describe the use of topical antipruritics.
4. Explain the use of fatty acid supplements.
5. Explain the use of astringents.
6. Explain the use of skin antiseptics.
7. Exhibit a basic understanding of wound healing.

INTRODUCTION

Dermatologic conditions are frequently seen in veterinary practice. From ectoparasitic problems to allergies, veterinarians are continually combating companion animal skin problems. As a veterinary technician, this is one area in which your expertise will be used because clients will ask many questions about shampoos, dips, conditioners, soaks, lotions, creams, ointments, sprays, powders, and topical products designed to have activity against fleas, ticks, and mosquitoes. Each of these products may be used to treat a full spectrum of dermatologic problems from parasites to **pyoderma.** Patients are often presented for examination of a skin disease when in reality they have an underlying systemic illness. Veterinarians use various diagnostic procedures (e.g., skin scrapings, allergy testing, and **dermatophyte** tests) to determine the cause of skin disease. Technicians play a vital role by obtaining a complete history, knowing how to perform the diagnostic procedures used in a dermatologic workup, and providing client education. Client education is essential when skin disease is treated because clients must understand the purpose of medications and how they should be properly used.

ANATOMY AND PHYSIOLOGY

The skin is a part of the **integumentary system** and constitutes the largest organ in the body. It is made up of three layers (Figure 11-1) and serves multiple functions. It provides a barrier against the outside world by preventing entry of pathogenic microorganisms and by protecting against physical and chemical insults. It senses heat, cold, pain, touch, pressure, and other sensations like **pruritus** and helps to regulate body temperature through mechanisms related to cutaneous blood flow, sweating, and the haircoat. The skin plays a role in immunologic defense through the actions of Langerhans (dendritic or antigen-presenting) cells and keratinocytes, produces vitamin D_3 from precursors in the skin, and acts as a reservoir for electrolytes and other substances. This organ may also play a limited role in the excretion of some substances from the body (Table 11-1).

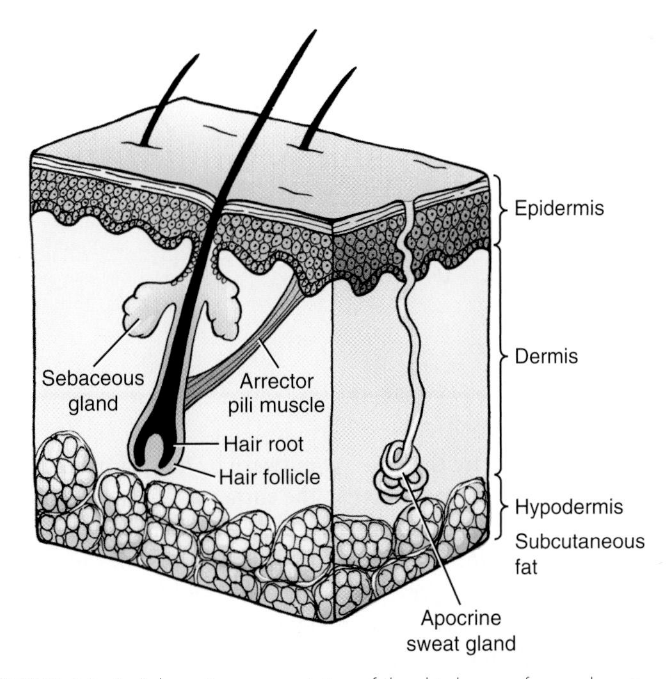

FIGURE 11-1 Schematic representation of the skin layers of normal canine skin.

TABLE 11-1 Common Skin Disorders With Suggested Treatments and Various Products Available

DISEASE	SULFUR	SALICYLIC ACID	COAL TAR	BENZOYL PEROXIDE	CHLORHEXIDINE	HYDROCORTISONE	THERAPEUTIC PRODUCTS
Seborrhea sicca	✓	✓					SebaLyt Shampoo Sebolux Shampoo Allerseb-T Shampoo
Seborrhea oleosa	✓	✓	✓	✓			LyTar Shampoo Pyoben Shampoo SulfOxyDex Shampoo
Hot spots				✓	✓	✓	ChlorHex Shampoo Pyoben Gel Gentocin Topical Spray
Skinfold dermatitis				✓			OxyDex Gel Pyoben Gel
Deep pyoderma				✓			Pyoben Shampoo SulfOxyDex Shampoo Systemic antibiotics
Superficial pustular dermatitis				✓			Pyoben Shampoo OxyDex Shampoo SulfOxyDex Shampoo
Superficial folliculitis				✓	✓		ChlorHex Shampoo Pyoben Shampoo SulfOxyDex Shampoo
Atopy/allergic contact dermatitis	✓	✓	✓			✓	Micro Pearls Advantage Seba-Moist Shampoo DermaCool-HC Spray
Schnauzer comedo syndrome				✓			Micro Pearls Advantage Benzoyl Plus Shampoo OxyDex Shampoo

The three primary layers of the skin are the epidermis, the dermis or corium, and the hypodermis or subcutis (also called the *panniculus*). The dermis provides most of the thickness of the skin. The epidermis comprises five distinct layers. These layers are the basal (deepest), spinous, granular, clear, and horny/cornified (superficial) layers. Epidermal cells are replenished in the basal layer and are pushed outward by newly forming layers. As these cells reach the surface, they are flattened and hardened to form a protective barrier. It normally takes 21 to 22 days for cells to reach the outer layer; this process is called the *epidermal turnover rate.* The epidermal turnover rate may be sped up in some disease processes. Continual shedding of these cells is called *desquamation.* When the process becomes excessive, scale or dandruff is seen. The epidermis includes a population of normal microorganisms that help to prevent overgrowth of pathogenic microorganisms.

The dermis or corium is located directly beneath the epidermis and is separated from and attached to it by the basement membrane. The dermis is a thick layer that comprises collagen fibers, blood vessels, nerves, lymphatics, and other structures such as hair follicles, sebaceous glands, and sweat glands. Sebaceous glands are found throughout haired skin, and their ducts empty into hair shafts. One type of sweat gland (eccrine) is found only in footpads and may play a role in body temperature regulation. The dermis gives stability and flexibility to the skin and acts to maintain and repair the skin.

The hypodermis is the deepest layer of the skin. It is made up of fat and connective tissue. Its functions are to provide padding and insulation and to serve as an energy store.

The skin produces hair and other keratinized structures like nail, horn, nasal pads, and footpads. Hair grows from follicles found in the dermis. In contrast to humans, who have one hair per follicle, dogs and cats have multiple hairs per follicle. Individual hair follicles have associated glandular structures (see earlier) and arrector pili muscles that are responsible for piloerection (hair standing on end). The hair follicle is frequently involved in bacterial, fungal, and demodectic infections. If a hair follicle loses the hair and becomes plugged with sebaceous secretions and keratin, a **comedo** (blackhead) results. There are three stages or phases of hair growth called *anagen* (growth), *telogen* (rest), and *catagen* (intermediate). Hair grows until it reaches a predetermined length, enters a resting phase, and then is shed. The hair cycle is controlled by day–night length (photoperiod), environmental temperature, hormones, and nutritional status. General illness, skin disorders, poor nutrition, overbathing, and stress are conditions that may result in excessive shedding.

WOUND HEALING

A wound is created when an insult—either purposeful, such as surgery, or incidental, such as trauma—disrupts the normal integrity of the tissue (McCurnin and Bassert, 2006).

> *TECHNICIAN NOTES* Normal wound healing can be divided into four stages: inflammation, débridement, repair, and maturation.

However, more than one phase of wound healing usually is occurring at any time (McCurnin and Bassert, 2006). The inflammatory phase usually begins with hemorrhage and is limited by vessel contraction and constriction. Serum leakage into the wound deposits fibrinogen and other clotting elements. Later, this serum provides enzymes, proteins, antibodies, and complement. The débridement phase begins about 6 hours after injury and is facilitated by the appearance of neutrophils and monocytes that migrate to the wound. Neutrophils phagocytize bacteria and then die. Monocytes become macrophages and phagocytize necrotic debris. The repair phase is marked by the formation of a blood clot and is usually active by 3 to 5 days post injury. During the repair phase, fibroblasts produce **collagen** and other connective tissue proteins. Capillaries infiltrate the wound to provide blood supply and oxygen. This process forms **granulation tissue.** Epithelial cells proliferate beneath the scab, and the wound begins to contract. The maturation phase is the end of wound healing and is a period of remodeling. During this time, the wound consolidates and strengthens. Many factors contribute to proper wound healing. These include patient factors (e.g., the age of the patient, nutritional status, rest, environment, and general health); wound factors, including wound characteristics (i.e., contaminated wounds versus noncontaminated wounds); external factors (e.g., temperature regulation [i.e., bandage]); whether lavage is performed; and how the wound is closed (e.g., primary or secondary closure). A veterinarian must consider all these factors when determining how to treat a wound and when anticipating how well it will heal.

TOPICAL ANTIPRURITICS AND ANTIINFLAMMATORIES

Noncorticosteroids

Aluminum Acetate Solution

This is also known as Burow's solution.

Clinical Uses

This is an **astringent** solution and an antipruritic agent that is useful for the treatment of superficial skin problems. It can be used to help with acute moist **dermatitis,** fold dermatitis, and contact dermatitis. Some doctors may use it to treat otitis externa. The exact manner in which this agent works is not fully known at this time.

Dosage Forms

- Cort/Astrin Solution
- Corti-Derm Solution
- Buro-O-Cort 2:1
- Hydro-B 1020
- Domeboro Powder (human label)
- Pedi-Boro Soak Paks (human label)
- Domeboro Tablets (human label)
- Burow's Solution (human label)

Adverse Side Effects

Do not use anything that prevents the evaporation of this solution from the skin. Avoid contact with the eyes. Clients should wash their hands after administration and should wear gloves when applying the solution.

Colloidal Oatmeal

Clinical Uses

Colloidal oatmeal has unique properties in that it can be used topically as both an antiinflammatory and antipruritic agent. At this time, however, scientists are concerned about its mechanism of action. It is thought that perhaps it inhibits prostaglandin production.

Dosage Forms

- DermAllay Oatmeal Spray
- DermAllay Conditioner
- Epi-Soothe Cream Rinse
- ResiSoothe Leave-On Lotion
- Aloe & Oatmeal Skin & Coat Conditioner
- DermAllay Oatmeal Shampoo
- Epi-Soothe Shampoo
- Cortisoothe Shampoo
- Aloe & Oatmeal Shampoo

Adverse Side Effects

Colloidal oatmeal is very safe.

Topical Essential Fatty Acids

Clinical Uses

These products are commonly used for their antipruritic and antiinflammatory properties. They tend to help skin problems such as atopic dermatitis, sebaceous adenitis, and **seborrhea.** Some of these products have natural oils in them, which also may help skin problems. Essential **fatty acids** affect arachidonic acid levels and also affect the production of prostaglandins in the body, which can reduce inflammation and pruritus. Essential oils also help to create healthy skin.

Dosage Forms

- Dermoscent ATOP 7
- Dermoscent Cicafolia
- HyLyt EFA Bath Oil
- Dermoscent Essential 6 Spot-On
- HyLyt EFA Shampoo
- Dermoscent EFA Treatment Shampoo
- DermaLyte Shampoo
- Hyliderm Shampoo
- Allermyl Shampoo
- Allerderm Spot-On
- HyLyt EFA Creme Rinse

Adverse Side Effects

These are uncommon.

Topical Diphenhydramine HCl

Clinical Uses

Diphenhydramine is a first-generation antihistamine that has some local anesthetic properties. This drug can be absorbed transdermally but not enough to cause systemic effects.

Dosage Forms

Most products are human label; the exception is ResiHist Leave-On Lotion.

- ResiHist Leave-On Lotion—veterinary label
- Benadryl
- Dermamycin
- Ziradryl

Adverse Side Effects

Avoid contact with eyes or mucous membranes. Diphenhydramine should not be applied to skin that is oozing. Client should wear gloves when applying.

TECHNICIAN NOTES Topical diphenhydramine should not be used 2 weeks before allergy testing.

Topical Lidocaine and Lidocaine/Prilocaine

Clinical Uses

This product can be applied topically as a skin anesthetic and also helps with pruritus. It may be used to treat acute moist dermatitis, pruritic lesions, or painful skin conditions.

Dosage Forms

- Allercaine
- Allerspray
- DermaCool with Lidocaine Spray
- Hexa-Caine
- Biocaine
- EMLA Cream (human label)

TECHNICIAN NOTES EMLA cream may be used before intravenous catheter placement to ease the minor discomfort of the procedure.

Adverse Side Effects

Avoid contact with the eyes and do not use in ears. Clients should wear gloves when applying these products.

Phytosphingosine

Clinical Uses

Phytosphingosine is useful in treating localized inflammatory and pruritic cases such as atopic dermatitis. It can also be sprayed on sutures postoperatively to aid in the wound healing process.

Dosage Forms

- Douxo Calm Gel
- Douxo Calm Micro-emulsion Spray
- Douxo Calm Shampoo
- Douxo Seborrhea Shampoo
- Douxo Chlorhexidine PS
- Douxo Seborrhea Micro-emulsion Spray
- Douxo Seborrhea Spot on

Adverse Side Effects

This product may cause skin redness or irritation.

Pramoxine HCl

Clinical Uses

This agent has the ability to cause surface and local anesthetic characteristics, which can affect the peripheral nerves. It may be combined with other products to reduce pain or itching. At this time, scientists are unclear of this drug's mechanism of action.

Dosage Forms

The following are all veterinary-label products.

- Micro Pearls Advantage Dermal-Soothe Anti-Itch Spray
- Relief Spray
- Relief HC Spray
- Pramoxine Anti-Itch Spray
- Pramosoothe HC Spray
- Resiprox Leave-On Lotion
- Micro Pearls Advantage Dermal-Soothe Anti-Itch Shampoo
- Pramoxine Anti-Itch Shampoo
- Relief Shampoo
- Micro Pearls Advantage Dermal-Soothe Anti-Itch Cream Rinse
- Pramoxine Anti-Itch Cream Rinse
- Relief Cream Rinse

The following are all human-label pramoxine HCl products.

- AmLactin AP
- Prax
- Tronothane
- Itch-X
- PrameGel

Adverse Side Effects

Avoid contact with the eyes. This agent is not for ophthalmic use. Clients should wear gloves before applying these products to their pets' bodies.

Phenol/Menthol/Camphor

Clinical Uses

These agents are used in equines for overexertion, soreness, or stiffness.

Dosage Forms

- White Liniment
- Choate's Liniment

- Cool Gel
- Ice-O-Gel
- Shin-O-Gel
- Scarlet Oil Pump Spray

Adverse Side Effects

These products may cause local irritation. Do not use near the eyes. Do not use these products on cats.

Topical Neutralized Zinc Gluconate

Clinical Uses

This product can be used for mild itching, mild bacterial infections, and dry skin. It works well for relief from insect bites, acute moist dermatitis, acral lick dermatitis, fold dermatitis, feline acne, and postsurgical wounds. The exact mechanism of action is unclear at this time. Zinc has **antiseptic** and astringent ability.

Dosage Form

- Maxi/Guard Zn7 Derm

Topical Corticosteroids

Clinical Uses

Topical corticosteroids are used in conjunction with other treatments for localized itching or inflammatory conditions. Products containing betamethasone should be used after other products have been tried because the risks associated with betamethasone use are greater than the risks involved with hydrocortisone use (Plumb, 2011).

Dosage Forms

- Gentocin Topical Spray
- GentaSpray
- Betagen Topical Spray
- Gentamicin Topical Spray
- GentaVed Topical Spray
- Otomax Ointment
- DVMax Ointment
- Vetromax Ointment
- MalOtic Ointment
- Fuciderm Gel
- Betamethasone Dipropionate Ointment
- Betamethasone Dipropionate Cream
- Betamethasone Dipropionate Lotion
- Diprosone
- Clotrimazole and Betamethasone Dipropionate
- Lotrisone

Adverse Side Effects

Do not use in pregnant animals. This agent may cause tuberculosis of the skin. Avoid contact with the eyes. The animal should not be allowed to lick or chew at the affected sites for at least 20 to 30 minutes after application (Plumb, 2011).

Topical Hydrocortisone

Clinical Uses

Topical hydrocortisone is useful in the treatment of localized pruritus and/or inflammatory conditions. Because topically applied corticosteroids reduce the ability of leukocytes and macrophages to attack infected skin, the area to which such agents are applied will have less redness, itching, and swelling.

Dosage Forms

- CortiCalm Lotion
- Sulfodene HC Anti-Itch Lotion
- Zymox Topical Cream
- Zymox Topical Wipes
- Malacetic HC Wipes
- Relief HC Spray
- Pramosoothe HC Spray
- Cortispray
- DermaCool HC Spray
- Zymox Topical Spray
- Malacetic Ultra Spray
- Cort/Astrin Solution
- Corti-Derm Solution
- Hydro-Plus
- Buro-O-Cort 2:1
- Hydro-B 1020
- Cortisoothe Shampoo
- Chlorhexidine 4% HC Shampoo
- Malacetic Ultra Shampoo
- Resicort Leave-on Lotion

Adverse Side Effects

These products may cause tuberculosis of the skin. Do not use in pregnant animals. Clients should wear gloves when applying these products to their pets' skin. Keep out of the eyes. Do not allow the animal to lick or chew the application site for at least 30 minutes. Stop using 2 weeks before allergy testing.

Topical Isoflupredone Acetate

Clinical Uses

This is a high-potency topical corticosteroid. It is used in the treatment of otic or skin itching or inflammation that may be associated with bacterial infections. These products should be used as a last resort because the risks associated with them are greater than those with hydrocortisone.

Dosage Forms

- Tritop
- Neo-Predef with Tetracaine Powder

Adverse Side Effects

These products may cause tuberculosis of the skin. Do not use in pregnant animals. Clients should wear gloves when applying these agents to their pets' skin. Do not allow the animal to lick or chew the affected site for 30 minutes after application. Allergic reaction to neomycin and/or tetracaine may happen.

Mometasone Furoate

Clinical Uses

Mometasone furoate is useful in the treatment of itching and inflamed skin that may be associated with bacterial or yeast infections. When hydrocortisone products do not produce desirable results, this may be used.

Dosage Forms

- MoMetaMax Otic Suspension—veterinary label
- Elocon—human label

Adverse Side Effects

These products may cause tuberculosis of the skin. Do not use these products in pregnant animals. Use caution when treating a large area of skin or when the drug is used on small patients. Mometasone may delay wound healing when used for more than 7 days (Plumb, 2011).

Topical Triamcinolone Acetonide

Clinical Uses

This agent is useful as an adjunct in the treatment of pruritus. It is best suited for small lesions that only need to be treated for a short duration.

Dosage Forms

The following are all veterinary-label products.

- Medalone Cream
- Cortalone Cream
- Genesis Spray
- Derma-Vet Cream
- Panalog Ointment
- Animax Ointment
- Quadritop Ointment
- Derma-Vet Ointment
- Dermalog Ointment
- Dermalone Ointment

The following are all human-label products.

- Triamcinolone Acetonide Ointment
- Triamcinolone Acetonide Cream
- Triamcinolone Acetonide Lotion
- Kenalog
- Nystatin and Triamcinolone Acetonide

Adverse Side Effects

These products may cause tuberculosis of the skin. Do not use on pregnant animals. Keep out of the eyes. Do not allow the animal to lick or chew for 30 minutes after application. Stop using 2 weeks before allergy testing is to be done.

TOPICAL ANTIMICROBIALS

Benzoyl Peroxide

Clinical Uses

Benzoyl peroxide products are used topically as gels or shampoos. The shampoo products are usually used in cases involving oily skin, **pyodermas**, **furunculosis**, generalized demodicosis, and Schnauzer comedo syndrome (Plumb, 2011). Gels are used for treating pyodermas, chin acne, and localized demodex lesions. Benzoyl peroxide has antimicrobial actions. Gels can be used up to twice daily, but shampoos should only be used once a day.

Dosage Forms

The following are all veterinary-label products.

- Pyoben Gel
- OxyDex Gel
- Micro Pearls Advantage Benzoyl Plus
- Benzoyl Peroxide Shampoo

- OxyDex Shampoo
- Pyoben Shampoo
- Vet Solutions BPO-3 Shampoo
- SulfOxyDex Shampoo
- Oxiderm Shampoo
- DermaBenSs Shampoo

TECHNICIAN NOTES All shampoos should remain lathered on the skin for a minimum of 10 minutes before rinsing.

Adverse Side Effects
Do not use around eyes or mucous membranes. Clients should wear gloves when applying these products to their pets. Benzoyl peroxide will bleach fabrics, jewelry, carpet, and the pet's fur.

Topical Clindamycin

Clinical Uses
This is used in the treatment of feline acne. ClinzGard may be used in the treatment of anal sac abscesses, other abscesses, and puncture wounds.

Dosage Forms
Most products are human label unless otherwise specified.
- ClinzGard—veterinary label
- Clindamycin Phosphate
- Cleocin T
- Clindamax
- Clindagel
- Clindets
- Evoclin

Adverse Side Effects
Avoid use in individuals allergic to clindamycin. Clients should wear gloves when applying to their pets. Rarely, **pseudomembranous colitis** may occur in some patients.

Topical Gentamicin Sulfate

Clinical Uses
This is used to treat primary and secondary bacterial infections. Topical gentamicin can be used to treat "hot spots." Products that contain betamethasone, mometasone, or clotrimazole can be used as otic treatments.

Dosage Forms
Most products listed are veterinary label unless otherwise specified.
- Gentocin Topical Spray
- GentaSpray
- Betagen Topical Spray
- Gentamicin Topical Spray
- GentaVed Topical Spray
- GenOne Spray
- Otomax Ointment
- DVMax Ointment
- Vetromax Ointment
- MoMetaMax Otic Suspension
- Gentamicin—human label

Adverse Side Effects
This agent may be absorbed systemically if used on ulcers or burned or denuded skin.

Mupirocin (Pseudomonic Acid A)

Clinical Uses
This agent is Food and Drug Administration (FDA)-approved for treating pyoderma, interdigital cysts and draining tracts, acne, and pressure point pyodermas.

Dosage Forms
The following are human-label products unless otherwise specified.
- Muricin—veterinary label
- Mupirocin
- Bactroban Ointment
- Centany
- Bactroban Cream

Adverse Side Effects
Do not use in patients who are allergic to mupirocin or products containing polyethylene glycol.

Topical Nitrofurazone

Clinical Uses
This can be used to treat or prevent superficial infections.

Dosage Form
- Nitrofurazone Soluble Dressing—veterinary label

> TECHNICIAN NOTES United States federal law prohibits the use of nitrofurazone products in (or on) food animals, including horses to be used for food.

Silver Sulfadiazine (SSD)

Clinical Uses

This is used for second- and third-degree burns. It can also be used to treat skin infections caused by *Pseudomonas* spp.

Dosage Forms

No veterinary-labeled products are available for use.

- Silvadene
- SSD AF cream
- Thermazene
- SSD cream

Adverse Side Effects

Patients that are hypersensitive to sulfonamides may react to SSD. SSD may reduce granulation, so it should not be used in nongranulated wounds.

ANTISEPTICS

Acetic Acid/Boric Acid

Clinical Uses

These products are used to treat skin infections caused by *Staphylococcus* spp., *Pseudomonas* spp., and *Malassezia* spp.

Dosage Forms

All of the following are veterinary-label products.

- MalAcetic Ultra Spray
- Mal-A-Ket Wipes
- MalAcetic HC Wipes
- MalAcetic Wet Wipes
- MalAcetic Spray
- MalAcetic Shampoo

Adverse Side Effects

These include skin redness and irritation.

Chlorhexidine

Chlorhexidine may be easier on patients who are unable to tolerate benzoyl peroxide. It may have residual effects and can remain active on the skin after rinsing.

Clinical Uses

Chlorhexidine is used as a topical antiseptic. It does not seem to have much efficacy against *Pseudomonas* or *Serratia* spp.

Dosage Forms

Chlorhexidine is available as a solution, scrub, shampoo, ointment, and spray. All of the following are veterinary-label products.

- Chlorhexidine Spray
- Malaseb Spray
- Douxo Chlorhexidine PS Micro-emulsion Spray
- Chlorhex 2X 4% Spray
- ChlorhexiDerm Spray
- Ketoseb-D Spray
- Mal-A-Ket Plus TrizEDTA Spray
- TrizChlor 4 Spray
- Chlorhexidine Solution
- Chlorhexidine Concentrate
- Douxo Chlorhexidine 3% PS Pads
- Ketoseb-D Wipes
- Mal-A-Ket Wipes
- TrizChlor 4 Wipes
- Malaseb Pledgets
- Malaseb Towelettes
- Chlorhexidine Flush
- TrizChlor Flush
- Mal-A-Ket Plus TrizEDTA Flush
- Dermachlor Flush Plus
- Hexadene Flush
- Malaseb Flush
- ChlorhexiDerm Flush
- Chlorhexidine 0.2% Solution
- Ketoseb-D Flush
- Chlorhexidine Ointment
- Nolvasan Shampoo
- Chlorhexidine Shampoo 2%
- Chlorhexidine Shampoo 4%
- KetoChlor Shampoo
- Malaseb Shampoo
- Malaseb Concentrate Rinse
- TrizChlor 4 Shampoo
- ResiKetoChlor Leave-On Conditioner
- Chlorhexidine Scrub
- ChlorhexiDerm Plus Scrub

Adverse Side Effects
This agent may damage the eyes. Chlorhexidine is safe to use on cats, although irritation and corneal ulcer have been reported (Plumb, 2011).

Chloroxylenol (PCMX)

Clinical Uses
Chloroxylenol is also known as p-chloro-m-xylenol (PCMX). It is an antimicrobial disinfectant that is effective against gram-negative and gram-positive bacteria. It is also effective against RNA and DNA viruses. It may be used as a preoperative scrub of the skin, for cleaning wounds, for the treatment of bacteria and fungi, and for the treatment of yeast infections.

Dosage Forms
All of the following are veterinary-label products.

- Chloroxylenol Scrub
- Medicated Shampoo
- Vet Solutions Sebozole Shampoo
- Vet Solutions Universal Medicated Shampoo
- VPS Medicated Shampoo

Adverse Side Effects
Chloroxylenol may cause skin irritation.

Topical Enzymes

These include lactoperoxidase, lysozyme, and lactoferrin.

Clinical Uses
These are effective against *Staphylococcus* spp., *Pseudomonas* spp., *Malassezia* spp., *Candida albicans,* and *Microsporum* spp. and can be used on the skin.

Dosage Forms
All of the following are veterinary-label products.

- Zymox Topical Spray
- Zymox Topical Cream
- Zymox Topical Wipes
- Zymox Enzymatic Shampoo

Adverse Side Effects
These are uncommon.

Ethyl Lactate

Clinical Uses
This is useful in treating bacterial skin infections and superficial pyodermas.

Dosage Form

- Etiderm Shampoo

Adverse Side Effects
Erythema, pain, and itching are possible.

ANTIFUNGALS

Enilconazole

Clinical Uses
No dosage forms are available for topical use in the United States. This drug has been used in the treatment of **dermatophytosis** in small animals and in horses.

Adverse Effects
When used topically in felines, hypersalivation, vomiting, anorexia, weight loss, muscle weakness, and increased alanine aminotransferase (ALT) levels have been reported (Plumb, 2011).

Topical Ketoconazole

Clinical Uses
Ketoconazole is used against dermatophytes and yeasts. Patients with severe infections may need systemic therapy.

Dosage Forms
The following are all veterinary-label products.

- Ketoseb-D Spray
- Mal-A-Ket Plus TrizEDTA Spray
- MalAcetic Ultra Spray
- Ketoseb-D Wipes
- Mal-A-Ket Wipes
- Mal-A-Ket Plus TrizEDTA Flush
- Ketoseb-D Flush
- Mal-A-Ket Shampoo
- Ketochlor Shampoo
- ResiKetoChlor Leave-On Conditioner

The following are all human-label products.
- Nizoral A-D
- Nizoral
- Ketaconazole

Adverse Side Effects
Skin irritation is possible.

Lime Sulfur
This is also known as sulfurated lime solution.

Clinical Uses
Lime sulfur is used in the treatment of dermatophytosis and for the treatment of *Malassezia*, *Cheyletiellosis*, chiggers, and mange. It is also used in the treatment of demodex in cats.

Dosage Forms
The following are all veterinary-label products.
- LymDyp
- LimePlus Dip
- Vet Solutions Lime Sulfur Dip
- Lime Sulfur Dip
- LymDyp Spray

Adverse Side Effects
Lime sulfur may stain porous surfaces and discolor jewelry, and it may stain light-colored fur. Lime sulfur may cause skin irritation. Oral ingestion may cause nausea and oral ulcers, especially in cats; so it is best to use an Elizabethan collar (i.e., E-collar) to prevent this.

Topical Miconazole
Clinical Uses
It is used in the treatment of dermatophytes and yeast.

Dosage Forms
The following are all veterinary-label products.
- Micro Pearls Advantage Miconazole 1% Spray
- Conofite Spray 1%
- MicaVed Spray 1%
- Malaseb Spray
- Micazole Spray
- Malaseb Flush
- Malaseb Concentrate Rinse
- Malaseb Pledgets
- Malaseb Towelettes
- Conofite Cream 2%
- MicaVed Lotion 1%
- Micazole Lotion 1%
- Sebazole Shampoo
- Dermazole Shampoo
- Malaseb Shampoo

The following are all human-label products.
- Micatin
- Neosporin AF
- Lotrimin AF
- Prescription Strength Desenex
- Tetterine
- Zeasorb-AF
- Miconazole Nitrate
- Micatin
- Monistat-Derm

Adverse Side Effects
Avoid contact with the eyes. Skin irritation may occur. Do not apply to eroded or ulcerated skin.

Nystatin
Clinical Uses
Nystatin is useful for treating topical lesions caused by yeast.

Dosage Forms
The following are all veterinary-label products.
- Derma-Vet Cream
- Panalog Ointment
- Animax Ointment
- Quadritop Ointment
- Derma-Vet Ointment
- Dermalog Ointment

The following are all human-label products.
- Nystatin
- Nystatin and Triamcinolone Acetonide
- Mycogen II
- Mycolog-II
- Myco-Triacet II
- Myconel

Adverse Side Effects
Allergic reactions may occur.

Selenium Sulfide

Clinical Uses

Selenium sulfide is used for treating seborrheic disorders and *Malassezia.*

Dosage Forms

The following are all human-label topical products.

- Selenium Sulfide
- Selsun Blue Medicated Treatment
- Head & Shoulders Intensive Treatment
- Selsun

Adverse Side Effects

Do not use on cats. This agent may discolor jewelry and may stain hair coats. Mucous membranes and scrotal areas may become irritated.

Topical Terbinafine HCl

Clinical Uses

Terbinafine is useful for treating local lesions caused by *Malassezia.*

Dosage Forms

The following are all human-label products.

- Lamisil AT
- Lamisil
- Lamisil Advanced

Adverse Side Effects

Skin irritation is possible but usually is rare.

Salicylic Acid

Clinical Uses

Salicylic acid is used to treat seborrheic disorders. It has some antipruritic activity, as well as antibacterial, **keratoplastic**, and **keratolytic** actions.

Dosage Forms

The following are all veterinary-label products.

- KeraSolv Gel
- Derma-Clens cream
- Dermazole Shampoo
- SebaLyt Shampoo
- Nova Pearls Medicated Dandruff Shampoo
- Keratolux Shampoo
- Sebolux Shampoo
- Oxiderm Shampoo
- Oxiderm Shampoo + PS
- Micro Pearls Advantage Seba-Moist Shampoo
- Micro Pearls Advantage Seba-Hex Shampoo
- Universal Medicated Shampoo
- NuSal-T

Adverse Side Effects

Skin irritation is possible.

Precipitated Sulfur

Clinical Uses

Precipitated sulfur is used to treat seborrhea.

Dosage Forms

The following are all veterinary-label products.

- SebaLyt Shampoo
- Micro Pearls Advantage Seba-Hex Shampoo
- Micro Pearls Advantage Seba-Moist Shampoo
- Sebolux Shampoo
- Oxiderm Shampoo
- Oxiderm Shampoo + PS
- Keratolux Shampoo
- DermaPet DermaSebS Shampoo
- Nova Pearls Medicated Dandruff Shampoo
- Paraguard Shampoo
- SulfOxyDex Shampoo
- Medicated Shampoo

Adverse Side Effects

Skin irritation is possible. Sulfur may cause drying, itching, and irritation. The residual odor of this product may be offensive to clients.

Coal Tar

Clinical Uses

The use of coal tar shampoos has been somewhat controversial in veterinary medicine (Plumb, 2011). Manufacturing of almost all veterinary-label products has been discontinued. Coal tar has been used in treating **seborrhea oleosa** for many years.

Dosage Form

- NuSal T Shampoo—veterinary label

Adverse Side Effects

The FDA believes that coal tar products with concentrations of 5% or less are safe for human use (Plumb,

2011). Carcinogenic risks may be associated with these products.

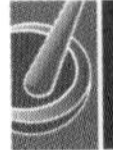

TOPICAL RETINOIDS

Tretinoin

Types of tretinoin include transretinoic acid and vitamin A acid.

Clinical Uses

These products are useful in treating acanthosis nigricans, idiopathic nasal and footpad hyperkeratosis, callous pyodermas, and chin acne.

Dosage Forms

All of the following are human-label products.

- Renova
- Retin-A
- Avita
- Altinac
- Renova

Adverse Effects

Avoid sun exposure. Products may cause allergic reactions or local irritation.

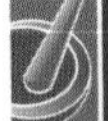

TOPICAL ANTIPARASITIC AGENTS

Amitraz

Clinical Uses

Amitraz is used in the treatment of generalized demodicosis. It is available as a topical spot-on treatment (ProMeris for dogs); a collar (Preventic) may also be used for flea and tick infestation prevention.

Dosage Forms

All of the following are veterinary-label products.

- Mitaban; availability may be undependable
- Taktic EC
- ProMeris for Dogs
- Preventic

Adverse Side Effects

Animals should not be stressed for at least 24 hours after application. Some animals may show signs of sedation, so owners should be warned. These products are not for use in dogs younger than 4 months. If the skin around the eyes needs to be treated, use a petrolatum-based ophthalmic ointment. Amitraz may be toxic to rabbits and cats. Yohimbine at an intravenous dose of 0.11 to 0.2 mg/kg may be used if an overdose occurs. Amitraz is contraindicated if an animal is taking monoamine oxidase inhibitors.

Crotamiton

Clinical Uses

This is a topical miticide and scabicide. It is used mainly for treating scaly leg mites in birds (*Knemidokoptes*).

Dosage Form

- Eurax—human label

Adverse Side Effects

Little is known about this product's safety. Irritation and allergic reactions are possible.

Deltamethrin

Clinical Uses

In the United States, deltamethrin-impregnated collars are labeled for killing fleas and ticks on dogs. In countries in which leishmaniasis is a problem, deltamethrin-impregnated collars may be used for repelling and killing sandfly vectors.

Dosage Form

- Scalibor Protector Band for Dogs—veterinary label

Adverse Side Effects

Do not use on dogs younger than 12 weeks. This product should be used very carefully around water because it is toxic to fish.

Dinotefuran Plus Pyriproxyfen (Plus Permethrin)

Clinical Uses

This is used for the control of adult and all immature flea stages. This product also contains permethrin to help kill and repel adult and immature fleas, ticks, and mosquitoes.

Dosage Forms

- Vectra for Cats and Kittens
- Vectra for Cats
- Vectra for Dogs and Puppies
- Vectra 3D

> **TECHNICIAN NOTES**
> - Do not use the dog product, which contains permethrin (i.e., Vectra 3D) on cats. Do not use this product on dogs that live in the same household as a cat.
> - This product should not be used on geriatric animals, animals that are debilitated, or nursing animals.

Fipronil or Fipronil/(S)-Methoprene

Clinical Uses

In the United States, fipronil is approved for the treatment of fleas, ticks, and chewing lice, which infest dogs and cats. It has also been used to treat chigger infestation and sarcoptic mange. Frontline Plus also has an insect growth regulator that kills flea eggs and flea larvae.

Dosage Forms

All of the following are veterinary-label products.

- Frontline Spray Treatment
- Frontline Top Spot for Cats and Kittens
- Frontline Plus for Cats and Kittens
- Frontline Top Spot for Dogs and Puppies
- Frontline Plus for Dogs and Puppies

Adverse Side Effects

These products are not to be used on puppies younger than 8 weeks. Do not use in rabbits. The product label states that the product is effective after bathing, but animals should not be bathed within 48 hours of application for best results. The product label also states that the product is effective after water immersion and exposure to sunlight. Areas of the skin to which the product has been applied may remain oily for up to 24 hours after application.

Imidacloprid, Imidacloprid with Permethrin, and Imidacloprid with Moxidectin

Clinical Uses

Imidacloprid topical solution (Advantage) is used for the treatment of adult and larval flea stages in dogs and cats. The combination product with permethrin (K9 Advantix) kills adult and larval forms of fleas, repels and kills ticks, and repels mosquitoes in dogs only. The canine combination product with moxidectin (Advantage Multi for Dogs in the United States and Advocate in Europe) is used for the prevention of heartworm disease, adult fleas, adult and immature hookworms, adult roundworms, and adult whipworms. It has also been successfully used in the treatment of sarcoptic mange, cheyletiellosis, and mild cases of demodicosis (Plumb, 2011). The feline combination product (Advantage Multi for Cats) is indicated for the prevention of heartworm disease, adult fleas, ear mites, adult and immature hookworms, and adult roundworms (Plumb, 2011).

Dosage Forms

- Advantage for Dogs
- Advantage for Cats
- K9 Advantix
- Advantage Multi for Dogs

Adverse Side Effects

For imidacloprid alone, do not use in puppies younger than 7 weeks or in kittens younger than 8 weeks. Do not use the combination product (K9 Advantix) on cats. Caution should be used in households with both dogs and cats, especially when cats are in close contact with or will groom dogs in the household.

When used as directed, adverse effects are unlikely. Most problems are seen after oral dosing of topical products (Plumb, 2011).

(S)-Methoprene Combinations

Clinical Uses

Methoprene is added to premise sprays and topical products to eliminate insects (usually fleas) because it prevents the maturation of eggs and larvae.

Dosage Forms

All of the following are veterinary-label products.

- Adams Spot On Flea and Tick Control
- Bio Spot On Flea and Tick Control for Dogs
- Frontline Plus for Cats and Kittens
- Frontline Plus for Dogs and Puppies

Adverse Side Effects
Methoprene can also be found in products that contain permethrin or phenothrin, which can be toxic to kittens.

Permethrin
Clinical Uses
This product acts as an adult insecticide and miticide.

Dosage Forms
All of the following are veterinary-label products.
- Adams Spot On Flea and Tick Control
- Bio Spot On Flea and Tick Control for Dogs
- K9 Advantix
- Proticall Insecticide for Dogs
- Vectra 3D
- Virbac Long Acting Knockout

Adverse Side Effects
This agent can be toxic to cats. Only use those products indicated for use in cats.

Topical Pyrethrins and Pyrethrin Combinations
Clinical Uses
These acts as adult insecticides and miticides. They have action against fleas, lice, ticks, and cheyletiella.

Dosage Forms
All of the following are veterinary-label products.
- Adams Flea and Tick Dust I
- Adams Flea and Tick Mist with IGR
- Adams Flea and Tick Mist for Cats
- Adams Plus Flea and Tick Shampoo with IGR
- Vet-Kem Ovitrol Plus Flea and Tick Shampoo
- EctoKyl 3X Flea and Tick Shampoo
- Ecto-Soothe 3X Shampoo
- Vet-Kem Ovitrol Plus Flea and Tick Shampoo
- Adams Pyrethrin Dip
- Pyrethrins Dip and Spray

Adverse Side Effects
Do not allow cats to groom themselves after products such as dips or sprays have been applied.

Topical Pyriproxyfen and Pyriproxyfen Combinations
Clinical Uses
This is a second-generation insect growth regulator (IGR) that is added to premise sprays and topical products to act against fleas.

Dosage Forms
All of the following are veterinary-label products.
- Adams Plus Flea and Tick Mist with IGR
- Adams Flea and Tick Mist for Cats
- Adams Plus Flea and Tick Shampoo with IGR
- Bio Spot Shampoo

Adverse Side Effects
When used alone, pyriproxyfen has low toxicity in mammals. Skin irritation or allergic reactions could occur.

Spinetoram
Clinical Uses
This is labeled for the prevention and treatment of flea infestations in cats and kittens 8 weeks of age or older.

Dosage Form
- Assurity

Adverse Side Effects
None are reported by the manufacturer.

REVIEW QUESTIONS

1. The skin consists of ________________ layers and is part of the ________________ system.
2. ________________ is essential for healthy skin.
3. Name seven functions of the skin.

   ____
4. Shampoos are more effective if left on the skin about ________ to ________ minutes before rinsing.

5. Keratolytics and keratoplastics are known as ______________________ agents.
6. Name the four stages of wound healing. ______________________
7. What does an astringent do to the skin? ______________________
8. Tissue irritation may be caused by counterirritants.
   a. True
   b. False
9. Patients are commonly presented for skin problems when in reality they may have a ______________________ illness.
10. Why are behavioral-type drugs used in treating skin illness? ______________________
11. All patients presented for dermatologic problems have an underlying systemic illness.
    a. True
    b. False
12. The _____ is the largest organ in the body.
    a. liver
    b. spleen
    c. skin
    d. stomach
    e. intestinal tract
13. Increased skin irritation may result in hyperpigmentation of the skin.
    a. True
    b. False
14. Humans have multiple hairs per follicle, but animals have one hair per follicle.
    a. True
    b. False
15. Shampoos should be left on the animal's skin for 5 to 10 minutes before rinsing.
    a. True
    b. False
16. The débridement stage of wound healing usually begins to occur about ___ hour(s) after injury.
    a. 2
    b. 3
    c. 1
    d. 6
17. During the repair phase of wound healing, fibroblasts produce _______ and other connective tissue proteins.
    a. angiogenesis
    b. collagen
    c. comedones
    d. hyperpigmentation
18. The maturation phase marks the beginning of wound healing.
    a. True
    b. False
19. _______ tissue is formed during healing of wounds of the soft tissue that consists of connective tissue cells and ingrown young vessels, which ultimately form a scar.
    a. Collagen
    b. Keratolytic
    c. Callus
    d. Granulation

REFERENCE

McCurnin DM, Bassert JM, editors: Clinical textbook for veterinary technicians, ed 6, Philadelphia, 2006, WB Saunders.

Plumb DC: Veterinary drug handbook, ed 7, Ames, Iowa, 2011, Wiley.

CHAPTER

12

Antiinfective Drugs

OUTLINE

KEY TERMS

- Antibacterial
- Antibiotic
- Antimicrobial
- Bacteria
- Bactericidal
- Bacteriostatic
- Beta-lactamase
- Detergent
- Disinfect
- Efficacy
- Fungicidal
- Fungistatic
- In vitro
- In vivo
- Iodophor
- Microorganism
- Nephrotoxic
- Ototoxic
- Sporicidal
- Tachypnea
- Teratogenic
- Thrombophlebitis

SULFONAMIDES
- Sulfachlorpyridazine
- Sulfadiazine/Trimethoprim and Sulfamethoxazole/Trimethoprim
- Sulfadimethoxine
- Sulfadimethoxine/Ormetoprim

ANTIBACTERIALS
- Aztreonam
- Chloramphenicol
- Clofazimine
- Dapsone
- Ethambutol
- Florfenicol
- Fosfomycin
- Isoniazid
- Methenamine
- Metronidazole
- Nitrofurantoin
- Novobiocin
- Potassium Iodide
- Rifampin
- Tiamulin
- Tinidazole
- Vancomycin

ANTIFUNGAL AGENTS
- Amphotericin B
- Caspofungin
- Fluconazole
- Flucytosine
- Griseofulvin
- Itraconazole
- Ketoconazole
- Nystatin
- Terbutaline HCl
- Voriconazole

ANTIVIRAL AGENTS
- Acyclovir
- Amantadine
- Famciclovir
- Interferon Alfa
- Interferon Omega
- Lysine
- Oseltamivir
- Zidovudine

DISINFECTANTS/ANTISEPTICS
- Biguanide Compounds
- Chlorines and Iodines
- Ethylene Oxide
- Formaldehyde
- Phenolics: Saponated Cresol and Semisynthetic Phenols
- Quaternary Ammonium Compounds: Cationic Detergents
- Other Disinfectants

LEARNING OBJECTIVES

After studying this chapter, you should be able to

1. Identify the classes of antiinfective drugs.
2. Describe the adverse side effects of antiinfective drugs.
3. Explain the clinical uses of antiinfective drugs.
4. Explain the clinical uses of antifungal agents.
5. Discuss antiviral drugs.
6. Explain how disinfectants and antiseptics are used.

INTRODUCTION

Microorganisms are ubiquitous in the environment. Some microorganisms have pathogenic potential, but others do not. Animals usually make initial contact with an infectious agent somewhere on the body's surface (e.g., mucous membranes, skin, respiratory tract, or digestive tract). In the fight against infection, several hundred **antimicrobial** drugs have been developed since the early 1900s. These drugs have been used to fight disease in both humans and animals.

Not all antimicrobials have the same degree of effectiveness against **microorganisms.** A determination can be made to distinguish different types of bacteria with the use of a Gram stain. The Gram stain is a laboratory procedure in which dyes are used to stain **bacteria** (Figure 12-1). Gram-positive bacteria stain dark blue to purple. Gram-negative bacteria stain pink to red. However, some bacteria cannot be identified through the Gram stain technique. For differentiating acid-fast bacilli, carbol fuchsin stain can be used and then decolorized with ethyl alcohol and hydrochloric acid. Other bacteria must be identified by special techniques such as dark-field examination or Gimenez stain. Giemsa and Wright stains may be used to identify parasites and intracellular microorganisms. Bacteria with similar staining properties tend to respond to the same antimicrobial therapy. Still other bacteria are classified by their ability to survive with or without oxygen. Aerobes are bacteria that must have oxygen to live and replicate. Other bacteria are able to live and multiply without oxygen; these are known as anaerobes. Anaerobes may be hardy and difficult to eradicate.

MECHANISM OF ACTION

Through analysis of the effects that a drug's action has on bacteria, antimicrobial drugs can be divided into two categories: **bactericidal** and **bacteriostatic.** However, some strains of mutant bacteria have greater resistance to some antimicrobials. Resistant strains of bacteria can make antimicrobial therapy difficult. Therefore, to prevent mutant strains from developing, antimicrobial drugs must not be used indiscriminately. Sometimes, it may be necessary to use two different types of antimicrobial drugs to treat patients with infections caused by two or more different organisms.

After a laboratory has identified the type of organism that is causing an infection, an **antibiotic** sensitivity test may be performed. Several tests are available for testing the susceptibility of an organism to a specific antimicrobial drug. Most commonly, the disk susceptibility test is used in small laboratories (Figure 12-2). With this test, an agar plate with a standard amount of cultured organism is used. Using

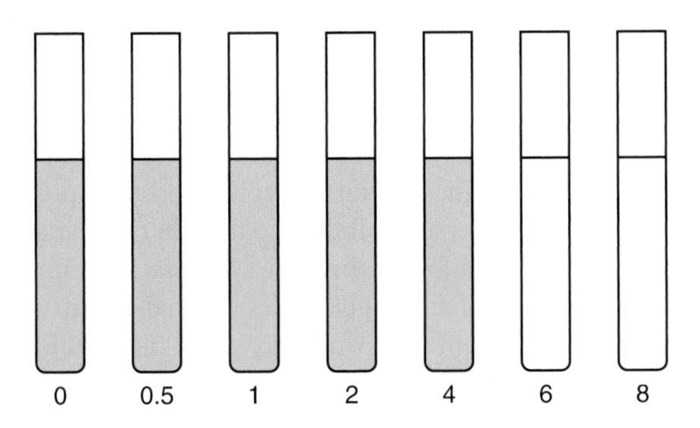

FIGURE 12-1 The broth dilution susceptibility test. Note that the organism grew in broth containing 0, 0.5, 1, 2, and 4 mg/mL of antibiotic. The organism was inhibited in the tube that contained 6 mg/mL. The minimum inhibitory concentration is 6 mg/mL.

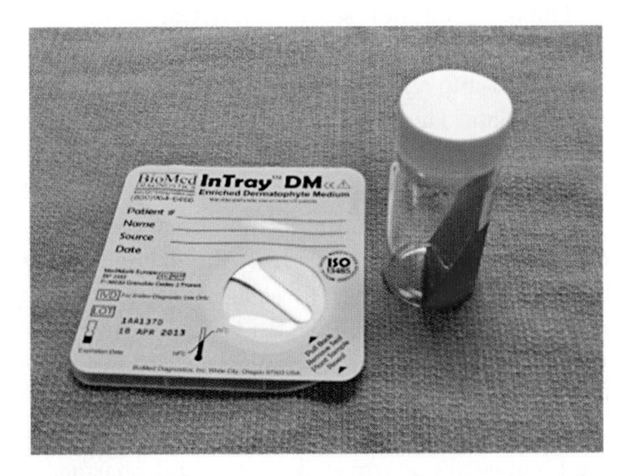

FIGURE 12-2 Dermatophyte test medium may be used to culture topical fungal infections. This medium contains a phenol red indicator that turns red as a dermatophyte grows and produces alkaline metabolic products.

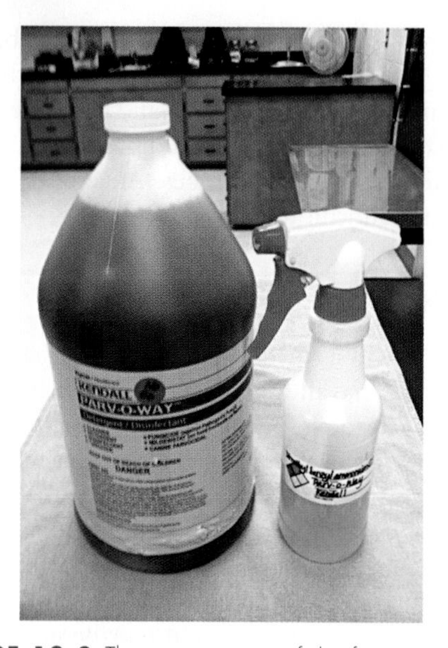

FIGURE 12-3 The concentrations of disinfectants vary from dilutions that are used for disinfecting kennels and floors to dilutions that are used as table sprays.

a dispenser, paper disks impregnated with various antimicrobial drugs are placed within the agar plate. Incubation is carried out, along with measurement of the zones of inhibition. These zones show which antimicrobial agents are susceptible or resistant to each particular antimicrobial and how effectively they may perform **in vitro.** The Kirby-Bauer procedure is commonly used in many laboratories.

The broth dilution susceptibility test is also used in many laboratories (Figure 12-3). An organism is inoculated into a series of tubes or wells in a microculture plate. These tubes or wells contain different concentrations of antimicrobials. The lowest concentration that macroscopically inhibits the growth of an organism is the minimum inhibitory concentration (MIC). The MIC represents the degree of susceptibility of an organism to a specific concentration of a particular antimicrobial drug. The antimicrobials that are effective in vitro may not always be the best choice for use **in vivo.** A clinician chooses which agent to use by considering the diagnosis and assessing each agent's pharmacodynamics and pharmacokinetics. This process allows a clinician to choose the most efficient and efficacious drug to treat a specific condition.

TECHNICIAN NOTES

Special Considerations When Antimicrobial Drugs Are Used

- Do not use antimicrobial drugs for mild infection.
- Antimicrobials should be used only for individuals at risk of severe infection.
- Do not dismiss the principles of asepsis just because there are many antibiotics from which to choose.
- The use of antimicrobials should be based on a definitive diagnosis.
- Do not use a broad-spectrum antibiotic if the infecting organism is sensitive to a specific antibiotic.
- Antimicrobial drugs should be administered in full therapeutic doses.
- If an antimicrobial can be used topically or locally, do so. This reserves the use of systemic drugs for serious disease.
- Be careful regarding antibiotic withdrawal times in animals to be slaughtered for human consumption and antibiotic withdrawal times in dairy cows.
- Penicillin G benzathine is long-acting (48 hours) and is not approved for use in dairy animals.

AMINOCYCLITOLS

Pharmacodynamics/Pharmacokinetics

Aminocyclitols belong to a class of drugs that are sugar-derived and that demonstrate important biologic value. Aminocyclitols are components that make up aminoglycoside-type antibiotics. Aminoglycoside antibiotics act on susceptible bacteria presumably by irreversibly binding to the 30S ribosomal subunit, thus inhibiting protein synthesis. Antimicrobial activity of aminoglycosides is enhanced in an alkaline environment. Aminoglycoside antibiotics are inactive against fungi, viruses, and most anaerobic bacteria (Plumb, 2011).

Aminoglycosides are not absorbed well after oral or intrauterine administration. They can be absorbed from topical administration when used in irrigations during surgical procedures. After intramuscular

TABLE 12-1 Aminoglycoside Preparations, Indications, and Antagonistic Drugs

DRUG	INDICATIONS	ANTAGONIST	COMMENTS
All aminoglycosides	Infections caused by susceptible pathogens, pneumonias, urinary tract infections, endometritis, and septicemias that are resistant to other antibiotics	Dimenhydrinate and ethacrynic acid affect hearing loss; methoxyflurane	Monitor patient for hearing loss; do not administer with methoxyflurane
Kanamycin, tobramycin, gentamicin, neomycin, streptomycin		Neuromuscular blocking agents	Administer calcium and anticholinergic agents as prescribed
Gentamicin		Amphotericin B and cephalosporins produce nephrotoxicity	Monitor renal function test results frequently when combining these agents
Neomycin		Digitalis glycosides, penicillin V	Doses may need to be adjusted when combining these agents
Gentamicin, tobramycin		Carbenicillin, ticarcillin, azlocillin, mezlocillin, piperacillin	Never mix these two types of antibiotics; if a patient is receiving combined therapy, administer the doses at least 1 hour apart

(IM) administration to dogs and cats, levels peak from 30 minutes to 1 hour later. After absorption, aminoglycosides are distributed primarily in the extracellular fluid. They do not readily cross the blood–brain barrier nor do they penetrate ocular tissue. Aminoglycosides tend to accumulate in the inner ear and kidneys, which explains their toxicity to those organs. Elimination of aminoglycosides after parenteral administration occurs almost entirely by glomerular filtration (Plumb, 2011). See Table 12-1.

> **TECHNICIAN NOTES** Aminoglycosides tend to take up residence in the ears and kidneys, making them **ototoxic** and nephrotoxic. Elimination mostly occurs by glomerular filtration.

Amikacin

Clinical Uses

Parenteral use is only Food and Drug Administration (FDA)-approved in dogs and is used to treat serious gram-negative infections. Amikacin is FDA-approved for intrauterine infusion in mares and for intraarticular injection in foals to treat septic arthritis.

Dosage Forms

All of the following are veterinary-label products.

- Amikacin Sulfate Injection (50 mg/mL)(sold in 50-mL vials)
- Amiglyde-V
- Amikacin Sulfate Intrauterine Solution (250 mg/mL)(sold in 48-mL vials)

Adverse Side Effects

This drug is ototoxic and nephrotoxic. Cats are very susceptible to the vestibular effects of amikacin. In the United States, amikacin is not FDA-approved for use in cattle or other food animals.

Storage of the Drug

Amikacin can be stored at room temperature and is stable for up to 2 years. Solutions over time may become pale yellow, but this does not decrease the drug's **efficacy.**

Apramycin

Clinical Uses

Some countries use this drug to treat bacterial enteritis, colibacillosis, and salmonellosis in pigs, calves, and poultry (Plumb, 2011).

Dosage Forms

- Apralan
- Apralan Soluble Powder

Adverse Side Effects

Do not use this drug in cats. Do not use in patients with myasthenia gravis.

Storage of the Drug

Apramycin powder should be stored in a cool dry place, in a tightly closed container. It should be protected from moisture. It should be stored at less than 25°C (or 77°F).

Gentamicin

Clinical Uses

This drug is used in the treatment of serious gram-negative infections.

Dosage Forms

All of the following are veterinary-label products.

- AmTech Gentamax 100
- Gentafuse
- Gentamax 100
- Gentaved 100
- Gentozen
- Garasol Injection
- AmTech Gentapoult
- Garacin Piglet Injection
- Gentamicin Sulfate Oral Solution
- Gen-Gard Soluble Powder
- Garacin Soluble Powder

Adverse Side Effects

Gentamicin should be used with extreme caution in patients with chronic renal failure (CRF). Do not use in patients that are debilitated, who have a fever, sepsis, or dehydration. Use this drug with caution in working dog breeds such as seeing-eye dogs, herding dogs, or dogs for the hearing impaired because it can cause ototoxicity. Do not use in animals with neuromuscular disorders or in patients with botulism. IM injections in horses may cause muscle irritation, so intravenous (IV) injections are preferred. Do not use gentamicin in rabbits.

Storage of the Drug

Gentamicin sulfate for injection and the oral solution should be stored at room temperature (15°C–30°C [59°F–86°F]). Do not store the drug in rusty containers, nor offer medicated-drinking water in rusty containers because the drug will be destroyed.

Neomycin

Clinical Uses

Neomycin is more **nephrotoxic** than the other aminoglycosides. It is also less effective against gram-negative organisms. Its use topically is mainly for the skin, eyes, and ears; orally, it is used to treat enteric infections, reduce microbe numbers in the colon before surgery, and reduce ammonia-producing bacteria in the treatment of hepatic encephalopathy.

Dosage Forms

All of the following are veterinary-label products.

- Neomycin Sulfate Oral Liquid
- Neo-325 Soluble Powder
- Neovet 325/100
- Neo Vet 325 Ag Grade
- Neo-Sol 50

Adverse Side Effects

Rarely, neomycin has caused ototoxicity, nephrotoxicity, severe diarrhea, and malabsorption of the intestines.

Storage of the Drug

Neomycin should be stored at room temperature, in tightly sealed, light-resistant containers. Neomycin (in the dry state) is stable for at least 2 years at room temperature.

Spectinomycin

Clinical Uses

This is sometimes used in dogs, cats, and horses. Spectinomycin only has FDA approval for cattle, chickens, turkeys, and swine.

Dosage Forms
All of the following are veterinary-label products.
- Adspec
- Spectam Injectable
- Spectinomycin Water Soluble
- Spectam Scour Halt
- SpectoGard Scour-Check
- L-S 50 Water Soluble Powder
- Linco-Spectin Sterile Solution

Adverse Side Effects
When spectinomycin is used correctly, adverse effects are uncommon. It probably has less ototoxicity and nephrotoxic activity than other aminoglycosides. Cattle that are injected subcutaneously (SC) have developed swelling at the site of injection.

Storage of the Drug
Store at room temperature. Avoid freezing.

Tobramycin

Clinical Uses
This drug is used for the prevention of cystine urolithiasis in patients that show no improvement after the use of dietary therapy combined with urinary alkalinization.

All of the following are veterinary-label products.
- Tobramycin Sulfate Injection
- Tobramycin Sulfate Powder for Injection
- Tobramycin Solution for Inhalation (TOBI)

Adverse Side Effects
According to Plumb (2011), increased liver enzymes, lethargy, dermatologic effects, aggressiveness, sulfur odor to the urine, or myopathy may be noted with this drug.

Storage of the Drug
Store tablets at room temperature in tightly sealed containers.

TECHNICIAN NOTES
- Because aminoglycosides enhance the effects of neuromuscular blocking drugs, it is best to refrain from using these drugs at the same time. Aminoglycoside blood levels should be determined before neuromuscular blocking drugs are used so that muscular collapse is prevented.
- Aminoglycosides are contraindicated in animals with renal insufficiency.
- Aminoglycosides are not approved for use in food-producing animals.
- Do not mix vials or syringes with other antibiotics.
- Aminoglycosides may cause problems such as ototoxicity or nephrotoxicity in animals, especially if the patient is receiving furosemide therapy when they are administered.

CARBAPENEMS

Pharmacodynamics/Pharmacokinetics
Carbapenems are a class of beta-lactam antibiotics with a wide range of **antibacterial** activity. Carbapenems inhibit bacterial cell wall synthesis, and they are usually bactericidal.

There are currently no pharmacokinetic data available for dogs and cats. In humans, these drugs are excreted in the urine or feces.

Ertapenem
Clinical Uses
Ertapenem may be useful in treating gram-negative bacterial infections and works well in the place of aminoglycosides when they should not be used.

Dosage Form
There are no veterinary label products available.
- Invanz—human label

Adverse Side Effects
The adverse effects in dogs and cats are unknown.

Storage of Drug
Ertapenem should be stored at room temperature.

Imipenem–Cilastatin
Clinical Uses
This drug combination is useful in equine or small animal medicine to treat serious infections when less expensive antibiotics perform poorly.

Dosage Forms

Only human-label products are available.

- ADD-Vantage
- Primaxin IV
- Primaxin IM

Adverse Side Effects

Gastrointestinal (GI) problems such as vomiting, anorexia, and diarrhea may be seen along with central nervous system (CNS) toxicity, pruritus, and anaphylaxis. It may cause seizures if the IV dose is given too rapidly.

Storage of Drug

Store at room temperature. After reconstitution, the solution is stable for 4 hours at room temperature or 10 hours if refrigerated. Do not freeze solutions.

Meropenem

Clinical Uses

Meropenem is useful in treating resistant gram-negative bacterial infections, especially when aminoglycosides may pose a risk.

Dosage Form

Only human-label products are available.

- Merrem IV

Adverse Effects

When given SC, meropenem may cause animals to have hair loss at injection sites.

CEPHALOSPORINS

Pharmacodynamics/Pharmacokinetics

Cephalosporins are a group of broad-spectrum, semisynthetic antibiotics derived from *Cephalosporium acremonium,* a species of soil-inhabiting fungi, which share the nucleus 7-aminocephalosporanic acid. Cephalosporins that were named before 1975 are spelled with *ph,* and those named after 1975 are spelled with *f.* First-generation cephalosporins are active mainly against gram-positive bacteria. Second-generation cephalosporins have a broader spectrum of activity, and third-generation cephalosporins are mainly used against gram-negative organisms. Fourth-generation cephalosporins have an extended spectrum and have increased resistance to hydrolysis and B-lactamases (Plumb, 2011). See Table 12-2.

Orally Active

- Cephalexin
- Cephradine
- Cefadroxil
- Cefaclor
- Cephaloglycin

Parenterally Active

Cephalosporins that are active by parenteral administration are placed into four groups.

Group I

This group has fair activity against gram-positive bacteria and moderate activity against gram-negative bacteria; the drugs show poor activity against *Pseudomonas.*

- Cefapirin
- Cefacetrile
- Cephaloridine
- Cephalothin
- Cefazolin

Group II

This group has high activity against *Enterobacteriaceae.*

- Cefamandole
- Cefmenoxime
- Cefotaxime
- Cefotiam
- Ceftiofur
- Cefuroxime
- Ceftriaxone

Group III

This group has high activity against *Pseudomonas* and other gram-negative bacteria.

- Cefsulodin
- Ceftazidime
- Cefoperazone

TABLE 12-2 Cephalosporin Preparations, Indications, and Antagonistic Drugs

DRUG	INDICATIONS	ANTAGONIST	COMMENTS
Cefadroxil	Infections caused by sensitive organisms in, for example, the respiratory tract, skin, urinary tract, soft tissue, bones, and joints	All cephalosporins: gentamicin	Ingestion of food does not impair absorption
Cephalexin	Urinary tract infections		Ingestion of food may delay absorption
Cephalothin	Infections caused by sensitive organisms in, for example, the respiratory tract, skin, urinary tract, soft tissue, bones, and joints		Intramuscular injection painful; inactivated in liver
Cefazolin	Same as for cephalothin		Highly protein-bound; very rarely nephrotoxic
Cephapirin	Same as for cephalothin		Intramammary infusion for mastitis
Cefamandole	Life-threatening, gram-negative infections		Dose should be reduced in patients with renal failure
Cefoxitin (a cephamycin)	Treatment of susceptible infections		Local reaction may occur at injection site
Ceftiofur HCl	Treatment of respiratory disease in cattle and swine; broad spectrum against gram-positive and gram-negative bacteria including beta-lactamase–producing strains		May be used in lactating dairy animals
Ceftiofur sodium	Treatment of respiratory disease in cattle, sheep, horses, and swine; urinary tract infections in dogs; and for control of early mortality associated with *Escherichia coli* organisms in day-old chicks and day-old turkey poults; broad spectrum against gram-positive and gram-negative bacteria including beta-lactamase–producing strains		May be used in lactating dairy animals

Group IV

This group is resistant to β-lactamase.

- Cefoxitin
- Moxalactam
- Cefmetazole
- Cefotetan

Cefaclor

Clinical Uses

Cefaclor is used to treat infections that are resistant to first-generation cephalosporins.

Dosage Forms

Only human-label products are available.

- Ceclor Pulvules (oral capsules)
- Raniclor (chewable tablets)
- Cefaclor Extended Release Oral Tablets

Adverse Side Effects

In humans, this drug can cause GI upset and hypersensitivity reactions. It may cause increases on liver function tests, as well as intermittent increases in blood urea nitrogen (BUN) and serum creatinine levels.

Storage of the Drug
Capsules, tablets, and powder for suspension should be kept at room temperature. After the oral suspension has been reconstituted, it should be refrigerated and discarded after 14 days.

Cefadroxil

Clinical Uses
Cefadroxil is useful in treating infections of the skin, soft tissue, and genitourinary tract in dogs and cats.

Dosage Forms
Products are human-label unless otherwise specified.
- Cefa-Drops (FDA-approved for use in dogs and cats)—veterinary label
- Cefadroxil Oral Tablets (1 g)
- Cefadroxil Oral Capsules (500 mg and 125 mg/5 mL, 250 mg/5 mL, 500 mg/5 mL)
- Cefadroxil Powder for Oral Suspension

Adverse Side Effects
These are usually not serious and occur rarely. They include hypersensitivity, GI effects, the potential for nephrotoxicity, and **tachypnea,** rarely.

Storage of the Drug
Cefadroxil should be stored at room temperature. After reconstitution, the suspension should be refrigerated and discarded after 14 days.

Cefazolin

Clinical Uses
In the United States, there are no FDA-approved cefazolin products for veterinary use. It may be used for surgical prophylaxis in humans.

Dosage Forms
Only human-label products are available.
- Cefazolin Sodium Powder for injection
- Cefazolin Sodium for IV infusion

Adverse Side Effects
These are usually not serious and do not often happen. Some signs that may be seen include hypersensitivity, fever, eosinophilia, and lymphadenopathy. Pain at the injection site may occur when given IM, and it may have the potential for nephrotoxicity.

Storage of the Drug
Cefazolin sodium powder and solutions for injection should be protected from light. The powder should be stored at room temperature. After reconstitution, the solution is stable for 24 hours when kept at room temperature or 96 hours if refrigerated. After reconstitution, if freezing is desired, the preparation is stable for at least 12 weeks.

Cefepime

Clinical Uses
Cefepime is useful in treating serious infections in dogs or foals when aminoglycosides are contraindicated.

Dosage Form
Only human-label products are available.
- Maxipime

Adverse Side Effects
Clinical signs that may be seen include loose stools in dogs. IM injections may be painful.

Storage of the Drug
The powder for injection should be stored between 35.6°F and 77°F.

Cefixime

Clinical Uses
Uses for cefixime in veterinary medicine are limited. It should be used when other cephalosporins or fluoroquinolones are contraindicated.

Dosage Form
Only human-label products are available.
- Suprax

Adverse Side Effects
GI upset, hypersensitivity, and possibly fever may occur.

Storage of the Drug
Cefixime powder for suspension should be stored at room temperature in tightly sealed containers. After reconstitution of oral suspension, refrigeration is not required. The solution should be discarded after 14 days regardless of whether it has been refrigerated.

Cefotaxime

Clinical Uses

Uses for this drug in veterinary medicine are limited. Its use should be reserved for cases in which other drugs are ineffective.

Dosage Form

Only human-label products are available.

- Claforan

Adverse Side Effects

GI distress, hypersensitivity, and possibly fever may occur.

Storage of the Drug

Cefotaxime's storage is the same as that used for Cefixime.

Cefotetan Disodium

Clinical Uses

Cefotetan is a good choice for treating serious infections.

Dosage Form

Only human-label products are available.

- Cefotetan Disodium Powder for Solution

Adverse Side Effects

This drug appears to be well tolerated. The following may be seen: hypersensitivity, pain at the injection site, and gut flora alteration. Cefotetan may cause nephrotoxicity.

Storage of the Drug

The sterile powder for injection should be stored below 22°C (71.6°F). Darkening of the powder over time does not harm its efficacy. After reconstituting with sterile water, the solution is stable for 24 hours if stored at room temperature or 96 hours if refrigerated.

Cefovecin

Clinical Uses

Cefovecin is FDA-approved to treat skin infections in dogs and in cats to treat wounds and abscesses.

Dosage Form

- Convenia—veterinary label

Adverse Side Effects

This drug is well-tolerated in dogs and cats. In dogs, it may cause some changes in laboratory results such as increases in gamma glutamyl transpeptidase (GGT) and alanine aminotransferase (ALT). In cats, changes in laboratory results include mild increases in ALT, increases in BUN, and moderately increased creatinine levels. In dogs, clinical signs including depression, lethargy, and vomiting may be seen.

Storage of the Drug

Store the powder and reconstituted product in the original container and keep refrigerated at 36°F to 46°F. Use the entire contents within 56 days after reconstitution. Protect from light. Solution that darkens over time does not adversely affect the drug's potency.

Cefoxitin

Clinical Uses

Cefoxitin can be used clinically when injectable cephalosporins are indicated.

Dosage Form

Only human-label products are available.

- Cefoxitin Sodium Powder for injection and infusion

Adverse Side Effects

These are usually not serious and rarely occur. Hypersensitivity and pain at the injection site may be seen, it may alter gut flora, and it has potential for nephrotoxicity.

Storage of Drug

Cefoxitin should be stored at temperatures less than 30°C.

Cefpodoxime Proxetil

Clinical Uses

This drug is used in the treatment of skin infections.

Dosage Forms

- Simplicef—veterinary label
- Vantin—human label

Adverse Side Effects
Cefpodoxime proxetil may cause diarrhea, vomiting, and allergic reactions.

Storage of the Drug
Store at 68°F to 77°F.

Ceftazidime

Clinical Uses
Ceftazidime is useful in treating gram-negative bacterial infections. It may be used in the treatment of gram-negative infections in reptiles.

Dosage Forms
Only human-label products are available.
- ADD-Vantage
- Fortaz
- Ceptaz
- Tazidime

Adverse Side Effects
Ceftazidime may cause GI disturbances, pain when administered by IM injection, and allergic reactions.

Storage of the Drug
The drug should be stored at 59°F to 86°F.

Ceftiofur Crystalline Free Acid

Clinical Uses
This drug is used in swine for the treatment of respiratory disease. It is used in cattle for the treatment of bovine respiratory disease (BRD), shipping fever, and pneumonia. In dairy cattle, it is used for the treatment of subclinical mastitis.

Dosage Forms
Only veterinary-label products are available.
- Miglyol
- Excede

Adverse Side Effects
Hypersensitivity reactions may occur.

Storage of the Drug
The ready-to-use injectable product should be stored at 68°F to 77°F.

Ceftiofur Sodium

Clinical Uses
Ceftiofur sodium is used in cattle for the treatment of respiratory disease and acute interdigital necrobacillosis. It is used in swine for the treatment of bacterial pneumonia. In sheep and goats, it is used for the treatment of pneumonia. In horses, it is used for the treatment of respiratory infections. It is used in dogs for the treatment of urinary tract infections and is used in chicks and poults for the control of early mortality. Withdrawal time in cattle is 4 days before slaughter. No milk discard time is needed. In sheep and goats, no withdrawal time for slaughter or withholding milk is needed. Do not use in horses intended for human consumption.

Dosage Form
- Naxcel

Adverse Side Effects
These are usually rare. Pain may follow injection. Administration to horses under stress may be associated with acute diarrhea that could be fatal. Hypersensitivity reactions may occur.

Storage of the Drug
Unreconstituted powder should be stored at room temperature. Protect from light. Color change will not affect efficacy. After reconstitution, the solution is stable for up to 7 days when refrigerated.

TECHNICIAN NOTES
- Naxcel is approved for use in lactating dairy animals.
- Remember to read package inserts regarding milk withholding time, withholding time in animals to be slaughtered, and milk withholding time after mastitis treatment.

Ceftriaxone

Clinical Uses
Ceftriaxone is used to treat serious infections. It has activity against *Borrelia burgdorferi*, which makes it an excellent choice for treating Lyme disease.

Dosage Form
Only human-label products are available.
- Rocephin

Adverse Side Effects
These include hematologic effects, "sludge" in bile, hypersensitivity reactions, increased liver enzyme, BUN, and creatinine levels, and urine casts. Pain on IM injection may occur.

Storage of the Drug
The powder for reconstitution should be stored at or below 77°F.

Cefuroxime

Clinical Uses
Cefuroxime may be a good choice in small animal medicine for treating bacterial infections that are not responsive to first-generation cephalosporins.

Dosage Forms
Only human-label products are available.
- Ceftin
- Zinacef

Adverse Side Effects
GI effects may occur.

Storage of the Drug
Store tablets in tightly sealed containers at room temperature. Store powder for suspension at 35.6°F to 46.4°F.

Cephalexin

Clinical Uses
Cephalexin is not FDA-approved for veterinary use in the United States. It has been used to treat dogs, cats, horses, rabbits, ferrets, and birds that are infected with *Staphylococcus*.

Dosage Forms
Only human-label products are available.
- Keflex
- Other generic brands

Adverse Side Effects
There is a low occurrence of problems associated with cephalexin. Cephalexin has been known to cause salivation, tachypnea, and excitability in dogs and emesis and fever in cats.

Cephapirin

Clinical Uses
An intramammary cephapirin sodium product is FDA-approved in the United States for the treatment of mastitis.

Dosage Forms
All of the following are veterinary-label products.
- Cefa-Lak
- ToMORROW
- Cefa-Dri
- Metricure

Adverse Side Effects
These rarely occur. Allergic reactions, rashes, fever, and lymphadenopathy may be seen.

Storage of the Drug
Cephapirin intramammary syringes should be stored at controlled room temperature.

MACROLIDES

Pharmacodynamics/Pharmacokinetics

Many of the macrolides inhibit protein synthesis by penetrating the cell wall and binding to the 50S ribosomes subunits in susceptible bacteria. Many of them are considered bacteriostatic antibiotics. They have a broad spectrum of activity. The majority of these drugs are excreted from the body in the bile.

Azithromycin

Clinical Uses
This is a good broad-spectrum agent. It may be used to treat *Bordetella* in canines.

Dosage Form
Only human-label products are available.
- Zithromax

Adverse Side Effects
Azithromycin can cause vomiting in dogs when given at high doses. It has fewer GI effects than erythromycin.

Storage of the drug
Store tablets at temperatures less than 86°F.

Clarithromycin
Clinical Uses
Clarithromycin is used to treat *Helicobacter* spp. infections in cats and ferrets. It is useful in treating *Rhodococcus equi* infections in foals.

Dosage Forms
Only human-label products are available.
- Biaxin and Biaxin XL
- Prevpak; a combination of lansoprazole, amoxicillin, and clarithromycin

Adverse Side Effects
Redness of the ears may occur when the drug is used in cats. GI disturbances may occur.

Storage of the Drug
Store the tablets at 59°F to 86°F.

Erythromycin
Clinical Uses
Erythromycin is FDA-approved to treat infections in swine, sheep, and cattle. It may be used to treat esophageal reflux in dogs and cats.

Dosage Forms
The following are human-label products unless otherwise specified.
- Gallimycin-100—veterinary label
- Ery-Tab
- Erythromycin Filmtabs
- E.E.S. 400
- E.E.S. Granules
- EryPed 400
- EryPed Drops
- Erythrocin
- Eryzole
- Pediazole

Adverse Side Effects
These occur rarely. When injected IM, pain at the injection site may occur. Oral dosing may cause GI problems. In swine, rectal prolapse and rectal edema have been reported. The use of erythromycin in adult equines remains controversial.

Storage of the Drug
Store in tightly sealed containers at room temperature.

Tulathromycin
Clinical Uses
Tulathromycin is used in non-lactating dairy cattle to treat upper respiratory infections, bovine foot rot, and infectious bovine keratoconjunctivitis.

Dosage Form
Only veterinary-label products are available.
- Draxxin

Adverse Side Effects
These are minimal in cattle and swine. Allergic reactions are possible. SC or IM injections may cause local tissue reactions.

Storage of the Drug
Store below 77°F. The agent is stable up to 36 months.

Tylosin
Clinical Uses
The injectable form of the drug is FDA-approved in dogs and cats. It is not used very often in those species. It is sometimes used to treat chronic colitis in small animals. Tylosin is commonly used in cattle and swine for treating infections.

Dosage Form
Only veterinary-label products are available.
- Tylan

Adverse Side Effects
These include pain at injection site and possible GI upset.

Storage of the Drug
Store in well-closed containers at room temperature.

PENICILLINS

History of Penicillin
Sir Alexander Fleming was born on August 6, 1881 in Scotland. He served as a captain during World War

I. After seeing many of his comrades dying of bacteria-infected wounds, he desperately wanted to find a cure that could save lives. The main problem was finding an antibacterial substance that would not be toxic to animal tissue. In 1928, he was studying influenza virus in his somewhat disorganized laboratory. He saw a mold that had developed in a petri dish after being discarded in the sink before being disinfected. He noticed that the culture plate was one that contained *Staphylococcus* and that this mold had created a zone of inhibition around itself. He named the substance (mold) penicillin. Dr. Fleming died on March 11, 1955 (nobelprize.org, 2013).

Pharmacodynamics/Pharmacokinetics for Penicillins

Penicillin is bactericidal against susceptible bacteria. It acts by inhibiting mucopeptide synthesis in the cell wall, which results in a defective barrier and an osmotically unstable spheroplast (Plumb, 2011). Some penicillins are not absorbed well when administered orally but are rapidly absorbed after IM injections. After being absorbed by the body, penicillin is present throughout the body except for the cerebrospinal fluid, joints, and milk. Penicillin G is mostly excreted into the urine (Table 12-3).

Amoxicillin

Clinical Uses

Amoxicillin is used to treat a wide range of infections in various species. Amoxicillin is a reasonable choice for treating abscesses in cats even before culture and susceptibility results are available.

Dosage Forms

All of the following are veterinary-label products.

- Amoxi-Tabs
- Amoxi-Drop
- Amoxi-Mast

All of the following are human-label products.

- Amoxil
- Trimox
- Moxatag

Adverse Side Effects

These rarely occur. Allergic reactions may occur. Amoxicillin may cause GI upset when administered orally. High doses or prolonged doses have been associated with neurotoxicity. Liver enzymes may rise.

Storage of the Drug

Store at room temperature. After reconstitution, the oral suspension should be refrigerated (preferably). Discard unused portions after 14 days. Product should be shaken well before administering.

Amoxicillin/Clavulanate

Pharmacodynamics/Pharmacokinetics

Clavulanic acid acts by irreversibly bonding to **beta-lactamases** and penicillinases produced by bacterial agents. Clavulanate potassium is readily absorbed after oral dosing. It can cross the placenta but is not considered **teratogenic**.

Clinical Uses

This combination drug is used in the treatment of urinary tract, skin, and soft tissue infections in dogs and cats. It can also be used for treatment of canine periodontal disease, bacterial cystitis in female dogs, and hepatobiliary infections in dogs or cats (sometimes with a fluoroquinolone as an adjunct).

Dosage Forms

- Clavamox Tablets—veterinary label
- Clavamox Drops—veterinary label
- Augmentin—human label

Adverse Side Effects

Allergic reactions and GI upset may occur.

Storage of the Drug

Store at temperatures less than 75°F. After reconstitution, suspensions are stable for 10 days if refrigerated. Unused portions should be discarded after 10 days.

Ampicillin

Clinical Uses

Ampicillin is commonly used as a parenteral dosage form.

Dosage Forms

- Polyflex—veterinary label
- Principen—human label

TABLE 12-3 Penicillin Preparations, Indications, and Antagonistic Drugs

DRUG	INDICATIONS	ANTAGONIST	COMMENTS
Narrow-Spectrum Penicillins			
Penicillin G sodium	Infections caused by penicillin-sensitive organisms: bacterial pneumonia, upper respiratory tract infections, equine strangles, blackleg, infected wounds, urinary tract infections (at high doses)	Tetracyclines, chloramphenicol, and paromomycin	May add to sodium load
Penicillin G potassium	Same as for penicillin G sodium	Same as for penicillin G sodium	May produce hyperkalemia (IV); delayed absorption in horses (IM); unreliable absorption
Penicillin G procaine	Same as for penicillin G sodium	Same as for penicillin G sodium	Never give IV; contraindicated in some exotics and horses that race; preslaughter withdrawal and milk withholding periods
Penicillin G benzathine	Same as for penicillin G sodium	Same as for penicillin G sodium	Never give IV; preslaughter withdrawal required, and may persist in dairy cattle milk for 2 weeks
Narrow-Spectrum, Acid-Resistant Penicillins			
Penicillin V	Mild infections already controlled by parenteral therapy	Same as for penicillin G sodium	Should not be administered with food; less active against gram-negative bacteria than penicillin G
Beta-Lactamase–Resistant Penicillins			
Methicillin	Pyodermatitis, otitis externa, and other conditions caused by *Staphylococcus aureus*	Same as for penicillin G sodium	Not stable in solution; many incompatibilities in vitro
Cloxacillin	Same as for methicillin	Same as for penicillin G sodium	Frequently used in dry-cow intramammary preparations
Dicloxacillin and floxacillin	Same as for methicillin	Same as for penicillin G sodium	Absorbed from GI tract better than cloxacillin
Oxacillin	Same as for methicillin	Sulfonamides	Not absorbed as well as cloxacillin
Broad-Spectrum Penicillins			
Ampicillin and hetacillin	Infection of organs and tissues caused by ampicillin-sensitive bacteria	Chloramphenicol, erythromycin, tetracyclines, cephaloridine	Incompatible with many drugs and solutions; food impairs absorption; milk withholding and preslaughter withdrawal times
Amoxicillin	Same as for ampicillin	Same as for ampicillin	Absorbed from GI tract better than ampicillin
Piperacillin	Same as for ampicillin	Aminoglycosides	
Carbenicillin sodium	Same as for ampicillin, but especially *Pseudomonas* infections	Same as for ampicillin	Freshly mixed solutions should be used

TABLE 12-3 Penicillin Preparations, Indications, and Antagonistic Drugs—cont'd

DRUG	INDICATIONS	ANTAGONIST	COMMENTS
Broad-Spectrum Penicillins			
Carbenicillin indanyl sodium	Same as for carbenicillin sodium	Same as for ampicillin	Absorbed rapidly from the GI tract
Ticarcillin	Same as for carbenicillin sodium	Same as for ampicillin	Used as an intrauterine infusion in mares
Potentiated Penicillins			
Amoxicillin-potassium clavulanate (4 : 1)	Wide range of infections when used in combination	Same as for ampicillin	Capsules/tablets that are not kept in air-tightly sealed containers lose activity; do not give to patients allergic to penicillins or cephalosporins
Inhibitor of Tubular Secretion of Penicillins			
Probenecid	Prolongs blood levels of penicillins that have very short plasma half-lives or that are extremely costly	Same as for ampicillin	

IV, Intravenous; *IM*, intramuscular; *GI*, gastrointestinal.

Adverse Side Effects
Hypersensitivity and GI upset may occur.

Storage of the Drug
Ampicillin can be stored at room temperature before reconstitution. After reconstitution, the drug is stable for 3 months if refrigerated.

Ampicillin/Sulbactam
Pharmacodynamics/Pharmacokinetics
Combining sulbactam with ampicillin extends its spectrum of activity to those bacteria that would otherwise cause ampicillin to be ineffective. This medication is best administered parenterally.

Clinical Uses
It is effective parenterally against beta-lactamase–producing bacterial strains of otherwise resistant bacteria.

Dosage Form
Only human-label products are available.
- Unasyn

Adverse Side Effects
IM injections are painful. IV injection may cause **thrombophlebitis**. Allergic reactions are possible.

Storage of the Drug
Unreconstituted powder should be stored at temperatures at or below 86°F.

Cloxacillin
Clinical Uses
Cloxacillin is used for intramammary infusions in dry and lactating dairy cattle. It is important to adhere to milk withdrawal times when using this drug.

Dosage Forms
- Orbenin-DC
- Dry-Clox
- Bovaclox
- Dariclox

Adverse Side Effects
Allergic reactions may occur.

Storage of the Drug
Store at temperatures less than 77°F.

Dicloxacillin

Clinical Uses
Dicloxacillin is administered per os (PO; by mouth) for the treatment of bone, skin, and other soft tissue infections in small animals.

Dosage Form
Only human-label products are available.
- Dicloxacillin Sodium Capsules

Adverse Side Effects
Allergic reactions may occur. This drug may cause GI upset when given orally.

Storage of the Drug
Store at temperatures less than 68°F.

Oxacillin

Clinical Uses
Oxacillin is used in the treatment of bone, skin, and other soft tissue infections in small animals.

Dosage Forms
Only human-label products are available.
- Oxacillin Sodium Powder for Oral Solution
- ADD-Vantage

Adverse Side Effects
These include allergic reactions and GI upset. Neurotoxicity can occur with prolonged use.

Storage of the Drug
Store at room temperature.

Penicillin G

Clinical Uses
Penicillin is the drug of choice for a variety of bacteria.

Dosage Forms
All of the following are veterinary-label products.
- Penicillin-G Procaine Injections
- Go-Dry (over-the-counter)
- Masti-Clear
- Albadry Plus
- Quartermaster

All of the following are human-label products.
- Pfizerpen
- Tubex
- Bicillin LA
- Permapen

> **TECHNICIAN NOTES**
> - Veterinary personnel who are allergic to penicillin should be careful when handling this drug.
> - Some species, such as snakes, birds, turtles, guinea pigs, and chinchillas are sensitive to procaine penicillin G.
> - Subcutaneous administration of penicillin G or benzathine penicillin should be avoided because of potential tissue injury and residue potential in food animals.
> - Penicillin should not be used in horses intended for food.
> - Carefully read labels concerning milk withholding times and the treatment of animals to be slaughtered for food.
> - Penicillin G benzathine is long-acting (48 hours) and is not approved for use in dairy cattle.

Adverse Side Effects
Do not use in individuals that are sensitive to penicillins.

Storage of the Drug
Store at room temperature. After powder for injection is reconstituted, the solution should be kept refrigerated. Penicillin G and benzathine penicillin G should be stored at 48°F or lower but not frozen.

Penicillin V
The aforementioned information regarding penicillin G closely resembles the efficacy of penicillin V. The main difference is that penicillin V is more readily absorbed when given PO than is penicillin G.

Dosage Form
Only human-label products are available.
- Veetids

Piperacillin and Piperacillin/Tazobactam

Clinical Uses

Veterinary experience is limited, but piperacillin/tazobactam is a good choice to use until results of culture and sensitivity testing are returned.

Dosage Forms

Only human-label products are available. Products are available generically.

Adverse Side Effects

All of the following may occur: hypersensitivity reactions, pain after IM injection, and GI upset.

Storage of the Drug

Store at controlled room temperature.

Ticarcillin/Clavulanate

Clinical Uses

Ticarcillin/clavulanate is used for serious systemic infections and works well when compounded and used as an otic preparation for *Pseudomonas* otitis.

Dosage Form

Only human-label products are available.

- Timentin

Adverse Side Effects

Do not use in patients with impaired renal function. Patients receiving high dosages may be more prone to developing platelet function abnormalities or CNS effects.

Storage of the Drug

Keep unused vials at room temperature.

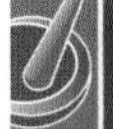

TETRACYCLINES

Pharmacodynamics/Pharmacokinetics

Tetracyclines usually act as time-dependent antibiotics and inhibit protein synthesis by reversibly binding to 30S ribosomal subunits of susceptible organisms, thereby preventing binding to those ribosomes of aminoacyl transfer-RNA (Plumb, 2011). Tetracyclines are generally considered to be bacteriostatic antibiotics. Tetracyclines have activity against most mycoplasma, spirochetes (including the Lyme disease organism), chlamydia, and rickettsia. With regard to gram-positive bacteria, the tetracyclines have activity against some strains of staphylococci and streptococci, but the resistance of these organisms is on the rise. Oxytetracycline and tetracycline have almost identical spectrums of activity and patterns of cross-resistance. Tetracyclines have antiinflammatory and immunomodulating effects. They can suppress antibody production and chemotaxis of neutrophils and inhibit lipases, collagenases, prostaglandin synthesis, and activation of complement component 3. Tetracyclines are readily absorbed after being administered orally. IM administration carries a lower ability to be absorbed. Tetracyclines can cross the placenta, enter fetal circulation, and can be distributed into milk. Tetracyclines are eliminated from the body by glomerular filtration. The elimination half-life of tetracycline is about 5 to 6 hours in dogs and cats. See Table 12-4.

> **TECHNICIAN NOTES** Tetracyclines given to young animals may cause yellow to brown discoloration of bones and teeth.

Chlortetracycline

Clinical Uses

Chlortetracycline is used mostly in water or feed treatments or topically for ophthalmic use.

Dosage Forms

The following are all veterinary-label products.

- Aureomycin
- CTC
- CLTC 100 MR

Adverse Side Effects

When given in high doses, this drug may cause an increased BUN level and hepatotoxicity; it should be used with caution in patients with renal disease. High doses in ruminants can cause ruminal microflora depression. In small animals, high doses may cause nausea, vomiting, anorexia, and diarrhea. Cats do not tolerate oral tetracycline well. Long-term use in dogs may cause urolith formation. Horses stressed by

TABLE 12-4 Tetracycline Preparations, Indications, and Antagonistic Drugs

DRUG	INDICATIONS	ANTAGONIST	COMMENTS
Oxytetracycline	Infections of organs or tissues caused by tetracycline-sensitive strains; anaplasmosis; often ineffective for endocarditis, empyema, meningitis, septic arthritis, and osteomyelitis	Antacids, milk, diuretics, methoxyflurane, penicillins, ferrous sulfate	Long withdrawal times in cattle; shock reaction may occur when given intravenously in horses; diarrhea also common in horses
Chlortetracycline	Same as for oxytetracycline	Antacids, milk, diuretics, methoxyflurane, penicillins	
Tetracycline	Same as for oxytetracycline	Same as for oxytetracycline	
Doxycycline, minocycline	Same as for oxytetracycline, but much better tissue penetration; doxycycline is especially useful for canine ehrlichiosis	Minocycline—same as for chlortetracycline; doxycycline—same as for oxytetracycline, barbiturates, and carbamazepine	These drugs are potent broad-spectrum tetracyclines

surgery, anesthesia, or trauma may develop severe diarrhea. Long-term tetracycline therapy can result in overgrowth (superinfections) of nonsusceptible bacteria or fungi.

Storage of the Drug

Keep tetracyclines in tightly sealed containers protected from light.

Doxycycline

Clinical Uses

Doxycycline is commonly used in small animals to treat *Borrelia,* leptospira, rickettsiae, chlamydia, mycoplasma, bartonella, and bordetella. Doxirobe is used in dogs as an oral application for the prevention/treatment of periodontal disease.

Dosage Forms

All of the following are human-label products unless otherwise specified.

- Doxirobe—veterinary label
- Periostat
- Alodox Convenience Kit
- Vibramycin and Vibra-Tabs
- Oraxyl
- Doryx
- Oracea
- Monodox
- Adoxa
- Atridox
- Doxy-100 and -200
- Medomycin

Adverse Side Effects

After oral administration, the most common effects seen in dogs and cats are vomiting, diarrhea, and anorexia. Giving the drug with food seems to help some of these problems. Oral doxycycline has been blamed for causing esophageal strictures in cats. Therefore, after giving an oral dose to cats, it should be followed by at least 6 mL water.

Storage of the Drug

Keep stored in tightly sealed, light-resistant containers at temperatures less than 86°F.

Minocycline HCl

Clinical Uses

Minocycline is useful for the treatment of brucellosis, especially when used in conjunction with aminoglycosides.

Dosage Forms

Only human-label products are available.

- Dynacin
- Myrac

- Solodyn
- Arestin

Adverse Side Effects
After oral administration in dogs and cats, nausea and vomiting are the most commonly reported side effects.

Storage of the Drug
Keep oral preparations in tightly sealed containers at room temperature. Do not freeze the oral suspension. The injectable form should be stored at room temperature and protected from light.

Oxytetracycline

Clinical Uses
Oxytetracycline is commonly used in large animal (bovine) medicine.

Dosage Forms
All of the following are veterinary-label products.

- Terramycin
- Liquamycin
- Bio-Mycin
- Biocyl
- Oxyject
- Oxytet
- Liquamycin LA-200
- Tetradure-30
- Terramycin Scours Tablets

Adverse Side Effects
Oxytetracycline may cause ruminal depression in ruminants.

Storage of the Drug
Store in tightly sealed, light-resistant containers at room temperature.

Tetracycline

Clinical Uses
Tetracycline is still used as an antimicrobial, although other forms are more commonly used in today's veterinary practices.

Dosage Forms
A variety of veterinary-label products are available.

- Delta Albaplex (a combination product with tetracycline, novobiocin, and prednisolone)

The following are human-label products.

- Sumycin-250 and -500
- Sumycin Syrup

> *TECHNICIAN NOTES*
> - Never give tetracycline intravenously to a horse.
> - Absorption of tetracyclines through the GI tract is dramatically decreased by the presence of food, milk products, and antacids.
> - Carefully read labels about use in animals to be slaughtered.
> - Tetracycline is not approved for use in lactating dairy animals or poultry that produce eggs for human consumption.

LINCOSAMIDES

Pharmacodynamics/Pharmacokinetics

Lincosamide antibiotics are broad-spectrum antibiotics that have activity against anaerobes, gram-positive aerobic cocci and toxoplasma parasites, among others. Horses, rodents, ruminants, and lagomorphs are hypersensitive to lincosamides. Lincosamides are distributed to milk and can cause diarrhea in nursing animals. The pharmacokinetics of lincosamides have not been extensively studied in veterinary species (Plumb, 2011). The following information is from studies on the effect of the drugs on humans. Lincosamides are rapidly absorbed after oral dosage. Peak serum levels are reached about 2 to 4 hours after oral dosing. IM administration peaks about twice as long as that reached after oral dosing. Lincosamides are distributed into most tissues. The drugs can cross the placenta. Lincosamides are partially metabolized in the liver. Unchanged drug and metabolites are excreted in the urine, feces, and bile. The elimination half-life of lincomycin is about 3 to 4 hours in small animals (Plumb, 2011).

> *TECHNICIAN NOTES*
> - Carefully read labels about use in animals for slaughter.
> - Lincosamides should not be administered to rabbits, hamsters, guinea pigs, or horses.

Clindamycin

Clinical Uses

Clindamycin is FDA-approved for use in dogs and cats. It is commonly used to treat wounds, abscesses, and osteomyelitis caused by *Staphylococcus aureus*. It may also be used to treat toxoplasmosis.

Dosage Forms

The following are all veterinary-label products.

- Antirobe Capsules
- Clintabs
- Antirobe Aquadrops
- Clinsol

The following are all human-label products.

- Cleocin
- Cleocin Pediatric
- ADD-Vantage; Cleocin Phosphate
- Cleocin Phosphate IV

Adverse Side Effects

Clindamycin may cause GI upset and esophageal strictures in cats when administered without food or a water bolus. Cats may have hypersalivation or lip smacking after oral administration. IM injections cause pain at the injection site.

Storage of the Drug

Store at room temperature.

Lincomycin

Clinical Uses

Lincomycin is FDA-approved for use in dogs, cats, swine, and in combination with other agents for chickens. It is used to provide treatment against anaerobes, gram-positive aerobic cocci, and toxoplasma parasites.

Dosage Forms

All of the following are veterinary-label products unless otherwise specified.

- Lincocin
- Lincocin Aquadrops
- Lincocin Sterile Solution
- Lincomix Injectable
- Lincocin—human label

> TECHNICIAN NOTES
> - Lincomycin is not for use in avians used for egg laying, breeders, or turkeys.

Adverse Side Effects

Lincomycin may cause GI upset and pain at the injection site when given as an IM injection. Rapid IV administration can cause hypotension and cardiopulmonary arrest.

Storage of the Drug

Store at room temperature.

Pirlimycin

Clinical Uses

Pirlimycin is used for intramammary infusion for dairy cattle.

Dosage Form

Only veterinary-label products are available.

- Pirsue Aqueous Gel

> TECHNICIAN NOTES Milk withdrawal time (when used at labeled doses) is 36 hours after the last treatment. Meat withdrawal time (when used at labeled doses) is 9 days.

Adverse Side Effects

No adverse effects have been reported at this time.

Storage of the Drug

Store syringes at or below 77°F.

Tilmicosin

Clinical Uses

Tilmicosin is used in the treatment of bovine or ovine respiratory disease caused by *Mannheimia (pasteurella) haemolytica*. It is also used in cattle, sheep, and rabbits, and it can be used in swine as a medicated feed agent.

Dosage Forms

Only veterinary-label products are available.

- Micotil 300 Injection
- Pulmotil 90

TECHNICIAN NOTES

- Micotil is not approved for use in lactating dairy animals.
- Carefully read labels about use in animals to be slaughtered.
- Do not use in automatically powered syringes.
- Do not give IV to camelids.

Adverse Side Effects
IM injections may cause local tissue irritation. When injected SC, tilmicosin may cause edema. Avoid contact with the eyes. Tilmicosin is potentially lethal to humans, swine, and horses. In case of human injection, contact a physician immediately.

Storage of the Drug
Store at room temperature. Protect from exposure to direct sunlight.

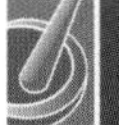

QUINOLONES

Pharmacodynamics/Pharmacokinetics

Quinolones are bactericidal agents. The mechanism of action is believed to be inhibition of bacterial DNA-gyrase (a type-II topoisomerase), which prevents DNA supercoiling and DNA synthesis (Plumb, 2011). These agents have activity against many gram-negative bacilli and cocci. They have variable activity against most streptococci, so they are not usually recommended for these infections. Bacterial resistance is a concern. These drugs are well absorbed after oral dosing. Quinolones are distributed throughout the body. Highest concentrations are found in the bile, kidney, liver, lungs, and reproductive system. Quinolones are eliminated from the body by both renal and nonrenal routes.

Ciprofloxacin

Clinical Uses
Ciprofloxacin may be used when a larger oral dosage of IV product is desired (as an alternative to enrofloxacin.) This drug differs from enrofloxacin in its pharmacokinetics. In dogs, enrofloxacin's bioavailability is almost twice that of ciprofloxacin after oral administration. Ciprofloxacin is one of the metabolites of enrofloxacin.

Dosage Forms
Only human-label products are available.

- Cipro
- Cipro XR

Adverse Side Effects
Ciprofloxacin may cause hypersensitivity. Its use is contraindicated in growing animals because it may cause cartilage abnormalities. Use with caution in patients with renal or hepatic insufficiency and in patients that are dehydrated. It is preferable to administer the drug PO on an empty stomach.

Storage of the Drug
Store in tightly sealed containers at temperatures less than 86°F, unless otherwise noted by the manufacturer.

Danofloxacin

Clinical Uses
Danofloxacin is labeled for use in cattle (not dairy or veal) to treat BRD. It can be used in cattle by administering two injections SC 48 hours apart. The FDA prohibits extralabel use in food animals.

Dosage Form
Only veterinary-label products are available.

- A180

Adverse Side Effects
Hypersensitivity may occur. Lameness in calves has been reported. SC injections in cattle may cause local irritation to tissue.

Storage of the Drug
Store at or below 86°F.

Difloxacin

Clinical Uses
Difloxacin is used in dogs for treatment of bacterial infections susceptible to the drug. It is not labeled for use in cats or other species.

Dosage Form
Only veterinary-label products are available.
- Dicural

Adverse Side Effects
This drug may cause hypersensitivity. Use caution in young growing animals because it may cause cartilage abnormalities. It may also cause seizure disorders, hepatic or renal insufficiency, dehydration, and GI distress.

Storage of the Drug
Store between 59°F and 86°F.

Enrofloxacin
Clinical Uses
Enrofloxacin is used effectively against a variety of pathogens, although it is not effective against anaerobes. It is somewhat contraindicated in growing animals because it may cause cartilage abnormalities. It is approved for use in cattle (not calves). Extralabel use is prohibited.

Dosage Form
Only veterinary-label products are available. Enrofloxacin is not recommended for use in humans because of CNS effects.
- Baytril
- Baytril 100

Adverse Side Effects
These include GI distress, CNS stimulation, crystalluria, and hypersensitivity. IV administration can be risky in small animals.

Storage of the Drug
Store in tightly sealed containers less than 86°F.

Ibafloxacin
Clinical Uses
Ibafloxacin is used in dogs and cats primarily in Europe. This drug is not available in the United States. It is labeled for treating dermal infections, deep pyoderma, wounds, abscesses, and upper respiratory tract infections.

Dosage Form
Only veterinary-label products are available.
- Ibaflin

Adverse Side Effects
Ibafloxacin may cause diarrhea, vomiting, dullness, anorexia, and salivation.

Storage of the Drug
Do not store at temperatures above 77°F.

Marbofloxacin
Clinical Uses
Marbofloxacin is effective against a variety of pathogens. It has no efficacy against anaerobes.

Dosage Form
Only veterinary-label products are available.
- Zeniquin

Adverse Side Effects
Marbofloxacin may cause hypersensitivity and GI distress. It is not for use in young growing animals because of the potential for cartilage abnormalities.

Storage of the Drug
Store at or below 86°F.

Orbifloxacin
Clinical Uses
This drug is used in dogs and cats for bacterial infections susceptible to orbifloxacin. It can help in the treatment of susceptible gram-negative infections in horses.

Dosage Forms
- Orbax—veterinary label
- Orbax Suspension—veterinary label

Adverse Side Effects
Orbifloxacin may cause GI upset.

Storage of the Drug
Store between 36°F and 86°F.

TECHNICIAN NOTES

- The safety of fluoroquinolones in breeding or pregnant dogs and cats has not been determined.
- Fluoroquinolones cannot be used in cattle intended for dairy production or in veal calves.
- Fluoroquinolones cannot be used in laying hens that produce eggs for human consumption.
- Carefully read labels regarding withdrawal periods for animals intended for slaughter.

SULFONAMIDES

Pharmacodynamics/Pharmacokinetics

Sulfonamides are bacteriostatic agents when used alone. It is thought that they prevent bacterial replication by competing with para-aminobenzoic acid (PABA) in the biosynthesis of tetrahydrofolic acid in the pathway to form folic acid. Only microorganisms that make their own folic acid are affected by sulfa drugs. Sulfonamides are readily absorbed from the GI tract of non-ruminant animals. Peak levels occur 1 to 2 hours after administration. Levels tend to be highest in the liver, kidney, and lungs and lower in muscle and bone. Sulfonamides are excreted from the body by the kidneys with some action by the liver (Plumb, 2011).

Sulfachlorpyridazine

Clinical Uses

Sulfachlorpyridazine is used in the treatment of diarrhea in calves caused by *Escherichia coli* in those patients younger than 1 month. It is used to treat colibacillosis in swine.

Dosage Forms

Only veterinary-label products are available.

- Vetisulid Powder
- Vetisulid Oral Suspension

Adverse Side Effects

Sulfachlorpyridazine may precipitate in the urine. It may cause keratoconjunctivitis sicca in dogs, bone marrow depression, hypersensitivity reactions, focal retinitis, fever, vomiting, and non-septic polyarthritis. It may be potentially teratogenic. IV injection given rapidly may cause muscle weakness, blindness, ataxia, and collapse. SC or IM injection may cause tissue irritation.

Storage of the Drug

Store at room temperature. Protect from light. Avoid freezing.

Sulfadiazine/Trimethoprim and Sulfamethoxazole/Trimethoprim

Clinical Uses

These combinations are used in dogs and horses to treat infections caused by susceptible organisms. They are effective for treating prostate infections and for infections caused by many strains of methicillin-resistant staphylococci.

Dosage Forms

All of the following are veterinary-label products.

- Tribrissen 400 Oral Paste
- Di-Biotic 48%
- Tribrissen 48% Injection
- Tucoprim Powder
- Uniprim Powder
- Trivetrin (Canada)
- Borgal (Canada)

All of the following are human-label products.

- Trimpex
- Bactrim
- Bactrim DS
- Septra DS
- Septra
- Cotrim Pediatric
- Sulfatrim

Adverse Side Effects

Keratoconjunctivitis sicca, hypersensitivity, acute neutrophilic hepatitis with icterus, vomiting, anorexia, diarrhea, fever, hemolytic anemia, urticaria, polyarthritis, facial swelling, polydipsia, crystalluria, hematuria, polyuria, cholestasis, hypothyroidism, anemias, agranulocytosis, idiosyncratic hepatic necrosis in dogs, and potentially teratogenicity are all possible.

Storage of the Drug

Store at room temperatures in tightly sealed containers.

Sulfadimethoxine

Clinical Uses

This drug is for use in dogs and cats for respiratory, genitourinary, enteric, and soft tissue infections. It is used in the treatment of coccidiosis in dogs, but the use of this drug is not FDA-approved for this indication. Sulfadimethoxine is used in horses to treat *Streptococcus equi.* It is used in cattle to treat shipping fever complex, calf diphtheria, bacterial pneumonia, and foot rot. In poultry, sulfadimethoxine is added to drinking water to treat coccidiosis, fowl cholera, and infectious coryza.

Dosage Forms

Only veterinary-label products are available.

- Albon Injection 40%
- Di-Methox Injection 40%
- Albon Tablets
- Albon SR

Adverse Side Effects

Sulfadimethoxine may precipitate in the urine, may contribute to the risk of crystalluria, hematuria, and renal tubule obstruction. It causes the same adverse effects as seen with other sulfonamides.

Storage of the Drug

Store at room temperature in tightly sealed containers.

Sulfadimethoxine/Ormetoprim

Clinical Uses

This combination is FDA-approved for the treatment of skin and soft tissue infections in dogs caused by *S. aureus* and *E. coli.*

Dosage Forms

The following are all veterinary-label products.

- Primor
- Rofenaid 40
- Romet 30

Adverse Side Effects

These are the same as seen with other sulfonamides.

Storage of the Drug

Store in tightly sealed containers at room temperature.

ANTIBACTERIALS

Aztreonam

Clinical Uses

Aztreonam is used in small animals to fight serious infections caused by a wide variety of bacteria.

Dosage Forms

- Azactam—veterinary label
- Cayston—veterinary label

Adverse Side Effects

In humans, known side effects include colitis, pain or swelling after IM injection, and phlebitis after IV administration.

Storage of the Drug

Store powder for reconstitution at room temperature.

Chloramphenicol

Clinical Uses

Chloramphenicol is used to treat a variety of infections in small animals and horses, especially those caused by anaerobic bacteria.

Dosage Forms

- Chloramphenicol Tablets and Capsules (various milligrams)—veterinary label
- Chloromycetin—veterinary label
- Chloromycetin Sodium Succinate—human label

TECHNICIAN NOTES

- Chloramphenicol is very stable and residual amounts of the drug can be left in meat, milk, or eggs. Therefore, the FDA has prohibited the use of chloramphenicol in food animals because of human public health implications.
- Chloramphenicol is not recommended for dogs maintained for breeding purposes.
- Chloramphenicol should not be administered simultaneously with penicillin, streptomycin, or the cephalosporins.

Adverse Side Effects

Chloramphenicol may cause aplastic anemia in humans.

Storage of the Drug
Store in tightly sealed containers at room temperature.

Clofazimine

Clinical Uses
In small animals, this drug is used against mycobacterial diseases such as leprosy-like or *Mycobacterium avium*-related disease states.

Dosage Form
There are no veterinary-label products available. Lamprene (human-label) is only available to physicians enrolled as investigators treating Hansen's disease (i.e., leprosy) or multidrug-resistant tuberculosis.

Adverse Side Effects
These include GI upset and skin, eye, and excretion discoloration.

Storage of the Drug
Store in tightly sealed containers protected from moisture at temperatures less than 86°F.

Dapsone

Clinical Uses
Dapsone is useful in the treatment of mycobacterial diseases in dogs and possibly cats. It may be useful in the adjunct treatment of brown recluse spider *(Loxosceles reclusa recluse)* bites.

Dosage Form
Only human-label products are available.
- Dapsone Oral Tablets

Adverse Side Effects
Dapsone may cause hepatotoxicity, dose-dependent methemoglobinemia, hemolytic anemia, thrombocytopenia, neutropenias, GI disturbance, neuropathies, cutaneous drug eruptions, and photosensitivity. It may possibly be a carcinogen.

Storage of the Drug
Store at room temperature.

Ethambutol

Clinical Uses
Ethambutol is useful in treating mycobacterial infections.

Dosage Form
Only human-label products are available.
- Myambutol

Adverse Side Effects
Because of public health risks, especially in immunocompromised people, treatment of mycobacterial infections in domestic or captive animals is controversial.

Storage of the Drug
Store below 104°F.

Florfenicol

Clinical Uses
Florfenicol is FDA-approved for use in cattle in the treatment of BRD.

Dosage Forms
Only veterinary-label products are available.
- NuFlor
- NuFlor Gold
- NuFlor Concentrate Solution
- Aquaflor
- Resflor Gold

TECHNICIAN NOTES
- Florfenicol is not approved for use in female dairy cattle 20 months or older and should not be used in veal calves, calves younger than 1 month old, or calves receiving an all-milk diet.
- Florfenicol is for intramuscular injection only. Injections should be administered into the neck, and no more than 10 mL should be given per site.

Adverse Side Effects
Florfenicol may cause anorexia, decreased water consumption, and diarrhea. Reactions may be severe if injected at sites other than the neck. Anaphylaxis and collapse have been reported in cattle.

Storage of the Drug
Store between 36°F and 86°F.

Fosfomycin
Clinical Uses
Fosfomycin is useful in the treatment of multidrug-resistant urinary tract infections in dogs.

Dosage Form
Only human-label products are available.
- Monurol

Adverse Side Effects
Very little information about adverse effects in animals is known. In humans, it may cause diarrhea. In cats, renal tubular damage may occur.

Storage of the Drug
Store at room temperature.

Isoniazid
Clinical Uses
Isoniazid is sometimes used for chemoprophylaxis in small animals that live in households with a human that has tuberculosis.

Dosage Forms
Only human-label products are available.
- Nydrazid
- Rifater
- Rifamate

Adverse Side Effects
Hepatotoxicity, CNS stimulation, peripheral neuropathy and thrombocytopenia, ataxia, seizures, salivation, diarrhea, vomiting, and arrhythmias have been reported.

Storage of the Drug
Store at temperatures below 104°F.

Methenamine
Clinical Uses
Methenamine is used for prophylaxis of recurrent urinary tract infections. It is not commonly used in veterinary medicine.

Dosage Form
Only human-label products are available.
- Urex

Adverse Side Effects
GI upset with nausea, vomiting, and anorexia are possible.

Storage of the Drug
Store at room temperature.

Metronidazole
Clinical Uses
Metronidazole is used in the treatment of *Giardia* in both dogs and cats. In horses, the drug has been used for the treatment of anaerobic infections.

Dosage Forms
Only human-label products are available.
- Flagyl
- Flagyl 375
- Flagyl ER
- Helidac

> TECHNICIAN NOTES Metronidazole is prohibited for use in food animals by the FDA.

Adverse Side Effects
Metronidazole may cause neurologic disorders, lethargy, weakness, neutropenias, hepatotoxicity, hematuria, anorexia, nausea, vomiting, and diarrhea. In horses, there have been reported cases of *Clostridium difficile* and *Clostridium perfringens* diarrhea and death after the use of metronidazole.

Storage of the Drug
Store at room temperature.

Nitrofurantoin
Clinical Uses
Nitrofurantoin is used to treat urinary tract infections.

Dosage Forms
Only human-label products are available.
- Macrodantin
- Macrobid
- Furadantin

> **TECHNICIAN NOTES**
> - Except for approved topical use, nitrofurantoin has been prohibited in food-producing animals.
> - Nitrofurantoin should not be used in veal calves.

Adverse Side Effects
Nitrofurantoin may cause GI disturbance and hepatopathy.

Storage of the Drug
Store at room temperature and protect from the light.

Novobiocin
Clinical Uses
When used in combination with penicillin G, these two drugs are used in dry dairy cattle as a mastitis tube.

Dosage Forms
The following are all veterinary-label products.
- Albadry Plus
- Delta Albaplex
- Delta Albaplex 3X

Adverse Side Effects
When used systemically, novobiocin may cause fever, GI disturbances, and blood dyscrasias.

Storage of the Drug
Store in tightly sealed containers at room temperature.

Potassium Iodide
Clinical Uses
This is primarily used in the treatment of actinobacillosis and actinomycosis in cattle.

Dosage Forms
Veterinary-label generic forms are available. The following, however, are all human-label products.
- SSKI
- Pima
- Thyrosafe
- Losat

Adverse Side Effects
Chronic use may cause iodism. Cats are more prone to this. Signs in cats include vomiting, inappetence, depression, twitching, hypothermia, and cardiovascular failure.

Storage of the Drug
Store at room temperature.

Rifampin
Clinical Uses
The principle use of rifampin in veterinary medicine is for treatment of *R. equi* infections in young horses. In small animals, it may be used in conjunction with antifungal agents in the treatment of histoplasmosis.

Dosage Forms
Only human-label products are available.
- Rimactane
- Rifadin

Adverse Side Effects
Rifampin may cause red-orange colored urine, tears, sweat, and saliva. There are no harmful consequences from this effect (Plumb, 2011).

Storage of the Drug
Store in tightly sealed containers at room temperature.

Tiamulin
Clinical Uses
Tiamulin is used in swine to treat pneumonia and swine dysentery.

Dosage Forms
Only veterinary-label products are available.
- Denagard 10
- TiaGard
- Denagard Liquid Concentrate

Adverse Side Effects
These are considered unlikely.

Storage of the Drug
Protect from moisture and store in a dry place.

Tinidazole

Clinical Uses

Tinidazole may be useful in treating anaerobic infections, particularly those associated with dental problems, has some antiprotozoal effects, and may be used in the treatment of giardiasis.

Dosage Form

Only human-label products are available.

- Tindamax; also generics

Adverse Side Effects

GI disturbances are possible. The drug has a very bitter taste.

Storage of the Drug

Store at controlled room temperature.

Vancomycin

Clinical Uses

Vancomycin is used to treat methicillin-resistant *Staphylococcus spp.* (MRSA).

Dosage Form

Only human-label products are available.

- Vancocin

Adverse Side Effects

Nephrotoxicity and ototoxicity are the most serious potential adverse effects.

Storage of the Drug

Store in tightly sealed containers at room temperature.

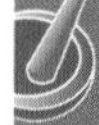

ANTIFUNGAL AGENTS

Pharmacodynamics/Pharmacokinetics

Ketoconazole is **fungistatic** against susceptible fungi. It is believed that some antifungal agents increase cellular membrane permeability and cause secondary metabolic effects and growth inhibition. Some antifungals are readily absorbed after oral administration, whereas other antifungal agents must be given IV.

Amphotericin B

Clinical Uses

Amphotericin B is a systemic antifungal used for serious mycotic infections. It must be administered IV.

Dosage Forms

Only human-label products are available.

- Amphotericin B for Injection
- Abelcet
- AmBisome
- Fungizone

> **TECHNICIAN NOTES**
>
> - Amphotericin B is administered intravenously through dilution in 5% dextrose.
> - Renal function should be monitored closely during treatment.

Adverse Side Effects

Amphotericin B is nephrotoxic. Renal function monitoring must be done.

Storage of the Drug

Vials of amphotericin B powder for injection should be stored in the refrigerator and protected from light and moisture.

Caspofungin

Clinical Uses

Caspofungin may be used in the treatment of invasive aspergillosis or disseminated *Candida* infections in companion animals. Very little information exists on its use in dogs and cats.

Dosage Form

Only human-label products are available.

- Cancidas

Adverse Side Effects

Adverse effects in animals have not been determined. In humans, the drug is generally well tolerated. A rash, facial swelling, pruritus, and anaphylaxis have been reported. Hepatic dysfunction has also been reported.

Storage of the Drug

Refrigeration is necessary.

Fluconazole

Clinical Uses

Fluconazole is useful in the treatment of systemic mycoses such as cryptococcal meningitis, blastomycosis, and histoplasmosis.

Dosage Forms

Only human-label products are available.

- Diflucan
- Viaflex Plus

Adverse Side Effects

There is only limited experience with this drug in domestic animals. So far, it seems safe for use in dogs and cats. Some side effects include inappetence, vomiting, and diarrhea.

Storage of the Drug

Store at temperatures less than 86°F in tightly sealed containers.

Flucytosine

Clinical Uses

This drug is active against strains of *Cryptococcus* and *Candida*.

Dosage Form

Only human-label products are available.

- Ancobon

Adverse Side Effects

Flucytosine may cause GI disturbances, dose-dependent bone marrow depression, cutaneous eruption, oral ulceration, and increased levels of hepatic enzymes.

Storage of the Drug

Store preferably at room temperature.

Griseofulvin

Clinical Uses

Griseofulvin is used in dogs and cats to treat dermatophytic fungal infections of the skin, hair, and claws. It is used to treat ringworm in horses. The oral tablets that are FDA-approved for dogs and cats are no longer marketed in the United States, but human dosage forms are available.

Dosage Forms

- Am Tech Griseofulvin Powder—veterinary label
- Grifulvin V—human label
- Gris-PEG—human label

> **TECHNICIAN NOTES**
>
> - Griseofulvin should not be administered to pregnant or breeding animals.
> - Absorption of griseofulvin is enhanced by administration with a fatty meal.

Adverse Side Effects

Griseofulvin may cause anorexia, vomiting, diarrhea, anemia, neutropenia, leukopenia, thrombocytopenia, depression, ataxia, hepatoxicity, dermatitis/photosensitivity, and toxic epidermal necrolysis. Cats are more susceptible to adverse side effects.

Storage of the Drug

Store at less than 104°F.

Itraconazole

Clinical Uses

Itraconazole may be used to treat systemic mycoses. It is probably more effective than ketoconazole but is much more expensive than ketoconazole. Itraconazole is considered by many to be the drug of choice for treating blastomycosis.

Dosage Forms

- Itrafungol—veterinary label (available in other countries; not in the United States)
- Sporanox—human label

Adverse Side Effects

Anorexia in dogs and hepatic toxicity may occur.

Storage of the Drug

Store between 59°F and 77°F.

Ketoconazole

Clinical Uses

Ketoconazole is used to treat fungal infections in dogs, cats, and other small species. Use of ketoconazole in cats is controversial, and some say it should never be used in that species. It can also be used for the medical treatment of hyperadrenocorticism in dogs.

Dosage Forms
There are no veterinary-label products available for systemic use.
- Ketoconazole tablets—human label

Adverse Side Effects
Ketoconazole may cause GI disturbances and hepatic toxicity. Ketoconazole may cause infertility in male dogs.

Storage of the Drug
Store in tightly sealed containers at room temperature.

Nystatin
Clinical Uses
Nystatin is used in the treatment of oral or GI tract *Candida* infections in dogs, cats, and birds.

Dosage Forms
There are no veterinary-label products available for oral use.
- Nilstat—human label
- Mycostatin—human label

Adverse Side Effects
Nystatin may cause GI upset and hypersensitivity.

Storage of the Drug
Store at room temperature in tightly sealed, light-resistant containers.

Terbutaline HCl
Clinical Uses
Terbutaline is used as a bronchodilating agent in the treatment of cardiopulmonary diseases such as tracheobronchitis, collapsing trachea, pulmonary edema, and allergic bronchitis. Occasionally, it is used in horses for bronchodilating effects.

Dosage Form
Only human-label products are available.
- Brethine

Adverse Side Effects
This drug may cause increased heart rate, tremors, CNS excitement, and dizziness.

Storage of the Drug
Store in tightly sealed containers at room temperature.

Voriconazole
Clinical Uses
Voriconazole is used to treat a variety of fungal infections in veterinary patients. There is some interest in treating birds for aspergillosis with this drug.

Dosage Forms
Only human-label products are available.
- Vfend
- Vfend I.V.

Adverse Side Effects
Accurate information in veterinary medicine is limited. Liver enlargement may occur. Cats tend to have many more side effects.

Storage of the Drug
Store below 86°F.

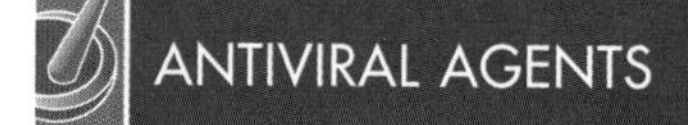

ANTIVIRAL AGENTS

Antiviral agents are used to treat viruses. The current drugs on the market are used in the treatment of herpes simplex types 1 and 2, cytomegalovirus, Epstein-Barr, and varicella-zoster viruses. Elimination half-lives in dogs, cats, and horses for acyclovir are about 3 hours.

Acyclovir
Clinical Uses
Acyclovir is useful in treating herpes infections in a variety of avian species and in cats with corneal or conjunctival herpes infections. It should be used with caution in veterinary patients because information about using this drug is not well established in animal patients. Acyclovir is being

investigated as a treatment for equine herpes virus type-1 myeloencephalopathy in horses, but its clinical efficacy has not been proven at this time (Plumb, 2011).

Dosage Forms
Only human-label products are available.
- Zovirax; generics also

Adverse Side Effects
Acyclovir may cause GI disturbances when given orally.

Storage of the Drug
Store in tightly sealed, light-resistant containers at room temperature.

Amantadine
Clinical Uses
In 2006, the FDA banned the extralabel use of amantadine and other influenza antivirals in chickens, turkeys, and ducks. It is useful in the treatment of chronic pain, especially pain that is untouched by the use of opioids.

Dosage Form
Only human-label products are available.
- Symmetrel

Adverse Side Effects
Very limited experience exists in domestic animals. Some reports include agitation in dogs, loose stools, flatulence, and diarrhea.

Storage of the Drug
Store in tightly sealed containers at room temperature.

Famciclovir
Clinical Uses
Famciclovir may be useful in the treatment of feline herpes infections.

Dosage Form
Only human-label products are available.
- Famvir

Adverse Side Effects
These are not well-documented. Famciclovir appears to be well-tolerated when used for up to 3 weeks.

Storage of the Drug
Store at room temperature.

Interferon Alfa
Pharmacokinetics/Therapeutics
Interferon has antiviral, antiproliferative, and immunomodulating effects. This is thought to occur by its effects on the synthesis of RNA, DNA, and cellular proteins. The mechanisms for its antineoplastic activities are not well understood but are probably also related to these effects (Plumb, 2011).

Dosage Forms
Only human-label products are available.
- Roferon-A
- Intron A
- Alferon N

Adverse Side Effects
In cats, no adverse effects are common.

Storage of the Drug
Refrigeration is necessary.

Interferon Omega
Clinical Uses
This drug is labeled in the European Union (EU) for dogs 1 month of age or older for the reduction in mortality and clinical signs of parvovirus (Plumb, 2011). In cats 9 weeks of age or older, it is labeled for treating feline leukemia virus (FeLV) and/or feline immunodeficiency virus (FIV) in non-terminal clinical stages. It may have some benefit in treating canine distemper, canine atopic dermatitis, acute feline calicivirus infections, feline infectious peritonitis, or feline herpetic keratitis, but data are still being gathered to determine its efficacy (Plumb, 2011).

Dosage Form
- None available in the United States
- Virbagen Omega—veterinary label; in the EU

Adverse Side Effects
Interferon omega may cause vomiting, slight decreases in red blood cell, platelet, and white blood cell counts. Increased ALT levels have been observed. Mild diarrhea and fatigue has been noted in cats. Dogs may develop antibodies to interferon omega if treatment is prolonged or repeated.

Storage of the Drug
Refrigeration is necessary. Protect from freezing.

Lysine
Clinical Uses
Lysine may be effective in suppressing feline herpesvirus (FHV-1) infections in cats. Lysine is an amino acid that is thought to compete with arginine for incorporation into many herpes viruses (Plumb, 2011).

Dosage Forms
All of the following are veterinary-label products unless otherwise specified.
- Viralys Gel
- Viralys Powder
- L-Lysine Powder-Pure
- Enisyl—human label

Adverse Side Effects
These are unlikely when mixed with food.

Storage of the Drug
Store at room temperature.

Oseltamivir
Clinical Uses
Oseltamivir has been suggested as a treatment for canine parvovirus infections. Some studies have been performed to ascertain the effectiveness of this drug in equines infected with equine influenza.

Dosage Form
In 2006, the FDA banned the extra-label use of oseltamivir and other influenza antivirals in chickens, turkeys, and ducks (Plumb, 2011).
- Tamiflu—human label

Adverse Side Effects
No information in animals is available.

Storage of the Drug
Store at or below 77°F.

Zidovudine
Clinical Uses
Zidovudine may be useful in treating FIV or FeLV.

Dosage Form
Only human-label products are available.
- Retrovir

Adverse Side Effects
In cats, reductions in red blood cells, packed cell volume, and hemoglobin are the most commonly reported adverse effects. Diarrhea and weakness have also been reported.

Storage of the Drug
Store at room temperature.

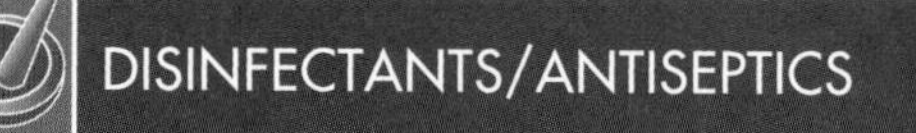

DISINFECTANTS/ANTISEPTICS

Biguanide Compounds
Chlorhexidine is the most common disinfectant in this group. In high dilutions, it is bactericidal, fungicidal, and active against enveloped viruses (e.g., feline infectious peritonitis virus and FeLV). Other viruses, spores, and mycobacteria are relatively resistant.

Clinical Uses
These include disinfecting surgical instruments, anesthetic equipment, and kennels. It is also available as a surgical scrub and a teat dip.

Dosage Forms
- Nolvasan Cap-Tabs
- Nolvadent oral solution
- Nolvalube (lubricating jelly)
- Nolvasan solution
- Nolvasan surgical scrub
- Virosan solution

Adverse Side Effects
Adverse side effects are uncommon.

Chlorines and Iodines

Chlorines and iodines are halogens that inactivate pathogens by oxidizing free sulfhydryl groups on bacterial enzymes. Chlorines are bactericidal, exhibit high levels of activity against viruses, and are **fungicidal** and tuberculocidal unless highly diluted. Iodines and **iodophors** are bactericidal, exhibit high levels of activity against viruses, are fungicidal and tuberculocidal, and are effective against bacterial spores.

Clinical Uses

Chlorines are recommended for floors, plumbing fixtures, spot disinfection, and fabrics not harmed by bleaching. Iodine tincture is used for skin preparations and thermometers. Iodophors are used to disinfect thermometers, utensils, rubber goods, and dishes and for presurgical skin preparation.

Dosage Forms

- Sodium hypochlorite
  - Clorox bleach
- Iodine tincture (7%)
- Betadine surgical scrub
- Povidone solution

Adverse Side Effects

The strong vapor of chlorines may irritate the eyes and mucous membranes. Skin irritation may result from failure to rinse a chlorine-disinfected surface. Chlorine bleaches colored fabrics and is corrosive to most metals. Tinctures of iodine contain alcohol and are drying to the skin. They stain and may corrode metal. Iodophors may corrode metal. Iodine solutions stain and may corrode metal, and high concentrations (3.5%) may irritate living tissue.

> **TECHNICIAN NOTES**
> - These compounds are inactivated by organic material.
> - Always check labels for dilution requirements (more is *not* better).
> - Iodophors are less staining and irritating than other iodine compounds.

Ethylene Oxide

Ethylene oxide works via substitution of cell alkyl groups for labile hydrogen atoms. It sterilizes against bacteria, fungi, and viruses. This gas, which should be handled carefully when used by veterinary personnel, may irritate the lungs and cause chemical burns if skin contact occurs. The gas is flammable and is considered to be a human carcinogen. When inanimate objects are sterilized, this gas must be used with proper ventilation and according to proper Occupational Safety and Health Administration (OSHA) standards. See Table 12-5.

Clinical Uses

Ethylene oxide is used to sterilize inanimate objects such as blankets, pillows, mattresses, instruments with lenses, rubber goods, thermolabile plastics, books, and papers.

Adverse Side Effects

Adverse side effects are uncommon if ethylene oxide is used according to proper OSHA standards and with good ventilation.

> **TECHNICIAN NOTES**
> - Special equipment is required when ethylene oxide is used as a sterilization gas.
> - After rubber boots are sterilized with this gas, it is best to let them "air" for several hours before donning them, to prevent chemical burns to the skin of the feet.
> - Proper ventilation (refer to OSHA standards) must be employed when this gas is used.

Formaldehyde

The mode of action for formaldehyde is the same as for ethylene oxide. It is noncorrosive and is effective against bacteria, fungi, spores, and viruses. It is considered to be carcinogenic to humans and must be used only in diluted amounts.

Clinical Uses

Formaldehyde is used as a disinfecting gas or solution. The gas can be used to **disinfect** large areas, such as a cabinet or incubator. The solution is appropriate for instrument disinfection. Delicate instruments may be vapor disinfected.

TABLE 12-5 Disinfectant Preparations and Their Activity

DISINFECTANT GROUP	PROPRIETARY PRODUCTS	RECOMMENDATIONS	BACTERICIDAL	VIRUCIDE	FUNGICIDAL	SPORICIDAL AT ROOM TEMPERATURE
Quaternary ammonium compounds	Q-Cide, Roccal-D Plus, D-128	Instruments, dairy equipment, rubber goods	M	M	M	N
Phenolics	Panteck Cleanser	Laundry rinse, floors, walls, equipment	M	M	H	N
	Lysol I.C. Disinfectant Spray					
	Beaucoup					
Halogens	*Chlorines:* Clorox, Purex	Floors, spot disinfection	M	H	H	S
	Iodophors: Betadine, Povidone solution	Presurgical skin preparation, thermometers, dairy operation	H	H	M	S
Glutaraldehyde	Cidex	Instruments	H	H	H	M
Chlorhexidine	Nolvasan, Virosan	Instruments, surgical scrub, dairy operation	M	M	M	N
Alcohols	Isopropyl alcohol 70%	Instruments, thermometers, skin preparation	H	N	S	N

H, High activity; *M*, moderate activity; *N*, no activity; *S*, slight activity.

TECHNICIAN NOTES

- For adequate disinfection, formaldehyde requires long contact time.
- Organic material inactivates its effectiveness.

Adverse Side Effects

These include toxicity to skin and mucous membranes because of its strong odor.

Phenolics: Saponated Cresol and Semisynthetic Phenols

The mode of action of phenolics is protein coagulation. They destroy selective permeability of cell membranes; leakage of cell constituents results. They are effective against bacteria, fungi, and some viruses, but they are not **sporicidal** and are only weakly effective against nonenveloped viruses (e.g., parvovirus). Cresol must be used in soft water and is slow-acting. Organic matter, soap, or hard water (except cresol) does not inactivate phenolics. They have high detergency and a residual effect if allowed to dry on surfaces.

Clinical Uses

These include use as a general disinfectant for laundry, floors, walls, and equipment.

Dosage Forms

- Beaucoup
- Lysol I.C. Disinfectant Spray

Adverse Side Effects

Adverse side effects are uncommon, but repeated and prolonged skin exposure may result in accumulation in tissue and eventual toxic effects such as neurotoxicity or teratogenicity.

TECHNICIAN NOTES Some phenolics have objectionable odors.

Quaternary Ammonium Compounds: Cationic Detergents

Cationic **detergents** concentrate at the cell membrane and are thought to act by dissolving lipids in cell walls and membranes. They are more active against gram-positive than against gram-negative organisms. They are bacteriostatic at high dilutions, but spores, viruses, mycobacteria, and *Pseudomonas aeruginosa* are relatively resistant. Organic debris, hard water, and anionic soaps and detergents inactivate quaternary ammonium compounds.

Clinical Uses

These include cleaning of instruments, utensils, inanimate objects, and rubber goods. They may be used for instrument soaks except for instruments with cemented lenses.

Dosage Forms

- Roccal-D Plus
- Q-Cide
- D-128

Adverse Side Effects

Adverse side effects are uncommon.

TECHNICIAN NOTES Read labels carefully because some quaternary ammonium compounds do not effectively disinfect against some common viruses (e.g., parvovirus).

Other Disinfectants

Soaps

Soaps, or anionic detergents, have only slight bactericidal activity but are effective in the mechanical removal of organisms. They are not sporicidal or tuberculocidal and have limited virucidal activity. They often contain germicides, such as triclosan, that decrease the number of resident flora after washing. Their mode of action is the same as that of cationic detergents.

Organic Mercury Compounds

These compounds such as merbromin (Mercurochrome) and thimerosal (Merthiolate) may be used as antiseptics. They have only slight bactericidal activity.

Alkalis

Alkalis such as lye and quicklime may be used for disinfecting stables and premises.

Hydrogen Peroxide

Hydrogen peroxide is an oxidizing agent that is available as a 3% aqueous solution and may be used for cleaning and disinfecting wounds and as a mouthwash for septic stomatitis.

Glutaraldehyde

Glutaraldehyde is a dialdehyde that is bactericidal, virucidal, fungicidal, and sporicidal. It is not inactivated by organic debris. Its uses include disinfecting surgical instruments, anesthetic equipment, floors, walls, and nonfood contact surfaces.

REVIEW QUESTIONS

1. Different types of bacteria can be distinguished with the use of a ________________ stain.
2. Gram-positive bacteria will stain what color? ________
3. Gram-negative bacteria will stain what color? ________
4. ________________ is approved for use in lactating dairy animals.
5. ________________ can cause staining of teeth in young animals.
6. ________________ should never be given intravenously to horses.
7. Some aminoglycosides may be ________________-toxic and/or ________________-toxic.
8. Griseofulvin is used to treat ________________.

9. A drug's ______________________ of activity is the range of bacteria affected by its action.
10. Aerobes are bacteria that require oxygen to live.
    a. True
    b. False
11. A fungicidal agent inhibits the growth of fungi.
    a. True
    b. False
12. A bacteriostatic agent inhibits the growth of bacteria.
    a. True
    b. False
13. Penicillin-G benzathine is a long-acting antibiotic that is approved for use in dairy animals.
    a. True
    b. False
14. All the following drugs are classified as penicillins, except ______________________.
    a. cephalexin
    b. amoxicillin
    c. ampicillin
    d. cloxacillin
15. Naxcel is not approved for use in lactating dairy animals.
    a. True
    b. False
16. Clindamycin is classified as a(n) ______________________.
    a. penicillin
    b. cephalosporin
    c. aminoglycoside
    d. tetracycline
17. Veterinarians commonly dispense aminoglycosides to patients with renal insufficiency.
    a. True
    b. False
18. Enrofloxacin is a ______________________.
    a. penicillin
    b. cephalosporin
    c. fluoroquinolone
    d. tetracycline
19. Amphotericin B may be used in the treatment of mycotic fungal infections.
    a. True
    b. False
20. A 4-month-old, 40-lb female Labrador retriever is presented to the veterinarian. The pup is diagnosed with deep pyoderma. The veterinarian orders cephalexin to be given at a dosage rate of 25 mg/kg PO, BID for 7 days. On hand in the pharmacy are cephalexin (250 mg) capsules and cephalexin (500 mg) capsules. What is the dose the patient should receive? Which size capsules should be chosen? How many capsules should be dispensed?
    a. 909 mg; 500 mg; 7 capsules
    b. 454 mg; 500 mg; 14 capsules
    c. 238 mg; 250 mg; 7 capsules
    d. 312 mg; 500 mg; 14 capsules
21. An Airedale terrier is diagnosed with Lyme disease. The dog weighs 75 lb. The veterinarian orders doxycycline for treatment at a dosage of 10 mg/kg PO q24h for 21 days. On hand in the pharmacy are doxycycline capsules (100 mg) and doxycycline capsules (250 mg). What is the dose for this patient? What size capsule is best to use? How many capsules need to be dispensed for this dog?
    a. 681 mg; 250 mg; 63 capsules
    b. 234 mg; 250 mg; 21 capsules
    c. 446 mg; 250 mg; 42 capsules
    d. 340 mg; 250 mg; 28 capsules
22. A Border collie pup weighing 15 lb is presented to the veterinarian. The dog is infected with *Isospora canis.* The veterinarian orders sulfadimethoxine for treatment. The dosage is 55 mg/kg PO initially on the first day of therapy, then 27.5 mg/kg PO for 9 days. On hand in the pharmacy are 250-mg tablets. How many tablets should be dispensed for this patient?
    a. 10.5 tablets
    b. 20.5 tablets
    c. 15.5 tablets
    d. 30.5 tablets
23. A Holstein cow diagnosed with bovine respiratory syncytial virus (BRSV) needs to be treated. The veterinarian orders tilmicosin at a dosage of 10 mg/kg SC. On hand in the pharmacy is a parenteral product with a concentration of 300 mg/mL. If the cow weighs

900 lbs, how many milliliters should be obtained for treatment?
a. 12.6 mL
b. 15.6 mL
c. 13.6 mL
d. 14.6 mL

24. A lagomorph is presented to the veterinarian with *Pasteurella multocida*. The rabbit weighs 4.5 lb. The veterinarian orders enrofloxacin at a dosage of 5 mg/kg PO for 14 days. On hand in the pharmacy is enrofloxacin injectable with a concentration of 22.7 mg/mL. How many milliliters should the rabbit get for one dose?
a. 0.90 mL
b. 0.75 mL
c. 0.55 mL
d. 0.45 mL

REFERENCES

Plumb DC: Veterinary drug handbook, ed 7, Ames, Iowa, 2011, Wiley-Blackwell.

Nobelprize.org: Sir alexander fleming–biographical (website). http://www.nobelprize.org/nobel_prizes/medicine/laureates/1945/fleming-bio.html. Accessed April 10, 2013.

CHAPTER

13 Antiparasitic Drugs

KEY TERMS

Anthelmintic
Bots
Ectoparasite
Endoparasite
Helminths
Microfilaria
Nematodes
Organophosphate
Parasitiasis
Parasitosis
Symbiosis

OUTLINE

LEARNING OBJECTIVES

After studying this chapter, you should be able to

1. Name the ingredients found in common anthelmintics and insecticides.
2. Explain the delivery systems of insecticides.
3. Educate clients about products covered in this chapter.
4. Explain the importance of reading and understanding product labels.
5. Identify the different classes of parasiticides and any contraindications for each particular class.

INTRODUCTION

Controlling parasites in companion animals is a high priority for veterinary medicine. Some people get squeamish when talking about worms, but once the subject is broached, most clients listen intently to what is being said. Veterinary technicians play an important role in educating clients about the life cycle of parasites and the drugs used to eradicate them, and in explaining how important the health of the public is to veterinary medicine in terms of the removal of those parasites with zoonotic potential. This interaction gets the point across and shows how important it is to keep pets free of parasites.

> *TECHNICIAN NOTES*
> - Veterinary technicians can educate both adults and children by allowing them to view parasite eggs under the microscope during their pet's physical examination.
> - Allowing a child to view parasite eggs under the microscope may be all it takes to spark the interest of a future veterinary technician.

A formalin-preserved heart infected with *Dirofilaria immitis* adults provides a great visual aid when the subject of heartworm prevention is discussed. Serum bottles with *Toxocara canis* or *Dipylidium caninum* adults also make good visual aids when client education is provided.

Parasites live on this earth in many diverse forms and relationships. Parasites lead a symbiotic life (**symbiosis**). Five types of symbiotic relationships have been identified: (1) predator–prey, (2) phoresis, (3) mutualism, (4) commensalism, and (5) parasitism (Hendrix, 2006). An example of a predator-prey relationship is that of a hawk that finds, captures, and eats a mouse that is running in a field. The word form *phore,* from which phoresis is derived, means *to carry.* An example of phoresis is the bacterium *Moraxella bovis,* the etiologic agent of infectious bovine keratoconjunctivitis, or pinkeye, being mechanically carried from the eyes of one cow to those of another on the sticky footpads of the face fly, *Musca autumnalis* (Hendrix, 2006). Mutualism occurs when both members of a symbiotic relationship gain from each other. An example of mutualism is the ciliated protozoa that live in the rumen of a cow. The cow benefits by having bulk and fiber digested more readily, and the ciliates benefit because the rumen provides a warm, liquid environment in which to live. Commensalism is a type of symbiotic relationship in which one symbiont benefits, but the other symbiont is not harmed. An example of commensalism is mistletoe growing in the top of a tree. Lastly, parasitism occurs when one species lives at the expense of another. An example of parasitism is *Trichuris vulpis* that live in the cecum of the canine.

Sometimes, an animal may harbor a parasite on or within its body that is potentially pathogenic, but the animal does not exhibit any outward signs (i.e., clinical disease) of parasitism. This is known as **parasitiasis.** If, however, the animal harbors a parasite on or within its body, and injury occurs to the animal because of the parasite, this is known as **parasitosis.** Parasites living on the outside of an animal's body are known as **ectoparasites** (e.g., fleas and ticks), and parasites living on the inside of an animal's body are known as **endoparasites** (e.g., canine heartworms). An animal with ectoparasites is said to be infested, and an animal with endoparasites is said to be infected. Sometimes, a parasite may wander from its normal location in the host's body to another location where it does not normally live. These parasites are said to be aberrant (erratic). Although most veterinary personnel use the lay term given to parasites when speaking with a client, it is also important for veterinary technicians to know the genus and species name of the most common parasites. The Linnaean classification scheme is fundamental in keeping parasites organized (i.e., kingdom, phylum, class, order, family, genus, and species).

Each parasite has its own individual life cycle, which may consist of several stages. Every parasite has at least a definitive host and, depending on the species, may have one or more intermediate hosts. The host that contains the adult (sexually mature) stage of the parasite is known as the definitive host, and the host that contains the immature (not sexually mature) stage of the parasite is known as the intermediate host. Knowing the life cycle of parasites helps veterinarians determine which drugs to use and how many doses will be needed to eradicate the parasite from the host animal's body.

Some parasites have zoonotic potential. This means they may be transmissible from animals to humans. Veterinary technicians should be familiar with which parasites have this ability so they can properly educate clients. Examples of parasites with zoonotic potential include *Toxoplasma gondii, Trichinella spiralis, Ancylostoma caninum,* and *Toxocara canis* (Hendrix, 2006).

The Companion Animal Parasite Council (www.capcvet.org) recommends fecal centrifugation techniques to accurately diagnose endoparasitism. Additionally, the amount of feces collected for evaluation is important and should consist of at least 1 g. The specific gravity of flotation solution is equally important, in that ideally it should be 1.18 to 1.20.

> TECHNICIAN NOTES Educating clients about how to collect a freshly voided fecal sample from a pet will result in more accurate fecal evaluations. (Tell them to bring a sample in a resealable plastic bag to each of their pets' appointments.)

Ectoparasites represent an ongoing problem faced by companion animal and livestock owners. Numerous products are manufactured for the removal of fleas and ticks from an animal's body. Because so many products are available, veterinary technicians play an important role in educating clients about the effectiveness of each product. Client education is important in the area of ectoparasites because misuse of over-the-counter insecticides can be fatal. Clients should be taught to ask veterinary personnel about the correct use of shampoos, dips, sprays, powders, and topical parasiticides (e.g., fipronil and imidacloprid) before a purchase is made.

Parasitology is a fascinating subject. However, for most clients, it is not fascinating at all because they just want their pet to be free of worms and bugs. It is up to veterinary personnel to have knowledge about available products and to remember that—as technology evolves—lifelong learning must be pursued so that professionals can remain current with how each drug or parasiticide works. Veterinary personnel have a double responsibility because it is up to them to protect both pets and their owners from those parasites with zoonotic potential and to educate clients accordingly. Veterinary medicine truly has a twofold purpose: the medical treatment of animals *and* protection of the public from health risks associated with zoonotic diseases and parasites. In some ways, veterinary medicine is more important than human medicine when it is considered from this standpoint because it represents the first defense in the protection of human health. Reading package inserts helps veterinary personnel to understand how a particular drug works. Tables 13-1 to 13-9 list products and their uses for various species.

ENDOPARASITES

Endoparasites found in the gastrointestinal (GI) tracts of animals benefit not only from the foodstuffs the animal ingests but also from body fluids (e.g., blood). Horses with increased numbers of endoparasites in the GI tract may develop colic. Puppies and kittens with increased numbers of intestinal parasites may develop fatal anemia if not treated early. Adult heartworms can cause disruption of the normal movement of blood within the heart chambers, resulting in clinical signs similar to congestive heart failure. Without treatment, a dog with active heartworm infection will die.

In the following section, some of the most common **anthelmintics** used in veterinary practice today are discussed. As a veterinary technician, you may come into contact with products not mentioned in this section. The charts in this section list various products, their trade names, and their effectiveness. Since anthelmintics are so numerous, many veterinarians keep only a few products to meet their needs and to limit inventory. Some products are available under many different names. Experience will provide familiarity with various available brands.

ANTINEMATODAL

Benzimidazoles

Benzimidazoles interfere with the worm's energy level on a cellular basis. They bind to beta tubulin and prevent its entry into microtubules that are needed for energy metabolism. Without energy, the worm dies.

TABLE 13-1 Parasiticides Used for Treatment and Control of Internal Parasites in Dogs and Cats

	PARASITE									
DRUG	*TOXOCARA, TOXASCARIS*	*ANCYLOSTOMA, UNCINARIA*	*STRONGYLOIDES*	*TRICHURIS*	*DIROFILARIA* ADULTS	*DIROFILARIA* MICROFILARIAE	*TAENIA*	*DIPYLIDIUM*	*GIARDIA**	COCCIDIA
Albendazole	+	+	–	+	–	–	+	–	+	–
Amprolium	–	–	–	–	–	–	–	–	–	+
Butamisole hydrochloride	–	+	–	+	–	–	–	–	–	–
Dichlorophen	–	–	–	–	–	–	+	+	–	–
Dichlorophen/toluene	+	+	–	–	–	–	+	+	–	–
Dichlorvos	+	+	–	+	–	–	–	–	–	–
Diethylcarbamazine	+	–	–	–	–	+	–	–	–	–
Epsiprantel	–	–	–	–	–	–	+	+	–	–
Febantel	+	+	–	+	–	–	+	–	–	–
Febantel/praziquantel	+	+	–	+	–	–	+	+	–	–
Fenbendazole	+	+	–	+	–	–	+	–	–	–
Furazolidone	–	–	–	–	–	–	–	–	+	–
Ivermectin	+	+	–	+	–	+	–	–	–	–
Mebendazole	+	+	–	+	–	–	+	–	–	–
Melarsomine dihydrochloride	–	–	–	–	+	–	–	–	–	–
Metronidazole	–	–	–	–	–	–	–	–	+	–
Milbemycin oxime	+	+	–	+	–	+	–	–	–	–
N-Butyl chloride	+	+	–	–	–	–	–	–	–	–
Nitroscanate	+	+	–	+	–	–	+	+	–	–
Oxibendazole/diethylcarbamazine	+	+	–	+	–	+	–	–	–	–
Piperazine salts	+	–	–	–	–	–	–	–	–	–
Praziquantel	–	–	–	–	–	–	+	+	–	–
Praziquantel/pyrantel pamoate	+	+	–	–	–	–	+	+	–	–
Praziquantel/pyrantel pamoate/febantel	+	+	–	+	–	–	+	+	–	–
Pyrantel pamoate	+	+	–	–	–	–	–	–	–	–
Quinacrine hydrochloride	–	–	–	–	–	–	–	–	+	–
Selamectin	+	+	–	–	–	+	–	–	–	–
Sulfadiazine/trimethoprim	–	–	–	–	–	–	–	–	–	+
Sulfadimethoxine	–	–	–	–	–	–	–	–	–	+
Thiabendazole	–	–	+	–	–	–	–	–	–	–

+, Indicated for use; –, not indicated for use.
*Paromomycin, an antibiotic, is being used to manage *Cryptosporidium* infections and resistant *Giardia* infections in dogs and cats.
From McCurnin DM, Bassert JM: Clinical textbook for veterinary technicians, ed 5, Philadelphia 2002, WB Saunders.

TABLE 13-2 Parasiticides Used to Treat Internal Parasites in Horses

	PARASITE						
DRUG	***GASTEROPHILUS***	**ASCARIDS**	***STRONGYLUS VULGARIS***	***STRONGYLUS EDENTATUS***	**SMALL STRONGYLES**	**PINWORMS**	***STRONGYLOIDES***
Cambendazole	–	+	+	+	+	+	+
Dichlorvos	+	+	+	+	+	+	–
Febantel	–	+	+	+	+	+	+
Fenbendazole	–	+	+	+	+	+	+
Ivermectin	+	+	+	+	+	+	+
Moxidectin	+	+	+	+	+	+	–
Oxibendazole	–	+	+	+	+	+	+
Oxfendazole	–	+	+	+	+	+	+
Phenothiazine	–	–	+	+	+	–	–
Piperazine salts	–	+	–	–	+	+	–
Pyrantel salts	–	+	+	–	+	–	–
Thiabendazole	–	–	+	+	+	+	+
Thiabendazole/piperazine	–	+	+	+	+	+	+
Thiabendazole/trichlorfon	+	+	+	+	+	+	+
Trichlorfon	+	+	–	–	–	+	–
Trichlorfon/phenothiazine/piperazine	+	+	+	–	+	+	–

+, Indicated for use; –, not indicated for use.
From McCurnin DM, Bassert JM: Clinical textbook for veterinary technicians, ed 5, Philadelphia, 2002, WB Saunders.

Clinical Uses

Benzimidazoles are used in the following species:

- *Horses.* Effective against strongyles, pinworms, and ascarids
- *Cattle.* Ascarids, several species of strongyles and other stomach worms; albendazole is also effective against adult liver flukes and tapeworms; fenbendazole is also effective against lungworms
- *Sheep and goats.* Ascarids, several species of strongyles and other stomach worms; fenbendazole is also effective against lungworms
- *Dogs.* Hookworms, roundworms, and whipworms; some are effective against *Taenia pisiformis* but not *D. caninum*
- *Swine. Strongyloides* and lungworms
- Many of the benzimidazoles are used as anthelmintics for exotics such as snakes and birds.

Dosage Forms

This class includes the following products:

- Thiabendazole (Equizole, TBZ, Omnizole)
- Oxibendazole (Anthelcide EQ)
- Mebendazole (Telmin, Telmintic)
- Fenbendazole (Panacur, Safeguard)
- Cambendazole (Camvet)
- Oxfendazole (Benzelmin, Synanthic)
- Albendazole (Valbazen)

Adverse Side Effects

These are uncommon but include vomiting and diarrhea. Mebendazole has clinically produced hepatotoxicity in dogs.

TABLE 13-3 Parasiticides Used to Treat Internal Parasites in Cattle, Sheep, and Goats

	PARASITE													
DRUG	***HAEMONCHUS***	***OSTERTAGIA***	***TRICHOSTRONGYLUS***	***COOPERIA***	***NEMATODIRUS***	***STRONGYLOIDES***	***BUNOSTOMUM***	***TRICHURIS***	***OESOPHAGOSTOMUM***	***CHABERTIA***	***DICTYOCAULUS***	***MONIEZIA***	***FASCIOLA***	***COCCIDIA***
Albendazole	+	+	+	+	+	–	+	–	+	+	+	+	+	–
Amprolium	–	–	–	–	–	–	–	–	–	–	–	–	–	–
Clorsulon	–	–	–	–	–	–	–	–	–	–	–	–	+	–
Decoquinate	–	–	–	–	–	–	–	–	–	–	–	–	–	+
Fenbendazole	+	+	+	+	+	+	+	+	+	+	+	–	–	–
Haloxon	+	+	+	+	–	–	–	–	–	–	–	–	–	–
Ivermectin	+	+	+	+	+	+	+	–	+	+	+	–	–	–
Lasalacid	–	–	–	–	–	–	–	–	–	–	–	–	–	+
Levamisole	+	+	+	+	+	+	+	+	+	+	+	–	–	–
Moxidectin	+	+	+	+	+	–	+	–	+	–	+	–	–	–
Monensin	–	–	–	–	–	–	–	–	–	–	–	–	–	+
Morantel tartrate	+	+	+	+	+	+	+	–	+	+	+	–	–	–
Phenothiazine	+	+	+	–	–	–	–	–	+	–	–	–	–	–
Sulfonamides	–	–	–	–	–	–	–	–	–	–	–	–	–	+
Thiabendazole	+	+	+	+	+	+	+	–	+	+	–	–	–	–

+, Indicated for use; –, not indicated for use.
From McCurnin DM, Bassert JM: Clinical textbook for veterinary technicians, ed 5, Philadelphia, 2002, WB Saunders.

TABLE 13-4 Parasiticides Used to Treat Internal Parasites in Swine

	PARASITE							
DRUG	***ASCARIS***	***STRONGYLOIDES***	***OESOPHAGOSTOMUM***	***TRICHURIS***	***HYOSTRONGYLUS***	***METASTRONGYLUS***	***STEPHANURUS***	***COCCIDIA***
Dichlorvos	+	–	+	+	+	–	–	–
Fenbendazole	+	–	+	+	+	+	–	–
Hygromycin B	+	–	+	+	–	–	–	–
Ivermectin	+	+	+	–	+	+	+	–
Levamisole	+	+	+	–	+	+	+	–
Piperazine salts	+	–	–	–	–	–	–	–
Pyrantel tartrate	+	–	+	–	–	–	–	–
Sulfonamides	–	–	–	–	–	–	–	+
Thiabendazole	–	+	+	–	+	–	–	–

+, Indicated for use; –, not indicated for use.
From McCurnin DM, Bassert JM: Clinical textbook for veterinary technicians, ed 5, Philadelphia, 2002, WB Saunders.

TABLE 13-5 Drugs Used to Treat Internal Parasites in Reptiles

	PARASITE						
DRUG	ECTOPARASITES	NEMATODES	TREMATODES	CESTODES	*CRYPTOSPORIDIUM*	COCCIDIA	AMOEBAE AND TRICHOMONADS
Metronidazole (Flagyl)	–	–	–	–	–	–	+
Paromomycin (Humatin 400)	–	–	–	–	–	–	+
Praziquantel (Droncit)	–	–	+	+	–	–	–
Febantel plus Praziquantel (Vercom)	–	+	+	+	–	–	–
Dichlorvos (Task)	–	+	–	–	–	–	–
Dichlorvos (Vapona Strip)	+	–	–	–	–	–	–
Levamisole (Tramisol, Ripercol)	–	+	–	–	–	–	–
Thiabendazole (Thibenzole)	–	+	–	–	–	–	–
Fenbendazole (Panacur)	–	+	–	–	–	–	–
Mebendazole (Telmin)	–	+	–	–	–	–	–
Ivermectin* (Ivomec)	+	+	–	–	–	–	–
Dithiazanine iodide (Dizan)	–	+	–	–	–	–	–
Sulfadiazine (many trade names)	–	–	–	–	–	+	–
Sulfamerazine (many trade names)	–	–	–	–	–	+	–
Sulfamethazine (many trade names)	–	–	–	–	–	+	–
Sulfadimethoxine (Albon)	–	–	–	–	–	+	–
Trimethoprim plus Sulfadiazine (Di-Trim, Tribrissen)	–	–	–	–	+	+	–

+, Effective; –, not effective.
*Do not use in chelonians. Contraindicated in animals that have been given diazepam or will receive diazepam within 10 days of administration of ivermectin.
Data from Frye FL: Reptile care, Neptune City, NJ, 1991, T.F.H. Publications.

TECHNICIAN NOTES

- Read labels carefully regarding use in lactating dairy animals and animals to be slaughtered.
- None of these products is approved for use in cats.

Organophosphates

Organophosphates consist of a group of insecticides that inactivate acetylcholinesterase. Without this enzyme, parasites (especially ectoparasites) are unable to move because these chemicals stop nerve transmission. Many of these pesticides tend to break

TABLE 13-6 Parasiticides Used for Control of External Parasites on Dogs and Cats

	PARASITE			
DRUG	FLEAS	LICE	MITES	TICKS
Allethrin	+	–	–	–
Amitraz	–	–	+	–
Carbaril	+	+	+	+
Chlorpyrifos	+	+	+	+
Cythioate	+	–	–	–
d-Limonene	+	+	–	–
Diazinon	+	+	–	+
Fenthion	+	–	–	–
Fipronil	+	+	–	+
Imidacloprid	+	+	–	–
Lime-sulfur	–	–	+	–
Lindane (not legal in United States)	+	+	+	+
Linalool	+	–	–	–
Lufenuron	+	–	–	–
Malathion	+	+	–	+
Methylcarbamate	+	+	–	+
Permethrin	+	+	–	+
Phosmet	+	+	+	+
Pyrethrins	+	+	–	+
Resmethrin	+	+	–	–
Rotenone	+	+	–	+
Selamectin	+	–	+	+

+, Indicated for use; –, not indicated for use.
From McCurnin DM, Bassert JM: Clinical textbook for veterinary technicians, ed 5, Philadelphia, 2002, WB Saunders.

TABLE 13-7 Parasiticides Used for Control of External Parasites on Horses

	PARASITE				
DRUG	LICE	FLIES	MITES	TICKS	MAGGOTS
Coumaphos	+	+	–	+	+
Malathion	+	+	+	+	–
Permethrin	+	+	–	+	–
Pyrethrins	+	+	–	–	–

+, Indicated for use; –, not indicated for use.
From McCurnin DM, Bassert JM: Clinical textbook for veterinary technicians, ed 5, Philadelphia, 2002, WB Saunders.

down when exposed to light, air, soil, and other environmental factors. However, some traces have been known to be residual in drinking water and food. Although they may degrade rather quickly, these substances have a high level of toxicity and may cause problems in people and animals exposed to large doses. SLUDGE is a good mnemonic to use for remembering the effects of toxic doses of these drugs: *s*alivation, *l*acrimation, *u*rination, *d*efecation, *G*I upset, and *e*mesis. Atropine may be used as an antidote.

Clinical Uses

Organophosphates are used in the following species:

- *Horses.* Effective against **bots,** roundworms, strongyles, and pinworms but less effective against *Strongyloides*
- *Cattle, sheep, and goats.* Strongyles
- *Dogs and cats.* Hookworms, roundworms, whipworms
- *Swine.* Ascarids, whipworms, nodule worms, strongyles

Dosage Forms

This class includes the following products:

- Trichlorfon (Combot, Dyrex T.F., Equibot TC)
- Coumaphos (Baymix, Dairy Dewormer BX Crumbles)
- Haloxon (Loxon)
- Dichlorvos (Task, Atgard)

Adverse Side Effects

Adverse side effects include those expected with any organophosphate poisoning: excessive salivation, vomiting, diarrhea, muscle tremors, and miosis.

TABLE 13-8 Parasiticides Used for Control of External Parasites on Cattle, Sheep, and Goats

DRUG	PARASITE											
	CATTLE GRUB	HORN FLY	FACE FLY	OTHER FLIES	MAGGOTS	CHEWING LICE	SUCKING LICE	PSOROPTIC MITE	OTHER MITES	EAR TICKS	OTHER TICKS	SHEEP KED
Carbaril	−	+	+	+	−	+	+	−	−	+	+	−
Coumaphos	+	+	+	+	+	+	+	+	−	+	+	+
Chlorpyrifos	−	+	−	−	−	+	+	−	−	−	−	−
Dichlorvos	−	+	+	+	−	−	−	−	−	−	+	−
Famphur	+	−	−	−	−	+	+	−	−	+	+	−
Doramectin	−	−	−	−	−	+	+	−	−	−	−	−
Fenthion	+	−	−	−	−	+	+	−	−	+	+	−
Fenvalerate	−	+	+	−	−	−	−	−	−	+	−	−
Ivermectin	+	−	−	−	−	−	+	+	+	+	+	−
Methoxychlor	−	+	+	+	−	+	+	−	−	+	+	−
Moxidectin	+	+	−	−	−	+	+	+	+	−	−	−
Permethrin	−	+	+	−	−	−	−	−	−	−	+	−
Phosmet	+	+	−	−	−	+	+	+	+	+	+	−
Pyrethrins	−	+	+	+	−	−	−	−	−	−	−	−
Rotenone	−	−	−	−	−	+	+	−	−	−	−	+
Trichlorfon	+	+	−	−	+	+	+	−	−	+	+	−

+, Indicated for use; −, not indicated for use.
From McCurnin DM, Bassert JM: Clinical textbook for veterinary technicians, ed 5, Philadelphia, 2002, WB Saunders.

TABLE 13-9 Parasiticides Used for Control of External Parasites on Swine

DRUG	PARASITE			
	LICE	FLIES	MITES	MAGGOTS
Coumaphos	+	+	–	+
Fenthion	+	–	–	–
Ivermectin	+	–	+	–
Malathion	+	–	+	–
Methoxychlor	+	–	–	–
Permethrin	+	+	+	–
Pyrethrins	–	+	–	–

+, Indicated for use; –, not indicated for use.
From McCurnin DM, Bassert JM: Clinical textbook for veterinary technicians, ed 5, Philadelphia, 2002, WB Saunders.

TECHNICIAN NOTES

- It is very important that these anthelmintics not be administered concurrently or within a few days of the use of other cholinesterase inhibitors, other organophosphates, succinylcholine, or phenothiazine derivative agents.
- Atropine and pralidoxime (2-PAM) are antidotal.
- Read labels carefully regarding use in lactating dairy animals and animals to be slaughtered.

Tetrahydropyrimidines

Clinical Uses

Tetrahydropyrimidines are used in the following species:

- *Horses.* Ascarids, strongyles, pinworms
- *Cattle, sheep, and goats.* Strongyles
- *Dogs and cats.* Hookworms, roundworms
- *Swine.* Roundworms, strongyles

Dosage Forms

This class includes the following products:

- Pyrantel pamoate (Nemex, Strongid-T, Anthelban)
- Pyrantel tartrate (Banminth 48)
- Morantel tartrate (Nematel, Rumatel)

Adverse Side Effects

These are uncommon but may include increased respiration, profuse sweating, and incoordination.

TECHNICIAN NOTES Read labels carefully regarding use in lactating dairy animals and animals to be slaughtered.

Imidazothiazoles

Clinical Uses

Imidazothiazoles are used in the following species:

- *Horses.* Ascarids, strongyles
- *Cattle, sheep, and goats.* Strongyles, lungworms
- *Dogs and cats.* Febantel—hookworms, roundworms, whipworms; levamisole has been used in dogs as a microfilaricide
- *Swine.* Strongyles, *Strongyloides,* lungworms, nodule worms
- These products also may be used effectively in some exotic species.

Dosage Forms

This class includes the following products:

- Febantel (Rintal)
- Levamisole

Adverse Side Effects

These include transient foaming at the mouth.

TECHNICIAN NOTES Read labels carefully regarding use in lactating dairy animals and animals to be slaughtered.

Avermectins

Avermectins are derived from the bacterium *Streptomyces avermitilis.* Avermectins kill by interfering with nervous system and muscle function, thus breaking down neurotransmission. The drug binds and activates glutamate-gated chloride channels that are present in neurons and myocytes, which results in neuromuscular paralysis and death. In mammals, glutamate-gated chloride channels are absent. Therefore, invertebrates are susceptible to these drugs. Avermectins do not cross the blood–brain barrier unless given at high doses.

Ivermectin

Clinical Uses

- *Horses.* Large and small strongyles, pinworms, ascarids, hairworms, large-mouth stomach

worms, neck threadworms, bots, lungworms, intestinal threadworms, and summer sores secondary to *Habronema* or *Draschia* spp
- *Cattle.* Gastrointestinal roundworms, lungworms, cattle grubs, sucking lice, and mites
- *Swine.* Gastrointestinal roundworms, lungworms, lice, and mange mites
- *Dogs.* Effective preventive for *D. immitis;* Heartgard Plus contains pyrantel pamoate and is effective against hookworms and roundworms
- *Cats.* Effective preventive for *D. immitis* and for the removal of hookworms
- *Birds and snakes.* Effective against some endoparasites and ectoparasites

Dosage Forms
- Heartgard
- Heartgard Plus
- Heartgard for Cats
- Eqvalan
- Ivomec)

Moxidectin
Clinical Uses
- *Horses.* Large and small strongyles, encysted cyathostomes, ascarids, pinworms, hairworms, large-mouth stomach worms, and bots
- *Cattle.* Gastrointestinal roundworms, lungworms, cattle grubs, mites, lice, and horn flies
- *Dogs.* Effective preventive for *D. immitis*

Dosage Forms
- Quest 2% Equine Oral Gel
- Cydectin Pour-On

Doramectin
Clinical Uses
- *Cattle.* Gastrointestinal roundworms, lungworms, eyeworms, grubs, biting and sucking lice, horn flies, and mange mites
- *Swine.* Gastrointestinal roundworms, lungworms, kidney worms, sucking lice, and mange mites

Dosage Forms
- Dectomax Injectable Solution
- Dectomax Pour-On

Eprinomectin
Clinical Uses
- Indicated for various GI roundworms, cattle grubs, lice, mange mites, and lungworms
- No meat or milk withdrawal times for this agent
- May also be useful in the treatment of ear mites in rabbits (*Psoroptes cuniculi*)

Dosage Form
- Eprinomectin (topically applied avermectin antiparasiticide for cattle)

Adverse Side Effects

These are uncommon. Toxic signs include mydriasis, ataxia, tremors, and depression.

TECHNICIAN NOTES
- Although not approved, Ivomec is sometimes used for the treatment of ear mites in cats and scabies in dogs.
- Because of the small amount of medication in heartworm preventives, crumbling or breaking of the tablets or use of a chewable version is not recommended.
- Read labels carefully regarding use in lactating dairy animals and animals for slaughter. Moxidectin is approved for use in dairy cattle of all ages and at all stages of lactation, except for veal calves.

Other Agents
Piperazine
Clinical Uses
- *Dogs and cats.* Roundworms
- Used effectively in exotics such as birds and snakes
- Commonly combined in large-animal dewormers to broaden its spectrum and enhance its efficacy

Dosage Forms
- Pipa-Tabs
- Pip-Pop 320

Praziquantel/Pyrantel Pamoate/Febantel
Clinical Uses
- *Dogs.* Effective for the removal of tapeworms, hookworms, roundworms, and whipworms

Dosage Form
- Drontal Plus

Adverse Side Effects
These are uncommon.

TECHNICIAN NOTES
- Do not use in dogs weighing less than 2 lb or in puppies younger than 3 weeks.
- Do not use in pregnant animals.

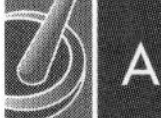

ANTICESTODAL

Drugs used for treating tapeworms have greatly improved over the years. These newer agents are more effective and do not necessitate fasting before their administration.

Bunamidine

Clinical Uses
- *Dogs. T. pisiformis, D. caninum, Echinococcus granulosus,* and *Echinococcus multilocularis*
- *Cats. D. caninum, Taenia taeniaeformis*

Dosage Form
- Scolaban

Adverse Side Effects
These are uncommon but include vomiting, anorexia, diarrhea, and lethargy.

TECHNICIAN NOTES
- No adverse reactions have been reported in pregnant or breeding animals.
- This product is not for use in puppies younger than 4 weeks or kittens younger than 6 weeks.

Epsiprantel

Clinical Uses
- *Dogs. T. pisiformis* and *D. caninum*
- *Cats. T. taeniaeformis* and *D. caninum*

Dosage Form
- Cestex

Adverse Side Effects
These are uncommon.

TECHNICIAN NOTES
- Safety in pregnant or breeding animals has not been established.
- This product is not for use in puppies or kittens younger than 7 weeks.

ANTITREMATODAL

Clorsulon

Clinical Uses
- *Cattle.* Liver flukes
- Effective against immature and adult flukes

Dosage Form
- Curatrem

Adverse Side Effects
These are uncommon.

TECHNICIAN NOTES
- This product is not approved for use in female dairy cattle of breeding age.
- Read label regarding use in animals to be slaughtered.

Albendazole

Clinical Uses
- *Cattle.* Liver flukes
- Effective against adult flukes and many intestinal worms

Dosage Form
- Valbazen

Praziquantel

Clinical Uses
- *Dogs and cats.* Lung flukes

Dosage Form
- Droncit

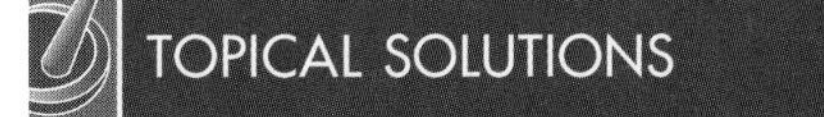

TOPICAL SOLUTIONS

Emodepside/Praziquantel

Clinical Uses
- A topical solution for the treatment and control of hookworms, roundworms, and tapeworms in cats 8 weeks of age or older

- Emodepside is a cyclic depsipeptide
- Praziquantel is an isoquinoline cestocide
- To be applied every 30 days for preventive purposes
- A client may use this product instead of oral medications, which may be difficult to administer to cats

Dosage Form
- Profender

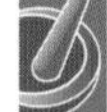

ANTIPROTOZOAL

Protozoa are single-celled organisms found at various body sites that have the ability to replicate rapidly. Coccidia and *Giardia* are the protozoa that are most commonly associated with diarrhea in many species of animals. Protozoa are most commonly transmitted via contaminated feed and/or water. Prevention of these parasites includes providing uncontaminated food and water and clean housing and avoiding overcrowding. A vaccine is also available for the prevention of giardiasis in dogs. *Babesia* is a hematozoan (i.e., a protozoan) that is transmitted by ticks and affects many species of animals. An injectable treatment for babesiosis is available for dogs.

Drugs for Treating Coccidia and Other Protozoa

Dosage Forms
- Monensin (Coban 60); turkeys and chickens
- Amprolium (Corid); calves
- Clopidol (Coyden 25); chickens
- Diclazuril (Clincox); horses
- Maduramicin ammonium (Cygro Type A Medicated Article); chickens
- Decoquinate (Deccox); cattle, calves, and goats
- Narasin/nicarbazine (Maxiban 72); chickens
- Ponazuril (Marquis); horses
- Robenidine hydrochloride (Robenz Type A Medicated Article); chickens
- Sulfadimethoxine (Albon); chickens, turkeys, dogs, and cats

Adverse Side Effects
These are uncommon.

> *TECHNICIAN NOTES* Read labels carefully regarding use in food-producing animals and animals to be slaughtered.

Drugs for Treating *Giardia*

Dosage Forms
- Metronidazole (Flagyl); dogs and cats
- Albendazole (Valbazen); dogs and cats

Adverse Side Effects
These are uncommon, but vomiting and diarrhea may occur in some animals treated with metronidazole.

> *TECHNICIAN NOTES* Metronidazole is not recommended for use in pregnant animals.

Drugs for Preventing *Giardia*

A vaccine for dogs is available to help prevent *Giardia lamblia* infection and to reduce the duration of cyst shedding. This vaccine is administered subcutaneously, and a booster is given 2 to 4 weeks after the first vaccination. Annual revaccination is recommended.

Dosage Form
- GiardiaVax

Adverse Side Effects
These are uncommon.

> *TECHNICIAN NOTES*
> - May be used in dogs 8 weeks of age.
> - After exposure to *Giardia*, some vaccinates may shed cysts. Clients should be educated regarding proper hygiene and sanitation practices to prevent zoonotic disease.

Drugs for Treating *Babesia*

Imizol is available for the treatment of clinical signs of babesiosis and/or evidence of *Babesia* organisms in the blood. This product is indicated for use in dogs, and treatment consists of two injections given over a 2-week interval.

Atovaquone is effective in treating dogs with *Babesia gibsoni* infections. When used in combination with azithromycin, it can be used to treat cytauxzoonosis in cats.

Diminazene aceturate is used in several species to treat for trypanosomiasis, babesiosis, or cytauxzoonosis. This drug is available in several countries but not the United States.

Imidocarb dipropinate can be used to treat *Babesia* and related parasites. It has also been used to treat cytauxzoonosis in cats, although results on its efficacy are not yet available (Plumb, 2011).

Dosage Forms

- Imizol
- Atovaquone
- Diminazene aceturate
- Imidocarb dipropinate

Adverse Side Effects

These may include injection pain and mild cholinergic signs such as salivation, nasal drip, and vomiting. Other less common side effects include panting, restlessness, diarrhea, and mild injection site inflammation.

> TECHNICIAN NOTES
>
> Severe cholinergic signs may be reversed with atropine sulfate.

HEARTWORM DISEASE

Heartworm disease is commonly found throughout the United States. This disease primarily affects dogs and wild Canidae, although cats and ferrets also may become infected. *D. immitis* is the filarial **nematode** that causes heartworm disease. *Acanthocheilonema reconditum* (formerly known as *Dipetalonema reconditum*) (Hendrix, 2006) is a subcutaneous filarial nematode that does not require treatment because it is nonpathogenic. *Prevention* is the key word for controlling heartworm disease. Dogs not undergoing an approved heartworm disease prevention program should be tested for the presence of adult heartworms before preventive treatment is begun. Clients should be educated about the importance of treating an existing infection if one exists, preventing infection or reinfection, and ensuring periodic testing that may be necessary. (Many veterinarians will not prescribe heartworm prevention without an annual heartworm antigen test.) Over the past several years, the number of cats in which heartworm disease has been diagnosed has increased. The treatment and justification for prevention of heartworms in cats continue to be controversial (Smith, 1999). Products for the prevention of *D. immitis* infection in cats are available. No adulticide products have been approved for use in cats. Table 13-10 provides a comparison of several heartworm preventives that are on the market at this time.

ADULTICIDES

Melarsomine Dihydrochloride

Melarsomine is an arsenic compound administered by deep intramuscular injection in the lumbar region. The administration schedule is based on classification of the severity of heartworm disease. Melarsomine appears to be more efficacious than thiacetarsamide (Caparsolate), less irritating to tissue, and does not cause hepatic necrosis (Plumb, 2011).

Dosage Form

- Immiticide

Adverse Side Effects

Some dogs experience reactions such as pain, swelling, and tenderness at the injection site. Firm nodules may form at the injection site. Coughing, gagging, depression, lethargy, anorexia, fever, lung congestion, and vomiting are common reactions.

> TECHNICIAN NOTES
>
> - The manufacturer recommends use of a 23-gauge, 1-inch needle for dogs up to 22 lb and a 22-gauge, 1½-inch needle for dogs larger than 22 lb.
> - Safety in breeding, lactating, or pregnant bitches has not been determined.
> - Melarsomine is contraindicated in dogs with severe heartworm disease (Class 4, according to manufacturer disease classification).
> - Clients must be informed of the potential for morbidity and mortality associated with heartworm treatment.
> - Exercise in dogs should be restricted after treatment has been provided.

TABLE 13-10 Comparison of Products Indicated for Heartworm Prevention

	MODE OF ADMINISTRATION	AGE PARAMETERS	SAFETY OF PRODUCT FOR PREGNANT ANIMALS	EFFECTIVENESS AFTER SWIMMING	ACTION FOR LATE DOSE	RESULT IF GIVEN MISTAKENLY TO HW+ DOGS	EFFECT ON OTHER PARASITES	HW LIFE CYCLE STAGE TARGETED
Heartgard Plus	Chewable tablet given PO on the same day every month	*Puppies:* 6 weeks *Kittens:* 6 weeks	Yes	N/A	15-day grace period (one dose protects against infection up to 45 days)	Not approved for such use; probably will not cause problems	*Dogs:* Roundworms Hookworms *Cats:* Hookworms	Third and fourth stage microfilaria larvae
Interceptor	Flavored tablet given PO on the same day every month	*Puppies:* 8 weeks *Cats:* Not approved for use in cats	Yes	N/A	Can pick up next dose when mistake is noted but should not wait longer than 2 to 3 weeks	Probably safe if microfilaria counts are not too high; may be dangerous if microfilaria counts are high	Hookworms Roundworms Whipworms	Microfilaria larvae stages, third, fourth and some fifth larvae stages
Revolution	Topical application on the same day every month	*Puppies:* 6 weeks *Kittens:* 6 weeks	Yes	No effect, but pet must be dry when product is applied	Up to 2 months is grace period	Is safe because product is FDA-approved for use in HW-positive dogs	Sarcoptic mange mites, ear mites, fleas, roundworms in cats, and hookworms in dogs	Microfilaria fourth stage larvae
Sentinel*	Flavored tablet given PO on the same day every month	*Puppies:* 8 weeks *Cats:* Not approved for use in cats	Yes	N/A	Can pick up next dose when mistake is noted but should not wait longer than 2 to 3 weeks	Probably safe if microfilaria counts are not too high; may be dangerous if microfilaria counts are high	Hookworms Roundworms Whipworms	Microfilaria fourth stage larvae
ProHeart	Tablet given PO on the same day every month; injection given by vet, which lasts 6 months	*Puppies:* 8 weeks *Cats:* Not approved for use in cats	Yes	N/A	Up to 84-day grace period	Safe because product is approved by FDA for use in HW+ dogs	*Tablets:* Heartworms only *Injectable:* Heartworms and hookworms	Microfilaria third stage larvae

FDA, U.S. Food and Drug Administration; HW, heartworm; PO, by mouth.
*Sentinel has lufenuron in it, which breaks down the chitin within the flea's shell, rendering it harmless.

Microfilaricides should be given 6 weeks after administration of the adulticide. They are used to kill circulating **microfilaria.** Although not approved as microfilaricides, ivermectin and milbemycin oxime have been used, as well as levamisole.

PREVENTIVES

Imidacloprid Plus Moxidectin

Clinical Uses

- *Dogs.* Must be 7 weeks or older and weighing at least 3 lb
- *Cats.* Must be 9 weeks or older and weighing at least 2 lb
- To be applied topically on a monthly basis

Dosage Form

- Advantage Multi

Ivermectin

Clinical Uses

- *Dogs.* Monthly preventive; the Plus formula contains pyrantel pamoate and is effective against hookworms and roundworms
- *Cats.* Monthly preventive for *D. immitis* and for the removal of hookworms
- Eliminates the tissue stage of heartworm larvae

Dosage Forms

- Heartgard
- Heartgard Plus
- Heartgard for Cats

Adverse Side Effects

These are uncommon. Toxic signs include mydriasis, depression, and ataxia.

> *TECHNICIAN NOTES*
> - If diethylcarbamazine citrate (DEC) is replaced, the first dose should be given within a month after cessation of DEC treatment.
> - This product is safe to use in pregnant and breeding animals.
> - Do not use in puppies or kittens younger than 6 weeks.

Milbemycin Oxime

Clinical Uses

- *Dogs.* Monthly preventive; also controls hookworms, roundworms, and whipworms
- Eliminates the tissue stage of heartworm larvae
- Sentinel product contains lufenuron for flea control

Dosage Forms

- Interceptor
- Sentinel

Adverse Side Effects

These are uncommon.

> *TECHNICIAN NOTES*
> - If diethylcarbamazine citrate (DEC) is replaced, the first dose should be given within 1 month after cessation of DEC treatment.
> - This product is safe to use in pregnant and breeding animals.
> - Do not use in puppies younger than 4 weeks.

Moxidectin

Clinical Uses

- *Dogs.* Monthly preventive used for *D. immitis.*
- Eliminates the tissue stage of heartworm larvae
- This drug has been taken off the market.

Dosage Form

- ProHeart

Adverse Side Effects

Adverse side effects may include lethargy, vomiting, ataxia, anorexia, diarrhea, nervousness, weakness, polydipsia, and itching.

> *TECHNICIAN NOTES*
> - If diethylcarbamazine citrate (DEC) is replaced, the first dose should be given within 1 month after cessation of DEC treatment.
> - This product is safe to use in pregnant and breeding animals.
> - Do not use in puppies younger than 8 weeks.

Selamectin

Clinical Uses

- *Dogs and cats.* Used as a monthly preventive
- Available as a solution for topical administration
- Indications include prevention of heartworm disease caused by *D. immitis,* prevention and control of flea infestations, treatment and control of ear mites *(Otodectes cynotis)* infestation, treatment and control of sarcoptic *(Sarcoptes scabiei)* mange in dogs, and hookworm and roundworm treatment in cats.

Dosage Form

- Revolution

Adverse Side Effects

These are uncommon but include transient, localized alopecia at the application site of some treated cats.

> *TECHNICIAN NOTES*
> - If diethylcarbamazine citrate (DEC) is replaced, the first dose should be given within 1 month after cessation of DEC treatment.
> - This product is safe to use in pregnant and breeding animals and in avermectin-sensitive collies.
> - Do not use on puppies or kittens younger than 6 weeks.
> - This product should not be applied if the haircoat is wet. Bathing the animal 2 or more hours after treatment will not reduce its effectiveness.

Diethylcarbamazine Citrate

Clinical Uses

- Daily preventive; also controls roundworms
- Filaribits Plus also contains oxibendazole for the control of hookworms, whipworms, and roundworms.
- Eliminates the tissue stage of heartworm larvae

Dosage Forms

- Carbam
- Filaribits
- Filaribits Plus

Adverse Side Effects

These include occasional vomiting. Filaribits Plus has been linked with hepatic dysfunction (Table 13-11).

> *TECHNICIAN NOTES*
> - Administering with food or directly after a meal reduces the possibility of vomiting.
> - This product is safe to use in pregnant and breeding animals.
> - Missing just 2 to 3 days can affect the efficacy of this product.
> - Do not use in puppies younger than 8 weeks.

ECTOPARASITES

Most ectoparasites are ubiquitous in the environment; therefore, control is often difficult. Environmental factors such as housing (indoor or outdoor) and geographic location may affect the incidence of many ectoparasites such as fleas and ticks. When trying to control ectoparasites, the veterinary technician must be familiar with the products used to eradicate these parasites and must be able to educate clients about how to properly combat their pet's infestation. Not only do ectoparasites cause misery to their host, but many dermatologic problems also arise from their infestation. Additionally, increased infestation of fleas may affect humans because fleas are not host specific. Table 13-12 provides a comparison of various topical products on the market at this time.

APPLICATION SYSTEMS

Prediluted Sprays

Consumers like the convenience of sprays, and sprays are available for animal and environmental use. These formulations are available only for the use specified on the label and should be used accordingly. Sprays are available as water-based and alcohol-based formulations. Water-based sprays do not penetrate oily coats or fabrics as well and do not dry as quickly as alcohol-based sprays. However, alcohol-based sprays may be irritating and drying to the skin. Alcohol-based sprays do usually kill ectoparasites quickly. Environmental sprays are usually residual. Most pet sprays require application daily or every 2 to 3 days for adequate parasite control.

Adverse Side Effects

These vary among products. Carefully read warning labels.

TABLE 13-11 Heartworm Preventive Products That Aid in the Treatment and Control of Other Parasites

PRODUCT	HEARTWORMS	HOOKWORMS	ROUNDWORMS	WHIPWORMS	FLEAS	EAR MITES	SARCOPTIC MANGE	TICKS
Heartgard Plus Chewables (ivermectin and pyrantel pamoate)								
Canine	+	+	+	–	–	–	–	–
Heartgard Chewables (ivermectin)								
Feline	+	+	–	–	–	–	–	–
Revolution (selamectin)								
Canine	+	–	–	–	Adults and eggs	+	+	*Dermacentor variabilis*
Feline	+	+	+	–	Adults and eggs	+	–	–
Interceptor (milbemycin oxime)								
Canine	+	+	+	+	–	–	–	–
Feline	+	+	+	–	–	–	–	–
Sentinel (Milbemycin oxime and lufenuron)								
Canine	+	+	+	+	Eggs and larvae	–	–	–
Trifexis (spinosad and milbemycin oxime)								
Canine	+	+	+	+	Adults	–	–	–

+, Indicated for use; –, not indicated for use.
From Bassert JM: McCurnin's Clinical textbook for veterinary technicians, ed 8, St. Louis, 2014, Saunders.

TECHNICIAN NOTES

- Spray the pet from head to tail, including the legs and abdomen. Avoid only the eyes, mouth, and nose. For best results, spray against the natural lay of the hair.
- Educate clients about environmental control and how to treat the pet.
- Read labels before applying to young, sick, or pregnant animals. Some products are not safe for certain species (e.g., cats).
- Water-based flea sprays are best used on young animals because alcohol-based sprays tend to evaporate quickly and may cause loss of body heat. It is best to apply water-based sprays only to the dorsal area and then to spread the spray by combing through the haircoat. In this way, the young animal does not lose body heat.

Emulsifiable Concentrates

Dips

Concentrates have to be diluted with water. Dips usually are used after a shampoo and generally are considered residual.

Adverse Side Effects

These vary among products. Read labels carefully for animal and user safety and precautions.

TECHNICIAN NOTES

- Removal of excess water or drying of the coat before dipping is recommended to prevent further dilution of the product.
- For best results, do not rinse after applying the dip.
- Organophosphate dips should *never* be applied to cats.

TABLE 13-12 Comparison of Products Indicated for Flea and Tick Control

	REVOLUTION	ADVANTAGE	FRONTLINE AND FRONTLINE PLUS	K9 ADVANTIX
Active ingredient	Selamectin	Imidacloprid	Frontline: fipronil Frontline Plus: fipronil and methoprene	Imidacloprid and Permethrin
Age animal must be for safe application	Puppies: 6 weeks Kittens: 6 weeks	Puppies: 7 weeks Kittens: 8 weeks	Puppies: 10 weeks Kittens: 12 weeks	Puppies: 7 weeks Cats: Do not use on cats
Safety in pregnant or lactating animals	Safe	Not safe (safety has been approved in other countries, but the U.S. EPA does not recognize this testing. No studies have been done in United States)	Not safe	Not safe
Time needed to kill all fleas after first application	42 hours	24 hours	42 hours	12 hours
Does product wash off easily?	No	Yes; can be washed off completely with a degreasing shampoo	No	No
How soon after a bath can the product be applied?	As soon as pet is dry	As soon as pet is dry	Wait 2 days	As soon as pet is dry
Effectiveness on ticks	Yes; *Dermacentor variabilis*	No	Yes; *Amblyomma americanum*; deer tick; *Dermacentor variabilis; Rhipicephalus sanguineus*	Yes; *Amblyomma americanum*; deer tick; *Dermacentor variabilis; Rhipicephalus sanguineus*
Other parasites affected	Ear mites; sarcoptic mange mites; roundworms and hookworms in cats	Fleas only	Fleas and ticks only	Fleas and ticks; repels mosquitoes
Duration of strength in one application	1 month	1 month	1 month for ticks; 1 month for fleas on cats; 1 to 3 months for fleas on dogs	1 month
Is a prescription needed?	Prescription drug	No; product is an insecticide, not a drug	No; product is an insecticide, not a drug	Can be obtained from a licensed veterinarian only
Manufacturer's website	www.revolutionpet.com	www.nofleasusa.com	www.frontline.com	www.bayerus.com

Yard and Kennel Sprays

These are designed for environmental use and should not be used on animals. These products are residual.

Adverse Side Effects

These vary among products. Directions for application should be followed carefully for the safety of the user and of animals.

Shampoos

These products may contain insecticides or medications, or they may be effective only for cleaning the coat. Some shampoos are available as concentrates and require dilution before use. Shampoos are not considered to be residual. Shampoos should be rinsed well; water hardness/softness affects how quickly some shampoos rinse away.

Adverse Side Effects

These vary among products. Shampoos that contain carbamates or organophosphates should not be used with other products of the same origin.

> **TECHNICIAN NOTES**
> - Read labels carefully. Shampoos may seem harmless, but they can be harmful if used improperly.
> - It is recommended that most shampoos be left on the haircoat for 5 to 10 minutes before rinsing.
> - If shampoo is not rinsed well, a hot spot may develop on the pet's skin.

Dusts

The popularity of these products has decreased with the availability of effective sprays. In addition, dusts do not provide a quick kill.

Adverse Side Effects

These include irritation to mucous membranes and drying of the skin and haircoat.

Foggers

Foggers work best in large, open rooms. Remind clients that foggers do not go around corners, under couches, or into closets. Combining foggers with a premises spray enhances results. Labels should always be read carefully.

Monthly Flea and Tick Products

Fipronil

Fipronil is a topical solution that provides flea and tick control; according to the manufacturer, the product collects in the oils of the skin and hair follicles. It controls less severe flea infestations for up to 3 months and ticks for 1 month. Fipronil kills newly emerged adult fleas and all stages of ticks (Table 13-13).

Dosage Forms

- Frontline Top Spot for Dogs
- Frontline Top Spot for Cats

Adverse Side Effects

Adverse side effects include hypersensitivity (rare) and possible irritation at the site of administration (Plumb, 2011).

> **TECHNICIAN NOTES**
> - The product remains effective after bathing, water immersion, or exposure to sunlight.
> - Do not use on kittens younger than 12 weeks or on puppies younger than 10 weeks.
> - This product may be harmful to debilitated, aged, pregnant, or nursing animals.
> - Do not use more often than once every 30 days.
> - It is recommended that gloves be worn when applying this product.

Imidacloprid

Imidacloprid is a topical solution that provides flea control and, according to the manufacturer, is not absorbed into the bloodstream or other internal organs. It controls less severe flea infestations for up to 4 weeks and kills newly emerged adult fleas. Table 13-14 lists various imidacloprid products.

Dosage Form

- Advantage

Adverse Side Effects

Adverse side effects are uncommon.

TABLE 13-13 Veterinary-Label Fipronil With and Without (s)-Methoprene Products

PRODUCT (COMPANY)	FORM: CONCENTRATION	LABEL STATUS	OTHER INGREDIENTS; COMMENTS; SIZE(S)
Frontline Spray Treatment (Merial)	Spray: 0.29% fipronil	OTC-EPA	Labeled for use on dogs, cats, puppies, kittens 8 weeks or older. 8.5, 17 oz
Frontline Top Spot for Cats and Kittens (Merial)	Solution: 9.7% fipronil	OTC-EPA	Labeled for use on cats or kittens 8 weeks or older. Single-dose 50-mL applicators in three or six packs
Frontline Plus for Cats and Kittens (Merial)	Solution: 9.8% fipronil, 11.8% (s)-methoprene	OTC-EPA	Labeled for use on cats or kittens 8 weeks of age or older. Single-dose 50-mL applicators in three or six packs
Frontline Top Spot for Dogs and Puppies (Merial)	Solution: 9.7% fipronil	OTC-EPA	Labeled for use on dogs or puppies 8 weeks or older. Single-dose 50-mL applicators in three or six packs
Frontline Plus for Dogs and Puppies (Merial)	Solution: 9.8% fipronil, 8.8% (s)-methoprene	OTC-EPA	Single-dose applicators in three or six packs. Labeled for dogs or puppies 8 weeks or older. For dogs weighing 0-22 lb: 0.67 mL For dogs weighing 23-44 lb: 1.34 mL For dogs weighing 45-88 lb: 2.68 mL For dogs weighing 89-132 lb: 4.02 mL

EPA, U.S. Environmental Protection Agency; OTC, over-the-counter.
From Plumb DC: Plumb's veterinary drug handbook, ed 7, Wiley-Blackwell, 2011.

TECHNICIAN NOTES

- This product remains effective after bathing, water immersion, or exposure to sunlight.
- Do not use on kittens younger than 8 weeks or on puppies younger than 7 weeks.
- This product should not be used in pregnant animals.
- This product may be used weekly for severe infestations.
- It is not necessary to wear gloves when applying this product.

Imidacloprid and Permethrin

This combination is a once-a-month topical product for dogs that is used to treat ticks and fleas and to repel mosquitoes. It can be used on puppies 7 weeks or older. K9 Advantix is effective after swimming.

Dosage Form

- K9 Advantix

Lufenuron

Lufenuron is a monthly flea control administered orally; it is absorbed into fatty tissue and slowly released into the bloodstream. Sentinel also contains milbemycin for the prevention of heartworms and the control of some intestinal parasites in dogs. Lufenuron controls fleas by preventing the development of chitin, the substance that makes up the flea's exoskeleton. This product does not kill adult fleas. Fleas must take a blood meal to ingest the product.

Dosage Forms

- Program Tablets
- Program 6 Month Injectable for Cats
- Program Suspension
- Sentinel

Adverse Side Effects

Adverse side effects are uncommon. Cats may develop a small lump at the injection site.

TECHNICIAN NOTES

- Do not use in puppies or kittens younger than 6 weeks. Sentinel is approved for use in puppies 4 weeks old.
- Oral products are considered to be safe for use in pregnant, breeding, or lactating animals.
- The safety of the injectable product in reproducing animals has not been established.

TABLE 13-14 Veterinary-Label Imidacloprid Topical Products

PRODUCT (COMPANY)	FORM: CONCENTRATION	LABEL STATUS	OTHER INGREDIENTS; COMMENTS; SIZE(S)
Advantage for Dogs (Bayer)	Topical solution: imidacloprid 9.1%	OTC-EPA	Flea adulticide/larvicide for use on dogs and puppies 7 weeks or older. In cards of four or six tubes: Under 10 lb: 0.4 mL (green) 11-20 lb: 1 mL (teal) 21-55 lb: 2.5 mL (red) Over 55 lb: 4 mL (blue)
Advantage for Cats (Bayer)	Topical solution: imidacloprid 9.1%	OTC-EPA	Flea adulticide/larvicide for use on cats and kittens 8 weeks or older. In cards of four or six tubes: 9 lb or less: 0.4 mL (orange) Over 9 lb: 0.8 mL (purple)
K9 Advantix (Bayer)	Topical solution: imidacloprid 8.8%, permethrin 44%	OTC-EPA	Flea adulticide/larvicide, tick and mosquito repellant and treatment. For use on dogs and puppies 7 weeks or older. In cards of four or six tubes: Under 10 lb: 0.4 mL (green) 11-20 lb: 1 mL (teal) 21-55 lb: 2.5 mL (red) Over 55 lb: 4 mL (blue)
Advantage Multi for Dogs (Bayer)	Topical solution: imidacloprid 10%, moxidectin 2.5%	Rx	Approved for use on dogs 7 weeks or older, and more than 3 lbs body weight
Advantage Multi for Cats (Bayer)	Topical solution: imidacloprid 10%, moxidectin 1%	Rx	Approved for use on cats 9 weeks or older and more than 2 lb body weight
Human-label imidacloprid products: none			

EPA, U.S. Environmental Protection Agency; OTC, over-the-counter; Rx, prescription.
From Plumb DC: Plumb's veterinary drug handbook, ed 7, Wiley-Blackwell, 2011.

Metaflumizone

Metaflumizone can be used on cats 8 weeks or older. It is a topical spot-on product that prevents flea infestation for up to 6 weeks. Metaflumizone attacks the flea's nervous system by blocking neuronal sodium channels, resulting in paralysis and death of the flea. It has been proven to kill *Ctenocephalides canis* and *Ctenocephalides felis.* Table 13-15 lists various metaflumizone products.

Dosage Form

- ProMeris

Metaflumizone/Amitraz

This combination product can be given to puppies 8 weeks or older for the prevention of flea infestation for up to 6 weeks. It prevents tick infestation for up to 4 weeks and has efficacy against *Ixodes ricinus, Ixodes hexagonus, Dermacentor variabilis,* and *Rhipicephalus sanguineus.* It disrupts the tick's normal nerve function, leading to reduced feeding and attachment, paralysis, and finally death. Metaflumizone/amitraz is a topical spot-on product.

Dosage Form

- ProMeris Duo

TABLE 13-15 Veterinary-Label Topical Metaflumizone Products

PRODUCT (COMPANY)	FORM: CONCENTRATION	LABEL STATUS	OTHER INGREDIENTS; COMMENTS; SIZE(S)
ProMeris for Cats (Pfizer)	Topical solution: metaflumizone 9.1%	OTC-EPA	For use on cats and kittens 8 weeks or older. Product comes in two sizes: for cats less than 9 lb and for those more than 9 lb
ProMeris for Dogs (Pfizer)	Spot-On Solution: amitraz 14.34%, metaflumizone 14.34% mg/mL	OTC-EPA	For dogs and puppies 8 weeks or older. Must not be used on cats. See the product label for more information. Packaged in five different sizes according to the dog's weight.
Human-label metaflumizone products: none			

EPA, U.S. Environmental Protection Agency; OTC, over-the-counter.
From Plumb DC: Plumb's veterinary drug handbook, ed 7, Wiley-Blackwell, 2011.

Permethrin

Permethrin is a topical solution that provides flea and tick control; according to the manufacturer, migration of permethrin occurs on the skin surface. It controls fleas, deer ticks, and brown dog ticks for up to 4 weeks and American dog ticks for 2 to 3 weeks. Dogs should be tested for heartworm disease before initial treatment is provided.

Dosage Form

- Defend ExSpot Insecticide for Dogs

Adverse Side Effects

Adverse side effects include skin sensitivity and lethargy.

> **TECHNICIAN NOTES**
> - Efficacy is reduced with bathing.
> - Do not use more often than once every 7 days.
> - Do not use on cats.

Selamectin

Selamectin is a topical solution applied monthly that prevents or controls flea infestation in dogs and cats. It kills adult fleas and prevents flea eggs from hatching. In addition, selamectin is also indicated for prevention of heartworm disease in dogs and cats, treatment and control of ear mite infestations in dogs and cats, and treatment of hookworm and roundworm infections in cats.

Dosage Form

- Revolution

Adverse Side Effects

These are uncommon but include transient, localized alopecia at the application sites of some treated cats.

> **TECHNICIAN NOTES**
> - This product is safe to use in pregnant and breeding animals and in avermectin-sensitive collies.
> - Do not use in puppies or kittens younger than 6 weeks.
> - This product should not be applied if the haircoat is wet; bathing the animal 2 or more hours after treatment will not reduce effectiveness.
> - Dogs should be tested for heartworm disease before initial treatment is provided.

Spinosad

This is a monthly tablet for prevention of flea infestations. It can be used on dogs 14 weeks or older.

Dosage Form

- Comfortis

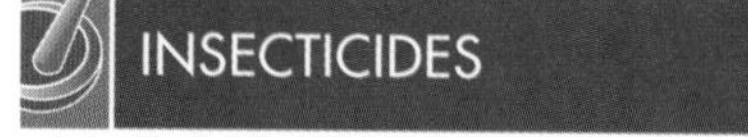

INSECTICIDES

Pyrethrins

These are extracted from pyrethrum or chrysanthemum flowers. They are generally considered safe for most mammals. Pyrethrins have a quick-kill effect and low residual activity (stabilized or microencapsulated pyrethrins have increased residual effects). They are commonly found in pet sprays, dips, shampoos, dusts, foggers, premises sprays, and yard and kennel sprays and are often used in conjunction with other insecticides. Pyrethrins are always used with synergists to maximize their effects.

Synthetic Pyrethroids

Kirk (1986) identifies pyrethroids as "synthesized chemicals modeled on the chrysanthemate molecule of natural pyrethrins, with various substitutions and modifications." Pyrethroids are commonly used in pet sprays, dips, foggers, premises sprays, and yard and kennel sprays. Most have a quick-kill effect, and some have limited residual effects. Their safety is comparable with that of natural pyrethrins. Synergists are not always needed with pyrethroids.

Dosage Forms

The following are common pyrethroids:

- D-trans allethrin (Duocide Spray; Mycodex Pet Shampoo)
- Resmethrin (Durakyl Pet Spray and Shampoo)
- Tetramethrin (Ectokyl IGR Pressurized Spray)
- D-Phenothrin (Duocide Spray; Mycodex Minifog)
- Permethrin (Defend EXspot; Permectrin Spray; Ectokyl IGR Total Release Fogger)

TECHNICIAN NOTES Read labels carefully; concentration affects the use of certain products in some species (e.g., cats).

Chlorinated Hydrocarbons

Once common, most have been banned because of their instability (e.g., dichlorodiphenyltrichlorethane [DDT]). They now have limited uses, and efforts to ban them completely are ongoing.

Dosage Forms

The following are common chlorinated hydrocarbons:

- Lindane (Happy Jack Kennel Dip)
- Methoxychlor (Purina Cattle Dust, Flea and Tick Powder)

Adverse Side Effects

Adverse side effects vary among products, but these products are considered very hazardous to humans and domestic animals. Read labels carefully before using.

TECHNICIAN NOTES Educate clients on the availability of safer products.

Carbamates

Carbamates act as cholinesterase inhibitors and should not be used with other cholinesterase inhibitors, phenothiazine derivatives, and succinylcholine. They are found in dusts, sprays, shampoos, and flea and tick collars.

Dosage Forms

The following are common carbamates:

- Carbaryl (Mycodex Pet Shampoo with Carbaryl, Sevin Dust, Adams Flea and Tick Dust II [used on birds])
- Bendiocarb (mainly large-animal products)
- Propoxur (mainly small-animal products)

Adverse Side Effects

These include excessive salivation, vomiting, diarrhea, muscle tremors, and miosis.

TECHNICIAN NOTES

- Read labels carefully.
- Atropine and 2-PAM (pralidoxime) are antidotal.

Organophosphates

Organophosphates act as cholinesterase inhibitors and should not be used with other organophosphates, carbamates, phenothiazine derivatives, or succinylcholine. They are found in dips, pet sprays, dusts, yard and kennel sprays, premises sprays, and systemics.

Dosage Forms

The following are common organophosphates:

- Chlorpyrifos (Adams Flea and Tick Dip, Yard & Kennel Spray)

- Dichlorvos (Vapona)
- Cythioate (Proban Tablets and Liquid—oral systemic flea control for dogs)
- Diazinon (Escort, Escort Plus, Terminator; used on snakes—Diazinon 25-E)
- Fenthion (Spotton)
- Phosmet (Paramite Dip for Dogs)

Adverse Side Effects

These include excessive salivation, vomiting, diarrhea, muscle tremors, and miosis.

> **TECHNICIAN NOTES**
> - These products should not be used in dogs prone to seizures.
> - Read labels carefully for user and animal safety.
> - Atropine and 2-PAM (pralidoxime) are antidotal.

Formamidines

Amitraz is the most commonly used formamidine in veterinary medicine. Of note, amitraz is not an organophosphate.

Dosage Forms

The following products contain amitraz:

- Mitaban (treatment for canine demodicosis)
- Preventic Tick Collar for Dogs
- Taktic (large-animal insecticide)

Adverse Side Effects

These include transient sedation, lowered rectal temperature, increased blood glucose level, and seizures.

> **TECHNICIAN NOTES**
> Read labels carefully.

Nitenpyram

These are oral tablets for canines and feline 4 weeks or older. Nitenpyram belongs to the chemical class neonicotinoids. It is used to kills adult fleas and starts working within 30 minutes of administration. It is safe for dogs or cats that are pregnant and/or nursing.

Dosage Form

- Capstar

Synergists

Synergists increase the efficacy of pyrethrins and some pyrethroids.

Dosage Forms

The following are common synergists:

- Piperonyl butoxide
- *N*-octyl bicycloheptene dicarboximide

Adverse Side Effects

Piperonyl butoxide has shown evidence of toxicity in cats and a low incidence of chronic neurologic side effects (e.g., tremors, incoordination, and lethargy); sprays have levels equal to or greater than 1.5% (Kirk, 1986).

Repellents

Repellants are commonly used in human, equine, and companion animal products. Most repel gnats, mosquitoes, and flies; when combined with pyrethrins and pyrethroids, they repel new fleas and ticks longer than the active ingredient alone.

Dosage Forms

The following are common repellents:

- 2,3,4,5-bis(2-butylene)tetrahydro-2-furaldehyde (MGK 11)
- Di-*n*-propyl isocinchomeronate (MGK 326)
- Butoxypolypropylene glycol

Insect Growth Regulators and Insect Growth Hormones

Maturation and pupation of flea larvae normally require a low level of natural insect growth regulators (IGRs). Products that contain IGRs mimic natural IGRs. They cause a high level of IGRs and interrupt the natural development of flea larvae. IGRs are found in pet sprays, flea collars, and premises sprays.

Dosage Forms

The following are common IGRs:

- Methoprene
- Fenoxycarb
- Pyriproxyfen (Nylar)

Other Insecticides

Rotenone

Rotenone is very toxic to fish and swine. It is commonly used in combination with other insecticides.

Dosage Forms

- Rotenone Shampoo
- Ear Mite Lotion

Ivermectin

Ivermectin is a systemic injectable for the control of ectoparasites and some **helminths.** Studies show efficacy against *S. scabiei* and *O. cynotis;* however, it is not approved for these uses in dogs or cats

Dosage Forms

- Ivomec 1% Injection for Cattle
- Ivomec 1% Sterile Solution for Swine

D-Limonene

This is an extract of citrus peel and is found in sprays, shampoos, and dips. It provides a quick kill but is not residual.

Dosage Forms

- VIP Flea Dip
- VIP Flea Control Shampoo

Benzyl Benzoate

Benzyl benzoate is effective against many ectoparasites and may be combined with other agents.

Petroleum Distillate

Petroleum distillate is usually added to pyrethrin and pyrethroid products as the solvent.

REVIEW QUESTIONS

1. Name five types of symbiotic relationships.
   ____
2. What is parasitiasis? ____________________
3. What is parasitosis? ____________________
4. What are ectoparasites?
   ____
5. What are endoparasites?
   ____
6. An animal with endoparasites is said to be ____________________, and an animal with ectoparasites is said to be ____________________.
7. What is an anthelmintic?
   ____
8. ____________________ dips should never be used on cats.
9. IGR is an acronym for ____________________.
10. Praziquantel is a drug that is used to rid the body of ____________________.
11. An example of __________ is the bacterium *Moraxella bovis,* the etiologic agent of infectious bovine keratoconjunctivitis, or pinkeye, that is mechanically carried from the eyes of one cow to those of another on the sticky footpads of the face fly *Musca autumnalis.*
    a. predator–prey
    b. commensalism
    c. mutualism
    d. phoresis
12. Ivermectin, moxidectin, and doramectin are in the ______________ class.
    a. avermectin
    b. ivermectin
    c. tetrahydropyrimidine
    d. microfilaricide
13. All the following are monthly heartworm preventives, except ______________.
    a. milbemycin oxime
    b. selamectin
    c. Heartgard Plus
    d. diethylcarbamazine
14. ______ is the most commonly used formamidine in veterinary medicine.
    a. Dichlorvos
    b. Propoxur
    c. Amitraz
    d. Selamectin

15. ____________________ is a topical solution that controls ascarids, hookworms, and tapeworms in felines.
    a. Selamectin (Revolution)
    b. Emodepside/praziquantel (Profender)
    c. Fipronil (Frontline)
    d. Lufenuron (Program)
16. An arsenic compound administered by deep intramuscular injection in the lumbar region is _____.
    a. caparsolate
    b. clorsulon
    c. melarsomine dihydrochloride
    d. Ivomec
17. Albendazole is the active ingredient found in _________.
    a. Droncit
    b. ProMeris
    c. Synanthic
    d. Valbazen
18. An organophosphate is a substance that can interfere with the function of the nervous system by inhibiting the enzyme cholinesterase.
    a. True
    b. False
19. Advantage has greater efficacy against _____, and Frontline has greater efficacy against _____.
    a. ticks; fleas
    b. fleas; ticks
20. _________ are parasitic worms, including intestinal roundworms, filarial worms, lungworms, kidney worms, heartworms, and others.
    a. Cestodes
    b. Trematodes
    c. Acanthocephalans
    d. Nematodes
21. A 1700-lb Angus bull needs to be dewormed with albendazole liquid. On hand in the pharmacy is albendazole (113.6 mg/mL). The dose is 10 mg/kg PO. How many milliliters should be obtained to treat this bull?
    a. 48 mL
    b. 68 mL
    c. 58 mL
    d. 38 mL
22. A herd of 55 Hereford cows need to be dewormed using Dectomax. The average weight of the individuals in the herd is 1200 lb. On hand in the pharmacy is Dectomax (10 mg/mL). The dose for this drug is 1 mL/110 lb of weight. How many total milliliters does the client need for deworming his herd?
    a. 600 mL
    b. 499.5 mL
    c. 799 mL
    d. 599.5 mL
23. A heifer-calf that weighs 120 lb is found to have *Eimeria zurnii.* The veterinarian orders amprolium for treatment of the calf. On hand in the pharmacy is Corid liquid (9.6%). The dosage is 10 mg/kg PO for 5 days. What is the dose? How many milliliters should be dispensed to the client to treat this calf?
    a. 5.6 mL; 28 mL
    b. 4.6 mL; 56 mL
    c. 4.6 mL; 16 mL
    d. 5.6 mL; 56 mL
24. A heifer-calf that weighs 120 lb is found to have *Eimeria zurnii.* The veterinarian orders amprolium for treatment of the calf. On hand in the pharmacy is Corid liquid (9.6%). The dosage is 10 mg/kg PO for 5 days. After the treatment, the veterinarian wants to use the drug for prophylaxis. The dosage for this is 5 mg/kg for 21 days. How many milliliters of the drug should be dispensed to provide prophylactic treatment for this calf?
    a. 59.65 mL
    b. 60 mL
    c. 49.65 mL
    d. 50 mL
25. A dog is found to have *Dipylidium caninum.* The dog weighs 22.4lb. The dosage is 68 mg for a dog this size. On hand in the pharmacy is the right drug to use, and it has a concentration of 34 mg per tablet. What drug should be used for this patient? How many tablets should be dispensed for one dose?
    a. doxycycline; 2 tablets
    b. praziquantel; 2 tablets
    c. diethylcarbamazine; 2 tablets
    d. furosemide; 2 tablets

REFERENCES

Hendrix CM, editor: Diagnostic veterinary parasitology, ed 2, St. Louis, 2006, Mosby.

Kirk RW: Current veterinary IX: small animal practice, Philadelphia, 1986, WB Saunders.

Plumb DC: Veterinary drug handbook, ed 7, Ames, Iowa, 2011, Wiley-Blackwell.

Smith P: New studies, products fuel heartworm debate, Vet Prod News 11(4):34–36, 1999.

CHAPTER 14

Drugs Used to Relieve Pain and Inflammation

KEY TERMS

Addison's disease
Analgesia
Cushing's disease
Histamine
Iatrogenic
Modulation
Multimodal analgesia
Nerve block
Neuropathic pain
Pathologic pain
Perception
Physiologic pain
Preemptive analgesia
Prostaglandin
Regional anesthesia
Somatic pain
Transdermal application
Transduction
Transmission
Visceral pain

OUTLINE

LEARNING OBJECTIVES

After studying this chapter, you should be able to

1. Define terms related to the pharmacology of drugs used to relieve pain and inflammation.
2. Describe the anatomy and physiology associated with pain production and relief.
3. List and discuss the four steps involved in the production of pain sensation.
4. Understand the difference between physiologic and pathologic pain.
5. Understand the concepts of preemptive and multimodal pain therapy.
6. List physical signs associated with the expression of pain in animals.
7. Describe the mechanism of action of the category of drugs known as nonsteroidal antiinflammatory drugs (NSAIDs).

8. List indications for the use of NSAIDs.
9. List potential adverse side effects of NSAIDs.
10. Describe the mechanism of action of the antihistamines.
11. Differentiate between the action of H_1 and H_2 histamine receptors.
12. List indications for muscle relaxants.
13. List the two major categories of corticosteroids and describe the effects of each.
14. Describe the hypothalamic–pituitary–adrenal axis, which controls the release of corticosteroids in the body.
15. List indications for the use of corticosteroids.
16. Describe potential adverse side effects of short-term and long-term corticosteroid use.
17. Describe the mechanism of action of local anesthetic agents.
18. List some indications for local anesthetic agents.

INTRODUCTION

Pain has been defined by the International Association for the Study of Pain as "an unpleasant sensory and emotional experience associated with actual or potential tissue damage." It may occur alone or in combination with inflammation. Pain sensation arises in the terminal ends of sensory nerve fibers called *nociceptors,* which are located in every tissue of the body. Nociceptors may be activated through mechanical, thermal, and chemical stimulation to create a nerve impulse. Chemical stimulation may be derived from an exogenous source or from endogenous chemicals such as eicosanoids (prostaglandins), bradykinin, serotonin, and others released in response to tissue damage. These substances may create a "sensitizing soup," which may create a lower threshold for nociceptors, amplifying the pain response (Muir, 2009)

Physiologic pain can be beneficial in that it can allow the animal to avoid damaging stimuli. **Pathologic pain** results from tissue or nerve damage and may be further classified according to its origin, severity, or duration. **Visceral pain** arises from hollow abdominal organs, peritoneum, heart, liver, and lungs while **somatic pain** arises from the musculoskeletal system. Somatic pain may be further described as superficial (arising from the skin) or deep (arising from periosteum, tendon, or joint tissues). **Neuropathic pain** can arise due to injury to the peripheral or central nervous system and is described in humans as "burning" or "shooting" (Gaynor, 2009). Pain can have varying degrees of severity (none, mild, moderate, or severe) and may be acute or chronic.

Severe or chronic pain may have an emotional content that activates sympathetic stimulation. It can be harmful because it can lead to stress and related problems such as gastrointestinal lesions, immunosuppression, delayed healing, hypertension, fatigue, abnormal behavior, and potential dysrhythmias. The ethical treatment of animals includes the "five freedoms": freedom from pain, freedom from hunger and malnutrition, freedom from discomfort, freedom from disease and injury, and freedom to express normal behavior.

Assessment of pain in animals can be very difficult because of the dependence on nonverbal communication in veterinary medicine. Furthermore, animals differ from people in their pain response. It is

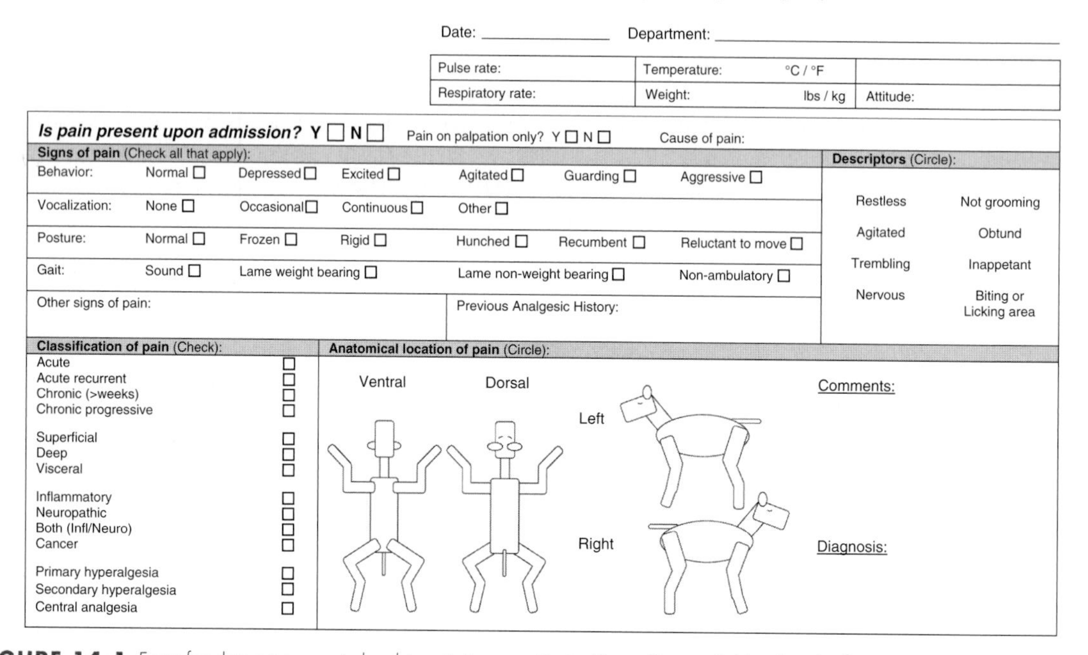

THE OHIO STATE UNIVERSITY VETERINARY TEACHING HOSPITAL

PAIN MANAGEMENT PLAN

PATIENT ID CARD

"Pain assessment is considered part of every patient evaluation, regardless of presenting complaint."

Date: ______________ Department: ______________

Pulse rate:	Temperature: °C / °F	
Respiratory rate:	Weight: lbs / kg	Attitude:

Is pain present upon admission? Y ☐ N ☐ Pain on palpation only? Y ☐ N ☐ Cause of pain:

Signs of pain (Check all that apply):

Behavior:	Normal ☐	Depressed ☐	Excited ☐	Agitated ☐	Guarding ☐	Aggressive ☐
Vocalization:	None ☐	Occasional ☐	Continuous ☐	Other ☐		
Posture:	Normal ☐	Frozen ☐	Rigid ☐	Hunched ☐	Recumbent ☐	Reluctant to move ☐
Gait:	Sound ☐	Lame weight bearing ☐		Lame non-weight bearing ☐		Non-ambulatory ☐

Other signs of pain: Previous Analgesic History:

Descriptors (Circle):

Restless	Not grooming
Agitated	Obtund
Trembling	Inappetant
Nervous	Biting or Licking area

Classification of pain (Check):

Acute ☐
Acute recurrent ☐
Chronic (>weeks) ☐
Chronic progressive ☐

Superficial ☐
Deep ☐
Visceral ☐

Inflammatory ☐
Neuropathic ☐
Both (Infl/Neuro) ☐
Cancer ☐

Primary hyperalgesia ☐
Secondary hyperalgesia ☐
Central analgesia ☐

Anatomical location of pain (Circle):

Ventral Dorsal Left Right

Comments:

Diagnosis:

FIGURE 14-1 Form for determining pain level in veterinary patients. (From Gaynor J: Handbook of veterinary pain management, St. Louis, 2008, Elsevier.)

important for wild animals to control the expression of pain to avoid predation or abandonment. Response to pain varies among individuals and may include increased heart rate, increased respiratory rate, mydriasis, salivation, vocalization, changes in facial expression, aggressive behavior, guarding of the painful site, restlessness, unresponsiveness, failure to groom, abnormal gait, and abnormal stance. A patient that is pain-free will be quiet and calm (Paddleford, 1999). Consult the *Handbook of Veterinary Pain Management* for pictures and descriptions of pain behaviors in animals. Pain scales and evaluation instruments (Figure 14-1) have been developed to make pain evaluation more objective.

Drugs used to control pain (analgesics) include nonsteroidal antiinflammatory drugs (NSAIDs), opioids, α-2 agonists, ketamine, and others. The body is able to produce its own opiate-like analgesic agents called *endorphins* and *enkephalins.* Efforts to synthesize these substances for commercial production have been unsuccessful.

At one time people believed that masking pain with analgesics could interfere with the diagnosis or treatment course of a disease. It is now known that animals in pain should be treated for humane reasons and so that the harmful side effects that accompany pain can be reduced. The treatment regimen may vary according to assessment of the severity and the origin of the pain. For best results, pain management intervention should be **preemptive** and include **multimodal analgesia** when possible.

Inflammation is a basic process that occurs in the body in response to tissue injury caused by physical, chemical, or biologic trauma. The objectives of this process are (1) to counteract the injury by removing or walling off the cause of the injury and (2) to repair or replace the damaged tissue. Clinical manifestations (cardinal signs) of inflammation include *redness, heat, swelling,* and *pain.* Although the process is designed to be protective, it can continue to become a source of further injury or damage (e.g., allergy, shock, or "proud flesh").

Damage to cells from any source results in the release of several chemical mediators that may initiate or prolong the inflammatory response. These chemicals include **prostaglandins,** leukotrienes, **histamine,** cytokines, and other mediators. These substances cause helpful responses such as dilation and increased permeability of blood vessels that result in increased blood flow to the injured tissue. Enhanced blood flow brings plasma to dilute the offending agent, fibrin to immobilize it, and phagocytic cells to remove it. Redness, heat, swelling, and, to some extent, the pain of inflammation result from increased amounts of blood in the damaged tissue. The chemical mediators serve other beneficial functions such as attracting phagocytic cells to the area of concern (chemotaxis) and several potentially harmful functions such as initiation of bronchoconstriction (histamine), anaphylactic shock, pain (histamine), cell death, platelet aggregation, and intestinal spasm. The inflammatory process can be acute (anaphylaxis) or chronic (flea allergy and arthritis).

Drugs that are used to minimize the inflammatory process include NSAIDs, glucocorticosteroids, and several miscellaneous agents such as dimethyl sulfoxide (DMSO). Another process mediated by a chemical (or chemicals) released from damaged cells is fever. Fever is an increase in body temperature to above normal; it is an important clinical indicator of disease. The purpose of fever may include destruction of invading microorganisms by heat inactivation and facilitation of biochemical reactions in the body. (Most chemical reactions are accelerated by increased heat.)

Heat is generated by the metabolic activity of muscles and glands and is dissipated through radiation or conduction loss from the skin, sweat evaporation, and evaporation during panting. A "thermostat" in the hypothalamus regulates these mechanisms, which control body temperature.

A substance that can initiate a fever is called a *pyrogen.* An exogenous pyrogen is a foreign substance (e.g., bacteria, viruses) that when introduced into the body causes the release of an endogenous pyrogen (a chemical mediator such as prostaglandin) from white blood cells; this endogenous pyrogen causes resetting of the hypothalamic thermostat. The hypothalamus then activates processes to generate or conserve body heat: shivering to generate more heat, constriction of blood vessels in the skin to prevent radiation and conduction loss, and decreased sweating or panting to reduce evaporation loss. Damaged cells in some instances may release endogenous pyrogens in the absence of exogenous pyrogens. Drugs used to control fever are primarily NSAIDs.

ANATOMY AND PHYSIOLOGY

The production of pain sensation arises through a four step process: **transduction, transmission, modulation,** and **perception** (Figure 14-2). The first step called *transduction* occurs in nociceptors, which are terminal sensory nerve endings found in almost every tissue of the body. The nociceptor creates action potentials (electric impulses) in peripheral sensory nerves when activated by noxious stimuli. The second step is the transmission of the impulses to the central nervous system (CNS) by two fiber systems: type C unmyelinated fibers are responsible for dull, poorly localized pain (in humans), and type A delta fibers are responsible for sharp, localized pain (Ganong, 2003). Type A and type C fibers carry impulses to the dorsal horn of the spinal cord (Figure 14-3). This information then, in the third step, undergoes modulation (suppression or amplification) and is transmitted up the cord via the spinothalamic tract through the thalamus to the cerebral cortex, where processing occurs and recognition results in pain perception. If any part of this neuronal chain or the cortical interpretive area is nonfunctional, pain sensation does not occur. Multimodal therapy takes advantage of this concept to intervene at different sites within the pathways. Because an active cortex is required, the perception of pain can occur only in a conscious animal. It should be remembered that reflexive activity (e.g., withdrawal reflex) without pain recognition can occur as a result of nociceptor stimulation (see Chapter 4).

The perception of pain can be enhanced by phenomena called *hyperalgesia* and *central sensitization* (Boothe, 2012). Hyperalgesia occurs when the area

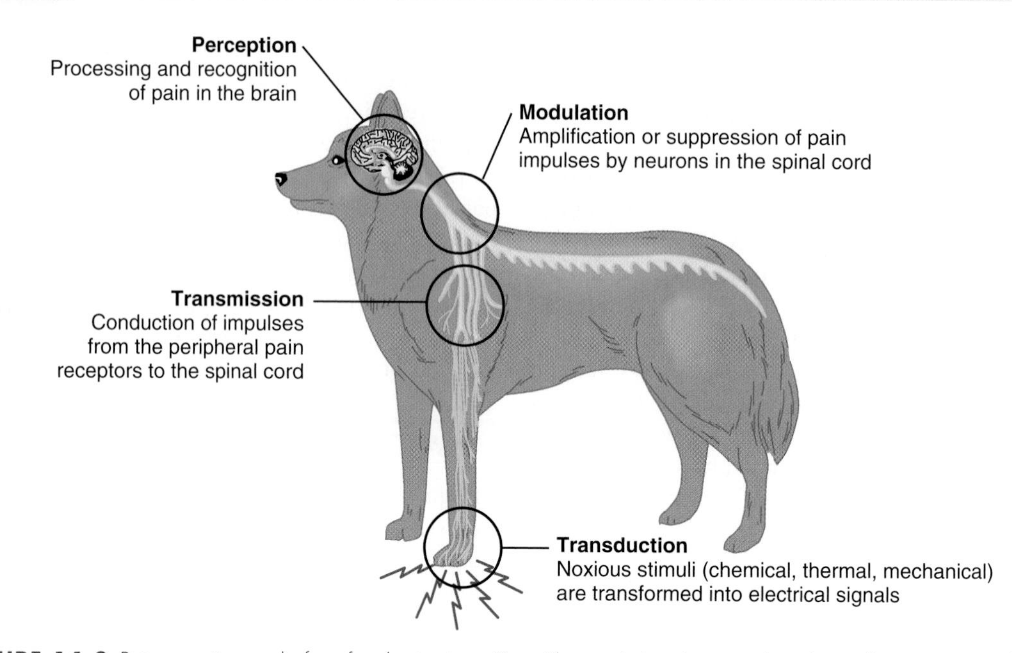

FIGURE 14-2 Pain sensation results from four basic steps. (From Thomas J: Anesthesia and analgesia for veterinary technicians, St. Louis, 2010, Elsevier.)

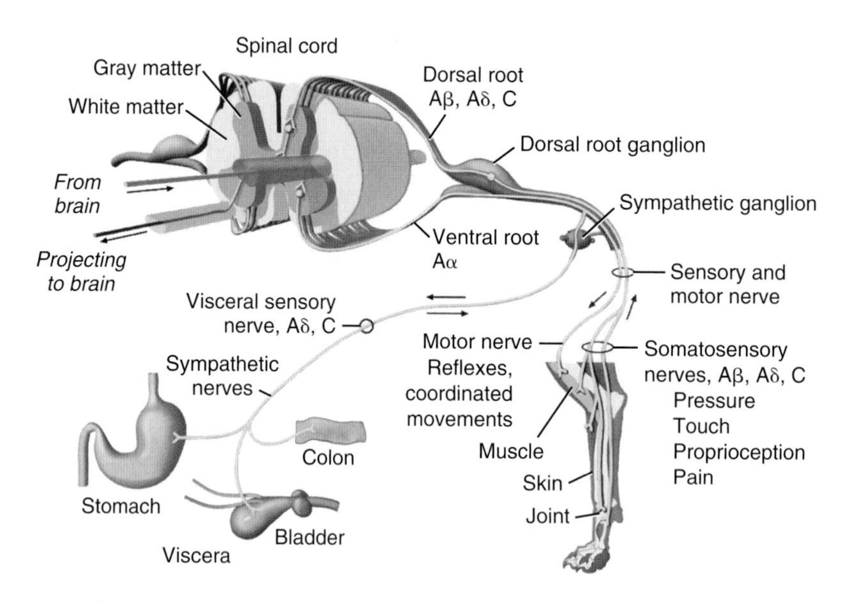

FIGURE 14-3 Pain pathways and relevant receptors. (From Gaynor J: Handbook of veterinary pain management, St. Louis, 2008, Elsevier.)

of tissue injury becomes more sensitive and the threshold for subsequent stimuli decreases. This sensitivity can spread to surrounding uninjured tissue (secondary hyperalgesia). When the neurons of the spinothalamic tract of the spinal cord are stimulated repeatedly, they apparently become sensitized and discharge at a much lower threshold. This activity is called *central sensitization,* or *"wind-up,"* and is the rationale for the idea that pain control is enhanced if an analgesic is given before pain is generated.

When spinal cord lesions occur, superficial pain is inhibited before deep pain or lesion severity worsens. The absence of deep pain is often a poor prognostic sign.

As mentioned previously, pharmacologic intervention for pain control may target a single or multiple points of intervention in the pain process. Transduction can be inhibited by local anesthetics, opioids, NSAIDs, and other substances. Transmission of nerve impulses can be inhibited by local anesthetics and alpha-2 agonists. Modulation of pain impulses can occur in the spinal cord through the effects of local anesthetics, opioids, alpha-2 agonists, tricyclic antidepressants, NSAIDs, anticonvulsants, and other drugs. Pain perception in the cortex can be inhibited by the use of anesthetics, opioids, benzodiazepines, and alpha-2 agonists.

NONSTEROIDAL ANTIINFLAMMATORY DRUGS

NSAIDs are very useful analgesic drugs that have been shown to work synergistically with opioids when used together. NSAIDs are thought to work by inhibiting an enzyme called cyclooxygenase (COX). Two forms (COX-1 and COX-2) of cyclooxygenase exist. COX-1 maintains physiologic functions such as modulation of renal blood flow and synthesis of gastric mucosa and is sometimes called the constitutive form (Paddleford, 1999). COX-2 is considered the induced (by tissue injury) form that promotes the formation of prostaglandin from cell membrane arachidonic acid (Figure 14-4). Generally, inhibition of COX-2 is responsible for effectiveness of NSAIDs whereas inhibition of COX-1 is associated with side effects. NSAIDs that selectively inhibit COX-2 are thought to produce fewer gastrointestinal side effects. Recent research has suggested that this scheme may be an oversimplification and that COX-2 may be constitutive in some tissues (Budsberg, 2009). COX-1

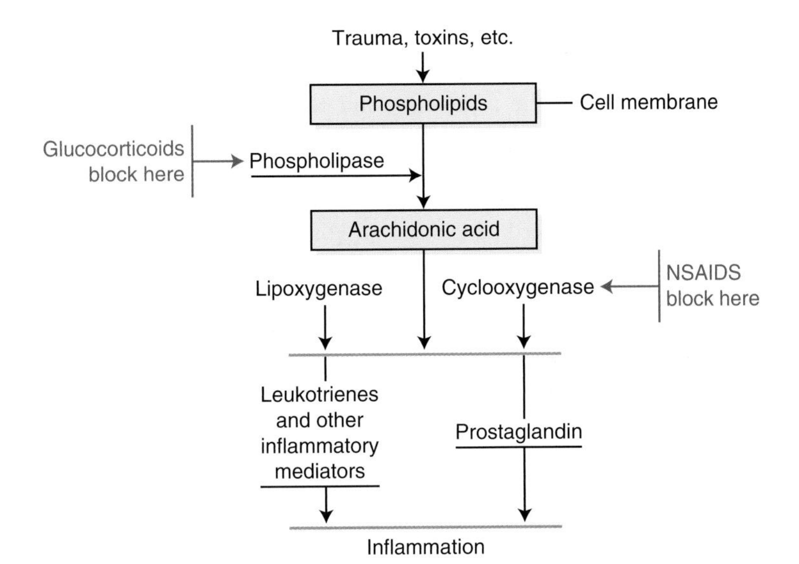

FIGURE 14-4 Actions of nonsteroidal antiinflammatory drugs (NSAIDs) and glucocorticoids that interrupt the inflammatory response.

versus COX-2 selectivity may depend on the drug, the dose, and the species (Claude, 2013). Because the degree of COX-1 and COX-2 inhibition for many of the newer NSAIDs is not well-defined, preferential COX-2 inhibitor may be chosen over selective COX-2 inhibitor because some inhibition of COX-1 and COX-2 may occur (Boothe, 2012). COX-1 sparing has the same connotation as preferential COX-2 inhibitor.

Glucocorticoids exert their effects by blocking phospholipase, an enzyme necessary for the production of both prostaglandins and leukotrienes (intervention is provided earlier in the sequence of the formation of inflammatory mediators). Because the inflammatory reaction is blocked earlier by glucocorticoids, they are more effective antiinflammatory agents than are NSAIDs (Langston and Mercer, 1988). NSAIDs are often preferred, however, because they have fewer side effects and they promote **analgesia** and fever reduction. At this time, it is not known why glucocorticoids do not induce the analgesic and antipyretic effects of NSAIDs. It is also unknown why some NSAIDs provide relief of only mild pain (aspirin) and others provide relief of moderate to severe pain (flunixin). Some clinicians speculate that NSAIDs may act to varying degrees centrally to modulate spinal transmission of pain impulses (Paddleford, 1999).

The most common side effects of the NSAIDs are gastrointestinal ulceration and bleeding, which probably result from interference with the normal mucous coating of the stomach. Other side effects may include hepatotoxicity, nephrotoxicity, inhibition of cartilage metabolism, bone marrow suppression, and bleeding tendencies (from reduced platelet aggregation).

All pets should undergo a thorough physical examination and history, as well as appropriate laboratory tests, before NSAIDs are initiated. Clients should be advised to stop the use of these drugs and to contact their veterinarian if they observe side effects in their pets that are receiving NSAIDs. Pets receiving long-term treatment with NSAIDs should have periodic evaluations of liver and kidney function performed. Clients should be advised to watch their pets for anorexia, vomiting, changes in bowel movements, bloody or tarry stools, lethargy or other changes in behavior, seizures, jaundice, changes in urination (frequency, color, or smell), or changes in the condition of the skin.

TECHNICIAN NOTES

- NSAIDs should be used with caution in geriatric animals.
- Combining NSAIDs or combining NSAIDs with corticosteroids should be done with great caution or avoided.

Salicylates

Aspirin, a salicylate, is also known as acetylsalicylic acid. Its actions include the following:

- Relief of pain (analgesia)
- Reduction in fever (antipyrexia)
- Inhibition of inflammation (antiinflammatory effect)
- Reduction in platelet aggregation (blood-thinning effect)

These effects are thought to occur as a result of the ability of aspirin to inhibit an enzyme (COX) that is responsible for the synthesis of prostaglandin. Prostaglandin is a chemical mediator of the processes that lead to pain, fever, inflammation, and platelet aggregation. Its inhibition results in diminishing of each process.

Clinical Uses

Clinical uses of aspirin exist for most animal species and may include the following:

- Relief of mild to moderate pain caused by musculoskeletal conditions such as arthritis and hip dysplasia
- Postadulticide treatment for heartworm disease
- Analgesia/antipyrexia
- Treatment of cats with cardiomyopathy
- Treatment of endotoxic shock

Dosage Forms

These include plain uncoated tablets, buffered uncoated tablets, enteric-coated forms, and boluses (large-animal applications). Many generic or brand names are available in many different strengths, including the following:

- Aspirin bolus; horses and cattle
- Aspirin tablets; dogs

- Aspirin gel; dogs
- Aspirin granules; horses

Adverse Side Effects

Adverse side effects of aspirin include gastric irritation, which can lead to ulceration and bleeding. *Cats are highly susceptible to aspirin overdosage because of their inability to metabolize it rapidly; they should receive this drug only under the supervision of a veterinarian.*

> TECHNICIAN NOTES
> - Enteric-coated aspirin, such as Ecotrin, may be used to prevent gastric irritation.
> - A 1-grain "baby" aspirin contains 65 mg; a 1.25-grain baby aspirin contains 81 mg.
> - Aspirin has no withdrawal time in food animals.

Pyrazolone Derivatives

Phenylbutazone

Phenylbutazone, a pyrazolone derivative, is an NSAID that is commonly used in veterinary medicine. Its actions include the following:

- Analgesia for mild to moderate pain
- Antiinflammatory action
- Antipyrexia

Clinical Uses

These include relief of inflammatory conditions of the musculoskeletal system of horses and dogs. Phenylbutazone is used extensively in horses for the treatment of lameness and for the relief of pain associated with colic. It sometimes is used in dogs and cattle for its antiinflammatory, analgesic, and antipyretic effects.

Dosage Forms

Dosage forms of phenylbutazone include parenteral injection, tablets, boluses, an oral paste, an oral gel, and powder.

- Phenylbutazone, tablets, boluses, paste, injection
- Phenylzone Paste
- Equi-Phar ButePaste
- ButaJect
- Phenylbute Paste

Adverse Side Effects

These include gastrointestinal bleeding and bone marrow suppression.

> TECHNICIAN NOTES
> - Phenylbutazone injection should be administered by the intravenous route only. Subcutaneous and intramuscular injection may lead to sloughing of tissue.
> - Prolonged use or an overdose can lead to bone marrow suppression in humans.
> - Prolonged use also may lead to ulcer formation.
> - Because of possible bone marrow suppression and potential ulcer formation, animals that are receiving long-term treatment with phenylbutazone should be monitored carefully.

Flunixin Meglumine

Flunixin is an NSAID that is labeled for use in horses and cattle. It has extralabel uses in other species. Its actions are related to its ability to inhibit COX and include the following:

- Analgesia
- Antipyrexia
- Antiinflammatory effects

Clinical Uses

Clinical uses of flunixin in horses include alleviation of pain associated with musculoskeletal disorders and colic. (Flunixin apparently has great ability to inhibit visceral pain.) Other uses in horses and other species include treatment of the following:

- Disk disease
- Endotoxic shock
- Calf diarrhea
- Parvovirus disease
- Heatstroke
- Ophthalmic conditions
- Postsurgical pain

Dosage Forms

Dosage forms of flunixin include injectable, oral paste, and oral granule formulations.

- Banamine Injection
- Banamine Oral Paste
- Banamine Oral Granules

- FlunixiJect
- Flunazine Injection

Adverse Side Effects

These are limited in horses but may include swelling at the injection site and sweating. In dogs, vomiting, diarrhea, nephrotoxicity, and gastric ulceration may occur with long-term use.

> TECHNICIAN NOTES
> - Flunixin is labeled for intravenous and intramuscular use in horses.
> - Some equine clinicians believe that flunixin relieves abdominal pain so well in horses that it may cause a sense of false security about the condition of an animal with colic.
> - Small-animal patients receiving flunixin should be well-hydrated and should be given intravenous fluids and ulcer prophylaxis (Paddleford, 1999).

Dimethyl Sulfoxide

DMSO is a clear liquid that was originally developed as a commercial solvent. It is noted for its antiinflammatory action and its ability to act as a carrier of other agents through the skin. Its antiinflammatory actions may be related to its ability to trap products associated with the inflammatory response. DMSO causes vasodilation when applied topically.

Clinical Uses

Clinical uses of DMSO are varied; however, the only labeled use for DMSO is for topical application to reduce acute swelling resulting from trauma in dogs and horses. DMSO has reportedly been used as the following:

- An adjunct to intestinal surgery (intravenously)
- A treatment for cerebral edema or spinal cord injury (intravenously)
- A treatment for perivascular injection of chemotherapeutic agents or other irritating substances (topical)
- A carrier of drugs across the skin

Dosage Forms

Dosage forms of DMSO include a solution (90%) and a gel (90%).

- DMSO Gel and Solution (90%)
- Synotic (DMSO and a steroid)

Adverse Side Effects

Adverse side effects of DMSO are probably minimal with limited use or exposure but may include the following: garlic taste, which occurs very shortly after the agent is applied to the skin; skin irritation accompanied by a burning sensation; and induction of birth defects (teratogenic) in some species.

> TECHNICIAN NOTES
> - Rubber gloves should be worn while applying DMSO.
> - Bandaging over an application of DMSO may cause skin irritation.
> - DMSO should be used carefully when cholinesterase inhibitors have also been used.

Buscopan Compositum

Buscopan Compositum is a product that contains butylscopolammonium bromide and metamizole sodium (dipyrone).

Clinical Uses

This product is used for the management of abdominal pain associated with equine colic.

Dosage Form

- Buscopan Compositum

Acetaminophen

Acetaminophen is an analgesic with limited antipyretic and antiinflammatory activities.

Clinical Uses

Clinical uses of acetaminophen are limited in veterinary medicine, and acetaminophen use should be discouraged because of the risk of potential toxicity and the availability of acceptable substitutes.

Dosage Forms

Dosage forms of acetaminophen include tablets, caplets, and liquid formulations. The following is a list of some of the human-label brand names:

- Tylenol
- Datril
- Tempra

TECHNICIAN NOTES

- Acetaminophen should never be given to cats.
- Over-the-counter products should be checked carefully for the presence of acetaminophen before they are used in cats.

Adverse Side Effects

Adverse side effects of acetaminophen use in cats include the formation of methemoglobinemia, cyanosis, anemia, and liver damage. *Cats have a limited ability to biotransform acetaminophen and may succumb to a single dose.*

Propionic Acid Derivatives

Carprofen

Carprofen is a propionic acid derivative NSAID that has been approved for oral use in dogs. Carprofen has been approved for oral and injectable use in dogs and cats in Europe. It has a half-life of 8 hours and is thought to work by inhibiting COX enzyme(s). An injectable form is now also available for use in the United States.

Clinical Uses

Uses include the relief of pain associated with degenerative joint disease and postoperative pain resulting from soft tissue or orthopedic repair.

Dosage Forms

- Carprofen (Rimadyl); available in tablets, caplets, injection, and chewable tablets
- Carprofen (Novox Caplets, Norocarp Caplets)

Adverse Side Effects

Side effects such as gastrointestinal ulceration and bleeding are apparently rare with this agent.

Ketoprofen

Ketoprofen is a propionic acid derivative with analgesic, antipyretic, and antiinflammatory activities. It is labeled for use in horses in the United States but has been used a great deal in dogs and cats in Europe and Canada.

Clinical Uses

In horses, ketoprofen is used for treatment of pain and inflammation associated with musculoskeletal disorders. It has been used for postoperative and chronic pain in dogs and cats.

Dosage Forms

- Ketofen (horses), injection
- Ketoprofen capsules, human label

Adverse Side Effects

Side effects may include gastrointestinal bleeding or ulceration, renal dysfunction, and generalized bleeding.

Naproxen

Naproxen is a propionic acid derivative that is similar to ketoprofen and ibuprofen. It is labeled for use in horses, although it has been used in dogs.

Clinical Uses

Naproxen is labeled for the "relief of pain, inflammation, and lameness associated with myositis and other soft tissue diseases of the musculoskeletal system of horses."

Dosage Forms

- Equiproxen (horses); no longer marketed in the United States
- Naprosyn (human)

Adverse Side Effects

Few side effects are reported in horses. Gastrointestinal ulceration has been reported in dogs.

Ibuprofen

Ibuprofen is reported to have the potential for serious side effects in dogs and cats and is not recommended for use in these species.

OTHER NONSTEROIDAL ANTIINFLAMMATORY DRUGS

Etodolac

Etodolac is an indole acetic acid derivative, COX-1–sparing NSAID that has been labeled for use in dogs.

Clinical Use

This drug is labeled for the management of pain and inflammation associated with osteoarthritis in dogs.

Dosage Form

- EtoGesic, tablets and injectable

Adverse Side Effects

Side effects include anorexia, vomiting, diarrhea, and lethargy.

Deracoxib

Deracoxib is an analgesic and a nonsteroidal antiinflammatory agent of the coxib (COX-1–sparing) class.

Clinical Use

Deracoxib is labeled for the control of pain and inflammation associated with orthopedic surgery in dogs with 4-lb body weight or greater and for the control of pain and inflammation associated with osteoarthritis in dogs weighing 14 lb or more.

Dosage Form

- Deramaxx

Firocoxib

Firocoxib is an NSAID that belongs to the coxib (COX-1–sparing) class.

Clinical Uses

The labeled use is for the treatment of pain and inflammation associated with osteoarthritis in dogs and horses.

Dosage Forms

- Previcox Chewable Tablets with once-daily dosing for dogs and Equioxx oral paste for horses.

Tepoxalin

Tepoxalin was previously marketed as an NSAID for the treatment of osteoarthritis in dogs. The manufacturer claims that this product is the only NSAID that blocks both arms of the arachidonic acid cascade (COX and lipoxygenase). It was manufactured as a "rapidly disintegrating" tablet that breaks down quickly on contact with the moisture of the animal's mouth and cannot be spit out. This dosage form was designed to improve owner/animal dosage compliance. This product is no longer commercially produced is the USA.

Clinical Use

Tepoxalin is labeled for the control of pain and inflammation associated with osteoarthritis in dogs.

Dosage Form

- Zubrin

Meloxicam

Meloxicam is a COX-2 receptor NSAID. It has antiinflammatory, analgesic, and antipyretic properties.

Clinical Uses

Meloxicam is used to control pain associated with surgical procedures, arthritis, and other causes. Metacam use in cats is limited to one-time subcutaneous injection for surgical pain.

Dosage Forms

- Metacam Oral Suspension, 1.5 mg/mL
- Metacam Injection for Cats, 5 mg/mL
- Metacam Injection for Dogs, 5 mg/mL
- OroCAM, oral spray for dogs

Adverse Side Effects

These are similar to other NSAIDs.

Robenacoxib

Robenacoxib is a coxib (COX-1–sparing) NSAID for the relief of pain and inflammation in dogs and cats.

Clinical Uses

Robenacoxib is used for the treatment of pain and inflammation associated with chronic osteoarthritis in dogs and cats and acute pain associated with musculoskeletal conditions in cats.

Dosage Form

- Onsior, tablets and injection

Adverse Side Effects

Side effects may include vomiting or diarrhea. The package insert should be consulted for potential interactions with some other drugs.

Polysulfated Glycosaminoglycan

This is a semisynthetic mixture of glycosaminoglycans derived from bovine cartilage. This drug reduces degenerative changes induced by noninfectious or traumatic joint disease and promotes activity in the synovial membrane. It is available in intraarticular and intramuscular forms and is labeled for use in horses and dogs.

Dosage Form

- Adequan

Hyaluronate Sodium

Hyaluronate sodium is a high viscosity mucopolysaccharide used for the treatment of synovitis in horses.

Dosage Forms

- Legend, approved for intraarticular and intravenous use in horses
- Hyalovet, intraarticular use in horses
- Hyvisc, intraarticular use in horses
- Conquer, oral gel for horses

Selenium and Vitamin E

This combination is labeled for relief of short-term symptoms of arthritic conditions in dogs.

Dosage Form

- Seletoc

Ketorolac

Ketorolac is an NSAID with efficacy similar to that of morphine. It carries a human label and may cause serious side effects.

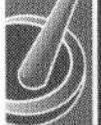

OPIOID ANALGESICS

Opioids and opioid receptors are discussed in a general fashion in Chapter 4. This section addresses only use of opioids to control pain.

Opioids relieve pain by binding with specific receptor sites in the brain, spinal cord, and peripheral tissue. By altering neurotransmitter release, they alter nerve impulse formation and transmission at many levels within the CNS. The ultimate effect is that the opioids block or inhibit pain impulses to higher CNS centers responsible for the perception of pain.

Opioid Agonists

Opioid agonists remain one of the most effective drug classes for relieving moderate to severe pain (Wagner, 2009). Opioid agonists are drugs that bind with all opioid receptor sites and produce opioid effects and respiratory depression, sedation, and addiction. Opioid agonists include alfentanil, carfentanil, codeine, etorphine, fentanyl, hydromorphone, meperidine, methadone, morphine, oxymorphone, and sufentanil. Even though some of these drugs are considered more potent than morphine, morphine is still considered to be one of the most effective of the opioids. All agonists are Class II controlled substances.

Clinical Uses

Opioid agonists are used to control moderate to severe pain in animals.

Dosage Forms

- Morphine sulfate (Infumorph, Astramorph PF, Morphine Sulfate for Injection)
- Oxymorphone (Opana and Numorphan)
- Hydromorphone (Dilaudid)
- Meperidine (Demerol)
- Codeine (codeine phosphate, codeine sulfate, Tylenol with codeine)
- Fentanyl, transdermal, tablets, and injectable

Adverse Side Effects

Side effects can include respiratory depression, sedation, excitement, and addiction. Cats are more sensitive to the excitatory effects of opioid agonists than are other species, and they tolerate low doses well.

Transdermal Fentanyl Use

Transdermal application of fentanyl has been successfully used in humans for control of chronic pain. This use has recently been adapted for control of postoperative and chronic pain in dogs and cats (extralabel).

Caution should be exercised when transdermal patches are used; the main concerns are to ensure that the animal does not eat or lick the patch (causing possible overdosage) and that accidental exposure to humans (especially children) does not occur. When the patch is applied, gloves should be worn; the skin over the dorsum of the neck should be clipped, cleansed, and allowed to dry well; good skin contact with the patch should be achieved; and a snug bandage should be applied to hold the patch in place.

The patch should never be cut because this interferes with the rate of release of fentanyl. The patch should be carefully disposed of after use.

Opioid Agonists–Antagonists

The opioid agonist–antagonist drugs bind with opioid kappa receptors but antagonize opioid mu receptors. Opioid agonists–antagonists include butorphanol (Class IV), pentazocine (Class IV), and nalbuphine. These drugs are considered effective for mild to moderate pain and have few side effects.

Clinical Uses

The primary use is for the relief of mild to moderate pain.

Dosage Forms

- Butorphanol (Torbugesic, Torbutrol, Stadol)
- Pentazocine (Talwin-V)
- Nalbuphine (Nubain)

Adverse Side Effects

Side effects include sedation, ataxia, and salivation (pentazocine).

Opioid Partial Agonists

The opioid partial agonists bind with the mu receptors but only partially activate them. Buprenorphine is the primary drug in this category. Recent studies have shown that buprenorphine may be effectively administered to cats by the sublingual/buccal route.

Clinical Uses

Uses include relief of mild to moderate pain in cats, dogs, horses and small mammals.

Dosage Form

- Buprenex; human label

Adverse Side Effects

Side effects include sedation and respiratory depression.

OTHER DRUGS USED AS PAIN CONTROL AGENTS

α-2 Adrenergic Agents

α-2 agonists are a group of sedative, analgesic drugs that exert their effects by interacting with α-2 adrenergic receptors in the CNS. Unlike primary analgesics like opioids and NSAIDs, α-2 agonists are considered adjuvant analgesics (Lamont, 2009). α-2 Agonists, unlike most primary analgesics, can have important cardiovascular side effects.

Clinical Uses

These agents may be used as a sedative–analgesic for short, noninvasive procedures, as a component of an injectable anesthetic protocol, as a preanesthetic sedative–analgesic agent, as a postoperative sedative–analgesic agent (bolus or constant rate infusion [CRI]), as a CRI during inhalation anesthesia, as an epidural or intrathecal agent, and others.

Dosage Forms

- Xylazine (Xylazine Injection, Rompun, AnaSed)
- Clonidine (Duraclon, human label)
- Dexmedetomidine (Dexdomitor)
- Medetomidine (Domitor)
- Romifidine (Sedivet)
- Detomidine (Dormosedan)

Adverse Side Effects

Side effects include bradycardia, transient hypertension, hypotension, muscle tremors, atrioventricular block, vomiting, and hypothermia.

Ketamine

Ketamine is classified as a dissociative anesthetic/N-methyl-D-aspartate (NMDA) receptor antagonist. NMDA receptors are involved in relaying pain information to the brain. NMDA receptor antagonism may help to prevent the "windup" phenomenon, allow use of lower doses of opioids, and prevent severe acute pain and chronic pain.

Clinical Uses

Microdoses of ketamine are used (primarily as a CRI) as a part of multimodal analgesic protocols.

Dosage Form

- Ketamine hydrochloride

Adverse Side Effects

At microdoses, there are few side effects, although tachycardia is possible.

Tramadol

Tramadol is a mu-receptor, opiate-like agonist (Plumb, 2011) that also inhibits the reuptake of norepinephrine and serotonin, causing it to act like an α-2 agonist (Gaynor, 2009).

Clinical Uses

Tramadol may be useful as an alternative analgesic agent or as an adjunct for postoperative or chronic pain in dogs and horses.

Adverse Side Effects

Side effects may include anxiety, tremor, vomiting, diarrhea, or sedation.

Miscellaneous Pain Control Agents

- *Lidocaine.* Lidocaine is used in all forms of local anesthesia including the transdermal patch, locally acting cream, and in injection and "splash" techniques. Lidocaine is also used as an intravenous antiarrhythmic and in combination with opioids, α-2 agents, and/or ketamine (e.g., morphine, lidocaine, ketamine [MLK], hydromorphone, lidocaine, ketamine [HLK], fentanyl, lidocaine, ketamine [FLK], and others) for analgesia or as an adjunct to inhalation anesthesia.
- *Amantadine.* Amantadine may be helpful with controlling "windup", neuropathic pain, and opioid tolerance.
- *Gabapentin.* Gabapentin is helpful in controlling pain related to neuropathic pain, osteoarthritis, and cancer.
- *Tricyclic antidepressants.* Agents like amitriptyline block the reuptake of serotonin and norepinephrine (possible α-2 effect) and may enhance opioid analgesia.
- *Benzodiazepines.* Diazepam has been used as an adjunctive analgesic in birds.

ANTIHISTAMINES

Antihistamines are drugs that are used to inhibit the effects or spreading of the inflammatory process. These drugs do not inhibit the formation of prostaglandins or other inflammatory mediators. They work by preventing histamine from combining with tissue receptors or by displacing histamine from receptor sites.

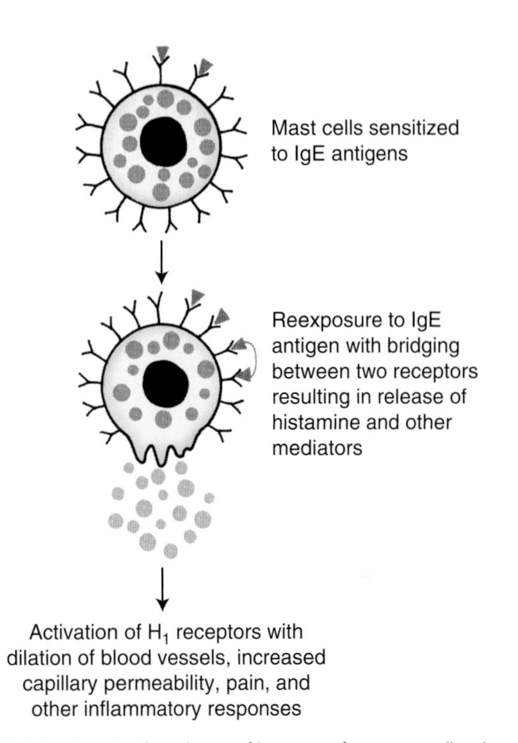

FIGURE 14-5 The release of histamine from mast cells when stimulated by immunoglobulin (Ig) E antibodies.

Because histamine is a major chemical mediator of the allergic response, antihistamines may be useful in controlling allergic responses.

Histamine is a chemical that is released from mast cells when they are adequately stimulated by immunoglobulin E (IgE) antibodies to allergens (Figure 14-5). Histamine then combines with tissue receptors and causes dilation of small blood vessels, increased permeability of capillaries, smooth muscle spasm, and increased secretion of glands. Two types of antihistamine receptors have been identified: H_1 and H_2.

Antihistamines competitively block the binding of histamine to H_1 receptors, which may block progression of the allergic response. Some antihistamines also block H_1 receptors that may contribute to motion sickness or nausea. Some antihistamines have a high affinity for H_1 receptors in the brain and cause a sedative effect.

Stimulation of H_2 receptors causes increased flow of hydrochloric acid by the gastric mucosa. H_2 blockers reduce the secretion of hydrochloric acid and may be used to treat gastrointestinal irritation and ulceration.

Clinical Uses

Antihistamines are used to treat the following:

- Pruritus
- Urticaria and angioedema associated with acute allergic reactions
- Laminitis in horses and cattle
- Downer cow syndrome
- Motion sickness
- Reverse sneeze syndrome
- Anaphylactic shock
- Upper respiratory tract conditions

Dosage Forms

These include injectables, oral preparations, and topical agents. Many brand names are available under veterinary and human labels. A partial list of the formulations follows.

H_1 Blockers

Dosage Forms

- Pyrilamine maleate (antihistamine injection)
- Pyrilamine maleate injection
- Pyrilamine maleate injection (Histavet-P)
- Tripelennamine hydrochloride (ReCovr Injection)
- Pyrilamine maleate, phenylephrine hydrochloride with a decongestant and an expectorant (cough syrup)
- Diphenhydramine HCl (Histacalm Shampoo, Spray)
- Diphenhydramine (Benadryl)
- Dimenhydrinate (Dramamine)
- Meclizine (Bonine)
- Promethazine (Phenergan)
- Cetirizine (Zyrtec)
- Loratadine (Claritin)
- Fexofenadine (Allegra)
- Chlorpheniramine maleate (Chlor-Trimeton)
- Clemastine (Tavist Allergy, Dayhist-1)
- Hydroxyzine (Atarax, Vistaril)
- Trimeprazine (Temaril-P)

H_2 Blockers

Dosage Forms

- Cimetidine (Tagamet)
- Ranitidine (Zantac)

Adverse Side Effects

Adverse side effects of the antihistamines include drowsiness, weakness, dry mucous membranes, urinary retention, and CNS stimulation on overdose.

> *TECHNICIAN NOTES* Antihistamines are not as effective in controlling pruritus in animals as they are in humans.

MUSCLE RELAXANTS

Skeletal muscle relaxants may be used as an aid in the treatment of acute inflammatory and traumatic conditions of muscle and the spasms that may result from these situations. They are thought to work by decreasing muscle hyperactivity without interfering with normal muscle tone. This action may be brought about by selective action on the internuncial neurons of the spinal cord.

Methocarbamol

Robaxin-V is labeled for use in dogs, cats, and horses.

Clinical Uses

This product is used to treat patients with the following:

- Intervertebral disk syndrome
- Strains and sprains
- Myositis and bursitis
- Muscle spasms
- Tying up in horses

Dosage Forms

- Robaxin-V tablets and Robaxin-V injectable

Other Muscle Relaxants

Dantrolene

Dosage Form

- Dantrium

Adverse Side Effects

These include excessive salivation, emesis, muscle weakness, and ataxia when overdosed. The package insert states that adverse side effects are seldom encountered.

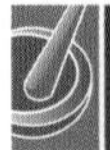

CORTICOSTEROIDS

Corticosteroid drugs are used in veterinary medicine to treat inflammatory, pruritic, and immune-mediated diseases. These drugs are also used to treat shock, laminitis, anorexia, adrenal insufficiency, and various other conditions. The technician should remember that corticosteroid therapy involves treatment of the signs of disease; it is seldom, if ever, curative.

Natural corticosteroids are hormones that are produced by the adrenal cortex, whereas corticosteroids used clinically are synthetic reproductions (analogues) of naturally occurring hormones. Corticosteroids are classified according to their activity as mineralocorticoids or glucocorticoids (Table 14-1) and according to their duration of action (Table 14-2) as short, intermediate, or long-acting. Mineralocorticoids such as aldosterone regulate electrolyte and water balance in the body. Glucocorticoids such as cortisone exert antiinflammatory and immunosuppressive effects and influence the metabolism of carbohydrate, fat, and protein. No corticosteroid has complete glucocorticoid or mineralocorticoid activity, but each has a predominant activity that determines its classification. Because mineralocorticoids are seldom used clinically, this discussion focuses on glucocorticoids.

Control of the release of naturally occurring corticosteroids (i.e., cortisol, corticosterone, and deoxycortisol) is complex and occurs through the hypothalamic–pituitary–adrenal axis (Figure 14-6). Control is exerted through this axis by two basic mechanisms. The first is a feedback mechanism that is related to the level of cortisol in the bloodstream. When the level of cortisol in the blood is lowered, the hypothalamus sends a chemical messenger called *corticotropin-releasing factor (CRF)* to the anterior pituitary gland. This causes the pituitary to release a

TABLE 14-1 Mineralocorticoid Versus Glucocorticoid Classification of Corticosteroids

DRUG	GLUCOCORTICOID POTENCY (ANTIINFLAMMATORY EFFECT)	MINERALOCORTICOID POTENCY
Hydrocortisone	1.0	1.00
Cortisone	0.8	0.80
Prednisone	4.0	0.25
Prednisolone	4.0	0.25
Methylprednisolone	5.0	0.00
Triamcinolone	5.0	0.00
Paramethasone	10.0	0.00
Flumethasone	15.0	0.00
Dexamethasone	30.0	0.00
Betamethasone	35.0	0.00

TABLE 14-2 Duration of Action of Corticosteroids

SHORT ACTING (<12 HOURS)	INTERMEDIATE ACTING (12-36 HOURS)	LONG ACTING (>48 HOURS)
Hydrocortisone	Prednisone	Betamethasone
Cortisone	Prednisolone	Dexamethasone
	Methylprednisolone	Flumethasone
	Triamcinolone	Paramethasone

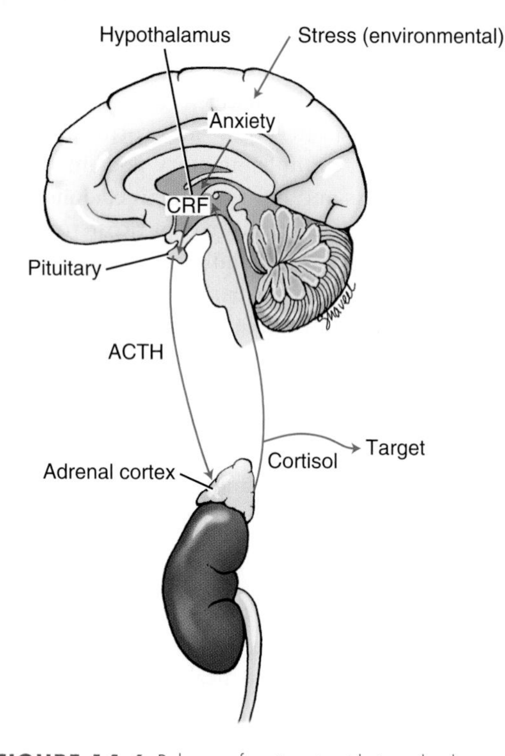

FIGURE 14-6 Release of corticosteroids is under the control of the hypothalamic–pituitary–adrenal axis. CRF, corticotropin-releasing factor; ACTH, adrenocorticotropic hormone.

substance called *adrenocorticotropic hormone (ACTH)* into the bloodstream. The blood then carries ACTH to the adrenal cortex, where it stimulates this structure to release cortisol to raise the amount in the blood to appropriate levels. On the other hand, a high level of blood cortisol inhibits release of CRF by the hypothalamus, and the blood level is thus prevented from reaching excessive levels. It should be noted that the hypothalamus cannot distinguish between naturally occurring cortisol and synthetic analogues administered by veterinarians.

The second mechanism for control of release of cortisol by the adrenal gland involves the stress response. External and internal stressors such as crowding, weaning, transporting, disease, surgery, trauma, pain, fear, anxiety, and many others can stimulate the hypothalamus—through impulses from higher brain centers—to release CRF. The control mechanism then proceeds in the fashion illustrated in Figure 14-6.

One of the major indications for the clinical use of corticosteroids is for their antiinflammatory effects. These effects are brought about by their ability to block the enzyme phospholipase, which promotes the reaction that results in the formation of prostaglandin—a primary mediator of the immune response. Corticosteroids also protect cells from inflammatory trauma by various mechanisms that include but are not limited to the following:

- Stabilizing cell membranes to help prevent their breakdown
- Stabilizing lysosomal membranes so they do not release their harmful enzymes
- Disrupting histamine synthesis
- Inhibiting interleukin synthesis
- Reducing exudative processes

Corticosteroids are also used clinically for their immunosuppressive effects. They are used to suppress the immune system in allergic conditions such as flea allergy dermatitis, atopy, autoimmune hemolytic anemia, rheumatoid arthritis, and uveitis. The immunosuppressive effect comes from the ability of corticosteroids to do the following:

- Inhibit antibody formation
- Decrease the concentrations of lymphocytes and eosinophils
- Suppress the migration of neutrophils
- Inhibit phagocytosis

Although immunosuppressive qualities are very useful clinically, they can also mask the signs of serious infection that are simultaneously present.

Corticosteroids are useful in the treatment of lymphoid tumors because they cause a direct lymphotoxic effect (Barton, 2012).

All steroid compounds are synthesized from a basic parent compound that has been described as resembling three rooms and a bath (Figure 14-7). Steroids are formed in three regions of the adrenal gland. Those regions and their respective products include the following:

- Zona glomerulosa—mineralocorticoids
- Zona fasciculata—glucocorticoids
- Zona reticularis—sex hormones (androgen and estrogen)

An increased number of double bonds in the parent compound, the addition of certain side chains, or the addition of fluorine atoms to the parent

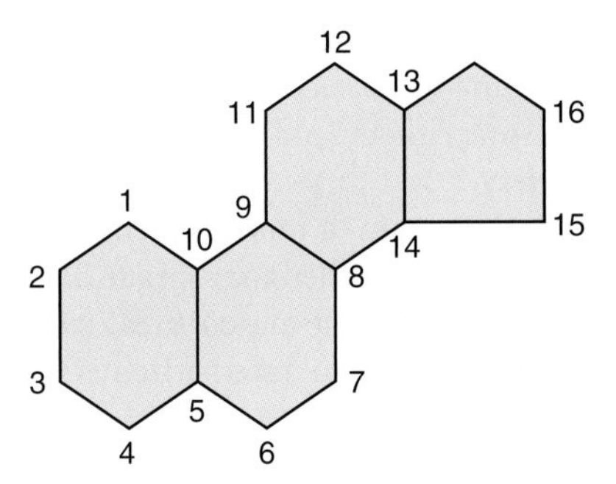

FIGURE 14-7 The configuration of the parent molecule of all steroid molecules, including corticosteroids.

molecule usually increases the antiinflammatory effects of corticosteroids.

Clinical Uses

Corticosteroids are used in treatment of the following conditions:

- Allergic reactions/conditions
- Inflammatory conditions of the musculoskeletal system
- Shock/toxemia
- Laminitis
- Inflammatory ocular conditions such as conjunctivitis and uveitis
- Addison's disease
- Autoimmune disease such as autoimmune hemolytic anemia, lupus, and rheumatoid arthritis
- Lymphocytic neoplasms

Dosage Forms

Corticosteroids are available in injectable, oral, and topical forms and in preparations that contain antibiotic, antifungal, and corticosteroid products. These products may be applied to the skin or mucous membranes, injected into lesions, given orally, or administered parenterally. When emergency conditions call for administration of corticosteroids, the intravenous route is normally used with a water-soluble product in a water-soluble vehicle. Water-soluble products can be injected via the intramuscular or subcutaneous route when life-threatening conditions do not exist. Long-acting depot (repositol) products are prepared in a poorly soluble vehicle to prolong their effects. The justification for these long-acting products has been questioned by some clinicians.

A list of some of the many available corticosteroid products follows here.

Injectables

- Azium solution (dexamethasone)
- Betasone (betamethasone)
- Cortisate-20 (prednisolone sodium phosphate)
- Depo-Medrol (methylprednisolone)
- Dexamethasone Injection
- Dexamethasone Sodium Phosphate
- Flucort Solution (flumethasone)
- Percorten-V (desoxycorticosterone)
- Predef 2x (isoflupredone)
- Solu-Delta-Cortef (prednisolone sodium succinate)
- Vetalog Parenteral (triamcinolone)

Oral

- Azium Powder (dexamethasone)
- Medrol (methylprednisolone)
- Methylprednisolone Tablets
- Temaril-P Tablets (prednisolone)
- Triamcinolone Tablets
- Vetalog Oral Powder/Tablets
- Prednisone generic tablets
- Prednisolone generic tablets

Topical

- Corticalm lotion
- Gentocin Topical Spray
- Cortispray
- Relief HC spray
- Synalar Otic Solution
- Kenalog spray

Adverse Side Effects

Adverse side effects of corticosteroids are numerous and include the following:

- Polyuria and polydipsia
- Thinning of the skin and muscle wasting that result from the ability of corticosteroids to convert protein into glucose (seen with long-term administration)
- Depressed healing
- Polyphagia and resultant weight gain

- **Iatrogenic** (caused by the veterinarian) hyperadrenocorticism, iatrogenic **Cushing's disease**
- Hypoadrenocorticism (iatrogenic) resulting from suppression of the hypothalamic–pituitary–adrenal axis by long-term administration of exogenous corticosteroids followed by sudden cessation of treatment (**Addison's disease**)
- Gastric ulcers with or without bleeding
- Osteoporosis (long-term)
- Abnormal behavior

Because administration of corticosteroids is fraught with many potential side effects, clinicians must give careful consideration to their use. Much information has been written about the appropriate use of corticosteroids in veterinary medicine, and a selection of the principles of use follows:

- Alternate-day dosing may help prevent iatrogenic hypoadrenocorticism.
- Administration should never be stopped abruptly but should be tapered off gradually.
- Very large doses may be used in emergency situations.
- Corticosteroids generally are not used for the treatment of corneal ulcers.
- When corticosteroids are injected into joint spaces, extreme care should be given to aseptic technique.

LOCAL, REGIONAL, AND TOPICAL ANESTHETIC AGENTS

Many clinical situations call for the use of local or topical anesthesia to prevent or relieve pain. These agents are discussed here in this chapter on pain relief rather than in the traditional context of anesthesia.

In some situations, general anesthesia is not available or is too dangerous for a client. In others, repair of a small laceration may not justify the use of general anesthesia. In equine medicine, lameness may be diagnosed by administering a **nerve block** to an area and then observing abatement of the lameness. In bovine medicine, it may be useful to administer a regional nerve block to prevent straining while replacing a prolapsed uterus. In cats, it may be useful to apply a local anesthetic to the larynx to facilitate placement of an endotracheal tube.

Local anesthetics work by preventing the generation and conduction of nerve impulses in peripheral nerves. These anesthetics are administered by the following routes:

- Topically to the skin or mucous membranes of the ear, eye, larynx, or other appropriate area
- By infiltration in a localized area, such as the margin of a wound, to anesthetize nerve endings (Figure 14-8).
- By dripping or "splashing" into a surgical site
- By injection into joint spaces
- For intravenous regional nerve block; may be used for foot surgery in cattle by applying a tourniquet to the proximal area of a limb and then infusing a local anesthetic into the limb
- Around nerve bodies
  - Epidural anesthesia—injection of a local anesthetic into the epidural space (Figure 14-8) of the spinal canal to provide anesthesia to the area around the anus and perineum for obstetric manipulations and to stop straining for the replacement of a prolapsed uterus
  - Nerve block—local anesthetic deposited around a specific nerve (Figure 14-9) to facilitate minor procedures (e.g., lameness diagnosis, dental procedures, declawing, dehorning, lid or lip suturing)
  - Paravertebral block—placement of a local anesthetic around a spinal nerve near where it leaves the intervertebral space; this procedure blocks a larger area and may be used for procedures such as cesarean section and rumenotomy

The onset and duration of action of the agents vary. Lidocaine has a rapid onset of action (5 to 10 minutes) and a somewhat short duration (1 to 2 hours). Lidocaine may cause a stinging sensation when injected. The onset of bupivacaine effect takes 20 minutes, but it lasts 4 to 6 hours. The effects of local anesthetics can be prolonged by adding epinephrine, which causes vasoconstriction, thereby prolonging absorption time by reducing blood supply in the area. Using ethyl alcohol as a local anesthetic agent may considerably prolong the duration of anesthesia. Some clinicians prefer to use xylazine or a narcotic agent for administering epidural anesthesia.

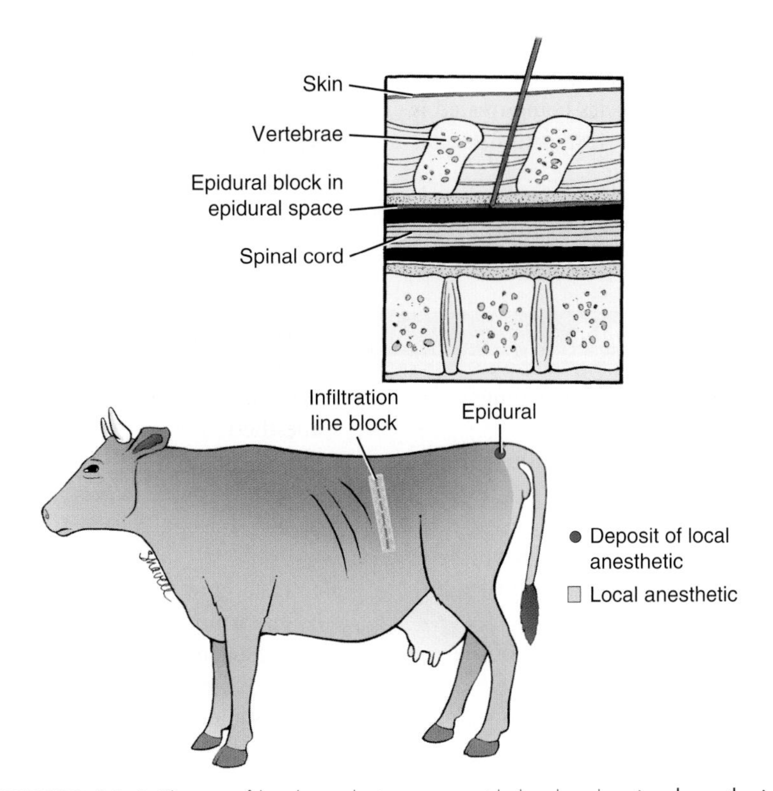

FIGURE 14-8 The use of local anesthetics can provide local and **regional anesthesia**.

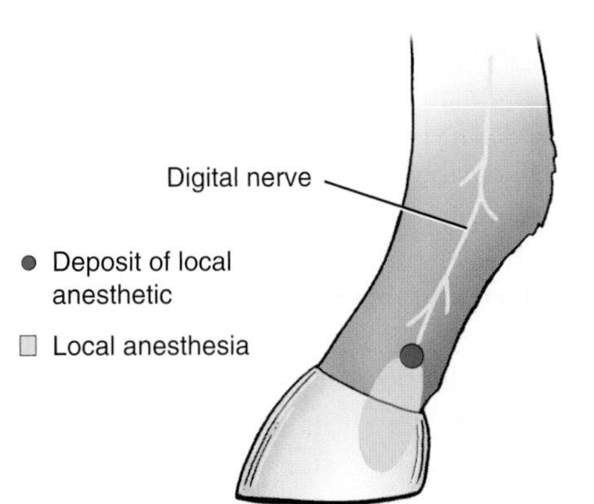

FIGURE 14-9 Local anesthesia for diagnosis of lameness in horses.

Clinical Uses

Local anesthetics are used for the following purposes:

- Infiltration of local areas
- Epidural anesthesia
- Topical application in the eye, ear, and larynx, among others
- Nerve block
- Antiarrhythmic effects

Dosage Forms

Local anesthetic agents are available in injectable and topical forms. A partial list of these agents follows here.

Injectable

- LidoJect (lidocaine)
- Marcaine (bupivacaine)
- Epidural Injection (procaine HCl)
- Lidocaine hydrochloride injection
- Carbocaine-V (mepivacaine)
- Other generic local anesthetics, including tetracaine and dibucaine

Topical

- Ophthaine (proparacaine)
- Ophthetic (proparacaine)

Adverse Side Effects

Local anesthetics can have adverse side effects if the total maximum dose for the species being treated is exceeded. Side effects may include restlessness, excitement, hypotension, and seizures.

TECHNICIAN NOTES

- Lidocaine with epinephrine should never be used if an antiarrhythmic is indicated.
- Exceeding the total recommended dose of local analgesics may cause toxicity.

REVIEW QUESTIONS

1. Pain sensation arises in free nerve endings called ________________.
2. List some signs associated with pain in animals.
   ____
3. NSAIDs that preferentially inhibit ________________ are thought to produce fewer gastrointestinal side effects.
4. What is the most common side effect of the NSAIDs? ________________
5. Why are cats so susceptible to aspirin overdose?
   ____
6. Phenylbutazone should be administered parenterally by the subcutaneous route only.
   a. True
   b. False
7. What Class II opioid is administered via transdermal patch? ________________
8. Corticosteroid therapy involves treatment of the signs of disease and often cures the disease as well.
   a. True
   b. False
9. What function do mineralocorticoids serve in the body? ________________
10. List some principles that should be followed concerning corticosteroid therapy.
    ____
11. What does the term *iatrogenic* mean?
    ____
12. Describe the side effects of short-term and long-term corticosteroid use.
    ____
13. What is the mechanism of action of local anesthetic agents?
    ____
14. What are some indications for the use of local anesthetics?
    ____
15. The body is able to produce its own opiate-like analgesic agents called ________________.
    a. histamine
    b. endorphins
    c. prostaglandins
    d. cytokines
16. A substance that can initiate a fever is called a(n) ________________.
    a. prostaglandin
    b. endorphin
    c. pyrogen
    d. pyometra
17. ________________ is also known as acetylsalicylic acid.
    a. Phenylbutazone
    b. Aspirin
    c. DMSO
    d. Acetaminophen
18. ________________ is a pyrazolone derivative.
    a. Phenylbutazone
    b. Carprofen
    c. Etodolac
    d. Deramaxx
19. Flunixin meglumine is a(an) ________________.
    a. propionic acid derivative
    b. antihistamine
    c. muscle relaxant
    d. NSAID
20. DMSO causes ________________ when applied topically.
    a. vasoconstriction
    b. vasodilation

21. ________________ is considered (even today) to be one of the most effective of the opioids.
   a. Fentanyl
   b. Morphine
   c. Tepoxalin
   d. Carprofen
22. ___________ is(are) a major chemical mediator(s) of the allergic response.
   a. Histamine
   b. Prostaglandins
   c. Pyrogens
   d. Hormones
23. All of the following are types of corticosteroids except ____________.
   a. dexamethasone
   b. Predef
   c. Vetalog
   d. ketoprofen
24. A local anesthetic such as lidocaine may be the drug of choice when an epidural is performed to replace a prolapsed uterus in a bovine.
   a. True
   b. False
25. List the four steps involved in the production of pain sensation ______________________________.
26. Define *windup* as it applies to pain production ______________________________.
27. Pain resulting from tissue injury is called ______________________pain.
28. Pain arising from abdominal or thoracic organs is called ________________pain.
29. List a class of drugs that would alter pain recognition and perception.________________
30. Pain control that utilizes a combination of drugs acting at different sites in the pain production pathways is called ______________________therapy.
31. An 80-lb dog will be treated with carprofen for osteoarthritis at 4.4 mg/kg once a day. Rimadyl chewable tablets (100 mg) will be used. How many tablets will you give with each dose? ________________
32. A 13-lb cat will be treated for acute musculoskeletal pain with robenacoxib at 1 mg/kg once a day for 5 days. Onsior tablets (6 mg/tablet) will be used. How many tablets will you dispense? ________________
33. An 8-lb cat will be treated for postsurgical pain with buprenorphine at a dosage of 0.02 mg/kg. Buprenex injectable (0.3 mg/mL) will be given by buccal administration. How much Buprenex will you draw up?
   ____
34. A 1200-lb horse will be treated for acute abdominal pain with flunixin meglumine at 1.1 mg/kg IV. Banamine injection (50 mg/mL) will be used. How much will you draw up?
   ____
35. Prepare a Morphine CRI for a 30-lb dog scheduled for an amputation. The morphine (15 mg/mL) will be given at a dosage of 2 mcg/kg/min. It will be added to a 500 mL bag of saline and the mixture infused at a rate of 30 mL/h. What volume of morphine will you draw up to add to the saline? Use the CRI formula from Chapter 3:

$$M = \frac{\{D \times W \times V\}}{\{R \times 16.67\}}$$

REFERENCES

Barton CL: Chemotherapy. In Boothe DM, editor: Small animal clinical pharmacology and therapeutics, Philadelphia, 2012, WB Saunders.

Boothe DM: Control of pain in small animals. In Boothe DM, editor: Small animal clinical pharmacology and therapeutics, Philadelphia, 2012, WB Saunders.

Budsberg SC: Nonsteroidal antiinflammatory drugs. In Gaynor JS, Muir WW, editors: Handbook of veterinary pain management, ed 2, St Louis, 2009, Elsevier.

Claude A: Acute pain management. In: The small animal practice: pharmaceutical options, in Proceedings, Tenn Vet Med Assoc, Murfreesboro, Tenn, 2013.

Ganong WF: Cutaneous, deep, and visceral sensation. In Ganong WF, editor: Review of medical physiology, ed 21, New York, 2003, McGraw-Hill.

Gaynor JS: Definitions of terms describing pain. In: Gaynor JS, Muir WW, editors: Handbook of veterinary pain management, ed 2, St. Louis, 2009, Elsevier.

Lamont LA: α-2 Agonists. In Gaynor JS, Muir WW, editors: Handbook of veterinary pain management, ed 2, St Louis, 2009, Elsevier.
Langston VC, Mercer HD: Non-steroidal anti-inflammatory drugs, in Proceedings. 17th Semin Vet Tech, West Vet Conf, Las Vegas, 1988.
Muir WW: Physiology and pathophysiology of pain. In Gaynor JS, Muir WW, editors: Handbook of veterinary pain management, ed 2, St. Louis, 2009, Elsevier.
Paddleford RR: Analgesia and pain management. In Manual of small animal anesthesia, Philadelphia, 1999, WB Saunders.
Plumb DC: Veterinary drug handbook, ed 7, Ames, Iowa, 2011, Wiley-Blackwell.
Wagner AE: Opioids. In Gaynor JS, Muir WW, editors: Handbook of veterinary pain management, ed 2, St. Louis, 2009, Elsevier.

CHAPTER 15

Therapeutic Nutritional, Fluid, and Electrolyte Replacements

OUTLINE

KEY TERMS

Buffer
Colloid
Dissociation
Electrolyte
Empirical
Hyperkalemia
Hypernatremia
Hypokalemia
Hyponatremia
Hypovolemia
Metabolic acidosis
Metabolic alkalosis
Oncotic pressure
Osmotic pressure
Solute
Total nutrient admixture
Transcellular fluid
Turgor

LEARNING OBJECTIVES

After studying this chapter, you should be able to

1. Define terms related to fluid, electrolyte, and selected therapeutic nutritional preparations.
2. Describe the distribution of water in the body.
3. Describe the composition of body and therapeutic fluids.
4. Define osmotic pressure and tonicity as they apply to fluids.
5. Discuss the basic principles of fluid therapy.
6. Describe fluid equipment and its use.
7. Categorize and provide examples of the fluids used in fluid therapy.
8. List and describe selected fluid additives.
9. List and describe selected oral electrolyte preparations.
10. List and describe selected parenteral vitamin–mineral products.

INTRODUCTION

Veterinary technicians often have an important role in fluid, electrolyte, and therapeutic nutritional therapy for patients. They administer parenteral or oral fluid or nutritional products and monitor patients' responses under the direction of a veterinarian. Because the use of these products can be critically important to the outcome of a case, technicians should have a thorough knowledge of the products and their use.

ANATOMY, PHYSIOLOGY, AND CHEMISTRY

Distribution of Body Water and Electrolytes

Measurements of total body water (TBW) have shown that water represents 50% to 70% of the total body weight in adult animals; 60% is often used as the average figure. As much as 80% of a neonatal animal's body weight may be water, which is a factor that makes fluid loss in young animals potentially very serious. An increase in body fat decreases the amount of TBW and makes it important to estimate fluid needs on the basis of lean body mass to avoid overhydration.

TBW is distributed in several compartments within the body (Figure 15-1). Sixty percent of TBW is found within cells and is called *intracellular fluid (ICF)*. ICF makes up 40% of total body weight. The other 40% of TBW is found outside the cells and is called *extracellular fluid (ECF)*. ECF accounts for 20% of total body weight.

ECF (discounting the relatively small **transcellular fluid** component) distributes itself between the interstitial fluid (15% of body weight) and the intravascular fluid or plasma (5% of body weight). The intravascular fluid volume is estimated at 90 mL/kg for dogs and 45 mL/kg for cats.

Body fluid compartments should be thought of as volumes of fluid and electrolytes in dynamic equilibrium, with fluids and electrolytes moving back and forth across semipermeable cell membranes. Changes in the quantity of fluid or electrolytes in one compartment usually result in changes in these quantities in other compartments. Fluids administered intravenously to an animal first enter the intravascular space of the ECF, move into the interstitial space, and then enter the ICF (Figure 15-2). In most cases, loss of fluid occurs first from the ECF and then from other compartments.

Composition of Body and Therapeutic Fluids

Body water contains an array of **solutes** that vary in quantity from compartment to compartment. A solute is a substance that dissolves in a solvent; this

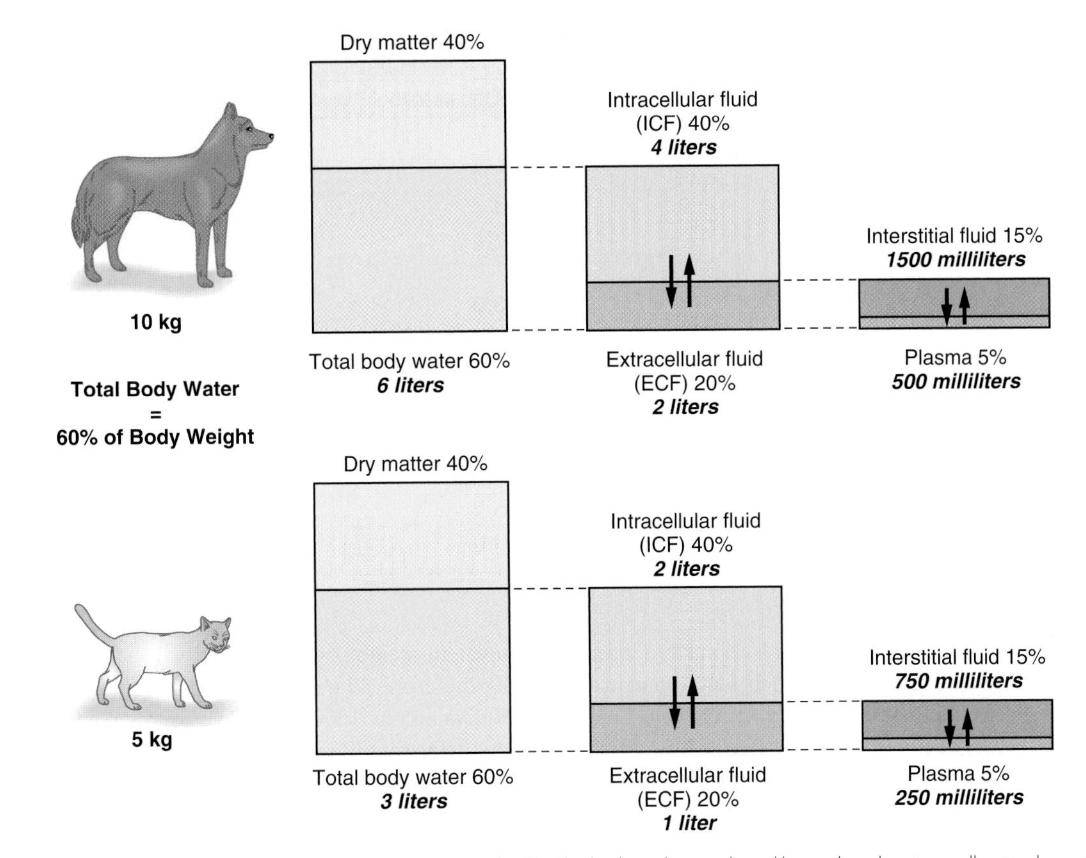

FIGURE 15-1 Body fluid compartments. (From DiBartola SP: Fluid, electrolyte and acid-base disorders in small animal practice, ed 3, St Louis, 2008, Saunders.)

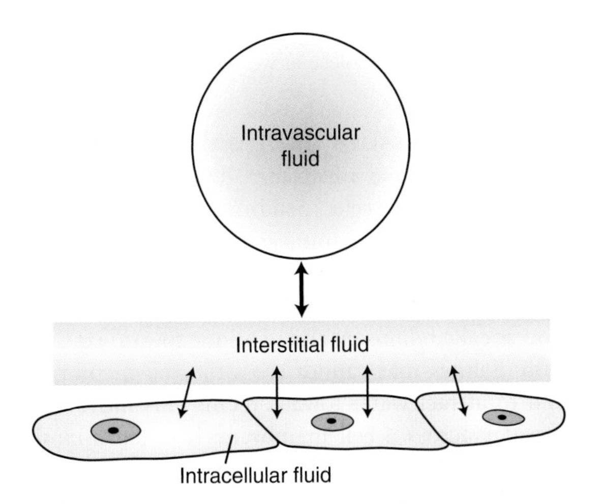

FIGURE 15-2 Schematic showing movement of fluid between compartments.

solvent is usually water in biologic systems. The molecules of substances called **electrolytes** break down (dissociate) into charged particles called *ions.* Electrolytes are positively charged (cations) or negatively charged (anions). The number of cations always equals the number of anions in healthy animals (Table 15-1). In the ECF, the most abundant cation is sodium, and the most abundant anions are chloride and bicarbonate. In the ICF, the major cations are potassium and magnesium, and the major anions are phosphates and proteins. Therapeutic fluids are described as balanced if they resemble ECF in composition and unbalanced if they do not. Lactated Ringer's solution (LRS) is an example of a balanced solution, and saline is an example of an unbalanced solution. Table 15-2 lists the composition of some of the solutions used in fluid therapy.

TABLE 15-1 Composition of Plasma, Interstitial Fluid, and Intracellular Fluid

ION	PLASMA (MEQ/L)	INTERSTITIAL FLUID (MEQ/L)	INTRACELLULAR FLUID (MEQ/L)
Cations			
Na^+	142	145.1	12.0
K^+	4.3	4.4	140
Ca^{2+}	2.5	2.4	4.0
Mg^{2+}	1.1	1.1	34
Total	**149.9**	**153.0**	**190**
Anions			
Cl^-	104	117.4	4
HCO_3^-	24	27.1	12
H_2PO_4	2	2.3	40
Protein	14	none	50
Other	5.9	6.2	84
Total	**149.9**	**153.0**	**190**

It is important for technicians to have a basic understanding of the way in which solute particles such as electrolytes are quantified in fluids. One of the oldest ways of measuring solute concentration is by describing the weight of the solute per 100 mL of solution (g%). A 0.9% sodium chloride (NaCl) solution (saline) would contain 0.9 g/100 mL or 900 mg/100 mL. Other clinically significant ways of describing the quantity of solute particles include the use of concepts of (1) the milliequivalent, (2) osmolality, (3) osmolarity, and (4) tonicity.

The milliequivalent is the unit of measurement that is used to express the concentration of electrolytes, such as sodium, potassium, and calcium, in solutions. The concentration of these substances is usually expressed as milliequivalents per liter (mEq/L) in fluids and milliequivalents per milliliter in supplements. The milliequivalent describes the tendency of a particle to combine with another particle and is defined as 1:1000 of an equivalent. An *equivalent weight* is defined as the weight in grams of an element that will combine with 1 g of hydrogen ion. For all practical purposes, the equivalent weight of a compound is equal to the gram molecular weight of the substance divided by the total positive valence of the material in question (Blankenship et al., 1976). For example, the equivalent weight of NaCl is 58.5/1 = 58.5, and 1 L of fluid containing 58.5 g of NaCl contains 1 equivalent weight or 1000 mEq of NaCl. The equivalent weight of sulfuric acid (H_2SO_4) is 98.1/2 = 49; therefore, 49 g of H_2SO_4 in 1 L of fluid contains 1 equivalent or 1000 mEq. The following formulas allow determination of milliequivalents of solute in a solution when the concentration in grams or milligrams is known:

$$\text{mEq/L} = \frac{\text{milligrams per liter}}{\text{molecular weight}} \times \text{valence}$$

or

$$\text{mEq/L} = \frac{\text{milligrams per deciliter} \times 10}{\text{molecular weight}} \times \text{valence}$$

Osmotic Pressure and Tonicity of Fluids

Body fluid compartments usually are separated by a semipermeable (cell) membrane that permits the passage of water and some solutes. Solutes that can cross the membrane tend to move from an area of higher to an area of lower concentration by the process called *diffusion* and continue toward equilibrium. Solutes that cannot cross the cell membrane tend to attract water toward them. This movement of water across a cell membrane is called *osmosis,* and the ability of particles to attract water is called **osmotic pressure.**

Osmolality is a determination of the osmotic pressure of a solution on the basis of the relative number of solute particles in 1 kg of the solution.

TABLE 15-2 Composition of Solutions Used in Fluid Therapy

	GLUCOSE* (G/L)	NA^{+} (MEQ/L)	CL^{-} (MEQ/L)	K^{+} (MEQ/L)	CA^{2+} (MEQ/L)	MG^{2+} (MEQ/L)	BUFFER† (MEQ/L)	OSMOLARITY (MOSM/L)	KCAL/L	PH
Dextrose Electrolyte Solution Composition										
5% Dextrose	50	0	0	0	0	0	0	252	170	4.0
10% Dextrose	100	0	0	0	0	0	0	505	340	4.0
2.5% Dextrose in 0.45% NaCl	25	77	77	0	0	0	0	280	85	4.5
5% Dextrose in 0.45% NaCl	50	77	77	0	0	0	0	406	170	4.0
5% Dextrose in 0.9% NaCl	50	154	154	0	0	0	0	560	170	4.0
0.45% NaCl	0	77	77	0	0	0	0	154	0	5.0
0.85% NaCl (normal saline)	0	145	145	0	0	0	0	290	0	5.0
0.9% NaCl	0	154	154	0	0	0	0	308	0	5.0
3% NaCl	0	513	513	0	0	0	0	1026	0	5.0
Ringer's solution	0	147.5	156	4	4.5	0	0	3.10	0	5.5
Lactated Ringer's solution	0	130	109	4	3	0	23(L)	272	9	6.5
2.5% Dextrose in lactated Ringer's solution	25	130	109	4	3	0	28(L)	398	94	5.0
5% Dextrose in lactated Ringer's solution	50	130	109	4	3	0	28(L)	524	179	5.0
2.5% Dextrose in half-strength lactated Ringer's solution	25	65.5	55	2	1.5	0	14(L)	263	89	5.0
Normosol-M in 5% dextrose‡	50	40	40	13	0	3	16(A)	364	175	5.5
Normosol-R‡	0	140	98	5	0	3	27(A) 23(G)	296	18	6.4
Plasma-Lyte§	0	140	103	10	5	3	47(A) 8(L)	312	17	5.5
Plasma-Lyte M in 5% dextrose‡	50	40	40	16	5	3	12(A) 12(L)	376	178	5.5
Plasma	1	145	105	5	5	3	24(B)	300	—	7.4
Additives and Solutions										
20% Mannitol	200(M)	0	0	0	0	0	0	1099	—	
7.5% $NaHCO_3$	0	893(B)	0	0	0	0	893(B)	1786	0	
8.4% $NaHCO_3$	0	1000(B)	0	0	0	0	1000(B)	2000	0	
10% $CaCl_2$	0	0	2720	0	1360	0	0	4080	0	
14.9% KCl	0	0	2000	2000	0	0	0	4000	0	
50% Dextrose	500	0	0	0	0	0	0	2780	1700	4.2

*All glucose, with one exception: *M*, mannitol.
†Buffers used: *A*, acetate; *B*, bicarbonate; *G*, gluconate; *L*, lactate.
‡CEVA Laboratories.
§Baxter Healthcare.
From Chew DJ, DiBartola SP: Saunders manual of small animal nephrology and urology, Philadelphia, 1986, WB Saunders Co.

The greater the number of particles, the greater the pressure generated. The unit of measurement of osmolality is the osmol (osm), and 1 osm of any substance is equal to 1 g molecular weight divided by the number of particles formed by the **dissociation** of that substance. A substance that dissociates into two particles in solutions creates twice as much osmotic pressure as one that does not dissociate. Because the quantities being measured are very small in biologic systems, the milliosmole (mOsm) is used when fluids are described. One kilogram of a solution containing 29.25 g (58.5/2 particles) of NaCl would generate 1 osm/kg, or 1000 mOsm/kg of osmotic pressure.

Osmolarity refers to the number of particles per liter of solvent rather than per kilogram of solvent, as with osmolality. Very little difference is observed, however, between osmolality and osmolarity of animal fluids, and the terms frequently are used interchangeably. A 1-L solution that contains a full gram molecular weight (58.5 g) of NaCl would generate 2 osm, or 2000 mOsm/L, of osmotic pressure.

Not all solutes contribute to osmotic activity (exert a "pull" on water molecules). Those particles that are capable of generating pressure are called *effective osmoles,* and those that are not are called *ineffective osmoles.* Sodium and glucose provide most of the effective osmoles in commercial fluid preparations. The total effective osmolarity/osmolality of a solution is called *tonicity.* The osmolality of dog and cat serum is approximately 300 mOsm/L. Commercial fluids with an osmolality of 300 mOsm/L are isotonic (e.g., Ringer's solution). Those with an osmolality greater than 300 mOsm/L are hypertonic (e.g., 10% dextrose), and those with an osmolality less than 300 mOsm/L are hypotonic (e.g., 0.45% saline).

An illustration of the importance of the osmolality of fluids is as follows: if a higher concentration of sodium exists than in the interstitial space, then water would be drawn from the intracellular space into the interstitial space. Once in the interstitial space, fluid would move between the intravascular space and the interstitial space to maintain balance between these two compartments. Flow into and out of the intravascular space occurs at the capillary level, whose membranes are permeable to small particles like sodium and glucose but are generally impermeable to large molecules like colloids and plasma proteins. A large amount of solute within the intravascular space will create high osmotic/**oncotic pressure** and cause water to be retained within or drawn into the vasculature. Another factor influencing the movement of fluids between compartments is the fluid hydrostatic pressure within the compartment. When the hydrostatic pressure of the fluid exceeds the osmotic/oncotic pressure (pull) of the solute, fluid leaves the compartment. Figure 15-3 illustrates the potential movement of water into and out of the vasculature based on the osmolality of the vascular fluid.

Because most therapeutic fluids are composed of solute concentrations similar to that found in body fluids, osmotic destruction of red blood cells by the fluids is avoided.

PRINCIPLES OF FLUID THERAPY

Fluid therapy is a critical but somewhat inexact component of veterinary medical care. It is critical because it is often lifesaving, but it is inexact because its application revolves around estimating the amount of fluid loss and, consequently, the amount of fluid that must be replaced. Fortunately, if the heart and kidneys and the processes that sense and control fluid balance are functioning normally, many errors of estimation are compensated for automatically.

Indications for Fluid Therapy

A basic factor in the decision to administer fluids is the animal's hydration status. Hydration status is determined by evaluation of the patient's history, physical examination status, and the results of basic laboratory tests. If it is determined that the animal has lost more water than it has taken in, it is said to be in a state of *dehydration,* and fluids must be administered to compensate. In addition, fluids often are administered to maintain normal hydration status in animals that are losing excessive fluid quantities, for the purpose of replacing electrolytes and nutrients in animals that are not eating properly, correcting **hypovolemia,** correcting acid–base and electrolyte imbalances, and maintaining an open intravenous line for administering medications.

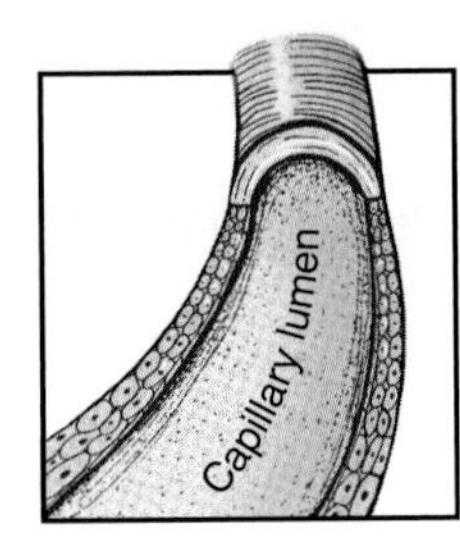

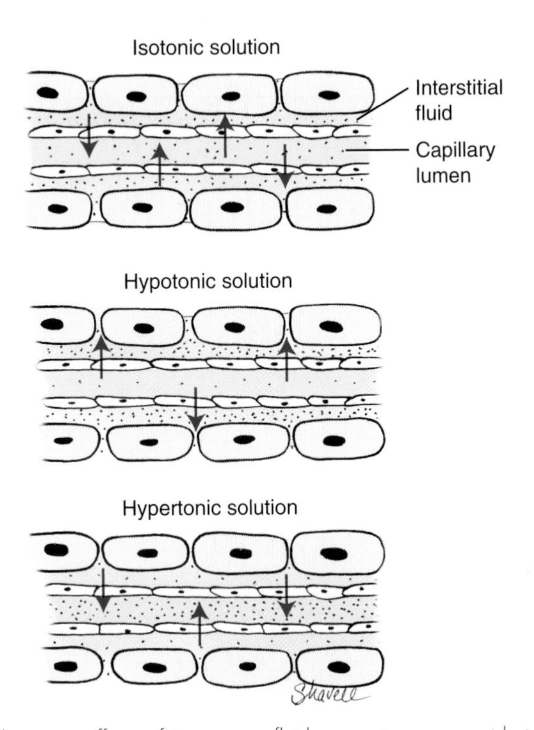

FIGURE 15-3 Schematic showing the potential osmotic effects of intravenous fluids on water movement between the interstitial space and the capillary lumen (intravascular space).

Fluid Balance

In healthy animals, the intake of fluid and electrolytes is adjusted to offset losses that occur. Sources of water intake include (1) water that is drunk, (2) water that is ingested in food, and (3) water that results from the metabolism of food (metabolic water). Normal routes of water loss include (1) urine, (2) fecal water, (3) sweat (horses), and (4) respiration. Respiratory loss potentially can be important in dogs because of panting, and sweating can be important in horses. Fluid losses are frequently characterized as sensible—those that can be measured easily (e.g., urine), and insensible—those that cannot be measured easily (e.g., fecal and respiratory losses).

> *TECHNICIAN NOTES* Insensible losses can be estimated at one third of maintenance requirements.

Decreased fluid intake often accompanies anorexia, and increased fluid loss occurs in disease states that cause polyuria, vomiting, and diarrhea. Third-space shifts or sequestrations of body water occasionally may cause quantities to be taken from circulation as they are trapped in body cavities or lost through skin lesions (e.g., intestinal obstruction, body cavity effusions, or hemorrhages). Extensive burns, which are uncommon in veterinary medicine, also can cause extensive fluid loss.

History, Physical Examination, and Laboratory Findings

A patient's history provides important information about the route and extent of water intake and loss. Knowing the route of loss can aid a clinician in determining the type of fluid to use to correct dehydration and electrolyte imbalances. For example, acute vomiting leads to loss of potassium and chloride ions, whereas acute diarrhea causes primarily a potassium

TABLE 15-3 Fluid and Electrolyte Disorders and Fluids Used in Their Correction

	SERUM					
CONDITION	**NA⁺**	**CL⁻**	**K⁺**	**HCO_3**	**VOLUME**	**FLUID OF CHOICE**
Diarrhea	D	D	D	D	D	Lactated Ringer's + KCl, Normosol-R
Pyloric obstruction	D	D	D	I	D	0.9% NaCl
Dehydration	I	I	N	N/D	D	Lactated Ringer's, 0.9% NaCl, 5% dextrose, Normosol-R
Congestive heart failure	N/D	N/D	N	N	I	0.45% NaCl + 2.5% dextrose, 5% dextrose
End-stage liver disease	N/I	N/I	D	D	I	0.45% NaCl + 2.5% dextrose + KCl
Acute renal failure						
Oliguria	I	I	I	D	I	0.9% NaCl
Polyuria	D	D	N/D	D	D	Lactated Ringer's + KCl, Normosol-R
Chronic renal failure	N/D	N/D	N	D	N/D	Lactated Ringer's solution, 0.9% NaCl
Adrenocortical insufficiency	D	D	I	N/D	D	0.9% NaCl
Diabetic ketoacidosis	D	D	N/D	D	D	0.9% NaCl (±KCl)

D, Decreased; *I*, increased; *N*, normal.
From Battaglia AM: Small animal emergency and critical care for veterinary technicians, St Louis, 2007, Elsevier.

loss. Table 15-3 illustrates the selection of crystalloid fluids to treat some common disease conditions.

The physical examination provides important information about the extent of fluid loss. The skin **turgor** test, along with other physical findings (see Table 15-4), is used to determine the percentage of body weight that has been lost via fluid (percent dehydration). The skin turgor test is performed by pinching up a fold of skin over the thoracic or lumbar area and then determining how long it takes to return to a normal position. If the neck area is used in small animals, the extra skin may cause misleading results. The point of the shoulder should be used in horses because the skin of the neck area can again be misleading. The longer the skin takes to return to normal, the greater the degree of dehydration. Animals with little body fat may appear to be more dehydrated than they really are (slow return to normal skin position) because of low body fat levels, whereas obese animals may appear to be well-hydrated when they are not because increased fat increases skin elasticity. Dehydrated animals may exhibit dry mucous membranes as well as increased skin tenting.

It is important to differentiate between dehydration and hypovolemia when assessing physical findings. *Hypovolemia* refers to what is occurring in the vascular system, whereas *dehydration* refers to changes in the intracellular and interstitial system. Because proper organ perfusion and function depend on adequate perfusion by the vascular system, correction of hypovolemia is often more urgent than treating mild to moderate dehydration. Signs used to detect hypovolemia are based on perfusion and include pale mucous membrane color, increased capillary refill time, hypotension, tachycardia, weak peripheral pulses, cool peripheral extremities, and hypothermia.

Because most of the evaluations mentioned earlier are subjective, simple laboratory tests may be

TABLE 15-4 Clinical Signs of Dehydration

	DRY ORAL MUCOUS MEMBRANES	INCREASED SKIN TENTING	TACHYCARDIA	DECREASED PULSE PRESSURE	SUNKEN EYES	ALTERATION OF CONSCIOUSNESS
5%	√	√				
7%	√	√	√			
10%	√	√	√	√		
12%	√	√	√	√	√	√

performed to aid in assessing hydration status. These tests include packed cell volume (PCV), total plasma protein (TPP), and urine specific gravity determination. Dehydration generally results in an increase in PCV, TPP, and urine specific gravity. Because anemia can make a dehydrated patient appear to be normally hydrated, PCV always should be evaluated with TPP. Plasma lactate levels may be elevated in cases with poor tissue perfusion. Technicians should consult more advanced references for interpretation of laboratory findings related to hydration status and hypovolemia.

Determining the Amount of Fluid to Administer

Three values that are calculated to determine the volume of fluid to administer are (1) the hydration deficit, (2) the maintenance requirement, and (3) the contemporary (ongoing) losses.

The hydration deficit, which is the amount of fluid that must be replaced to bring the animal back to a normal hydration status, is calculated by multiplying the percentage of dehydration by the patient's normal body weight. The percentage of dehydration is estimated from the history, physical examination, and laboratory findings. For example, if a 10-kg beagle is determined to be 5% dehydrated, the hydration deficit is calculated as follows:

$$10\text{ kg} \times 0.05\,(5\%) = 0.5\text{ kg of fluid loss}$$

$$0.5\text{ kg} \times 1000\text{ mL/kg} = 500\text{ mL of replacement fluid}$$

The second value needed to calculate the volume of fluids to administer is the maintenance value. Daily maintenance volumes are related to the daily energy requirement and can be read from the graph in Figure 15-4. A formula that also may be used to calculate maintenance needs is

$$\text{mL/day} = (30 \times \text{kg}) + 70$$

When the formula is used, our 10-kg beagle would need the following:

$$(30 \times 10\text{ kg}) + 70 = 370\text{ mL/day}$$

The final calculation to be made is that for ongoing losses. If it is estimated that the beagle is losing 100 mL of fluid per day through vomiting, then an additional 100 mL of fluid would have to be added to the total calculated volume.

The total volume that the beagle would need to be given in 24 hours is as follows:

500 mL to correct the hydration deficit
+ 370 mL for normal maintenance
+ 100 mL for ongoing vomiting losses
970 mL total

Abbott Animal Health provides a poster (Figure 15-5) that allows rapid estimation of fluid volumes based on maintenance needs as well as maintenance plus varying degrees of dehydration. The animal's weight is found, and the appropriate column is then consulted for the volume of fluid needed. This poster does not take ongoing losses into account but provides a quick determination of fluid volume needed as well as administration rates.

Routes of Fluid Administration

The route by which fluids are administered depends on several factors such as the nature of the condition being treated, its duration, and its severity. The routes that may be used include (1) intravenous, (2) subcutaneous, (3) intraperitoneal, (4) intraosseous, and

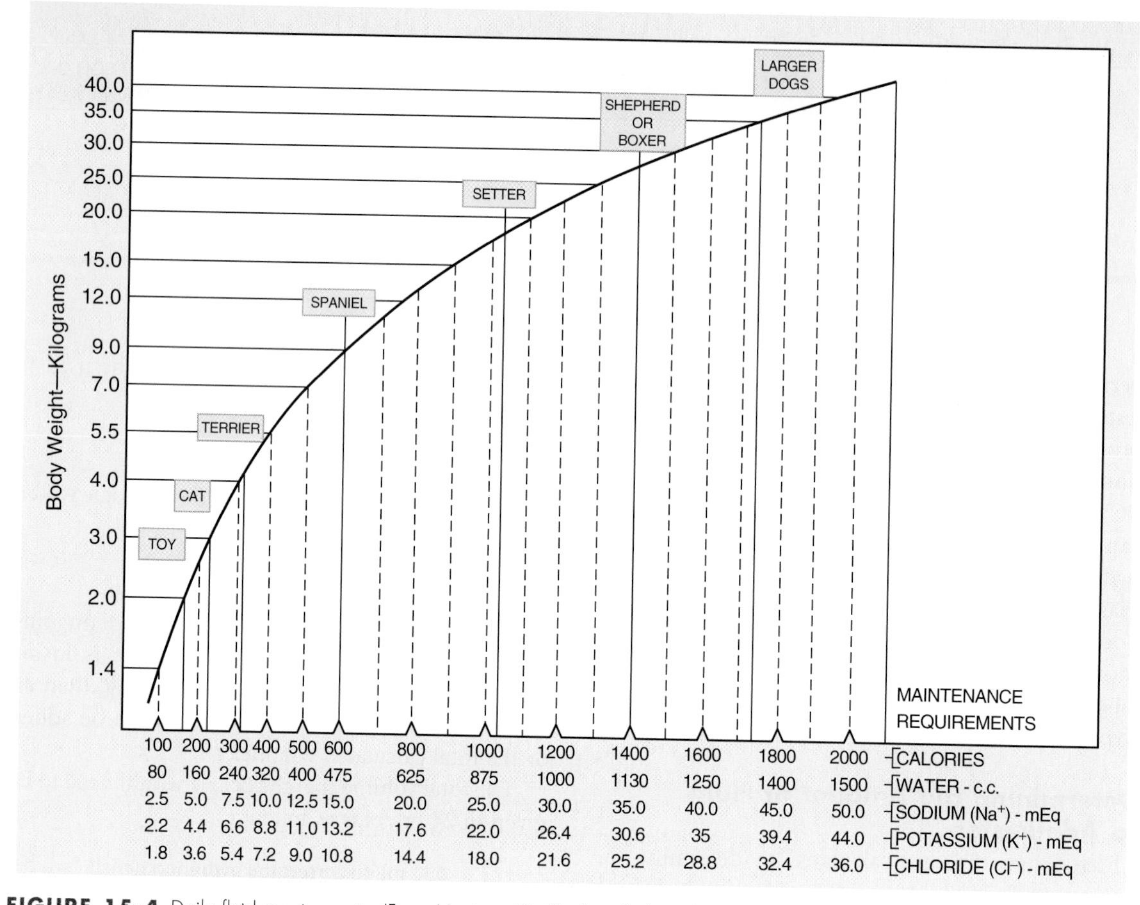

FIGURE 15-4 Daily fluid requirements. (From Harrison JB: Fluid and electrolyte therapy in small animals. J Am Vet Med Assoc 137:637–645, 1960.)

(5) oral. Fluids given by routes one, two, three, or four are administered by the parenteral route and may be referred to as parenteral fluids.

The intravenous route is preferred when the loss has been great or the disorder is severe. The intravenous route allows quicker, more precise delivery of fluids than the other routes. This route does require placement of an intravenous catheter and closer monitoring because of potential complications such as obstruction or kinking of the catheter, septicemia, embolism, and phlebitis. Catheters should be flushed with saline or heparinized saline (5 U/mL of 0.9% saline) every 8 to 12 hours and should be removed and replaced every 72 to 96 hours so that complications are minimized.

The subcutaneous route is useful when a patient's needs are not severe. The amount of fluid that can be administered subcutaneously depends on the size of the animal and the amount of loose skin that it has. Between 50 and 200 mL generally can be infused at a subcutaneous site. Great care should be taken not to administer enough fluid to dissect the skin loose from its blood supply because this can cause sloughing of skin over the site. Hypertonic or irritating fluids should not be given by the subcutaneous route.

The oral route is a practical means of administering fluids as long as an animal has no severe disorders of the gastrointestinal system. This route allows normal physiologic processes to control the amount of fluid and the amount and type of electrolytes

How much fluid should I give?

Maintenance Only

1. Estimate patient's **body weight** in pounds (or kilograms).
2. Go to **Maintenance Only** column (this gives total volume of fluids [in **mL/24 hrs**] that the patient requires based on his or her metabolic water requirements over 24 hrs [(30 x body weight in kilograms) + 70]).
3. If using a fluid pump or in-line regulator, use the **mL/hr** figure. If using a gravity-fed IV set, use the **drops/min** figure.
4. If patient is less than 5 kg, use a micro-drip infusion set that is calibrated to deliver 60 drops per milliliter of fluid. The drip rate **(drops/min)** is denoted in blue
5. If patient is over 5 kg, use a macro-drip infusion set that delivers 15 drops per milliliter of fluid. The drip rate **(drops/min)** is denoted in brown.

Maintenance and Dehydration

1. Estimate patient's **body weight** in pounds (or kilograms).
2. Estimate patient's **% Dehydration** deficit based on clinical signs as listed in boxes and choose appropriate data column. The figures in these columns include both the fluid volume required to replenish hydration in a 24-hour period and the patient's maintenance fluid requirements.
3. Proceed per the instructions from #3 in the **Maintenance Only** section above.
4. After 24 hours, the patient's hydration status should be reassessed and a fluid plan for the next 24 hours determined.

Overhydration

- Serous nasal discharge
- Increased respiratory rate
- Pulmonary crackles
- Chemosis
- Bloody frothy fluid from trachea or nose
- Peripheral or dependent edema

5% Dehydration
- Dry mucous membranes
- Mild skin tenting

7% Dehydration
- Increased skin tenting
- Dry mucous membranes
- Mildly increased heart rate
- Normal blood pressure and pulses

10% Dehydration
- Increased skin tenting
- Dry mucous membranes
- Increased heart rate
- Weak pulses

12% Dehydration
- Increased skin tenting
- Dry mucous membranes
- Sunken eyes, dry cornea
- Weak to absent pulses
- Low blood pressure
- Altered mentation and level of consciousness

Body Weight		Maintenance Only			Maintenance + 5% Dehydration			Maintenance + 7% Dehydration			Maintenance + 10% Dehydration			Maintenance + 12% Dehydration		
lb	kg	mL/24 hrs	mL/hr	drops/min	mL/24 hrs	mL/hr	drops/min	mL/24 hrs	mL/hr	drops/min	mL/24 hrs	mL/hr	drops/min	mL/24 hrs	mL/hr	drops/min
2	1	100	4	4	150	6	6	170	7	7	200	8	8	220	9	9
4	2	130	5	5	230	10	10	270	11	11	330	14	14	370	15	15
7	3	160	7	7	310	13	13	370	15	15	460	19	19	520	22	22
9	4	190	8	8	390	16	16	470	20	20	590	25	25	670	28	28
11	5	220	9	9	470	20	20	570	24	24	720	30	30	820	34	34
13	6	250	10	3	550	23	6	670	28	7	850	35	9	970	40	10
15	7	280	12	3	630	26	7	770	32	8	980	41	10	1,120	47	12
18	8	310	13	3	710	30	7	870	36	9	1,110	46	12	1,270	53	13
20	9	340	14	4	790	33	8	970	40	10	1,240	52	13	1,420	59	15
22	10	370	15	4	870	36	9	1,070	45	11	1,370	57	14	1,570	65	16
26	12	430	18	4	1,030	43	11	1,270	53	13	1,630	68	17	1,870	78	19
31	14	490	20	5	1,190	50	12	1,470	61	15	1,890	79	20	2,170	90	23
35	16	550	23	6	1,350	56	14	1,670	70	17	2,150	90	22	2,470	103	26
40	18	610	25	6	1,510	63	16	1,870	78	19	2,410	100	25	2,770	115	29
44	20	670	28	7	1,670	70	17	2,070	86	22	2,670	111	28	3,070	128	32
48	22	730	30	8	1,830	76	19	2,270	95	24	2,930	122	31	3,370	140	35
53	24	790	33	8	1,990	83	21	2,470	103	26	3,190	133	33	3,670	153	38
57	26	850	35	9	2,150	90	22	2,670	111	28	3,450	144	36	3,970	165	41
62	28	910	38	9	2,310	96	24	2,870	120	30	3,710	155	39	4,270	178	44
66	30	970	40	10	2,470	103	26	3,070	128	32	3,970	165	41	4,570	190	48
79	36	1,150	48	12	2,950	123	31	3,670	153	38	4,750	198	49	5,470	228	57
88	40	1,270	53	13	3,270	136	34	4,070	170	42	5,270	220	55	6,070	253	63
101	46	1,450	60	15	3,750	156	39	4,670	195	49	6,050	252	63	6,970	290	73
110	50	1,570	65	16	4,070	170	42	5,070	211	53	6,570	274	68	7,570	315	79
123	56	1,750	73	18	4,550	190	47	5,670	236	59	7,350	306	77	8,470	353	88
132	60	1,870	78	19	4,870	203	51	6,070	253	63	7,870	328	82	9,070	378	94
143	65	2,020	84	21	5,270	220	55	6,570	274	68	8,520	355	89	9,820	409	102
154	70	2,170	90	23	5,670	236	59	7,070	295	74	9,170	382	96	10,570	440	110
165	75	2,320	97	24	6,070	253	63	7,570	315	79	9,820	409	102	11,320	472	118
176	80	2,470	103	26	6,470	270	67	8,070	336	84	10,470	436	109	12,070	503	126
187	85	2,620	109	27	6,870	286	72	8,570	357	89	11,120	463	116	12,820	534	134
198	90	2,770	115	29	7,270	303	76	9,070	378	94	11,770	490	123	13,570	565	141
209	95	2,920	122	30	7,670	320	80	9,570	399	100	12,420	518	129	14,320	597	149
220	100	3,070	128	32	8,070	336	84	10,070	420	105	13,070	545	136	15,070	628	157

Abbott
A Promise for Life

FIGURE 15-5 How much fluid should I give? (Courtesy Abbott Animal Health.)

absorbed. This route is not satisfactory when large volumes of fluid must be given rapidly.

The intraperitoneal route allows for administration of large volumes of fluid, but absorption is slow. Peritonitis is a potential complication, and this route is not commonly used.

The intraosseous (femur, ilium, or humerus) route is sometimes used in very small animals or in those with poor access to veins. This route allows rapid delivery of fluids and blood but requires greater technical expertise for placing the delivery needle. Careful attention should be paid to sterile technique when this route is used so that osteomyelitis does not occur.

Rate of Administration

Once the volume of fluid needed and the route of administration have been decided, the time frame must be established for delivering the fluids. Rapid losses of fluid usually call for rapid replacement. Flow rates may depend on the type of fluid being administered (crystalloid vs. colloid), the conditions being treated, and the equipment available.

For treatment of patients with shock, crystalloid fluids may be administered rapidly (90 mL/kg/h in dogs and 40 mL/kg/h in cats). The use of a pressure administration cuff may allow more rapid infusion in these cases (Figure 15-6). Colloids and mixtures of crystalloids and colloids are generally administered at a slower rate than crystalloids alone. Advanced references should be consulted for specific rates.

Fluids ideally should be infused continuously during a 24-hour period. One method of determining fluid flow rate is to calculate the hydration deficit, add maintenance and ongoing losses, and set the drip rate to administer the total during a 24-hour period. Some clinicians prefer to administer the hydration deficit during the first few hours and then to give the remainder over a longer period. Some divide the total calculated volume into three equal parts and administer each in an 8-hour period. In many practices, fluid administration can be monitored for a part of the day only. In this case, the total 24-hour fluid volume can be administered during the period that the patient can be monitored. (Common sense and medical judgment, however, must be exercised.) Portions of the total volume may be administered subcutaneously when appropriate.

Fluids are administered from plastic bags through intravenous administration sets (Figures 15-7 and 15-8). Two sizes of administration sets that are commonly used in veterinary medicine are the standard macrodrip set (15 drops/mL) and the minidrip/microdrip set (60 drops/mL). Other sizes (10 drops/mL and 20 drops/mL) are also available. Microdrip sets are suited for use in administering fluids to cats and small dogs. The size of the administration set must be known to calculate the drip or flow rate.

To calculate the drip rate, first divide the total number of milliliters to be administered by the total number of minutes for administration to determine the number of milliliters per minute to deliver. Then, multiply the milliliters per minute by the drops per

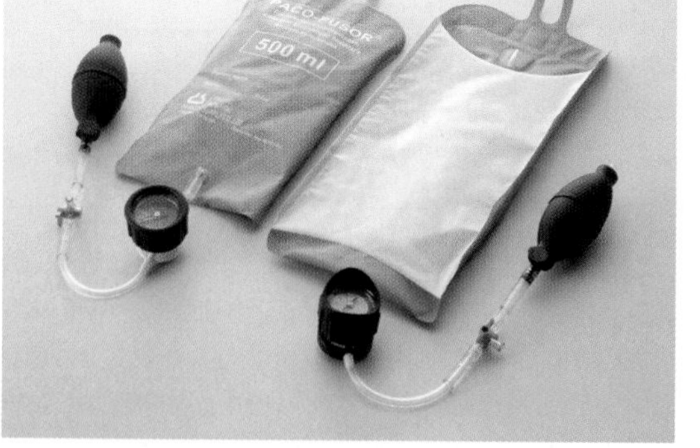

FIGURE 15-6 Pressure administration cuff.

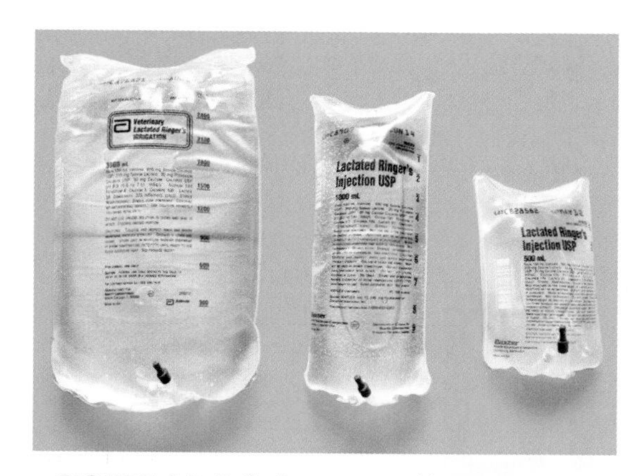

FIGURE 15-7 Fluid containers. Abbott IV Solutions.

milliliter of the administration set that has been chosen to arrive at the number of drops (gtt) per minute (gtt/min). For example, if the beagle needs 1200 mL of fluid during a 24-hour period and a standard (15 gtt/mL) administration set is used, then the calculation is as follows:

$$\frac{\text{Volume of infusion (mL)}}{\text{Time of infusion (min)}} \times \text{drop factor (gtt/mL)} = \text{gtt/mL}$$

$$\frac{1200 \text{ mL}}{24 \text{ hours} \times 60 \text{ min/hour}} = \frac{1200 \text{ mL}}{1440 \text{ min}} = 0.83 \text{ mL/min} \times 15 \text{ gtt/mL} = 12.5 \text{ gtt/min}$$

A rate of 12.5 gtt/min can be thought of as 1 drop approximately every 5 seconds.

$$\left(\frac{60}{12} = 5\right)$$

When standard gravity flow bags or bottles are used, drip rates are controlled by devices that are placed on the administration sets to adjust the diameter of the line (e.g., roller clamps, slide clamps, and screw clamps) (Figure 15-9). The flow rate is simply dialed in on the machine when fluid infusion pumps (mL/h) (Figure 15-10, *A*) or controllers (mL/min) are used (Figure 15-10, *B*).

Monitoring Fluid Administration

Fluids administered too rapidly or in too great a volume can be life threatening. Careful monitoring of the physical status of the animal is essential. Lung sounds, skin turgor, and the overall status of the animal should be monitored regularly, along with the PCV and the TPP. When a large volume of fluids is administered rapidly, it is prudent to insert a urinary catheter to monitor urine output and establish that the kidneys are functioning normally. Some clinicians also choose to insert a jugular catheter to monitor central venous pressure as a way of preventing fluid volume overload.

Signs of overhydration may include restlessness, serous nasal discharge, increased lung sounds (crackles), tachycardia, dyspnea, pitting subcutaneous edema, and an increased "Jello-like" feel in the subcutaneous tissue (Haskins, 2000). Fluid infusion should be slowed or stopped and the veterinarian contacted at the first appearance of these signs.

Labeled tape may be placed vertically on fluid bottles or bags to allow monitoring of the volume delivered (Figure 15-11). Bottles or bags also should be labeled with all pertinent information, including the presence of any additives. It may be helpful to place a horizontal piece of tape across the fluid container to indicate when fluid delivery is to be stopped.

A volume control system or Buretrol device may be used for administering small volumes of fluid (Figure 15-12). A clamp allows the volume control chamber to be filled with a predetermined amount of fluid from the bag or bottle. The line then is clamped off to prevent entry of additional fluid from the bag. The chamber can be refilled if desired.

Discontinuation of Fluid Therapy

Fluid therapy is discontinued when clinical signs improve and laboratory test results return to normal. When repeated evaluations of body weight, urine output, PCV, TPP, urine specific gravity, and central venous pressure show progressive improvement, fluid therapy may be tapered or discontinued. As the animal recovers, fluid therapy may be cut back by decreasing the fluid volume given by 25% to 50% per day.

Preparing Fluid Administration Equipment

When preparing to administer intravenous fluids, follow a standard protocol. After gathering supplies and preparing the injection site, check to see that the fluid type is correct and that it is not out of date. Then, determine that the container is not cracked or chipped and that the solution is clear. Fluids should never contain precipitates or appear cloudy. After inspecting the container's cap to make sure that it is intact, remove the metal cap (bottle) or insertion port cover (bag), while taking care not to contaminate the port. Close the flow clamp on the administration set, and remove the cover from the administration set spike. Wipe the port with an alcohol swab, and insert the administration set spike into the rubber stopper (bottle) or insertion port (bag). Hang the bottle or bag, and fill the administration set line by opening the flow clamp and allowing fluid to run through the line until all bubbles are cleared. Close the flow clamp and attach the adapter to the

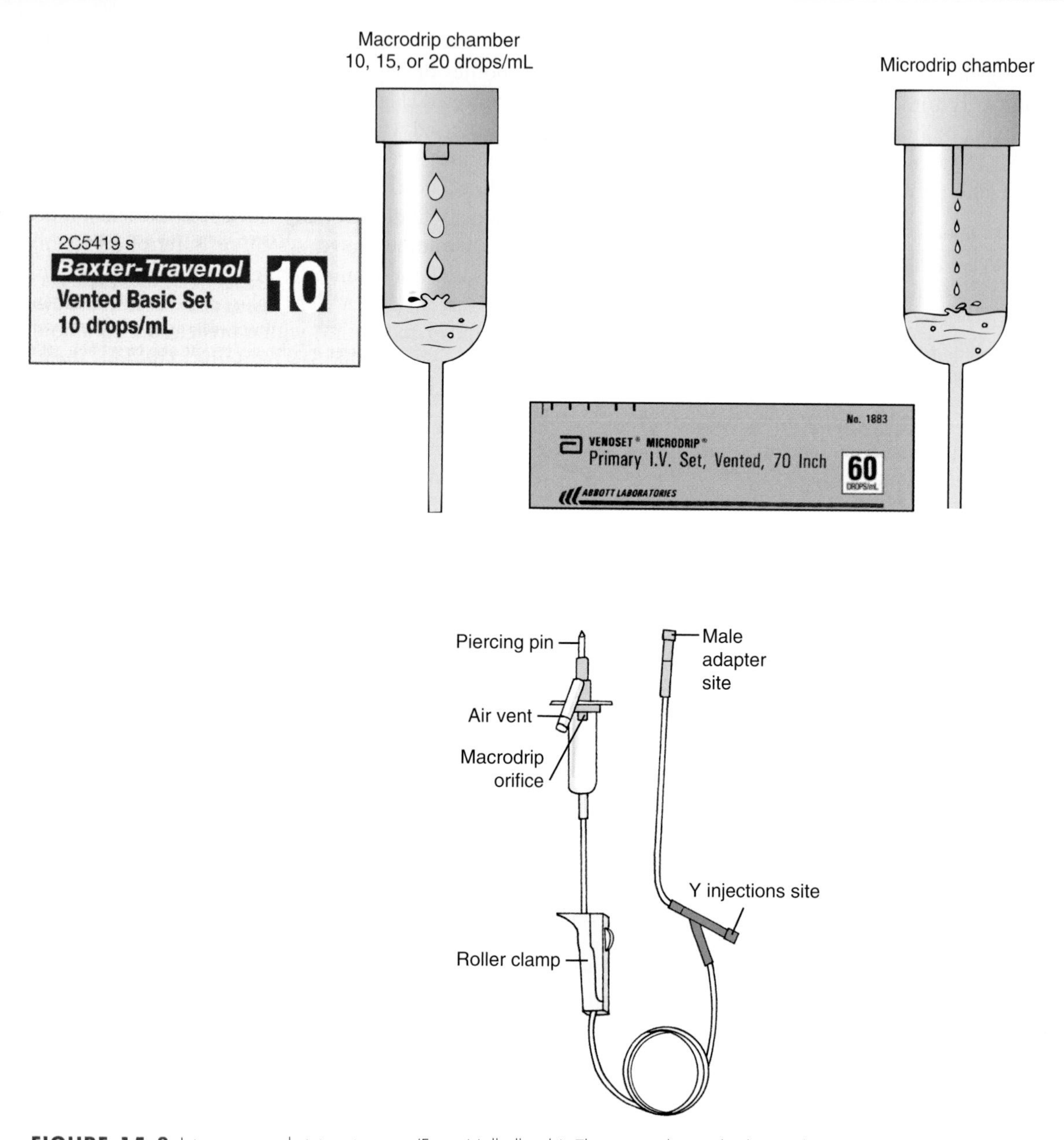

FIGURE 15-8 Intravenous administration set. (From Mulholland J: The nurse, the math, the meds, St Louis, 2011, Elsevier.)

intravenous catheter using sterile technique. After the flow clamp is opened to determine that the catheter and the line are patent, the drip rate may be adjusted as required.

If at any time the flow rate slows or stops, check the following: (1) the catheter for correct placement and patency, (2) the position of the patient to determine whether limb position or flexion has occluded the flow, (3) the flow clamp to see whether it is in the open position, (4) the tubing to determine whether it is kinked or crimped, and (5) the fluid level in the bottle.

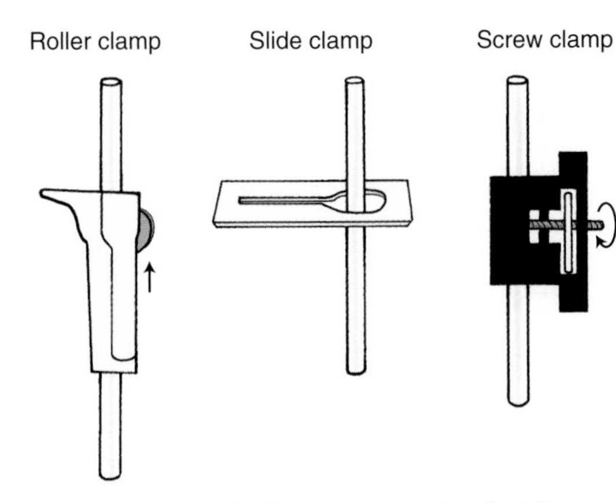

FIGURE 15-9 Clamps for controlling fluid flow.

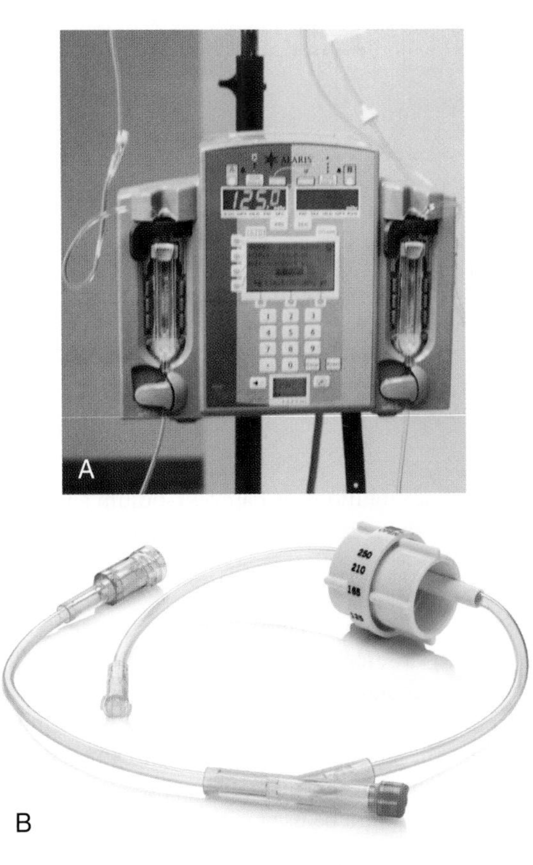

FIGURE 15-10 A, Intravenous infusion pump. B, Intravenous infusion controller. (A, From Kee JL, Marshall SM: Clinical calculations: with applications to general and specialty areas, ed. 6, St. Louis, 2009, Saunders. B, Courtesy Hospira, Inc., Lake Forest, IL. In Mulholland J: The nurse, the math, the meds, St Louis, 2011, Elsevier.)

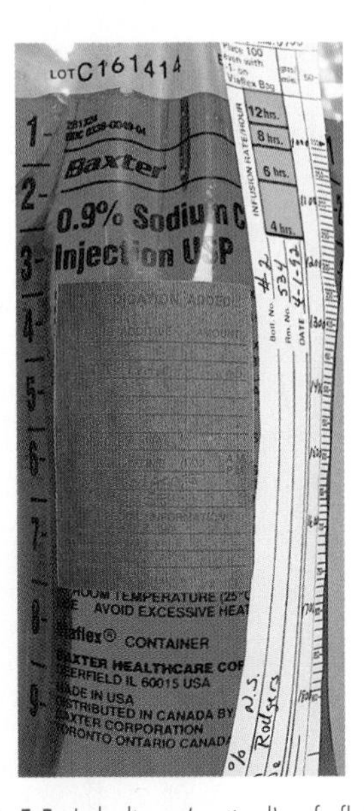

FIGURE 15-11 Labeling (vertical) of fluid bag. (From Potter PA, Perry AG, Stockert PA, Hall A: Basic nursing, ed 6, St. Louis, 2011, Mosby, p 511.)

Two fluid solutions may be administered simultaneously with the use of a piggyback setup of the containers (Figure 15-13). The secondary bag is hung higher than the primary bag, and the secondary administration set line is connected to the Y port of the primary administration set.

Technicians should understand the use of a three-way valve. The three-way valve permits three-way connections to be made. Flow of fluid through the valve depends on the position at which the control handle is placed. The handle points toward the line that is closed. Figure 15-14 illustrates the operation of a three-way valve.

TYPES OF SOLUTIONS USED IN FLUID THERAPY

Parenteral fluids can be broadly classified as crystalloids or colloids. Crystalloids may be further classified as isotonic high-sodium, hypotonic low-sodium, or hypertonic saline solutions. Colloids can be subdivided into synthetic starch-based colloids and natural colloids.

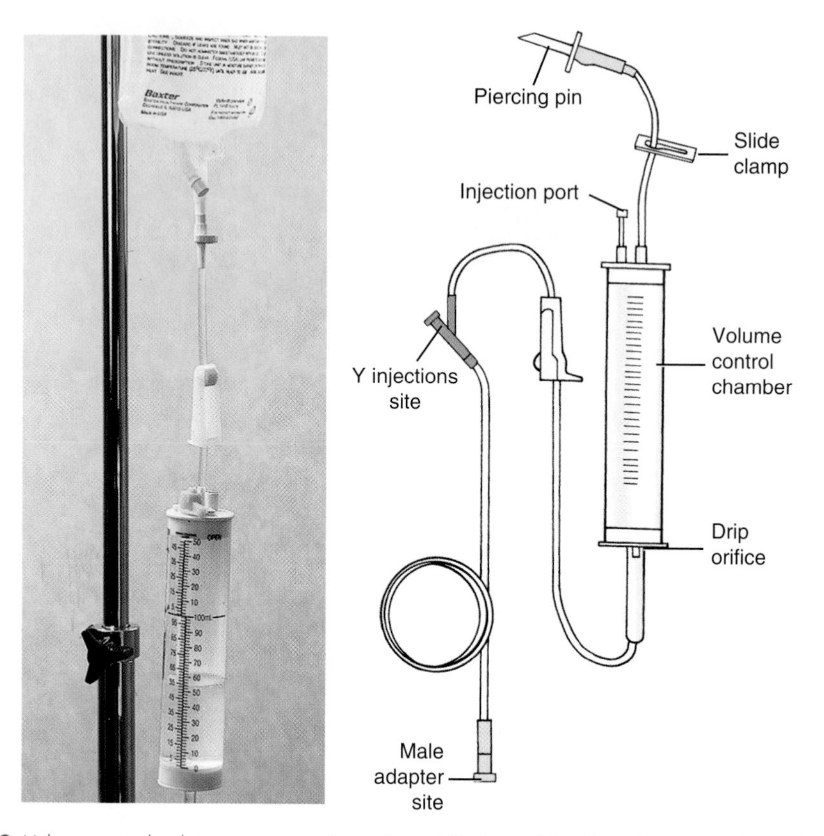

FIGURE 15-12 Volume control administration set. (From Perry AG, Potter PA: Clinical nursing skills and techniques, ed 7, St. Louis, 2010, Mosby.)

CRYSTALLOID SOLUTIONS

Crystalloids are solutions that contain electrolyte and nonelectrolyte substances capable of passing through cell membranes, therefore entering all body fluid compartments. Administration of crystalloid solutions results in rapid equilibration (within ½ to 1 hour) of fluid between the intravascular and interstitial spaces. Crystalloid solutions are used routinely in veterinary medicine because of their versatility and relatively low cost. Crystalloid solutions can be classified further as isotonic high-sodium (replacement solutions), hypotonic low-sodium (maintenance solutions), or hypertonic saline solutions. Replacement solutions resemble ECF in content, whereas maintenance solutions contain less sodium and more potassium than are found in replacement fluids.

Clinical Uses

Isotonic crystalloids have a sodium content and osmolality close to ECF (approximately 300 mOsm/L). A large percentage of the fluid infused will leave the intravascular space within 30 minutes. These fluids are versatile and may be used for treating shock, vomiting, diarrhea, pancreatitis, and other conditions. They should be used with caution or not used at all in patients in which sodium retention may be a problem (e.g., heart disease or renal disease).

Hypotonic crystalloids have a sodium content and an osmolality less than ECF, so infused fluid tends to hydrate the extracellular space. This occurs because

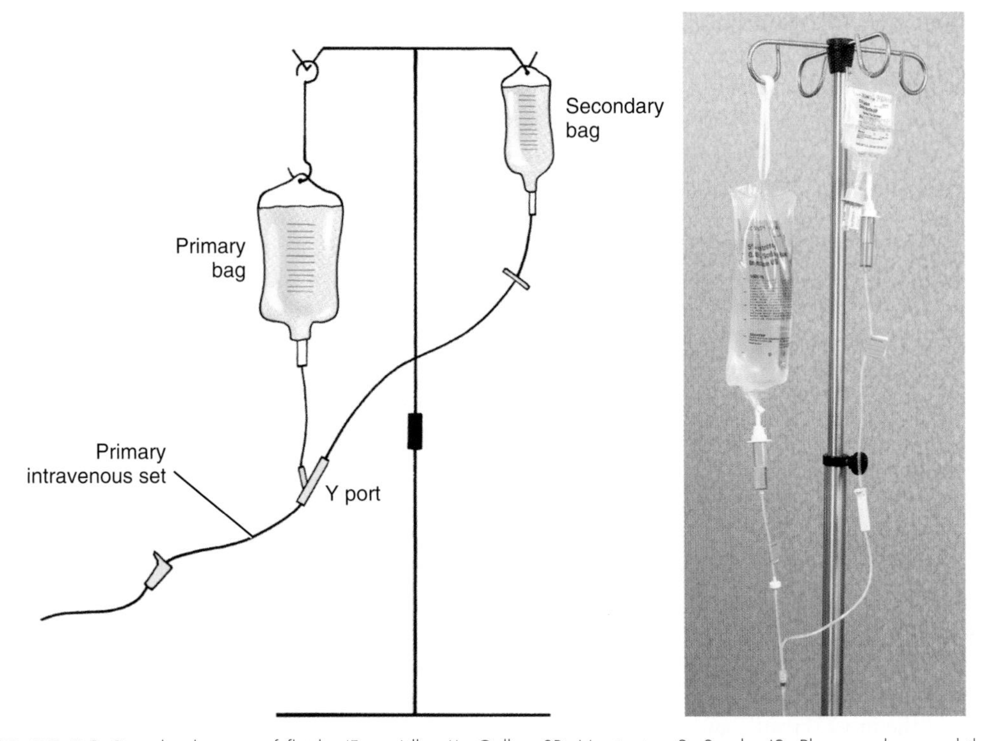

FIGURE 15-13 Piggyback setup of fluids. (From Lilley LL, Collins SR, Harrington S, Snyder JS: Pharmacology and the nursing process, ed 7, St. Louis, 2014, Mosby.)

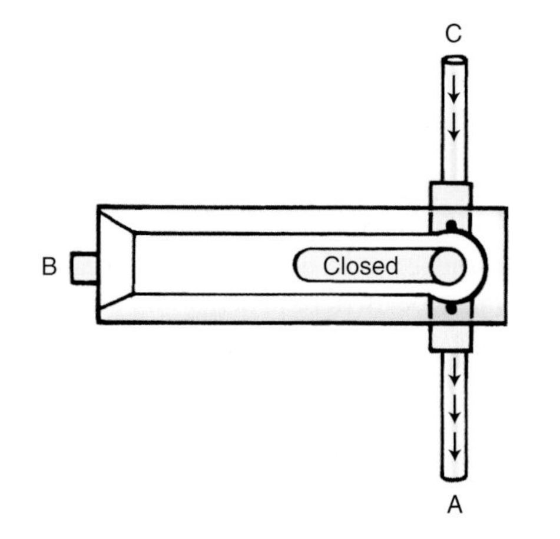

FIGURE 15-14 Operation of a three-way valve. The handle points toward the closed port allowing fluid to flow in through port C and out through port A. The handle may be positioned toward each of the ports to change the direction of entry and exit.

the extracellular space has a higher osmolality that pulls the fluid out of the vasculature into this space (see Figure 15-3). These fluids are used to treat hypernatremia or conditions in which sodium retention is a problem.

Hypertonic crystalloids have an osmolality greater than that of ECF and cause fluid to move out of the intracellular/interstitial space and into the intravascular space. They are used to treat shock (by increasing intravascular volume) and may be beneficial in treating intracranial edema (by "pulling" excess fluid out of the brain into the vasculature).

Dosage Forms

Dosage forms are numerous. Fluids are available in glass bottles, plastic bottles, and plastic bags that hold

250, 500, and 1000 mL. Containers that hold 3000 and 6000 mL are available for some solutions (see manufacturer product guides). The following section briefly describes the commonly used crystalloid solutions. See Table 15-2 for a listing of the composition and other characteristics of each.

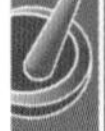

ISOTONIC HIGH-SODIUM CRYSTALLOIDS

Physiologic Saline

Physiologic saline is a 0.9% solution of NaCl and is also called *normal saline.* It also may be called *isotonic saline* because it has an osmolarity of 308 mOsm/L. Saline is used to increase plasma volume or to correct a sodium deficiency **(hyponatremia).** It also may be used to bathe tissues during surgery to prevent them from drying out. Because of its high sodium content, saline should not be used in animals with known heart disease.

Lactated Ringer's Solution

LRS is one of the most versatile and commonly used fluids in veterinary medicine. It is a balanced electrolyte replacement solution that can be administered by any route that is available. It contains 28 mEq/L of lactate, which is converted by the liver to bicarbonate to act as a **buffer** against acidosis. Theoretically, LRS should not be administered with blood because the calcium contents could cause clotting to occur. LRS is not currently considered appropriate for use in critical patients (Crowe, 2007). It is not appropriate to use LRS in liver disease because the lactate may not be metabolized to bicarbonate. LRS should not be used when hypercalcemia or cancer is present.

Ringer's Solution (Injection)

Ringer's solution contains slightly more sodium, chloride, and calcium than LRS. It contains no buffer. It is used in similar situations to LRS. This solution appears to have limited use in veterinary medicine.

Normosol R

Normosol R is a balanced, multiple-electrolyte solution with a dual buffering system (acetate and gluconate). Acetate and gluconate are metabolized outside the liver, which is a factor that may confer advantages in conditions such as liver disorders. Normosol is calcium free and thus may help to prevent potential incompatibilities with transfused blood or added sodium bicarbonate.

Plasma-Lyte

Plasma-Lyte R is a balanced replacement solution with 47 mEq/L of acetate and 8 mEq/L of lactate as buffers. It contains calcium. Plasma-Lyte A is a similar solution except that it contains no calcium or lactate.

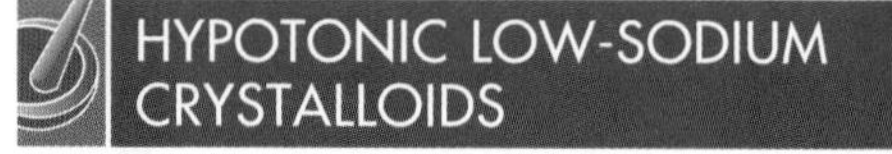

HYPOTONIC LOW-SODIUM CRYSTALLOIDS

Dextrose 5% in Water

Dextrose 5% in water (D_5W) is a nonbalanced solution that contains only dextrose (50 g/L) and water. Administering dextrose 5% is equivalent to administering pure water because the dextrose is metabolized to carbon dioxide and water. Dextrose 5% provides approximately 170 kcal/L (a quantity that cannot be relied on to meet the daily caloric needs of most small animals), although it may supplement other caloric sources. Dextrose 5% generally should not be given by the subcutaneous route because it may osmotically "draw" fluid from the vascular space. Dextrose in water should not be used as a maintenance solution because overdilution may cause an electrolyte imbalance. It is often mixed with a saline solution when hypotonic low-sodium solutions are indicated.

Dextrose 2.5% With 0.45% Saline

This solution contains 77 mEq/L each of sodium and chloride and 25 g/dL of dextrose (85 kcal/L). This solution may be used for patients who may be at risk if they take in too much sodium or for those with potential fluid retention.

Half-Strength Lactated Ringer's Solution With 2.5% Dextrose

This solution is a hypotonic low-sodium solution (66 mEq/L) containing small amounts of chloride (55 mEq/L) along with small amounts of potassium, calcium, dextrose, and lactate. It provides a slightly more balanced approach to the use of hypotonic low-sodium fluids.

Adverse Side Effects

Adverse side effects of fluid administration are primarily associated with overhydration. Signs of overhydration may include restlessness, shivering, serous nasal discharge, coughing, and pulmonary edema. High-sodium fluids should not be used in patients with heart disease, renal disease, inflammation, and/or edema.

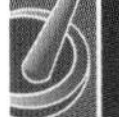

HYPERTONIC SALINE SOLUTIONS

Hypertonic saline solutions are available from commercial sources in 3%, 4%, 5%, 7%, 7.5%, and 23.4% preparations. These solutions are especially useful in treating hypovolemic shock with the use of small volumes of the solution. The 7.5% solution is considered the upper limit of concentration to avoid phlebitis.

Adverse Side Effects

These may include phlebitis, tissue irritation, rehemorrhage in traumatic shock, electrolyte imbalances, and—when the administration rate is too fast—hypotension, bronchoconstriction, and bradycardia.

> *TECHNICIAN NOTES*
> - Fluids that contain preservatives such as benzyl alcohol should never be given to cats because of the likelihood of toxic reactions.
> - Some clinicians warn against administering fluids with preservatives to puppies and adult dogs.

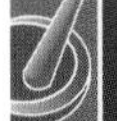

COLLOID SOLUTIONS

Colloid solutions contain large molecular weight particles that are unable to cross cell membranes and therefore are confined to the vascular space. Unlike crystalloid solute, these colloid particles are effective osmoles that are able to hold fluid in the vascular space and draw fluid from the interstitial space into the vascular space (expand the plasma volume).

Colloids include synthetic, starch-based colloids and natural colloids.

Clinical Uses

Colloid solutions are used for expansion of the plasma volume in the treatment of patients with hypovolemia not due to dehydration, septic shock, or hypalbuminemia. Colloids are useful in treating patients prone to edema because smaller fluid volumes are required for effective treatment.

Colloid administration can provide great patient benefit in select cases, but because of potential harmful side effects, they should be given judiciously.

Synthetic Colloids

Dextrans

Dextran 70 is a large molecular weight branched polysaccharide solution with osmotic effects similar to albumin. It is available as a 6% solution in 0.9% saline (Dextran 70, Gentran 70, Macrodex) or as a 6% solution in 5% dextrose (Macrodex). Dextrans remain in the vascular space for 4 to 8 hours. These products should be used with caution in patients subject to vascular overload. Dextran 70 is contraindicated in patients with coagulopathies.

Hydroxyethyl Starch

Hydroxyethyl starch (HES) or hetastarch is a large molecular weight starch that is used in the treatment of hypovolemia and hypoproteinemia. It may also reduce intravascular inflammation and reduce vascular permeability and leakage. Hetastarch expands the plasma volume longer (12 to 36 hours) and has fewer side effects than the dextrans. It is prepared as a 6% HES solution in 0.9% saline (Hespan) and a 6% HES solution in lactated electrolyte (Hextend). These products also can cause volume overload, coagulopathies, and hypersensitivity reactions. The primary disadvantage of hetastarch is its expense.

Oxyglobin

Oxyglobin is a purified solution of bovine hemoglobin in altered LRS. It provides a substitute for hemoglobin and enhances oxygen carrying capacity for up to 40 hours. It is useful in anemic patients and those with reduced oxygen carrying capacity. Oxyglobin has been shown to act as an effective plasma volume expander as well as a carrier of oxygen. It has an extended shelf life and does not require crossmatching because intact red blood cells are not present. Oxyglobin may cause vasoconstriction and increased blood pressure, and care should be taken when choosing the volume and rate of administration. It is an expensive product that has faced limited availability problems.

Natural Colloids

The natural colloids are high molecular weight solutions obtained from species-specific donor animals. Natural colloids act in a similar way to synthetic colloids by causing an increased intravascular volume and may contribute clotting factors in coagulopathies and provide blood cells in large volume loss. They include albumin (canine or human origin), fresh frozen plasma, frozen or stored plasma, and whole blood.

Albumin

Albumin provides over 75% of the oncotic pressure of plasma. Administration of albumin may be useful in critically ill patients needing intravascular volume expansion, especially if that animal is hypoalbuminemic, edematous, or suffering from vascular leakage of fluid. Human (Albuminar, Albutein, Flexbumin, Albuminate, and Plasbumin) and canine (Albumin, Canine) commercial albumin products are available. Caution should be used when administering the human albumin product because of "significant concerns with adverse effects," (Plumb, 2011). Few reports are available on the clinical use of the canine product.

Fresh Frozen Plasma

If the plasma is collected from centrifuged whole blood and frozen within 6 hours of collection, it is considered to be fresh frozen. Fresh frozen plasma contains albumin (and other plasma proteins) and clotting factors. It may be used to treat rodenticide coagulopathies, patients needing factor VII or von Willenbrand's factor, or disseminated intravascular coagulation. Fresh frozen plasma can be stored up to a year with preservation of the unstable clotting factors. After 1 year of storage fresh frozen plasma becomes stored plasma because of the loss of clotting factors. Freezing of plasma destroys the platelets.

Frozen or Stored Plasma

When frozen after 6 hours of collection plasma may not be suitable for treating factor VII or von Willenbrand's coagulopathy; however, it can be used to treat rodenticide coagulopathy (Rudloff, 2013) and patients with decreased protein levels.

Whole Blood

The primary use of whole blood is the treatment of patients with anemia. Because fresh whole blood contains all the coagulation factors and platelets, it can also be used in patients with coagulation or platelet disorders. Transfusions are generally given in cases of anemia when the PCV drops below 20% or the hemoglobin level drops below 7 g/dL. Transfusions should be started slowly, and the patient should be monitored closely for signs of transfusion reactions like panting, urticaria, or vomiting. Blood should be warmed to body temperature before administering through a line with a filter to remove small clots. The quantity of blood to transfuse can be calculated by determining the percent change in PCV that is desired and multiplying that number by 2 mL/kg for each kilogram of the animal's weight. For example, if a 20-kg animal has a PCV of 15% and the desired PCV is 25%, one would administer 400 mL of blood.

$$\text{Desired change in PCV: } 25\% - 15\% = 10$$

$$\text{Volume of blood to transfuse: } 10 \times 2 \text{ mL/kg} \times 20 \text{ kg} = 400 \text{ mL}$$

Adverse Side Effects

Adverse side effects of colloid administration include volume overload, coagulopathies, and hypersensitivity reactions. Allergic reactions may be seen in concentrated albumin or blood transfusions.

> **TECHNICIAN NOTES**
> - Colloids are not intended for maintenance or long-term use.
> - References should be checked when the appropriate flow rate for colloid solutions is determined.

TECHNICIAN NOTES

- The rate of administration of hypertonic saline solution is a very important consideration because exceeding this rate may cause serious side effects.
- Hypertonic saline should be infused through a well-secured intravenous catheter to prevent extravasation of irritating fluids.

FLUID ADDITIVES

In some instances, special substances may be added to intravenous fluid solutions to enhance the solutions' therapeutic effects. These substances may be added to correct acid–base abnormalities and electrolyte imbalances, to supplement calories, and to provide supplemental vitamins to replace those washed out by fluid therapy.

Sodium Bicarbonate

Sodium bicarbonate is an alkalizing agent that may be added to correct **metabolic acidosis** and certain other conditions. Because lactate or acetate in fluid preparations often cannot correct severe metabolic acidosis, supplementation becomes necessary. Normal serum bicarbonate is 24 mEq/L. Required amounts for supplementation may be calculated by measuring a patient's bicarbonate level and subtracting that value from 24 (normal). The difference is called the *bicarbonate deficit.* The bicarbonate deficit is multiplied by 0.3 and then by the animal's weight in kilograms to determine the number of milliequivalents of sodium bicarbonate to administer:

$$\text{Bicarbonate supplementation (mEq)} = \text{Bicarbonate deficit} \times 0.3 \times \text{weight (kg)}$$

A 20-kg dog with a bicarbonate level of 14 mEq/L would require 60 mEq bicarbonate supplementation.

$$\text{Bicarbonate supplementation (mEq)} = 24 - 14 = 10 \times 0.3 \times 20 = 60$$

When access to laboratory measurement of bicarbonate or carbon dioxide is not available, **empirical** estimations of supplementation levels are made on the basis of clinical judgment.

Bicarbonate concentration in commercial products is measured in milliequivalents per milliliter.

Clinical Uses

These include the treatment of metabolic acidosis and as an adjunctive therapy for the treatment of hypercalcemia or **hyperkalemia.** Sodium bicarbonate use is contraindicated in patients with metabolic or respiratory alkalosis and should be used with caution in patients with congestive heart failure, hypertension, oliguria, hypocalcemia, or hypokalemia.

Dosage Forms

Veterinary-approved forms include the following:

- An 8.4% (1 mEq/mL) solution for injection, which is available in 50-, 100-, and 500-mL vials (veterinary label)
- A choice of 4%, 4.2%, 5%, 7.5%, and 8.4% solutions for injection (human label)

Adverse Side Effects

These may include **metabolic alkalosis,** hypokalemia, hypocalcemia, and **hypernatremia.**

TECHNICIAN NOTES

- Sodium bicarbonate is incompatible with several solutions and should be mixed only after consulting product inserts or appropriate references.
- Some references indicate that sodium bicarbonate should not be added to solutions that contain calcium because of the potential for precipitates to form.
- Replacement of the total number of milliequivalents should be made over several hours.

Potassium Chloride

Potassium chloride is a solution that is used to supplement potassium deficits (**hypokalemia**). Anorexia, diuresis, and diarrhea are some of the common causes of hypokalemia. Normal serum potassium levels are between 3.5 and 5.5 mEq/L. Signs of hypokalemia include weakness, lethargy, muscle weakness and vomiting. Table 15-5 provides a guide for potassium supplementation that is based on the measured serum level of potassium. Intravenous potassium supplements must be diluted before administering and given slowly.

TABLE 15-5 Potassium Supplementation Guide*

SERUM K^+ (MEQ/L)	MEQ K^+ (TO ADD TO 250 ML FLUID)	MEQ K^+ (TO ADD TO 1 L FLUID)	MAXIMUM INFUSION RATE OF INTRAVENOUS FLUIDS (0.5 MEQ/KG/H)
<2.0	20	80	6
2.1–2.5	15	60	8
2.6–3.0	10	40	12
3.1–3.5	7	28	18
>3.5, <5.0	5	20	25

*For dogs or cats with hypokalemia or for those with potassium depletion and normal serum potassium levels. This regimen is designed to be infused in maintenance volume of fluids.

Clinical Uses
Potassium chloride is used for the treatment or prevention of potassium deficits.

Dosage Forms
Dosage forms for intravenous use include the following:
- Potassium chloride for injection (2 mEq/mL) in 10- and 20-mL vials (veterinary label)
- Potassium chloride for injection (2 mEq/mL) in a variety of vial sizes (human label)

Adverse Side Effects
These may include hyperkalemia, which is manifested by muscle weakness, and cardiac conduction disturbances, which can be life threatening. Potassium supplements may be contraindicated in hyperkalemia, renal failure, Addison's disease, or acute dehydration.

TECHNICIAN NOTES
- Potassium chloride solutions must be diluted before administration.
- The rate of infusion of potassium is critical. Consult product inserts or other references for appropriate rates.

Calcium Supplements
Calcium gluconate or calcium chloride is given as an intravenous infusion to correct hypocalcemia. Intravenous calcium must be administered slowly to avoid possible cardiac arrhythmias, cardiac arrest, or hypotension.

Clinical Uses
Calcium supplements are used for the treatment of hypocalcemia that may result from various conditions, which may include parathyroid gland disorders, milk fever, eclampsia, and excessive sweating in horses. Calcium in combination with phosphorus, magnesium, potassium, and dextrose is used to treat cattle with conditions such as grass tetany, milk fever, and downer cow syndrome.

Dosage Forms
A variety of veterinary-label and human-label products are available. The following is a partial list.
- Calcium gluconate injection (generic and proprietary) 10%, in ampules, syringes, vials, and bottles (veterinary label)
- Calcium gluconate (various proprietary names) 23%, in 100- and 500-mL bottles (veterinary label)
- Calcium chloride injection (generic and proprietary) 10%, in ampules, vials, and syringes (human label)
- Numerous combination products (Cal Dextro, Norcalciphos) that contain calcium, phosphorus, magnesium, potassium, and dextrose

Adverse Side Effects
Adverse side effects that result from hypercalcemia may include hypotension, cardiac arrhythmias, and cardiac arrest. These effects are usually a result of a too rapid infusion of calcium.

TECHNICIAN NOTES

- Any product that contains calcium should be given by slow intravenous administration to prevent cardiac complications.
- Products that contain 23% calcium are labeled for large-animal use.

50% Dextrose

When caloric supplementation is indicated, 50% dextrose often is used as a stock solution to be added to other fluids to provide a desired percent solution of dextrose. It usually is not possible to meet the total caloric needs of a small animal patient through dextrose supplementation of intravenous fluids. Supplementation often is indicated, however, in patients that are hypoglycemic because of fever, sepsis, insulin overdose, insulinoma, liver disease, and other conditions. Varying amounts of dextrose may be added in an attempt to keep the blood glucose level near the normal range (80 to 100 mg/dL).

Intravenous administration of 50% dextrose is used in ruminants as a treatment for uncomplicated ketosis.

To prepare a 2.5% solution of dextrose, add 50 mL (25 g) of 50% dextrose to 1 L of fluids. Fifty milliliters of the original fluid solution should be removed before 50% dextrose is added to keep the dilution correct. To prepare a 5% solution, add 100 mL of 50% dextrose to 1 L of fluids. A formula that may be used to determine the quantity of a stock solution to be used in the preparation of percent solutions follows:

$$\frac{\text{Desired strength}}{\text{Available strength}} = \frac{\text{How much you are going to use}}{\text{How much you are going to make}}$$

or

$$V_1 \times C_1 = V_2 \times C_2$$

For example, to make 250 mL of a 5% solution of dextrose using a stock supply of 50% dextrose, set up the formula in the following way:

$$\frac{5\%}{50\%} = \frac{X}{250}$$

$$\text{Cross multiplying} \quad 50X = 1250$$

$$X = 25 \text{ mL}$$

Therefore, to prepare 250 mL of 5% solution, draw up 25 mL of 50% dextrose and add 225 mL of a diluting fluid.

Clinical Uses

These include caloric supplementation in small animal patients and treatment of ketosis in ruminants.

Dosage Forms

Various manufacturers supply 50% dextrose. The most commonly used package is a 500-mL plastic bottle.

Adverse Side Effects

These are few if the product is used according to directions.

TECHNICIAN NOTES A 50% solution of dextrose contains 500 mg/mL.

Vitamin Supplements

Patients that have been given large amounts of fluid undergo diuresis, which may cause a corresponding loss of water-soluble vitamins (B complex and C), which makes fluid supplementation desirable. Animals with polyuria resulting from renal failure also lose water-soluble vitamins and benefit from supplementation of their parenteral fluids. Recommendations for supplementation vary from 0.5 to 2 mL per liter of fluids.

Clinical Uses

Vitamin supplements are used for restoration of normal levels of the water-soluble vitamins.

Dosage Forms

Several manufacturers produce vitamin B complex. Care should be taken to ensure that the form selected may be given intravenously. Many are labeled for intramuscular or subcutaneous use only.

Adverse Side Effects

These include hypersensitivity reactions to thiamine in the complex.

ORAL ELECTROLYTE PREPARATIONS

In severely dehydrated animals, fluids must be given by the intravenous route to be effective. In mild to moderate cases of dehydration, however, the oral route is a practical alternative to replenish water and electrolytes.

Oral electrolytes are packaged as powders that are mixed with water to form a solution that can be given free choice or by stomach tube. In some instances, oral pastes or fluids packaged for intravenous use may be given orally. The oral route of administration is especially useful for cases in which the veterinarian wishes to direct the pet or livestock owner in the home or farm treatment of the animal.

Diarrhea in young dairy calves, commonly called *calf scours,* is caused by bacteria, viruses, or nutritional factors and is a condition often treated with oral electrolyte solutions. The diarrhea is commonly a result of the type or amount of milk replacer that the calf is being fed. A calf is treated by eliminating the milk replacer from its diet and by giving it an oral electrolyte solution with glucose or glycine for 24 to 48 hours. Glucose and glycine provide a source of calories and may enhance absorption of the electrolytes. The solution may be administered via an esophageal feeder—a device that has a plastic bag (for mixing the electrolyte solution) attached to a rigid delivery tube (Figure 15-15). The tube has a ball of sufficient diameter on the distal end to prevent introduction of the tube into the trachea.

Oral electrolyte solutions or pastes often are given to performance horses to replace electrolytes lost through sweating. Horses participating in endurance races, 3-day events, and other athletically demanding events benefit from electrolyte replenishment.

Administration of oral electrolyte solutions also may be helpful as a follow-up to intravenous fluid therapy for dogs recovering from viral enteritis or other diseases that cause prolonged vomiting or diarrhea. Hypokalemia in dogs and cats may be treated with oral potassium products.

Clinical Uses

These include electrolyte and water replenishment.

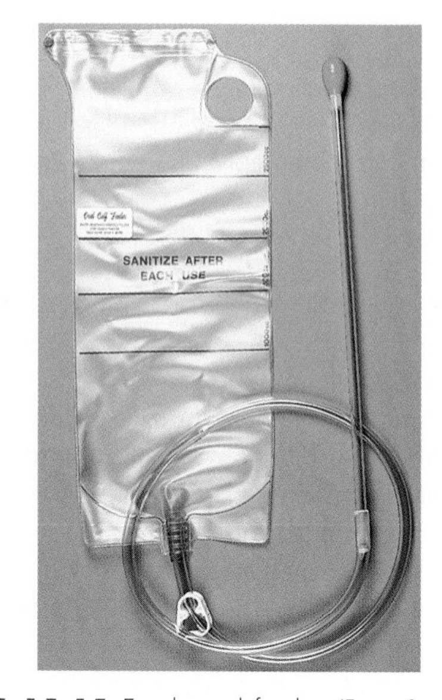

FIGURE 15-15 Esophageal feeder. (From Sonsthagen T: Veterinary instruments and equipment, St Louis, 2010, Elsevier.)

Dosage Forms

Dosage forms are numerous, and the following is only a partial listing:

- Avian Bluelite (powder)
- Calf Quencher
- Dexolyte
- Entrolyte (powder)
- Equi-Phar
- K9 Restart
- OraLyte (powder)
- Re-Sorb (powder)
- Tumil-K (powder, gel, and tablets for dogs and cats)
- Vedalyte 8× (powder)

Adverse Side Effects

These are rare if care is taken not to cause inadvertent administration into the respiratory system.

TECHNICIAN NOTES Some of the oral electrolyte products for farm animals also contain antibiotics.

PARENTERAL NUTRITION

The term *parenteral* indicates the administration of nutrients by a route other than the gastrointestinal tract. Parenteral nutrition is described in human medicine as total or partial in reference to whether all nutrient requirements are supplied. Diseased and debilitated patients require a daily intake of adequate calories and protein to maintain good immune function, tissue synthesis, and normal metabolic activities. Those patients that are unable or have no desire to eat normally may need parenteral nutrition.

The term *total parenteral nutrition* does not apply to veterinary patients because there is no need to meet the needs for all essential fatty and amino acids, fat- and water-soluble vitamins, and macro and trace minerals, as there is in people (Remillard et al., 2000). In veterinary medicine, an attempt is made to meet the animal patient's resting energy requirement and most of the requirements for amino and fatty acids and to provide some of the required vitamins and minerals.

Parenteral nutrition solutions must be compounded for the individual patient. A mixture of all required nutrients, called a ***total nutrient admixture*** (TNA), can be prepared for the veterinary patient in one fluid bag for convenience. The preparation of these solutions is beyond the scope of most veterinary clinics, but they may be available through human hospitals, veterinary schools, or specialty practices. For a list of products used in the formulation of the TNA, consult an article entitled "Parenteral Nutrition Products" by Miller and Bartges in Kirk's *Current Veterinary Therapy, XIII.*

PARENTERAL VITAMIN/MINERAL PRODUCTS

Parenteral vitamin/mineral products are used to prevent or treat various conditions in veterinary medicine. They are used as therapeutic agents in large animal medicine more often than in small animal medicine. White muscle disease, "tying up," polyneuritis, pinkeye, reproductive problems, bracken fern poisoning, and polioencephalomalacia are only a few of the conditions prevented or treated with vitamin products in large animal practice. In small animal practice, routine vitamin and mineral supplementation is not considered necessary if the animal receives a balanced diet. Many small animal clinicians regard overuse of vitamin/mineral products as a bigger problem than vitamin/mineral deficiencies. Warfarin poisoning (vitamin K) and certain dermatologic conditions (zinc) are exceptions.

Oral multivitamin/mineral products are numerous and are not listed here.

WATER-SOLUBLE VITAMINS

Vitamin B Complex

B-complex vitamins consist of a group of water-soluble vitamins that include thiamine, riboflavin, niacinamide (niacin), d-panthenol (pantothenic acid), pyridoxine, cyanocobalamin (B_{12}), biotin, choline, and folic acid. B vitamins serve as coenzymes for many metabolic reactions in the body. B complex often is added to intravenous fluids (discussed earlier) and may be given parenterally in an attempt to enhance the biochemical response of stressed or debilitated animals.

Clinical Uses

These vitamins are administered to replace or supplement a deficiency of B-complex vitamins.

Dosage Forms

- B-Complex Plus
- Vitamin B Complex
- Vitamin B Complex Fortified
- Vitamin B Complex Injectable

Adverse Side Effects

These can include allergic reactions and pain at the injection site.

TECHNICIAN NOTES

- Check the label before giving B complex intravenously.
- Observe the animal for allergic reactions.
- B-complex injections may cause pain at the injection site.

Thiamine Hydrochloride (Vitamin B_1)

Thiamine is a water-soluble B-complex vitamin that acts as a coenzyme for biochemical reactions involved in carbohydrate metabolism. Deficiency of thiamine may occur as a consequence of decreased intake or synthesis or from increased destruction, which may result from bracken fern poisoning, thiamine-destroying factors in the rumen, or thiaminase in raw fish. Polioencephalomalacia of ruminants also has been associated with thiamine deficiency.

Clinical Uses

Thiamine is administered for the treatment of thiamine deficiency in all domestic species and as an aid in the treatment of lead poisoning in cattle.

Dosage Forms

- Thia-Dex
- Thiamine Hydrochloride Injection (generic)
- Vitamin B_1 Powder

Adverse Side Effects

These may include hypersensitivity reactions and muscle soreness at intramuscular injection sites.

Cyanocobalamin (Vitamin B_{12})

Vitamin B_{12} is a B-complex vitamin that contains cobalt and is thought to act as a coenzyme in protein synthesis. Pernicious anemia is a condition that occurs in humans as the result of a failure to absorb B_{12} adequately. A deficiency in any case results in anemia because red blood cells fail to mature properly in the absence of B_{12}. B_{12} deficiencies are rare in veterinary medicine.

Clinical Uses

Vitamin B_{12} is administered for the management of B_{12} deficiencies.

Dosage Forms

- Vita-Jec Vitamin B_{12}
- Vitamin B_{12} injection

Adverse Side Effects

These may include allergic reactions to administration.

FAT-SOLUBLE VITAMINS

Vitamin A

Vitamin A is an organic alcohol that is converted from plant substances called *carotenoids* (e.g., beta carotene) in the intestine and liver and is stored primarily in the liver. It is needed for proper growth and maintenance of surface epithelium, for proper bone growth, and for maintenance of visual pigments in the retina. A deficiency of vitamin A may be associated with many clinical signs, including poor growth and reproductive performance, susceptibility to infectious disease, and poor vision in dim light. Many of the commercial vitamin A products are combined with vitamin D or E.

Clinical Uses

Vitamin A is administered for the prevention or treatment of vitamin A deficiencies.

Dosage Forms

- Vitamin A-D Injectable
- Vitamin A-D Injection
- Vita-Ject A-D 500
- Vitamin A-D

Adverse Side Effects

These are uncommon if label directions are followed.

Vitamin D

Vitamin D exists in two forms: D_2 and D_3. Vitamin D_2 is formed when a plant substance (ergosterol) is exposed to sunlight; D_3 is formed when a provitamin precalciferol in the skin is converted by sunlight. A deficiency of vitamin D is characterized by the development of rickets in young animals or osteomalacia in adults. Vitamin D often is combined commercially with vitamin A or E.

Clinical Uses

Vitamin D is administered for the treatment or prevention of vitamin D deficiencies.

Dosage Forms

Refer to the dosage forms for vitamin A.

Adverse Side Effects
These are uncommon if label directions are followed.

Vitamin E
Vitamin E (alpha-tocopherol) is involved (with selenium) in the metabolism of sulfur and acts as an antioxidant. Vitamin E is used in the prevention or treatment of selenium/vitamin E deficiency syndromes, such as white muscle disease (ewes, lambs, and calves), mulberry heart disease (sows and pigs), and myositis (horses).

Clinical Uses
Vitamin E is administered for the prevention and treatment of vitamin E deficiencies.

Dosage Forms
- Bo-Se; selenium, vitamin E injection (approved for use in calves, swine, and sheep)
- E-SE; selenium, vitamin E injection (approved for use in horses)
- Mu-Se; selenium, vitamin E injection (approved for use in nonlactating dairy cattle and beef cattle)
- L-Se; selenium, vitamin E injection (approved for use in lambs and baby pigs)
- Seletoc; selenium, vitamin E injection (approved for use in dogs)

Adverse Side Effects
These include allergic reactions and soreness at injection sites.

Vitamin K
Vitamin K is a fat-soluble vitamin required for the formation of prothrombin; for this reason, it is very important to the clotting process. Vitamin K is discussed in Chapter 18.

REVIEW QUESTIONS

1. Define hyperkalemia.
   ____
2. Intravascular fluid (plasma) makes up approximately ______________________ of body weight.
   a. 2%
   b. 5%
   c. 15%
   d. 40%
3. Explain the concept of a balanced solution for fluid therapy. ______________________
4. What are three units of measurement used for quantifying electrolytes in fluids?
   ____
5. Therapeutic fluids with an osmolality of approximately ______________________ mOsm/L are isotonic.
   a. 100
   b. 200
   c. 300
   d. 500
6. Give examples of sensible and insensible fluid losses. ______________________
7. Underestimation of the degree of dehydration is sometimes a problem in ______________________ animals.
8. One pound of fluid is equivalent to ______________________ milliliters, and 1 kg is equivalent to ______________________ milliliters.
9. The three volumes that are calculated to arrive at the total fluid therapy volume are ______________________.
10. Calculate the fluid needed for a 44-lb dog that is 6% dehydrated and is losing 100 mL of fluid daily through vomiting.
    ____
11. What drip rate should be used to deliver (over a 24-hour period) the fluid for the dog in question 10 (using a standard administration set)? ______________________

12. Describe how you would set up the first bag of fluids for the dog in question 10.
____
13. Tell how you would prepare 500 mL of 5% dextrose from a 50% stock solution.
____
14. What is the purpose of the lactate in lactated Ringer's solution? _______________
15. Describe the use of an esophageal feeder.
____
16. What type of fluid (tonicity) should not be given subcutaneously?
____
17. Give an example of a balanced solution and an example of an unbalanced solution.
____
18. _______________ is a determination of the osmotic pressure of a solution based on the relative number of solute particles in 1 kg of the solution.
19. The osmolality of dog and cat serum is approximately _______________ mOsm/L.
20. Commercial fluids with an osmolality of 300 mOsm/L are _______________.
21. How often should intravenous catheters be flushed? _______________
22. What is the longest time an IV catheter should remain in place before it is replaced?
____
23. What precaution should be observed when fluids are administered subcutaneously?
____
24. What fluid can be used to bathe tissues during surgery to prevent them from drying out?
____
25. Any product that contains the electrolyte _______________ should be given by slow IV administration to prevent cardiac complications.
26. Water represents _______________% to _______________% of the total body weight in adult animals.
   a. 10; 30
   b. 50; 70
   c. 50; 80
   d. 10; 50
27. Hyperkalemia is an excess of _______________ in the blood.
   a. Ca
   b. Ph
   c. K
   d. Cl
28. _______________ is decreased body pH caused by excess hydrogen ions in the extracellular fluid.
   a. Metabolic acidosis
   b. Metabolic alkalosis
   c. Hypernatremia
   d. Hyponatremia
29. Electrolytes with a positive charge are known as _______________.
   a. anions
   b. cations
   c. solutes
   d. ion
30. All the following may be signs of dehydration, except _______________.
   a. dry mucous membranes
   b. otitis externa
   c. reduced jugular distention (especially in horses)
   d. tachycardia
31. _______________ are solutions containing electrolyte and nonelectrolyte substances that are capable of passing through cell membranes and therefore capable of entering all body fluid compartments.
   a. Colloids
   b. Hypertonics
   c. Ca supplements
   d. Crystalloids
32. All the following statements about physiologic saline are true, except it _______________.
   a. is also called normal saline
   b. is also called isotonic saline
   c. is used to correct a sodium deficiency
   d. should not be used during surgery to bathe tissues
33. All the following statements about colloids are true, except they _______________.
   a. contain large molecular weight particles that are unable to cross cell membranes
   b. affect osmoles

c. are unable to hold fluid in the vascular space
d. are able to hold fluid in the vascular space

34. *Scours* is a medical term that is used to describe diarrhea in what species?
a. canines
b. felines
c. bovines
d. avians

35. Vitamin A is an organic alcohol that is converted from plant substances called *carotenoids* in the intestine and liver and is stored primarily in the ______________________. It is needed for maintenance of visual pigments in the retina.
a. liver
b. pancreas
c. stomach
d. intestines

Use Figure 15-5 and information provided to answer the remaining questions.

36. An adult dog weighing 44 lb needs maintenance fluids given. What is the volume of fluids needed for one day? What is the drip rate in drops/minute?

____

37. What volume of fluid is needed for 1 day for an 11-lb cat that is 5% dehydrated? What flow rate in mL/h would you use?

____

38. An 88-lb dog is seen with vomiting and diarrhea with 7% dehydration. The estimated fluid loss as vomitus and diarrhea is 200 mL/day. What is the fluid volume needed for a 24-hour period? What drip rate in gtt/s would you use to administer one fourth of the total volume over a 4-hour period?

____

39. What is the fluid volume needed for 1 day for a 9-lb puppy that is 5% dehydrated and losing 50 mL per day as diarrhea? What flow rate in mL/h would you use?

____

40. What is the fluid volume needed for 24 hours for a 220-lb dog that is seen with 10% dehydration and no ongoing fluid loss? What flow rate would you use in gtt/s to deliver one fourth of the total volume over a 12-hour period? ______________________________

REFERENCES

Blankenship J, Campbell JB: Solutions. In Blankenship J, Campbell JB, editors: Laboratory mathematics: medical and biological applications, St. Louis, 1976, Mosby.

Crowe DT: Emergency medicine, in Proceedings. Tenn Vet Med Assoc Annu Conf, Brentwood, Tenn, 2007.

Haskins SC: Fluid overload: how to identify and manage, in Proceedings. Int Vet Emerg Crit Care Symp, Orlando, Fla, 2000.

Plumb DC: Veterinary Drug Handbook, ed 7, Ames, Iowa, 2011, Wiley-Blackwell.

Remillard RL, Armstrong PJ, Davenport DJ: Assisted feeding in hospitalized patients: enteral and parenteral nutrition. In Hand MS, Thatcher CD, Remillard RL, et al, editors: Small animal clinical nutrition, Marceline, Mo, 2000, Walsworth Publishing Co.

Rudloff, E. Fluid therapy series: colloids in-depth. http://abbottanimalhealthce.com/. Accessed February 24, 2013.

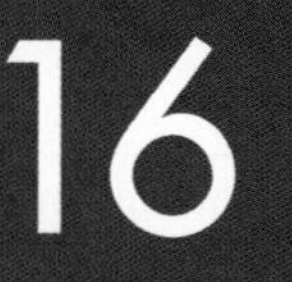

CHAPTER 16

Blood-Modifying, Antineoplastic, and Immunosuppressant Drugs

KEY TERMS

Alkylation
Cell cycle–nonspecific
Cell cycle–specific
Cytotoxic
Disseminated intravascular coagulation (DIC)
Endothelial layer
Erythropoietin
Fibrinolysis
Hybridoma
Metastasis
Myeloma
Myelosuppression
Thrombocytopenia
Thromboembolism
Thrombus
Vesicant

OUTLINE

LEARNING OBJECTIVES

After studying this chapter, you should be able to

1. Explain the role of erythropoietin in red blood cell formation.
2. Describe the significance of iron in the hemoglobin molecule.
3. Give an example of iron deficiency anemia that occurs in veterinary medicine.
4. List the potential indications for and limitations of hematinics and oxygen-carrying solutions.
5. Describe the clotting mechanism in general terms.
6. List four anticoagulants and discuss their methods of action.
7. List examples of topical hemostatics.
8. Name the antagonist for heparin overdose.
9. List the indications for the use of vitamin K_1 and discuss the possible adverse side effects of its use.

10. Define fibrinolysis and name a fibrinolytic agent.
11. Describe the phases of the cell cycle.
12. List six categories of antineoplastic drugs and give an example of each.
13. Define *biologic response modifier* (BRM) and list two examples of BRMs.
14. List indications for the use of immunosuppressive drugs and provide five examples.
15. Discuss the safety precautions involved in the use of antineoplastic drugs.

INTRODUCTION

In the first section of this chapter, drugs or agents that influence blood formation or its processes (e.g., clotting and **fibrinolysis**) such as hematinics, anticoagulants, anticoagulant antagonists/hemostatics, and fibrinolytic agents are discussed. Because anticoagulants are used routinely in veterinary practice, veterinary technicians should have a complete working knowledge of their applications and their potential misuse.

The second section covers antineoplastic and immunosuppressant drugs. Antineoplastic drug categories include alkylating agents, antimetabolites, mitotic inhibitors (vinca alkaloids), antibiotics, hormones, and miscellaneous agents. Safe handling techniques for these potentially dangerous agents are listed. Select immunosuppressant drugs and their clinical applications are discussed at the conclusion of this section.

BLOOD-MODIFYING DRUGS/AGENTS

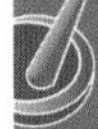

HEMATINICS

Red blood cells are formed in the bone marrow in response to stimulation by **erythropoietin,** a chemical released by the kidneys when hypoxia is present in this organ (Ganong, 2003) (Figure 16-1). Their primary function is to carry oxygen to the tissues. This activity is greatly enhanced by the hemoglobin component of red blood cells. Only a small portion of oxygen is carried in solution in the plasma.

Hemoglobin is made up of a protein and an iron-containing pigment (Figure 16-2). The iron in

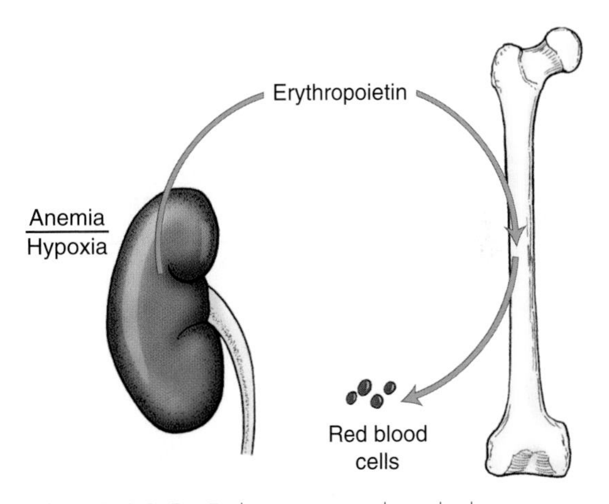

FIGURE 16-1 Erythropoietin stimulates the bone marrow to produce red blood cells.

hemoglobin must be in the ferrous (Fe^{2+}) state to combine with oxygen in the most efficient way. If the iron in hemoglobin is in the ferric (Fe^{3+}) state, hemoglobin cannot combine with oxygen and is called *methemoglobin.* Adequate amounts of iron, cobalt, copper, B vitamins, trace minerals, and protein are needed for normal hemoglobin and red blood cell formation.

Anemia can result from excessive loss of red blood cells, formation of inadequate numbers of red blood cells, or inadequate amounts of hemoglobin in the red blood cells. Iron deficiency anemia, a relatively common form in humans, is rare in animals that consume balanced diets. One exception, however, is baby pig anemia, a condition that results from inadequate assimilation of iron from the placenta of the sow for future hemoglobin formation by the piglet. The piglet is born without adequate stores of iron for

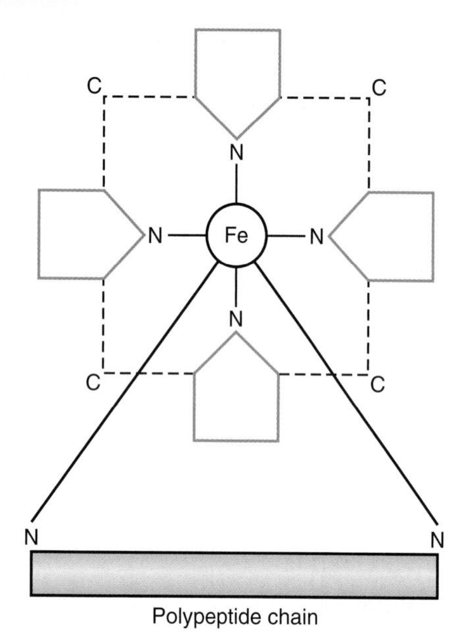

FIGURE 16-2 The structure of hemoglobin.

its rapid growth phase, and sow's milk is relatively low in this element. Baby pig anemia is a problem of pigs raised in confined environments (concrete or slatted floors) because those raised outdoors usually obtain adequate iron from the soil.

Hematinics are substances that tend to promote an increase in the oxygen-carrying capacity of the blood. Hematinics are used to prevent or treat anemia, and the primary ingredient in most of these products is iron, a vital component of hemoglobin. Some also contain copper and B vitamins to enhance red blood cell formation. The response to hematinic administration is relatively slow, and this factor makes use of hematinics ancillary to whole blood transfusion in acute anemia.

Iron Compounds

Many injectable and oral iron preparations are available for veterinary use under generic and proprietary labels. The form of iron in these products may be iron dextran, ferrous sulfate, peptonized iron, gleptoferron, ferric hydroxide, and others, and the form apparently has little effect on use. Copper, B vitamins, liver fraction (an iron source), and palatability enhancers often are also added to the oral products. Injectable forms are labeled for intramuscular injection and contain only iron. They may cause discoloration of muscle tissue at the site of injection.

Clinical Uses

Iron compounds are used for prevention or treatment of baby pig anemia or as a nutritional aid, depending on the form.

Dosage Forms

- Iron dextran complex
- FerroSul
- Ferrous Sulfate Oral Elixir
- CosmoFer
- Lixotinic
- Pet Tinic
- Gleptosil

Adverse Side Effects

These are rare but may include muscle weakness, prostration, or muscle discoloration.

> *TECHNICIAN NOTES* Pork quality assurance programs often recommend that iron injections be given in neck muscle rather than in the ham (a higher quality cut) because of potential meat staining and subsequent condemnation.

Erythropoietin

Erythropoietin, a protein produced in the kidneys, stimulates the division and differentiation of committed erythroid precursors in the bone marrow. A synthetic product, Epogen, has the same properties as erythropoietin and is available commercially. It is approved for human use and is produced by recombinant DNA technology. It is labeled for the treatment of anemia related to chronic renal failure or for that associated with azidothymidine treatment in patients with human immunodeficiency virus infection. No veterinary-approved product is available.

Clinical Uses

Erythropoietin is used in dogs and cats for the treatment of anemia associated with chronic renal failure or other causes.

Dosage Forms

- Epogen
- Procrit
- Epoetin Alfa for Injection
- Darbepoetin alfa (Aranesp)

Adverse Side Effects

In humans, adverse side effects may include hypertension, iron deficiency, polycythemia, and seizures. The use of human-coded proteins in dogs or cats could potentially cause allergic reactions.

Androgens

The treatment for anemia associated with chronic renal failure has traditionally been androgen therapy. Results obtained with the use of androgens for chronic anemia have been inconsistent.

Clinical Uses

Androgens are used for the treatment of chronic (nonregenerative) anemia.

Dosage Forms

- Winstrol-V
- Equipoise

Adverse Side Effects

These have included enlargement of the prostate, hepatic toxicity, and sodium and water retention.

Blood Substitutes

Researchers have looked for an oxygen-carrying substitute for red blood cells practically since it was learned that the hemoglobin in those cells was the transporting vehicle.

Oxyglobin is a red blood cell substitute that consists of a polymerized bovine product with a hemoglobin concentration of 13 g/dL in a modified lactated Ringer's solution. This solution has obvious benefits over blood products that include availability, a long shelf life, universal compatibility, and freedom from disease-producing agents.

This hemoglobin solution picks up and distributes oxygen in a manner similar to red blood cells, but the oxygen-carrying function is shifted to cross-linked hemoglobin molecules in the plasma. Because oxygen is carried by molecules in the plasma, diffusion of this gas across cell membranes occurs more efficiently than when it is carried by red blood cells because one fewer membrane must be crossed.

This product is stable for 3 years when unwrapped at room temperature or in the refrigerator but it should not be frozen. Once the wrapper has been removed, the product must be used within 24 hours. It is compatible with any other IV fluid, but other solutions should not be mixed in the same bag. A separate line should be used for these other solutions. No consideration is needed regarding blood typing or crossmatching when this product is used.

Oxyglobin also has osmotic properties similar to dextran 70 and hetastarch.

Clinical Uses

This product is labeled for the treatment of anemia in dogs regardless of the cause. It has been used in cats and foals but is not labeled for such use.

Dosage Form

- Oxyglobin (hemoglobin glutamer-200)

Adverse Side Effects

Potential side effects include pulmonary edema, discolored urine, discolored membranes, ventricular arrhythmias, fever, and coagulopathy. Oxyglobin can cause volume overload or vasoconstriction and should not be used in patients with cardiac or renal disease.

> **TECHNICIAN NOTES**
> - The recommended administration rate should not be exceeded.
> - Do not administer with other fluids or drugs through the same intravenous set.
> - Do not combine with other fluids in the same bag.

ANTICOAGULANTS

Blood coagulation is an obviously essential process that is designed to inhibit the loss of vital blood constituents from the circulatory system. Two separate systems or pathways may initiate the clotting mechanism—the intrinsic (intravascular) and extrinsic (extravascular) systems.

The intrinsic pathway is activated by injury to the **endothelial layer** of a blood vessel, which disrupts blood flow and causes a chain of chemical reactions leading to a **thrombus,** or clot. This process helps to repair damage to blood vessel walls that occurs from routine wear and from pathologic processes.

The extrinsic pathway is activated by injury to tissue and vessels, which release tissue thromboplastin. Thromboplastin stimulates the clotting mechanism. Vasoconstriction occurs in damaged blood vessels, causing a slowing of blood flow and facilitating clot formation. Platelet aggregation and adherence are also important steps in the clotting process.

The intrinsic and extrinsic pathways converge into a common pathway in the final steps of clot formation (Figure 16-3). At least 13 clotting factors participate in this series of reactions (called a *cascade*) in which the product of the preceding reaction promotes the next reaction (Table 16-1). The final step in the process is the conversion of fibrinogen to fibrin by thrombin. If any of the clotting factors in the

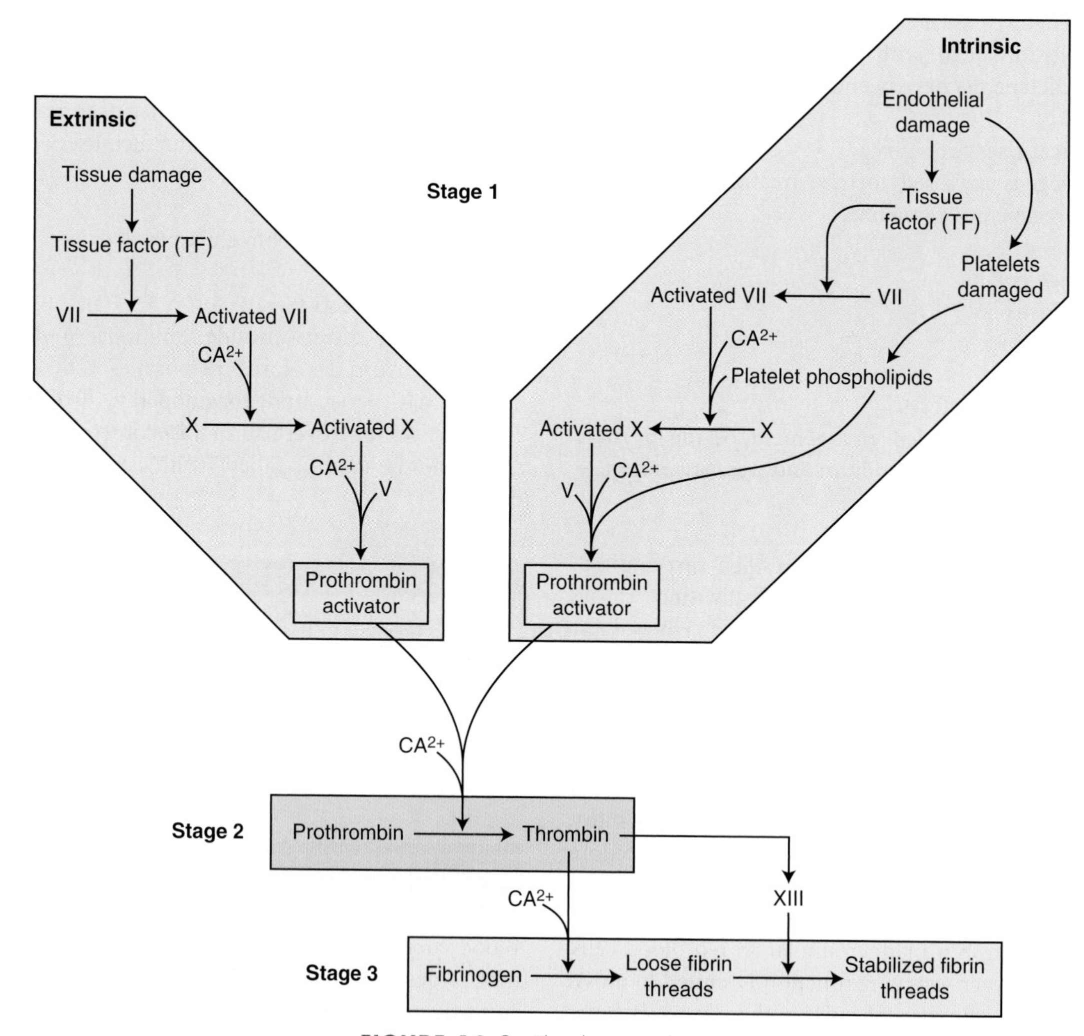

FIGURE 16-3 The clotting pathways.

TABLE 16-1 The Clotting Factors

COAGULATION FACTOR	SYNONYM
I	Fibrinogen
II	Prothrombin
III	Tissue factor (thromboplastin)
IV	Calcium ions
V	Proaccelerin, labile factor, or accelerator globulin
VI	Activated factor V
VII	Serum prothrombin conversion accelerator (SPCA), stable factor, or proconvertin
VIII	Antihemophilic factor (AHF), antihemophilic factor A, or antihemophilic globulin factor B
IX	Christmas factor, plasma thromboplastin component (PTC), or antihemophilic factor B
X	Stuart-Prower factor, thrombokinase
XI	Plasma thromboplastin antecedent (PTA) or antihemophilic factor C
XII	Hageman factor, glass factor, or contact factor
XIII	Fibrin-stabilizing factor (FSF) or fibrinase

cascade are deficient or missing, clotting does not occur.

A balance must be maintained in the body between clot formation and clot breakdown. Destruction of clots—fibrinolysis—occurs through the action of an enzyme called *plasmin.* Plasmin digests fibrin threads and other clotting products to cause clot lysis and the release of fibrin degradation products into the circulation.

Anticoagulants inhibit clot formation by tying up or inactivating one of the clotting factors to interrupt the cascade reaction. They are used clinically to prevent coagulation of blood (or other body fluid) samples that are collected for testing, to preserve blood for transfusions, to inhibit clotting in intravenous catheters, and to prevent or treat thromboembolic disorders (e.g., thromboembolic cardiomyopathy in cats).

Heparin may be used paradoxically to treat the bleeding disorder **disseminated intravascular coagulation (DIC).**

Heparin

Heparin is an anticoagulant that is found in many tissues of the body and is thought to be stored in mast cells. It is obtained from pig intestinal mucosa, and its strength is expressed in terms of heparin units. Heparin acts as an anticoagulant by preventing the conversion of prothrombin (factor II) to thrombin. Without thrombin, fibrinogen is not converted to fibrin and a clot does not form. Heparin does not break down clots but can prevent clots from increasing in size. It is administered therapeutically by intravenous or subcutaneous injection.

Clinical Uses

Heparin has various uses in veterinary medicine. It is used in vitro as an anticoagulant to preserve blood samples for testing by heparinizing (drawing heparin into the syringe and then forcing all visible quantities out) a syringe before the blood sample is drawn. It also is diluted in saline or sterile water for injection to form a flush solution for preventing clots in intravenous catheters. Heparin is sometimes used to preserve donated blood for transfusions when small quantities are needed (e.g., for cats or small dogs). It is used in vivo to aid in the treatment of DIC and **thromboembolism** and has been advocated for the treatment of laminitis in horses.

Dosage Forms

Forms approved for use in humans are used in veterinary medicine:

- Heparin sodium injection, 1000 U/mL
- Hep-Lock flush solution (10 or 100 U/mL)

Adverse Side Effects

These usually manifest as bleeding or **thrombocytopenia.**

TECHNICIAN NOTES

- Heparin should not be used as an anticoagulant when blood is collected for performing a differential count because white blood cell morphology may be adversely affected.

- A heparin flush solution may be prepared by diluting heparin in saline at a concentration of 5 U/mL (Crow et al., 1987).
- Approximately 750 U of heparin should be drawn into a 60-mL syringe to act as an anticoagulant when blood is collected for transfusion (Norsworthy, 1992).
- Heparin blood collection tubes have a green top.
- Protamine sulfate is the antidote for heparin overdose.

Ethylenediaminetetraacetic Acid

Ethylenediaminetetraacetic acid (EDTA) is an anticoagulant that prevents clotting by chelation of calcium (factor IV). With calcium ions tied up by EDTA, clotting cannot occur. It is used in vitro to preserve blood samples and is the anticoagulant of choice when a differential count is needed (it preserves white cell morphology well). EDTA is prepared in lavender-topped collection tubes.

The calcium salt of EDTA (calcium disodium versenate) is also used in vivo as a chelating agent to treat lead poisoning. This function does not involve the clotting mechanism (see Chapter 18).

Coumarin Derivatives

Coumarin derivatives such as dicumarol and warfarin are oral anticoagulants that bind vitamin K, therefore inhibiting the synthesis of prothrombin (factor II) and factors VII, IX, and X. These compounds are indicated for long-term treatment of thromboembolic conditions. They are used clinically to a greater extent in human medicine than in veterinary medicine.

Dicumarol may be found in moldy sweet clover and has been associated with fatal hemorrhagic disease in cattle. Warfarin and related compounds are used in many rat poisoning products.

Clinical Uses

Coumarin derivatives are used for the long-term management of thromboembolic conditions.

Dosage Form

- Coumadin tablets or injection
- Jantoven

Adverse Side Effects

Adverse side effects are related to hemorrhages.

TECHNICIAN NOTES Vitamin K_1 is the antidote for warfarin or dicumarol toxicity.

Acid Citrate Dextrose Solution and Citrate Phosphate Dextrose Adenine

Acid citrate dextrose (ACD) solution contains dextrose, sodium citrate, and citric acid and prevents clotting by chelating calcium. It is prepared in bottles or plastic bags for blood collection under both veterinary and human labels. Bottles are available for collecting 250 and 500 mL of blood. ACD solution preserves blood for 3 to 4 weeks.

Citrate phosphate dextrose adenine (CPDA-1) solution is available in plastic bags for collection of 450 mL of blood. CPDA-1 also prevents clotting by chelating calcium and preserves blood for as long as 6 weeks.

Eight milliliters of ACD or CPDA-1 can be drawn into a syringe to collect 50 mL of blood when small quantities are needed (Norsworthy, 1992).

Antiplatelet Drugs

Antiplatelet drugs such as aspirin appear to impair clotting through inhibition of platelet stickiness and clumping. This activity is thought to be mediated through inhibition of the proaggregatory prostaglandin called *thromboxane* (Pugh, 1991).

Aspirin has been used both to prevent thromboembolism associated with heartworm treatment in dogs and to treat cardiomyopathy in cats.

HEMOSTATICS/ANTICOAGULANT ANTAGONISTS

Substances that promote blood clotting—hemostatics—may be divided into two categories: (1) those applied topically and (2) those given parenterally.

Topical Agents

Topical agents act by providing a framework in which a clot may form or by coagulating blood protein to initiate clot formation. Framework substances used in topical hemostatics include gelatins and collagens, whereas styptics, hemostatic powders, and solutions are substances that initiate clotting through coagulation. The framework substances are absorbed after clot formation. Topical hemostatics are used to control capillary bleeding or bleeding from other small vessels.

Clinical Uses
These include the control of capillary bleeding at surgical sites or in superficial wounds.

Dosage Forms
- Gelfoam absorbable gelatin sponge
- Hemopad Absorbable Collagen Hemostat
- Surgicel Absorbable Hemostat
- Hemostat Powder (ferrous sulfate powder)
- Clotisol (ferric sulfate)
- Silver nitrate sticks
- Thrombogen topical thrombin solution
- Celox; Celox granules represent a new generation of hemostatic agents. Celox is made of chitosan, a natural polysaccharide that is broken down by naturally occurring enzymes. Celox granules are reported to control bleeding in hypothermic conditions and in heparinized blood.
- QuikClot Gauze Dressings; QuikClot gauze dressings are kaolin-impregnated gauze dressings used to control traumatic bleeding in conjunction with compression.

Adverse Side Effects
These are usually minimal but may include delayed wound healing.

Parenteral Agents
Parenterally administered hemostatic agents act as anticoagulant antagonists because they do not directly activate clotting. These substances promote the synthesis of clotting factors that have been depleted through poisoning or disease, or they tie up (inactivate) anticoagulants that have been overdosed. These drugs are not used to control surgical or traumatic bleeding.

Protamine Sulfate
Protamine sulfate is a protein that is produced from the sperm or testes of salmon or related species (Plumb, 2011). Protamine has a strongly basic pH, and heparin has a strongly acidic pH. Protamine combines with heparin to form inactive complexes (salt).

Clinical Uses
Protamine sulfate is used for the treatment of heparin overdose. Slow intravenous administration is recommended.

Dosage Form
- Protamine sulfate injection, USP

Adverse Side Effects
Hypotension and bradycardia can occur if given too rapidly.

Vitamin K_1 (Phytonadione)
Phytonadione is a synthetic substance that is identical to naturally occurring vitamin K_1. Vitamin K is necessary for the production (in the liver) of active prothrombin (factor II), proconvertin factor (factor VII), plasma thromboplastin component (factor IX), and Stuart factor (factor X). It is used clinically for treating cases in which vitamin K has been tied up or destroyed and in bleeding disorders associated with poor formation of vitamin K–dependent clotting factors. Immediate coagulant effect should not be expected after administration of vitamin K because several hours may pass before synthesis of new clotting factors occurs.

Clinical Uses
In veterinary medicine, vitamin K_1 is used for the treatment of rodenticide toxicity, for bleeding disorders related to faulty synthesis of vitamin K–dependent clotting factors, and for unknown anticoagulant toxicity.

Dosage Forms
- Aqua-Mephyton (human label)
- Konakion (human label)
- Vita-Jec

Adverse Side Effects
These include anaphylactoid reactions (intravenous use) and bleeding at the injection site.

TECHNICIAN NOTES Because of the possibility of anaphylactoid reactions, many consider intravenous administration of phytonadione to be contraindicated.

Aminocaproic Acid

Aminocaproic acid inhibits fibrinolysis through its effects on plasminogen activator and possibly via antiplasmin activity. It may be used to inhibit bleeding in certain conditions like thrombocytopenia. It is contraindicated in patients with active intravascular clotting.

Dosage Form

- Amicar

FIBRINOLYTIC (THROMBOLYTIC) DRUGS

Thrombolytic drugs are used to break down or dissolve thrombi. Occlusion of an artery by a thromboembolus can cause necrosis of tissue distal to the blockage if the obstruction is not removed quickly. In humans, damage to heart muscle that occurs when a coronary artery is occluded in a heart attack is a classic example of this process. Pulmonary thromboemboli sometimes occur in dogs after heartworm treatment and may accompany cardiomyopathy in cats.

Thrombolytic agents may help to remove or reduce the size of the occluding thromboembolus and minimize tissue damage. This action is brought about by stimulating conversion of plasminogen to the enzyme plasmin, which lyses the clots. The sooner the therapy is initiated after thromboembolism has occurred, the better the chances of success. Thrombolytic activity of one of the products (alteplase) is activated by the presence of fibrin so that recent clots are targeted.

The expense of these drugs often precludes their use in veterinary medicine.

Clinical Uses

Clinical uses include treatment of pulmonary embolism, treatment of arterial thrombosis and emboli, treatment of coronary thrombosis, and intravenous catheter clearance.

Dosage Forms

- Streptokinase (Streptase)
- Urokinase (Abbokinase)
- Alteplase (Activase)

Adverse Side Effects

These are related to bleeding episodes, especially if anticoagulants have also been used.

ANTINEOPLASTIC DRUGS

Antineoplastic drugs are administered to animals in an attempt to cure or lessen the effect of neoplasms. Neoplasia is the abnormal growth of tissue into a mass that is not responsive to normal cellular control mechanisms. The term *tumor* by definition indicates any tissue mass or swelling that may or may not be neoplastic. *Tumor* is often used broadly in common discussion to indicate a neoplasm. A neoplasm may be benign or malignant. In general, benign tumors (neoplasms) do not cause high mortality because they grow locally and do not invade adjacent tissue. These tumors may cause morbidity, however, by compressing or occluding organs. The term *cancer* is used to indicate a malignant neoplasm that is capable of causing destruction of the tissue of origin and is also capable of **metastasis** to other tissue. Malignant tumors are very damaging to tissue and often lead to the death of the patient if treatment is not provided. A third type of neoplasm is an in situ tumor, which is a small tumor in epithelial tissue that appears to contain cancer cells but does not cross the basement membrane and invade adjacent tissue. Treatment of neoplasia involves several methods, including the use of drugs (chemotherapy), surgery, radiation, and immune modulation. Regardless of the method used, the goals of treatment are to keep the neoplasia under control, increase survival time, and improve the quality of life of the patient.

If one is to understand the use of chemotherapy drugs, a basic understanding of cancer formation is in order. Cancer has been called a "complex mutagenic disease" (Withrow and Vail, 2007) in which genetic mutations give a cell or cells the ability to

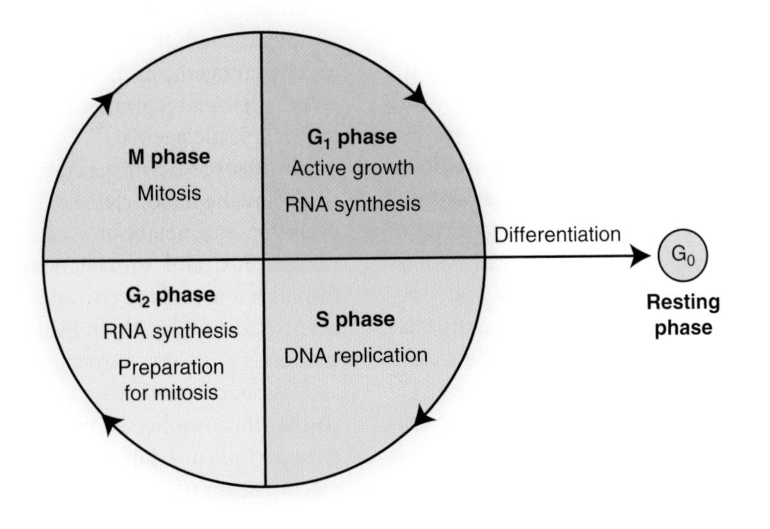

FIGURE 16-4 The cell cycle.

replicate in an unlimited way (initiation), form a mass of cells (promotion), and invade adjacent tissue (progression). Oncologists speculate that five to six genetic mutations are the minimum number that must occur to give a cell the six fundamental characteristics of cancer. These six characteristics are (1) self-sufficiency in the production of cell growth signals, (2) insensitivity to antigrowth signals, (3) the ability to evade programmed cell death (apoptosis), (4) unlimited potential to replicate, (5) sustained ability to promote angiogenesis (blood vessel formation for the cancer mass), and (6) the capacity to invade tissue and metastasize.

Several mechanisms are thought to be involved in the production of the six hallmarks of cancer. Proto-oncogenes are genetic elements in all normal cells that are capable of causing cancer if they are enhanced through abnormal regulation. The ability of the cancer cell to replicate in an unlimited way may be facilitated by activation or upregulation of an enzyme called *telomerase.* Defects in suppressor oncogenes or antioncogenes like the *p53* gene may take away the ability to control the normal cell cycle. Factors that may promote the mechanisms leading to cancer include viruses and chemical, physical, and hormonal influences.

PRINCIPLES OF CHEMOTHERAPY

Proliferating cells, whether they are found in normal tissue or in neoplasms, contain resting and dividing cells that are involved in phases of the cell cycle (Figure 16-4). These phases of the cell cycle include the S phase (DNA synthesis), the M phase (mitosis), the G1 and G2 phases (RNA synthesis), and the G0 (resting) phase. Chemotherapy can be directed toward a specific phase of the cell cycle or can be cycle nonspecific. Chemotherapy is most effective against rapidly growing tumors because actively dividing cells are more sensitive to DNA damage and cell cycle processes (Withrow & Vail, 2007). All rapidly dividing cells like those found in the bone marrow, gastrointestinal tract, reproductive organs, and hair follicles are affected by antineoplastic drugs. Chemotherapy may be used to treat a tumor with a known sensitivity to a drug or drugs, to make cancer cells more sensitive to radiation or other therapy methods, to reduce or eliminate metastases, to reduce tumor size for the purpose of relieving pain or improving function, and to reduce tumor size to facilitate surgical removal.

The effectiveness of chemotherapy depends on many factors. One of the most important is the length of time that a tumor is exposed to an effective dose of the drug. Another significant factor is the development of specific resistance to a drug by the tumor. A traditional way of using chemotherapy is to give the maximum tolerated dose (MTD) for the shortest time possible. Most of these drugs are dosed on the basis of estimated body surface area (Table 16-2). Many oncologists believe that accuracy of dosing is improved if the dosage is based on body weight rather than surface area for cats and dogs weighing less than 10 kg. Another way of giving chemotherapy drugs is by a frequent low dose over a longer time (metronomic method).

Chemotherapy drugs are often given in combinations to increase their overall effectiveness. Different tumors are treated with specific combinations of drugs at doses, durations, and intervals determined by carefully designed treatment protocols. Chemotherapy agents indiscriminately target rapidly dividing cells and often have a high therapeutic index. Consequently, toxicity is a possibility and side effects are often seen. The side effects can be self-limiting, but constant monitoring of the patient for persistent and/or severe toxic side effects is indicated. Side effects are most often related to the gastrointestinal and hemopoietic systems. Anorexia, nausea, vomiting, and diarrhea may be seen soon after treatment is started because of effects on the chemoreceptor trigger zone (CRTZ), or 3 to 5 days later because of injury to gastrointestinal epithelium. Bone marrow depression **(myelosuppression)** also may occur, resulting in a moderate to severe reduction in circulating neutrophils and/or platelets. Dogs with continuously growing hair like poodles, terriers, and Old English Sheepdogs may lose their hair as a result of chemotherapy. Cats may lose their whiskers and guard hairs. Other side effects may include cystitis, cardiomyopathy, anaphylactic reactions, and tissue damage due to extravasation of the drug(s). Many chemotherapy drugs are **vesicants** that cause inflammation and potential sloughing of tissue if leakage outside the vein occurs when the agents are administered. Some protocols call for pretreatment of the patient with drugs like antihistamines, steroids, antiemetics, and analgesics to reduce the severity of side effects.

Great care should be taken to prevent accidental exposure to chemotherapy drugs by technicians, veterinarians, and other employees because of the ability of these drugs to be teratogenic, mutagenic, and carcinogenic at therapeutic doses. Box 16-1 provides a list of recommendations for the safe use of antineoplastic agents.

Antineoplastic drugs have been categorized into the following major classes: alkylating agents, anthracyclines, antimetabolites, antitubulin agents, corticosteroids, and miscellaneous agents. Table 16-3 provides a list of the commonly used antineoplastic agents, as well as their indications, toxicities, and dosages.

Cancer chemotherapy can be a long, emotional, costly, and complicated process. Patients may experience periods of relapse and remission, harmful drug reactions can occur, and treatments can fail. Technicians should be prepared to counsel owners about the potential risks and the high level of commitment they will need to see the process through to completion. They should be able to make the animal owner aware that successful treatment can mean a longer and/or a better quality of life for their pet and a strengthening of the human–companion animal bond.

ALKYLATING AGENTS

Alkylating agents are **cell cycle–nonspecific** drugs that are able to cross-link strands of DNA to change its structure and inhibit its replication. This brings protein synthesis and cell division to a halt; cell death often follows.

Clinical Uses

Clinical uses include treatment of various neoplastic disorders, including lymphoproliferative neoplasms, osteosarcoma, hemangiosarcoma, and squamous cell carcinoma, and treatment of certain immune-mediated diseases (immunosuppression).

Dosage Forms

- Cytoxan, cyclophosphamide injection
- Leukeran, chlorambucil tablets
- Alkeran, melphalan tablets
- Nitrosoureas, lomustine, and carmustine
- Dacarbazine
- Ifex, ifosfamide

TABLE 16-2 Body Surface Area Conversion Charts (Body Weight in kg to m^2)

KG	M²	KG	M²	KG	M²
Weight to Body Surface Area Conversion Chart—Dogs					
0.5	0.064	17.0	0.668	34.0	1.060
1.0	0.101	18.0	0.694	35.0	1.081
2.0	0.160	19.0	0.719	36.0	1.101
3.0	0.210	20.0	0.744	37.0	1.121
4.0	0.255	21.0	0.769	38.0	1.142
5.0	0.295	22.0	0.785	39.0	1.162
6.0	0.333	23.0	0.817	40.0	1.181
7.0	0.370	24.0	0.840	41.0	1.201
8.0	0.404	25.0	0.864	42.0	1.220
9.0	0.437	26.0	0.886	43.0	1.240
10.0	0.469	27.0	0.909	44.0	1.259
11.0	0.500	28.0	0.931	45.0	1.278
12.0	0.529	29.0	0.953	46.0	1.297
13.0	0.553	30.0	0.975	47.0	1.302
14.0	0.581	31.0	0.997	48.0	1.334
15.0	0.608	32.0	1.018	49.0	1.352
16.0	0.641	33.0	1.029	50.0	1.371
Weight to Body Surface Area Conversion Chart—Cats					
0.1	0.022	3.0	0.208	6.8	0.360
0.2	0.034	3.2	0.217	7.0	0.366
0.3	0.045	3.4	0.226	7.2	0.373
0.4	0.054	3.6	0.235	7.4	0.380
0.5	0.063	3.8	0.244	7.6	0.387
0.6	0.071	4.0	0.252	7.8	0.393
0.7	0.079	4.2	0.260	8.0	0.400
0.8	0.086	4.4	0.269	8.2	0.407
0.9	0.093	4.6	0.277	8.4	0.413
1.0	0.100	4.8	0.285	8.6	0.420
1.2	0.113	5.0	0.292	8.8	0.426
1.4	0.125	5.2	0.300	9.0	0.433
1.6	0.137	5.4	0.307	9.2	0.439
1.8	0.148	5.6	0.315	9.4	0.445
2.0	0.159	5.8	0.323	9.6	0.452
2.2	0.169	6.0	0.330	9.8	0.458
2.4	0.179	6.2	0.337	10.0	0.464
2.6	0.189	6.4	0.345		
2.8	0.199	6.6	0.352		

From Withrow SJ, Vail DM: Withrow & MacEwan's small animal clinical oncology, ed 4, St. Louis, 2007, Saunders.

BOX 16-1 Chemotherapy Safety Recommendations

SAFETY ISSUE	RECOMMENDATIONS
To minimize the risk of topical contamination	• Wear approved chemotherapy administration gloves. Latex examination gloves are not impermeable to chemotherapeutic agents. If chemotherapy administration gloves are not available, double-glove with latex examination gloves. • Wear a nonabsorbent chemotherapy administration gown or, at minimum, wear a buttoned-up laboratory coat. • Do not push air bubbles out of the syringe. • The use of commercially available chemotherapy dispensing systems (e.g., PhaSeal) can decrease the risk of exposure. • Use safety goggles or other protective eyewear.
To avoid the oral route of contamination	• Never eat or drink in the chemotherapy administration room. • Never smoke or apply makeup in the chemotherapy administration room. • Never store chemotherapeutic drugs with food or other drugs. • Caution clients (and veterinary staff) always to wear gloves when administering chemotherapeutic drugs by the oral route.
Chemotherapy waste disposal	• Separate chemotherapy waste from other sharps and biohazards, including needles, syringes, catheters, gloves, and masks. • Contact a local human hospital for aid in disposal of all chemotherapy-associated waste.
Precautions for patient care and cleanup (although the amount of active drug eliminated from the patient is minimal, it is prudent to take precautions)	• Chemotherapeutic drugs are excreted in feces and urine: wear chemotherapy gloves when cleaning up after patients for 48 hours after drug administration. • No guidelines have been established for the disposal of pet waste; however, caution clients about cleaning up after their pets. If the patient urinates or defecates inside the home within 48 hours of receiving chemotherapy, owners should wear gloves to clean up waste and should double-bag all waste.

From Withrow SJ, Vail DM: Withrow & MacEwan's small animal clinical oncology, ed 4, St. Louis, 2007, Saunders.

Adverse Side Effects

Adverse side effects of the alkylating agents may include neutropenia, nephrotoxicity, thrombocytopenia, vomiting, and hemorrhagic cystitis.

TECHNICIAN NOTES Cyclophosphamide is also used as an immunosuppressant.

ANTHRACYCLINES

Many of the anthracycline antineoplastic agents are derived from soil fungi of the *Streptomyces* genus. They are cell cycle–nonspecific and exert their effects by binding with DNA and interfering with RNA and protein synthesis. Doxorubicin is the most commonly used drug in this class in veterinary medicine. It is widely used for various neoplastic conditions.

Clinical Uses

These agents are used for the treatment of lymphoproliferative neoplasms and various carcinomas and sarcomas.

Dosage Forms

- Adriamycin, doxorubicin hydrochloride for injection

TABLE 16-3 Commonly Used Chemotherapeutic Drugs

DRUG	MAIN INDICATIONS	TOXICITIES	DOSAGE
Alkylating Agents			
Cyclophosphamide	Lymphoma, carcinoma, sarcoma	Marrow, gastrointestinal (GI) tract, sterile hemorrhagic cystitis	Given orally (PO) or intravenously (IV); many dosing regimens can be used, depending on concurrent anticancer drugs
Chlorambucil	Lymphoma, chronic lymphocytic leukemia, mast cell tumor, IgM myeloma Substitute for cyclophosphamide if hemorrhagic cystitis occurs.	Mild marrow toxicity	Given PO only; many dosing regimens can be used, depending on concurrent anticancer drugs
CCNU (lomustine)	Relapsed lymphoma or mast cell tumor, brain tumor	Myelosuppression and idiosyncratic, potentially fatal hepatotoxicity	Dogs: 60–90 mg/m^2 PO every 3 weeks Cats: 50–60 mg/m^2 PO every 3–6 weeks
Dacarbazine	Lymphoma	Myelosuppression, vomiting during administration, perivascular irritation on extravasation	Dogs: 200 mg/m^2 IV daily for 5 days every 3 weeks *or* 1000 mg/m^2 IV every 3 weeks
Ifosfamide	Lymphoma	Hemorrhagic cystitis, myelosuppression	Dogs: 275–350 mg/m^2 IV with saline diuresis and mesna, every 3 weeks
Melphalan	Multiple myeloma, anal sac adenocarcinoma	Myelosuppression, potential cumulative thrombocytopenia	Dogs: 0.1 mg/kg every 24 hours for 10 days, then 0.05 mg/kg daily *or* 7 mg/m^2 PO daily for 5 days every 3 weeks Cats: 0.1 mg/kg every 24 hours
Anthracyclines			
Dactinomycin	Lymphoma	Myelosuppression, GI upset, perivascular damage with extravasation	0.75–0.8 mg/m^2 IV every 3 weeks
Doxorubicin	Lymphoma, carcinoma, sarcoma	Myelosuppression, GI upset, hypersensitivity during administration, perivascular damage with extravasation, cumulative (180 mg/m^2) myocardial toxicity, nephrotoxicity (cats)	Dogs: ≥10 kg: 30 mg/m^2 IV every 2–3 weeks Dogs <10 kg: 1 mg/kg IV every 2–3 weeks Cats: 1 mg/kg IV every 3 weeks

Continued

TABLE 16-3 Commonly Used Chemotherapeutic Drugs—cont'd

DRUG	MAIN INDICATIONS	TOXICITIES	DOSAGE
Doxorubicin HCl liposome injection	Lymphoma, carcinoma, sarcoma	Mild myelosuppression and/or GI upset, hypersensitivity during administration, perivascular damage with extravasation, palmar plantar erythrodysesthesia (PPES) nephrotoxicity (cats)	Dogs and cats: 1 mg/kg IV every 3 weeks
Idarubicin	Unclear	Mild myelosuppression and/or GI upset, perivascular damage with extravasation	Cats: 2 mg/day for 3 days every 3 weeks
Mitoxantrone	Lymphoma, transitional cell carcinoma	Myelosuppression, GI upset, perivascular damage with extravasation	Dogs: 5–5.5 mg/m^2 IV every 3 weeks Cats: 6 mg/m^2 IV every 3 weeks
Antimetabolites			
Methotrexate	Lymphoma	Mild myelosuppression and/or GI upset	Given PO or IV Dogs and cats: 0.8 mg/kg in combination with other chemotherapeutic drugs
Cytosine arabinoside	Lymphoma (myeloproliferative)	Mild myelosuppression and/or GI upset	Given subcutaneously (SQ), intramuscularly (IM), or IV; several different regimens can be used, depending on concurrent anticancer drugs.
Antitubulin Agents			
Paclitaxel	Under investigation	Hypersensitivity during administration	Dogs: 132 mg/m^2 IV every 3 weeks; must premedicate to minimize hypersensitivity
Vinblastine	Mast cell tumor	Myelosuppression, perivascular vesicant	Dogs: 2 mg/m^2 IV every 1–2 weeks
Vincristine	Lymphoma, mast cell tumor, transmissible venereal tumor, immune-mediated thrombocytopenia	Myelosuppression, perivascular vesicant, peripheral neuropathy, constipation in cats	Dogs and cats: 0.5–0.7 mg/m^2 IV weekly or as dictated by concurrent anticancer drugs
Vinorelbine	Primary lung tumor	Myelosuppression, perivascular vesicant	Dogs: 15–18 mg/m^2 IV every 1–2 weeks
Corticosteroids			
Prednisone	Lymphoma, mast cell tumor, myeloma, chronic lymphocytic leukemia Noncytotoxic indications: brain tumor, insulinoma, appetite stimulant	Polyuria, polyphagia, polydipsia, muscle wasting, behavioral changes	Dogs and cats cytotoxic dose: 2 mg/kg/day, taper according to protocol Dogs and cats noncytotoxic dose: 0.5 mg/kg/day

TABLE 16-3 Commonly Used Chemotherapeutic Drugs—cont'd

DRUG	MAIN INDICATIONS	TOXICITIES	DOSAGE
Miscellaneous Drugs			
Asparaginase	Lymphoma	Hypersensitivity reaction after administration	Dogs and cats: 400 IU/kg SQ or IM, maximum dose of 10,000 IU
Carboplatin	Osteosarcoma, carcinoma, sarcoma	Myelosuppression; potentially severe GI effects (small dogs)	Dogs: 300 mg/m^2 IV every 3 weeks Cats: 240–260 mg/m^2 IV every 3 weeks
Cisplatin	Osteosarcoma, carcinoma, sarcoma	Nephrotoxic—must be given with saline-induced diuresis; highly emetogenic; fatal to cats	Dogs: 70 mg/m^2 IV every 3 weeks Cats: Do not use
Hydroxyurea	Polycythemia vera, myeloproliferative diseases	Myelosuppression	Dogs: 50 mg/kg/day, tapering to every other day with remission Cats: 10 mg/kg/day, tapering to every other day with remission
Procarbazine	Lymphoma	GI upset, myelosuppression	Dogs: 50 mg/m^2 daily for 14 days on and 14 days off as part of mechlorethamine, Oncovin (vincristine), procarbazine, and prednisone (MOPP) protocol

From Withrow SJ, Vail DM: Withrow & MacEwan's small animal clinical oncology, ed 4, St. Louis, 2007, Saunders.

- Bleomycin
- Dactinomycin
- Mitoxantrone
- Idarubicin

Adverse Side Effects

These include bone marrow suppression, cardiotoxicity (cardiomyopathy), gastroenteritis, and anaphylaxis.

TECHNICIAN NOTES

- Some clinicians use antihistamines to premedicate animals to be treated with doxorubicin to suppress allergic reactions.
- Doxorubicin is a strong vesicant. Tissue sloughing can follow extravasation, and skin irritation can result from contact with the drug.
- Doxorubicin is commonly used in combination with other antineoplastic agents.
- Dexrazoxane is a drug that may be used to block doxorubicin-induced cardiac toxicity.

ANTIMETABOLITES

The antimetabolites are **cell cycle–specific** drugs that affect the S phase (DNA synthesis) of the cycle. These drugs are analogues of purines and pyrimidines—naturally occurring bases in DNA—that may be incorporated into the DNA molecule to inhibit protein and enzyme synthesis. Cellular functions needed for normal activity are thus blocked.

Clinical Uses
Clinical uses include treatment of lymphoproliferative neoplasms, treatment of gastrointestinal and hepatic neoplasms, and treatment of central nervous system lymphoma.

Dosage Forms
- Methotrexate, oral tablet or injection
- Cytosar-U, cytosine arabinoside injection
- 5-Fluorouracil cream or solution

Adverse Side Effects
These may include anorexia, nausea, vomiting, diarrhea, bone marrow suppression, hepatotoxicity, and neurotoxicity.

> **TECHNICIAN NOTES** Fluorouracil is contraindicated in cats because of adverse side effects.

ANTITUBULIN AGENTS

The plant alkaloids are cell cycle–specific for the M phase, inhibiting mitosis and causing cell death. They are thought to bind microtubular proteins and inhibit formation of the mitotic spindle, thus suspending mitosis in metaphase.

The two drugs in this category—vincristine and vinblastine—are natural alkaloids derived from the periwinkle plant (*Vinca rosea,* Linn). Protective clothing should be worn when these drugs are administered so that possible skin contact irritation does not occur.

Clinical Uses
Clinical uses include treatment of lymphoproliferative neoplasms, carcinomas, mast cell tumors, and splenic tumors.

Dosage Forms
- Oncovin, vincristine sulfate injection
- Alkaban-AQ, vinblastine sulfate for injection
- Paclitaxel, investigational drug
- Navelbine, vinorelbine

Adverse Side Effects
These may include gastroenteritis, bone marrow suppression, stomatitis, alopecia, and peripheral neuropathy.

> **TECHNICIAN NOTES**
> - Extravasation of plant alkaloids may cause tissue necrosis.
> - Skin contact causes irritation.

MISCELLANEOUS ANTINEOPLASTIC DRUGS

Platinum Drugs
The platinum drugs (carboplatin and cisplatin) are thought to act in a manner similar to the alkylating agents, which interrupt the replication of DNA in tumor cells (Papich, 2002).

Clinical Uses
These products are used for a variety of solid tumors, including osteosarcomas and carcinomas.

Dosage Forms
- Cisplatin (Platinol)
- Carboplatin (Paraplatin)

Adverse Side Effects
These include renal toxicity, nausea, anorexia, and vomiting (cisplatin). Dyspnea, pulmonary edema, and death may occur in cats. Carboplatin causes less nephrotoxicity, nausea, and vomiting than cisplatin.

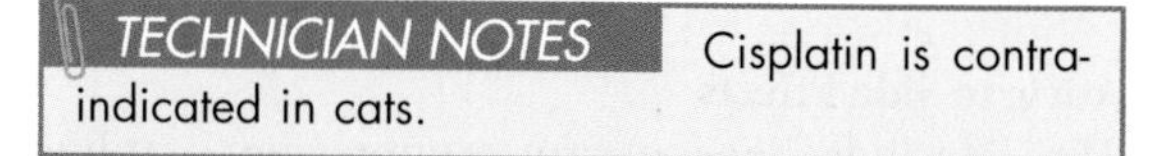
TECHNICIAN NOTES Cisplatin is contraindicated in cats.

Asparaginase
Asparaginase is the most commonly used miscellaneous agent. It is a cell cycle–specific (G1) enzyme extracted from *Escherichia coli* bacteria. Asparaginase acts as a catalyst in the breakdown of asparagine, an amino acid required by cancer cells. Deprived of a needed amino acid, the cancer cells die. Asparaginase has no effect on normal cells, and it is usually used in combination protocols.

Clinical Uses
Asparaginase is used for the treatment of lymphoproliferative neoplasms.

Dosage Form
- Elspar, asparaginase for injection

Adverse Side Effects
The adverse side effects of this drug include immediate hypersensitivity and gastrointestinal disturbances.

Glucocorticoids
The glucocorticoids prednisone and prednisolone are sometimes used for the treatment of neoplastic disorders. They are cell cycle–nonspecific. Corticosteroids have a lympholytic action, which makes them useful for treating lymphoid neoplasms. They are also helpful in the management of secondary complications of neoplastic diseases such as hypercalcemia and immune-mediated (thrombocytopenia) problems. In addition, they can increase appetite and the overall feeling of well-being in patients being treated for neoplasm. They usually are used in combination protocols with other antineoplastic drugs.

Piroxicam
Piroxicam is a nonsteroidal antiinflammatory agent that has been shown to be very effective in the treatment of transitional cell carcinoma of the bladder and squamous cell carcinoma in the dog. Piroxicam's antitumor effects are thought to be due to effects exerted on the immune system rather than on tumor cells.

Dosage Form
- Feldene

Adverse Side Effects
All nonsteroidal antiinflammatory drugs are capable of causing significant GI effects.

Hydroxyurea and procarbazine are two other agents in the miscellaneous category. See Table 16-3 for information about these two agents.

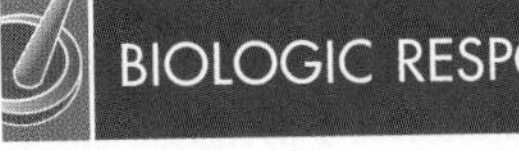

BIOLOGIC RESPONSE MODIFIERS

Biologic response modifiers (BRMs) are agents that alter the relationship between the tumor and the host animal in a way that improves the host's ability to mount an antitumor response (Grant et al, 1989). BRMs are used as an adjunct to conventional chemotherapy protocols, not as the sole agent of treatment.

Cancer develops in many animals because of an immunosuppressed state, and chemotherapy exacerbates the immunosuppression. BRMs may be used to stimulate or restore the compromised immune response of the host.

Examples of BRMs include bacterial agents, chemical agents, interferons, thymosins, cytokines/lymphokines, and monoclonal antibodies.

Monoclonal Antibodies
Monoclonal antibodies are identical immunoglobulin molecules formed by a single clone of plasma cells. They are produced by a **hybridoma,** a fusion of a specific antibody-producing B cell with **myeloma** cells (Figure 16-5). Hybridomas secrete large quantities of a very specific (for the tumor) antibody. Monoclonal antibodies may have direct **cytotoxic** effects on tumor cells, or they may be attached (conjugated) to chemotherapeutic agents such as radioisotopes, BRMs, or other agents for direct delivery to the tumor cells. In this way, they become a "magic bullet" directed at cancer cells (Figure 16-6).

Clinical Uses
A monoclonal antibody product for the treatment of canine lymphoma that was previously available is no longer being produced. Monoclonal antibody use is a valuable tool in diagnostics and research and has potential value in clinical therapy.

Interferon
Interferons are chemicals produced by leukocytes, fibroblasts, and epithelial cells. Interferons can exert antitumor, antiviral, and immunoregulatory effects. Several categories of interferons have been identified. Products that are available are approved for use in humans and have been used in humans to treat hairy cell leukemia, Kaposi's sarcoma, genital warts, and certain granulomatous diseases. In veterinary medicine, they have been used to attempt to prevent the development of fatal disease in feline leukemia virus (FeLV)–infected cats and to attempt to extend the survival time of cats infected with feline infectious peritonitis (FIP).

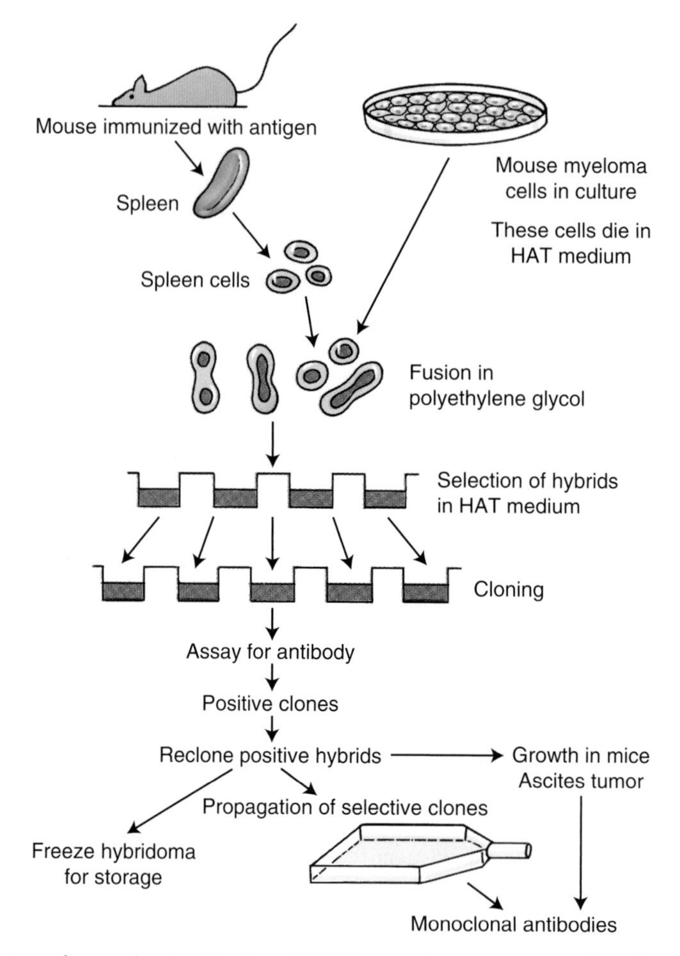

FIGURE 16-5 Production of monoclonal antibodies. *HAT,* Hypoxanthine–aminopterin–thymidine. (From Tizard I: Veterinary immunology: an introduction, ed 3, Philadelphia, 1987, WB Saunders.)

Clinical Uses

These may include the amelioration of FeLV- and FIP-related conditions.

Dosage Forms

- Roferon-A injection, recombinant interferon alfa-2a
- Intron A, recombinant interferon alfa-2b for injection
- Alferon N injection, human leukocyte–derived interferon alfa-n3
- Virbagen Omega, recombinant interferon of feline origin
- Actimmune gamma-1b, recombinant interferon

Adverse Side Effects

Adverse side effects in humans have included fever and flu-like symptoms.

Other Biologic Response Modifiers

- Acemannan. This product is licensed for the treatment of fibrosarcoma in dogs and cats.
- Interleukins. Seventeen interleukins have been identified. Their functions include various activities in the immune system such as cell enhancement or suppression, hemopoietic growth, and regulation of leukocyte function.
  - Interleukin-2. This substance's primary function is promotion of the clonal expansion of

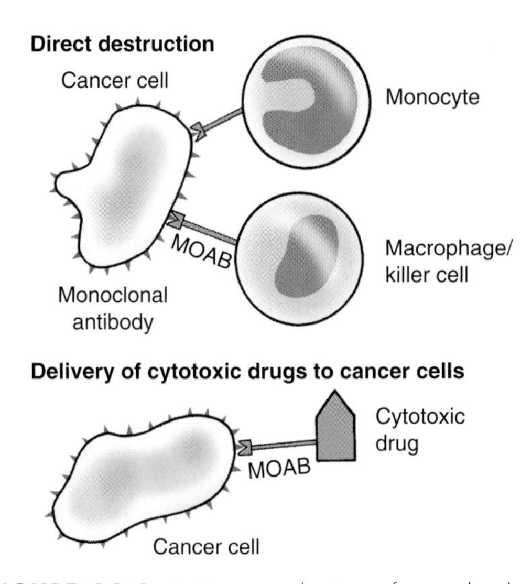

FIGURE 16-6 Antitumor mechanisms of monoclonal antibodies. *MOAB*, Monoclonal antibody.

antigen-specific T cells; it may be useful in treating certain canine and feline neoplasias (Kruth, 1998).

- Granulocyte colony-stimulating factor (G-CSF)—Filgrastim. These growth factors affect specific myeloid cell lines and may have some use in the treatment of neutropenia associated with the chemotherapy of canine or feline neoplasia or in the management of feline panleukopenia.
- Bacillus Calmette-Guérin (BCG). BCG is a live, attenuated strain of *Mycobacterium bovis* that activates B and T cells.
- Levamisole. Use of levamisole as an immunostimulant is controversial.
- *Propionibacterium acnes.* Immunoregulin is a killed suspension of *P. acnes* approved for use in veterinary medicine. It causes nonspecific immunostimulation.
- Staphylococcal protein A. This product initiates T- and B-lymphocyte proliferation.
- *Parapox ovis* virus immunomodulator—Zylexis. This product is used to treat horses with viral upper respiratory disease.
- Lymphocyte T-Cell Immunomodulator. This agent was developed to aid in the treatment of cats with feline leukemia or feline immunodeficiency virus infection.
- Canine Melanoma Vaccine. This vaccine carries a conditional U.S. Department of Agriculture approval for the treatment of melanoma in dogs.

IMMUNOSUPPRESSIVE DRUGS

Immunosuppressive drugs are used in veterinary medicine to treat various immune-mediated disorders. Some of the diseases related to an overactive or improperly responding immune system include lupus erythematosus, lymphocytic–plasmacytic enteritis, rheumatoid arthritis, immune-mediated skin disease, and hemolytic anemia. Many of the immunosuppressive drugs work by interfering with one of the stages of the cell cycle or by affecting cellular messengers.

Azathioprine

Azathioprine is an antimetabolite that affects cells in the S phase of the cell cycle. It inhibits both T lymphocytes and B lymphocytes to bring about immunosuppression. It has fewer side effects than cyclophosphamide and some of the other immunosuppressants. It is often used in combination with prednisone or prednisolone. Because cats are more likely to be affected by the side effects of this drug, it should not be used in this species.

Clinical Uses

Azathioprine is used primarily for the treatment of immune-mediated disease in dogs.

Dosage Forms

- Imuran tablets, azathioprine (50 mg)
- Imuran, azathioprine injection

Adverse Side Effects

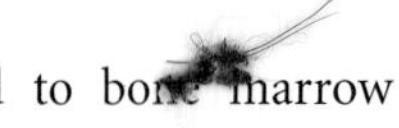

Adverse side effects are related to bone marrow suppression. Long-term use may predispose to infection.

Cyclosporine

Cyclosporine is a substance isolated from a fungus that inhibits proliferation of T lymphocytes (Boothe, 2012). It was approved for use in humans for prevention of organ transplant rejection; however, it has also been used to treat several immune-mediated diseases (e.g., uveitis, Graves' disease, psoriasis, pemphigus). It has been used in veterinary medicine for the prevention of organ transplant rejection, for treating immune-mediated skin disorders, and for the management of keratoconjunctivitis sicca (KCS) in dogs.

Clinical Uses

Clinical use of cyclosporine in practice is limited mainly to ophthalmic application for treatment of KCS and atopic dermatitis in dogs.

Dosage Forms

- Optimmune ophthalmic ointment
- Atopica capsules (dogs), atopica oral solution (cats)
- Restasis ophthalmic emulsion
- Sandimmune, cyclosporine gelatin capsules
- Sandimmune, cyclosporine oral solution
- Sandimmune, cyclosporine for injection

Adverse Side Effects

In humans, these may include nephrotoxicity, hepatotoxicity, nausea, vomiting, anaphylaxis (intravenous form), and others.

> *TECHNICIAN NOTES* Monitor the eyes for irritation or infection if cyclosporine is being used for KCS.

Metronidazole

Metronidazole is a substance that has antibacterial, antiprotozoal, and immunosuppressive activities. It may be used in conjunction with corticosteroids to enhance its immunosuppressive effects.

Clinical Uses

Clinical uses include treatment of lymphocytic–plasmacytic enteritis in dogs, treatment of giardiasis, and treatment of anaerobic bacterial infections.

Dosage Forms

- Flagyl, metronidazole tablets
- Flagyl, metronidazole powder for injection
- Flagyl IV, injectable

Adverse Side Effects

These may include gastrointestinal upset, neurologic disturbances, and lethargy.

> *TECHNICIAN NOTES* Clients must be warned about the potential severe side effects of Metronidazole.

Cyclophosphamide

Cyclophosphamide is an alkylating agent that is used as an antineoplastic agent and an immunosuppressant (see the earlier section on antineoplastic agents). Cyclophosphamide may produce serious side effects (e.g., hemorrhagic cystitis, bone marrow suppression, and gastroenteritis). It is an injectable agent.

Clinical Uses

Cyclophosphamide is used primarily as an immunosuppressant.

Dosage Form

- Cytoxan

Adverse Side Effects

These include bone marrow suppression, gastrointestinal signs, alopecia, and hemorrhagic cystitis.

Corticosteroids

Corticosteroids exert antiinflammatory and immunosuppressive effects through their inhibitory influence on neutrophils, T lymphocytes, blood vessels (decreased permeability), and cellular messengers (e.g., prostaglandin). They are generally considered to be antiinflammatory at lower doses and immunosuppressive at higher doses. Corticosteroids are often used in combination with other immunosuppressant/antineoplastic agents.

Other Immunosuppressive Agents

- Tacrolimus (Protopic). This is a topical agent that may be used in the treatment of atopic dermatitis and other dermatologic conditions.
- Pimecrolimus (Elidel). This is a topical agent similar to tacrolimus.
- Oclacitinib (Apoquel). This agent is a Janus kinase inhibitor labeled for the control of pruritus in dogs less than 12 months of age.
- Mycophenolate mofetil. This is an immunosuppressive drug that may be used for treating immune-mediated hemolytic anemia, inflammatory bowel disease, or myasthenia gravis in dogs.

REVIEW QUESTIONS

1. Anemia in baby pigs can be treated by the administration of ______________________.
2. A 10-year-old cocker spaniel is brought to the veterinary clinic with polyuria/polydipsia and mild anemia. What is a potential cause of these signs, and what may be used to treat the anemia? ______________________
3. Why are hematinics not indicated for cases of acute blood loss?

   ____
4. What is the anticoagulant of choice for collecting blood for hematologic studies?

   ____
5. How can you explain the fact that clots may form in the vascular system with no external trauma to blood vessels?

   ____
6. You have accidentally cut the quick of a Rottweiler puppy's nail. What would you use to stop the bleeding, and how does this agent work? ______________________
7. A 3-month-old chow is brought to the pet emergency clinic because it has eaten a box of rat poison. What drug would the veterinarian use to treat this condition, and by what route would it be administered?

   ____
8. An 8-year-old male Persian cat is brought to the veterinary clinic with an early onset of apparent rear leg paralysis and tachycardia. What agent may be used to treat this condition? ______________________
9. Briefly describe the phases of the cell cycle.

   ____
10. List the six categories of antineoplastic drugs, and give an example of each.

    ____
11. A 12-year-old Labrador retriever has been through a treatment protocol for lymphoma, and the owner has opted for the use of a BRM. What agent could be used in this case?

    ____
12. List four indications for the use of immunosuppressive agents.

    ____
13. Why should you be very careful to avoid extravasation of antineoplastic drugs?

    ____
14. List eight precautions that should be taken when antineoplastic drugs are handled.

    ____
15. Where in the body is erythropoietin produced?

    ____
16. What drug may be used to treat the anemia associated with chronic renal failure?

    ____
17. ______________________ digests fibrin threads and other clotting products to cause clot lysis and the release of fibrin degradation products into the circulation.
18. Which anticoagulant may be used to treat DIC?

    ____
19. Why should heparin not be used as an anticoagulant when blood is collected for performance of a differential count?

    ____
20. How does EDTA work as an anticoagulant?

    ____
21. What are some potential adverse side effects associated with the use of antineoplastic drugs?

    ____
22. On what dosage are most antineoplastic agents based? ______________________
23. Corticosteroids have a lympholytic action, which makes them useful for treating

    ______________________.
24. A substance with antitumor, antiviral, and immunoregulatory effects is

    ______________________.
25. Cardiomyopathy is a potential side effect of what antineoplastic agent?

    ____
26. Erythrocytes are formed in the ______________ in response to stimulation by erythropoietin.
    a. spleen
    b. bone marrow
    c. liver
    d. heart

27. The primary function of erythrocytes is to ____________________.
    a. ensure that the blood has a red color
    b. absorb erythropoietin
    c. absorb as much CO_2 as possible
    d. carry O_2 to the tissues
28. ____________________ are used to prevent or treat anemia.
    a. Vesicants
    b. Propionic acid derivatives
    c. Hematinics
    d. NSAIDs
29. All of the following are androgens, except ____________________.
    a. Winstrol-V
    b. Equipoise
    c. Deca-Durabolin
    d. Regu-Mate
30. The intrinsic and extrinsic pathways of blood coagulation do not converge into a common pathway in the final steps of clot formation because the endothelial layer of blood vessels has the ability to regenerate itself.
    a. True
    b. False
31. A heparin flush solution may be prepared by diluting heparin in saline at a concentration of ____________________.
    a. 2 U/mL
    b. 10 U/mL
    c. 5 U/mL
    d. 12 U/mL
32. Heparin test tubes have a ____________________ top.
    a. blue
    b. gray
    c. lavender
    d. green
33. Vitamin ____________________ is an antidote for warfarin or dicumarol toxicity.
    a. B_{12}
    b. C
    c. D
    d. K_1
34. ____________________ is the anticoagulant of choice when a WBC differential is performed.
    a. Heparin
    b. Diatomaceous earth
    c. Sodium citrate
    d. EDTA
35. Fluorouracil is contraindicated in __________ because of adverse side effects.
    a. caprines
    b. ovines
    c. avians
    d. felines
36. A 40-lb dog with lymphoma is being treated with a chemotherapy protocol that includes doxorubicin. The dosage of doxorubicin is 30 mg/m^2 IV. The concentration of the doxorubicin is 2 mg/mL. How many milliliters would you draw up and what precautions should be used in its administration?

    ____
37. A 60-lb dog with a mast cell tumor is being treated with a protocol that includes vincristine at a dosage of 0.5 mg/m^2. The concentration of the vincristine is 1 mg/mL. How many milliliters would you draw up?

    ____
38. A 12-lb cat with lymphosarcoma is being treated with a protocol that includes asparaginase at a dosage of 10,000 $units/m^2$. The concentration of the asparaginase solution is 1000 U/mL. How many milliliters would you draw up?

    ____
39. A 10-lb cat with rodenticide toxicity needs Vitamin K_1 treatment at a dosage of 5 mg/kg. The concentration of the vitamin K_1 is 10 mg/mL. How much would you draw up?

    ____
40. How many milliliters of heparin (1000 U/mL) would you add to a 250-mL bag of saline to prepare a concentration of 5 U/mL?

    ____

REFERENCES

Boothe DM: Immunodulators or biologic response modifiers. In Boothe DM, editor: Small animal clinical pharmacology and therapeutics, Philadelphia, 2012, WB Saunders.

Crow SE, Walshaw SO: Placement and care of intravenous catheters. In Crow SE, Walshaw SO, editors: Manual of clinical procedures in the dog and cat, Philadelphia, 1987, JB Lippincott.

Ganong WF: Endocrine function of the kidneys, heart, and pineal gland. In Ganong WF, editor: Review of medical physiology, ed 21, New York, 2003, McGraw-Hill.

Grant CK, Shelton GH: Biological response modifiers. In Kirk RW, Bonagura JD, editors: Current veterinary therapy X: small animal practice, Philadelphia, 1989, WB Saunders.

Kruth SA: Biologic response modifiers: interferons, interleukins, recombinant products, liposomal products. In Boothe DM, editor: The veterinary clinics of North America, small animal practice, Philadelphia, 1998, WB Saunders.

Norsworthy GD: Clinical aspects of feline blood transfusions. Compend Contin Educ Pract Vet 14:470, 1992.

Papich MG: Handbook of veterinary drugs, Philadelphia, 2002, WB Saunders.

Plumb DC: Veterinary drug handbook, ed 7, Ames, Iowa, 2011, Wiley-Blackwell.

Pugh DM: Blood formation, coagulation, and volume. In Brander GC, Pugh DM, Bywater RJ, et al, editors: Veterinary applied pharmacology and therapeutics, ed 5, London, 1991, Bailliere Tindall.

Withrow SJ, Vail DM, editors: Small animal oncology, ed 4, St. Louis, 2007, Saunders Elsevier.

CHAPTER

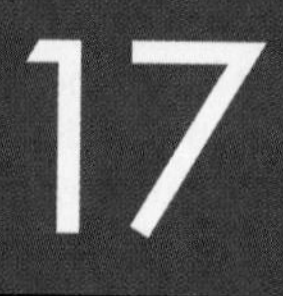

Immunologic Drugs

KEY TERMS

Active immunity
Adjuvant
Anaphylaxis
Antibody
Antigen
Avirulent
Bacterin
Monovalent
Passive immunity
Polyvalent
Preservative
Recombinant DNA technology
Virulence

OUTLINE

LEARNING OBJECTIVES

After studying this chapter, you should be able to

1. Explain the principles associated with vaccination.
2. Describe the differences between vaccine types.
3. Discuss the advantages and disadvantages of the different types of vaccines.
4. List common diseases that have available vaccines.
5. Describe the different routes of administration of vaccines.
6. List drugs used in immunotherapy.

PRINCIPLES OF VACCINATION

Keeping animals healthy through the proper use of immunization programs is an important aspect of veterinary medicine. Veterinary technicians must have knowledge concerning vaccine types and the diseases against which animals are vaccinated. Clients ask many questions regarding this area of their pet's care. It should be remembered that immunization should never take the place of regularly scheduled, routine veterinary checkups (McCurnin and Bassert, 2006). As animals enter into their geriatric years, regular laboratory profiles should be done to determine the health of major organ systems. Preventive medicine also includes a good physical examination as well as procurement of a complete history on the animal. Therefore, immunization programs are only one aspect of the overall health care that should be afforded companion animals. Livestock should be properly immunized to achieve a healthy herd.

Vaccinations are an important part of the preventive health care program for companion animals and food animals alike. Vaccines are given to lessen the chance of a particular disease occurring. A patient's response is determined by (1) health and age, (2) the type of vaccine given, (3) the route of administration, (4) concurrent incubation of infectious disease, (5) exposure to an infectious disease before complete immunity is reached, and (6) drug therapy. The ideal vaccine is safe and effective on challenge and has no undesirable side effects. Immunology is a very complex field of study. This chapter outlines only the basics of common vaccines and immunostimulants. Referencing an immunology textbook may be helpful if further information is desired.

In properly vaccinated females, antibodies are passed to their offspring in the form of maternal antibodies found in colostrum. It is important not to vaccinate very young animals when maternal antibodies are still present. The neonate's immune system is not capable of producing an immune response when maternal antibodies are blocking this mechanism. (See the charts within this chapter for specific times that various species should be vaccinated.)

Because of the risk of vaccine-associated sarcomas when inactivated feline vaccines are administered, it is becoming increasingly important that each vaccine be given at a certain place on a cat's body. Although the prevalence of sarcomas after vaccination has been reported at 1 case per 10,000 vaccines administered (McCurnin and Bassert, 2006), caution is warranted. The National Vaccine-Associated Sarcoma Task Force studying vaccine site tumors recommends that no vaccine be given in the intrascapular space. Rabies vaccine should be administered in the distal right rear leg, feline leukemia virus (FeLV) vaccine should be administered in the distal left rear leg, and all other vaccines should be administered in the right shoulder. It is also recommended that any vaccine lump present 3 months after the time of vaccination be removed, after a biopsy has been performed to reveal the extent of surgery that may have to be performed. Rear-leg amputation for sarcoma removal provides a better cure rate than surgery on the intrascapular space (McCurnin and Bassert, 2006). Some veterinarians follow the same vaccine site administration for dogs as is observed in cats.

In cattle, the location of vaccine administration is also important. With the advent of the Meat Quality Assurance Program, proper administration of injections and vaccines is critical in all food animal species. All intramuscular and subcutaneous injections in cattle should be given in the neck, if possible. Administration of most vaccines requires observation of a slaughter withdrawal, sometimes up to 60 days postvaccine (Figure 17-1).

The future of vaccination involves development of protocols that individualize vaccine schedules instead of having every animal vaccinated for every disease. Much discussion is ongoing in the veterinary community regarding vaccination of dogs and cats every 3 years rather than yearly. However, some state and county regulations may still mandate the yearly rabies vaccine regimen, and other states may legislate every 3 years. It is hoped that additional research will yield optimal revaccination intervals. Some studies have suggested that with some vaccines, protective immunity may last for years and annual revaccination may not be necessary. With new information and technology, the twenty-first century will see many changes in vaccines.

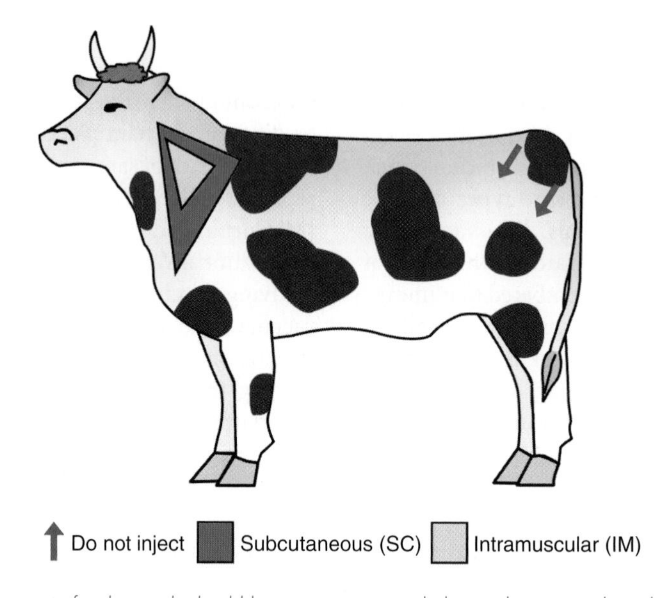

FIGURE 17-1 All injections in food animals should be given intramuscularly or subcutaneously in the neck region, as outlined in this figure. (From McCurnin DM, Bassert JM: Clinical textbook for veterinary technicians, ed 6, St. Louis, 2002, WB Saunders.)

COMMON VACCINE TYPES THAT PRODUCE ACTIVE IMMUNITY

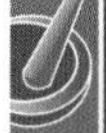

INACTIVATED

Manufacture of inactivated vaccines involves killing the organisms with chemicals that leave the **antigens** mostly unchanged. The antigens stimulate protective immunity. Inactivated vaccines are also referred to as *killed,* or *dead,* vaccines.

Advantages

- Inactivated vaccines are usually very safe.
- They are stable in storage.
- They are unlikely to cause disease through residual virulence.

Disadvantages

- Inactivated vaccines require repeated doses to achieve adequate protection.
- Adjuvants may cause severe local reactions.
- If repeated doses are required, costs may be higher.
- Inactivated vaccines contain **preservatives** such as penicillin, streptomycin, and fungistats.

Dosage Forms

- Leukocell 2: FeLV
- Duramune Cv-K: rabies virus
- Vibo-5/Somnugen: *Campylobacter fetus,* leptospirosis, *Haemophilus somnus* **bacterin**

See the vaccine charts within this chapter for a more comprehensive listing of the various vaccine types associated with each disease.

LIVE

A live vaccine is prepared from live microorganisms or viruses. These organisms may be fully **virulent** or **avirulent.** Few vaccines of this origin are in use, with the exception of several poultry vaccines.

Advantages

- Live vaccines necessitate fewer doses to achieve an immune response.

- Adjuvants are unnecessary, but the vaccine may contain preservatives.
- Live vaccines pose less risk of allergic response.
- They are inexpensive.

Disadvantages

- Live vaccines may be contaminated with unwanted organisms.
- They require careful handling. For example, accidental injection, ingestion, or exposure through a cut or the mucous membranes of brucellosis vaccine can cause undulant fever in humans.
- They do not store as well as inactivated vaccines.
- They may possess residual virulence.

Dosage Forms

- *Brucella abortus* Vaccine: *Brucella abortus* strain RB-51
- Ovine Ecthyma Vaccine: ovine ecthyma virus or sore mouth infection
- Chick Ark Bronc: infectious bronchitis (Massachusetts and Arkansas types)
- Protex-Bb: *Bordetella bronchiseptica*

See vaccine charts within this chapter for a more comprehensive listing of the various vaccine types associated with each disease.

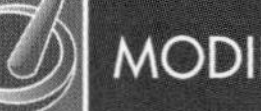

MODIFIED LIVE

In modified live vaccines, organisms undergo a process (attenuation) to lose their virulence so that when introduced to the body via inoculation, they cause an immune response instead of disease.

Advantages

- Effective vaccines for many viruses can be developed through attenuation of the causative virus.
- Immunity is comparable in response and longevity to killed products.

Disadvantages

- Modified live vaccines may cause abortion when given to pregnant animals.
- Some vaccines can cause mild immunosuppression.
- Residual virulence can cause a mild form of the disease.
- These vaccines contain preservatives such as penicillin, gentamicin, thimerosal, or a fungistat.

Dosage Forms

- Eclipse 3: feline rhinotracheitis, calicivirus, and panleukopenia
- Bovi-Shield 4: infectious bovine rhinotracheitis (IBR) virus, bovine virus diarrhea (BVD), parainfluenza 3 (PI3) virus, bovine respiratory syncytial virus

See vaccine charts within this chapter for a more comprehensive listing of the various vaccine types associated with each disease.

RECOMBINANT

In recent years, vaccines produced by **recombinant DNA technology** have become available for veterinary medicine. These vaccines are recognized as being safe, highly specific, potent, pure, and efficacious. These attributes may be the reason why recombinant vaccines are more desirable than any other vaccine type. Recombinant vaccines are divided into three categories:

Type I recombinant (subunit) vaccines—These vaccines are derived by inserting a foreign gene from a specific pathogen into a recombinant organism (e.g., yeast, bacterium, a virus). The recombinant organism multiplies, and the product of the gene is extracted, purified, and prepared for administration as a vaccine.

Type II recombinant (gene-deleted) vaccines—The manufacturing of these vaccines involves deletion of specific genes from a pathogenic organism. This manipulation produces a vaccine that has a low risk of producing disease but can still stimulate a protective immune response.

Type III recombinant (vectored) vaccines—These vaccines are derived from the insertion of specific pathogenic genetic material into a nonpathogenic or gene-deleted organism (e.g., poxvirus). This altered organism then is propagated in vitro and is used to manufacture the vaccine (Van Kampen, 1998).

Advantages
- These vaccines produce fewer adverse effects.
- They provide effective immunity.
- Type I and Type III vaccines cannot revert to virulence because of the way they are manufactured.
- Some of these vaccines can be administered orally.

Disadvantages
- Currently, few recombinant vaccines are available.
- New technology often brings with it a higher cost.

Dosage Forms
- Type I: RM Recombitek Lyme: *Borrelia burgdorferi*
- Type III: RM Recombitek C4: canine distemper, adenovirus type 2, parainfluenza, and parvovirus
- Type III: Raboral V-RG: oral vaccine for rabies virus (used in baiting devices for wildlife)
- Type III: Newcastle disease–fowl pox vaccine (recombinant): Newcastle disease and fowl pox
- Type III: Trovac-AIV H5: avian influenza subtype H5 and fowl pox

See vaccine charts within this chapter for a more comprehensive listing of the various vaccine types associated with each disease.

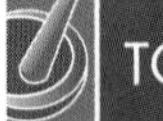

TOXOID

A toxoid is a vaccine that is used to produce immunity to a toxin rather than a bacterium or a virus. The toxin is treated with heat or chemicals to destroy its damaging properties without eliminating its ability to stimulate **antibody** production.

An anaculture combines toxoid and killed bacteria in a single dose prepared from highly toxigenic cultures and culture filtrates.

Characteristics
- Toxoids and anacultures provide protection for up to 1 year.
- Toxoids may contain adjuvants.
- Many toxoids contain preservatives such as phenol, thimerosal, and formaldehyde solution.

Dosage Forms
- Tetanus Toxoid: *Clostridium tetani*
- Tetnogen: *C. tetani*
- Fermicon CD/T: *Clostridium perfringens* types C and D, and *C. tetani*

COMMON VACCINE TYPES THAT PRODUCE PASSIVE IMMUNITY

ANTITOXIN

An antitoxin is a specific antiserum aimed at a toxin that contains a concentration of antibodies extracted from the blood serum or plasma of a hyperimmunized, healthy animal (usually a horse).

Characteristics
- An antitoxin neutralizes toxins produced by microorganisms.
- It may contain preservatives such as thimerosal, phenol, or oxytetracycline.
- Antitoxins produce immediate **passive immunity.**
- Immunity is short lived (about 7 to 14 days).
- Biologic products of equine origin may be associated with the development of equine serum hepatitis (Theiler's disease). This link has not been proven, but clients should be made aware of the possible risk before these products are administered.

Dosage Forms
- Clostratox BCD: *C. perfringens* types C and D
- Tetanus Antitoxin: *C. tetani*

ANTISERUM

An antiserum is a serum that contains specific antibodies extracted from a hyperimmunized animal (usually a horse) or an animal that has been infected with microorganisms that contain antigen.

Characteristics
- An antiserum kills living, infectious antigens.
- It may contain preservatives such as phenol, thimerosal, or oxytetracycline.

- An antiserum produces immediate passive immunity.
- Do not vaccinate within 21 days after antiserum is given. For example, if a calf is treated with a *Corynebacterium–Escherichia coli–Pasteurella–Salmonella* antiserum, then that calf should not be vaccinated with BVD, IBR, PI3, *H. somnus*, or *Pasteurella haemolytica* within 21 days of receiving the antiserum.
- Immunity is short lived.

Dosage Forms

- *Erysipelothrix rhusiopathiae* Serum Antibodies: *E. rhusiopathiae*
- Escherichia-Colicin-B: *E. coli*
- Septi-Serum: *Salmonella typhimurium*

OTHER TYPES OF VACCINES

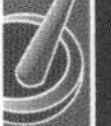

AUTOGENOUS VACCINE

An autogenous vaccine contains organisms isolated from an infected animal on a farm where a disease outbreak is occurring. This carefully prepared vaccine contains antigens needed for protection at that particular location.

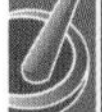

MIXED VACCINE

A mixed vaccine contains a mixture of different antigens. It is also referred to as a **polyvalent** vaccine. Each component of a mixed vaccine is required to achieve an immune response comparable with that of a vaccine containing a single antigen (**monovalent** vaccine).

ADMINISTRATION OF VACCINES

The intramuscular and subcutaneous routes are by far the most common methods for vaccine administration. These routes are easily accessible and provide systemic immunity, which is important in many diseases. Some diseases also respond well to local immunity. Vaccines against feline rhinotracheitis and calicivirus, canine infectious tracheobronchitis, and infectious bovine rhinotracheitis may be administered intranasally, or, in some cases, intraocular administration may be used to provide local immunity. After administration of these vaccines, the animal may experience a slight bout of watery eyes and occasional sneezing for a few days.

All of the previously mentioned routes of vaccine administration necessitate that each animal be handled individually. When a large number of animals require vaccination, these routes may not be feasible. Some vaccines may be mixed with drinking water or feed. Others can be aerosolized and inhaled by the animal. For example, on mink ranches, vaccine for canine distemper and mink enteritis may be administered in this manner, or poultry houses may vaccinate for Newcastle disease by aerosolization. The margin for incomplete vaccination is greater when aerosolization or mixing with feed or water is used. Some animals may not drink or eat enough to acquire adequate protection, or the aerosolized vaccine may not distribute equally throughout the room. Vaccine failure may be implicated if these animals contract the disease, whereas in reality, the animal did not receive enough vaccine to gain adequate immunity.

When conventional measures are used for vaccination, it is very important to carefully read the insert provided with the vaccine. Some vaccines may be administered intramuscularly or subcutaneously, but others may be administered by only one route. For example, some rabies vaccines require administration by an intramuscular route to be most effective. Subcutaneous injections should be given according to the manufacturer's instructions. Care should be used when one is vaccinating a cat to prevent vaccine-induced tumors.

If a vaccine requires reconstitution, this should be done with the diluent provided by the manufacturer. The vaccine should not be reconstituted until just before it is administered (see Chapter 2 for the proper reconstitution procedure). The full recommended dose should be given. Splitting a vaccine dose may result in an animal's failure to develop an adequate immune response and may lower its protection.

Mixing different vaccines to minimize the number of injections the animal receives is not recommended. This procedure can cause antigen blocking, resulting in one component interfering with the action of another; in this case, the animal does not receive adequate antigen to attain an effective immune response. Mixing of different vaccines may cause an increased chance of an allergic response. When different types of vaccines are administered, each vaccine should be administered at a separate site. It is also advisable to note the locations of administration and vaccine lot numbers on the patient's medical record. If a reaction or a problem develops later, a reference will be available to aid in evaluation of the problem.

When food animals are vaccinated, several factors must be considered. Almost all vaccine labels contain information advising not to vaccinate within 21 days of slaughter. Vaccines such as those for *B. abortus* are subject to federal limitations and regulations, and complete records are maintained on administration of these vaccines. Brucellosis vaccines are restricted to use by or under the direction of a licensed veterinarian. Carcass destruction is also a factor that involves food animal producers. Injection site lesions may cause damage to muscle tissue, requiring that area to be trimmed and discarded. If a vaccine may be administered intramuscularly or subcutaneously, the subcutaneous route would produce less tissue reaction and would eliminate muscle damage. This is important when one is dealing with animals used for meat consumption. Most vaccines on the market today can be given subcutaneously.

BIOLOGIC CARE AND VACCINE FAILURE

Biologics (especially modified live and live vaccines) are sensitive to inactivation by heat or sunlight. Clients purchasing vaccines should be provided with a cold pack if needed and should be warned against leaving such biologics in vehicles or in sunlight, where they may become warm and inactivated. Even the performance of killed products can be altered if proper handling and storage measures are not practiced. When these vaccines are shipped from the manufacturer, cold packs are put in the box to provide some refrigeration during shipment. In some areas, it may be advisable to anticipate how much vaccine may be needed during the hot summer months and to stock up on that amount during early spring to prevent shipments from overheating during summer transportation. Once a shipment is received, it should be quickly unpacked and placed under refrigeration. Vaccines should never be frozen because cells may rupture when the vaccine thaws, releasing toxins that can damage tissue or cause tissue death.

Inappropriate care of vaccines may lead to inactivation of the vaccine and may be perceived as a vaccine failure. Actual vaccine failure is relatively uncommon. If vaccines are purchased from a reputable manufacturer, one can be fairly sure that the vaccine provided will be effective. Failure usually occurs because of improper handling, storage, or administration.

Live vaccines are especially affected by concurrent antibiotic therapy. Live and modified live vaccines can be inactivated by chemicals used to clean or sterilize syringes and by the use of excessive alcohol or other disinfectants to swab the skin before injection. As was mentioned earlier, the route of administration may affect the ability of an animal to achieve an adequate immune response. Immunosuppressed, parasitized, stressed, or malnourished animals and those incubating disease are not able to mount an adequate immune response to prevent disease. Clients should always be advised that such problems can occur. In most cases, an adequate immune response is not achieved before 10 to 14 days. An 8-week-old puppy may not develop a strong immune response to protect against an infectious disease if challenged by maternal antibodies because it is not feasible to check immune titers to determine the presence of maternal antibodies. Therefore, it is recommended that puppies receive boosters every few weeks until they are about 4 to 5 months of age. Boosters allow vaccines to produce an optimum immune response. Clients often find it difficult to understand why they need to bring their pet in for boosters. If the reasons are explained and if clients are advised about why they should isolate their pet from animals with questionable vaccination histories, many cases of infectious disease would be prevented among young animals. Clients often perceive one vaccine to be enough or do not understand that their animal is not protected immediately after an injection has been received. Technicians should include this information when educating clients on animal and pet care.

ADVERSE VACCINATION RESPONSES

The most notable risks involving vaccination include residual virulence and toxicity, allergic reactions resulting from hypersensitivity, disease in immunosuppressed animals, possible effects on a fetus, and abortion. The veterinarian assesses these risks before a vaccine is administered. In most cases, the benefits of vaccination far outweigh the risks, but it may occasionally be necessary to omit or delay vaccination because of some of the factors just mentioned.

One of the most common reactions noted with vaccine administration is the sting felt by the animal after injection. This is most often caused by inactivating agents used in manufacturing the vaccine. Manufacturers are constantly researching ways to decrease these undesirable effects while still producing a quality product. This stinging reaction is short lived and does not usually cause a problem unless the animal reacts violently. Other common but not usually serious reactions include a slight fever, lethargy, and soreness at the injection site. These usually subside within 1 day. Hypersensitivity may be caused by several factors, including immunizing antigens, antigens acquired during the manufacture of the vaccine, and reactions to **adjuvants** used in the vaccine. Some animals may experience an anaphylactic shock reaction after receiving a vaccine, although this is uncommon. Clinical signs of **anaphylaxis** include vomiting, salivation, dyspnea, and incoordination. Epinephrine is usually the antidote of choice in cases of anaphylactic shock and should always be on hand when horses are vaccinated (McCurnin and Bassert, 2006). Other possible adverse side effects include vaccine-associated fibrosarcoma in cats and immune-mediated hemolytic anemia in dogs (Ford, 1998). The possible causes for these effects are under investigation.

VACCINATIONS FOR PREVENTIVE HEALTH PROGRAMS

Canine

As was stated earlier, vaccination is an important part of any preventive health program. Many vaccines may be available as a monovalent or polyvalent product. For dogs, a common polyvalent vaccine includes canine distemper (D), respiratory diseases caused by adenovirus type 2 (A_2), canine parainfluenza (P), leptospirosis (L), canine parvovirus (P), and coronavirus (C). It should be noted that vaccination with the A_2 virus also protects the dog against infectious canine hepatitis (ICH). This vaccine may be referred to as *DA₂PPL/C*. Many different combinations and product names are available. Most veterinarians choose a particular manufacturer from which to buy vaccine products. This helps to lessen the confusion caused by different names used to designate the manufacturers' products. Other available canine vaccines include those given for canine infectious tracheobronchitis *(B. bronchiseptica)*, rabies, and Lyme disease *(B. burgdorferi)*. Manufacturer recommendations should be followed regarding age, route of administration, and follow-up boosters needed for each individual vaccine. Box 17-1 provides an example of a vaccination program for dogs.

An exciting new therapeutic-type vaccine has been developed by Merial. Known as canine (oral) melanoma vaccine, it is indicated for use in dogs in which local disease has occurred. At present, the vaccine will only be sold to veterinarians who specialize in oncology.

Canine Vaccines

Canine distemper
Canine parvovirus
Rabies vaccine
Canine adenovirus
Infectious tracheobronchitis
Canine leptospirosis
Canine coronavirus
Canine *Giardia*
Canine Lyme borreliosis

Equine

Many horse vaccines are available, including those for tetanus, equine encephalomyelitis (may include Eastern, Western, and/or Venezuelan strains), equine rhinopneumonitis, equine influenza, *Streptococcus* (strangles), equine viral arteritis, equine monocytic ehrlichiosis (Potomac horse fever), anthrax spore, and rabies. Tetanus antitoxin is used in wounded

BOX 17-1 General Outline of a Preventive Health Program for Dogs

First Office Visit for Health Program—Usually at 6 Weeks of Age

A. Conduct a general physical examination and record body weight
B. Check for external parasites and dermatophytes, and initiate appropriate therapy
   1. Fleas, ticks, ear mites *(Otodectes cynotis)*
   2. Mange mites, especially *Demodex canis* and *Sarcoptes scabiei*
   3. Dermatophytes, particularly *Microsporum* spp. and *Trichophyton mentagrophytes*
C. Conduct a fecal examination including both direct smear and flotation
D. Initiate administration of heartworm preventive management
E. Administer an anthelmintic for hookworms and roundworms and, if tapeworms are present, administer praziquantel or epsiprantel
F. Vaccinate with DA_2PLPC* and, possibly, with kennel cough vaccine,[†] canine Lyme borreliosis vaccine, and *Giardia* vaccine
G. Advise on nutrition and routine grooming
H. Provide the owner with client education pamphlets on topics such as the following:
   1. Identification, treatment, and control of fleas, ticks, and ear mites
   2. Benefits of preventive management for canine heartworm disease
   3. Management of normal and abnormal puppy behaviors
   4. Skin, nail, and ear care
   5. "How to" on grooming and nutrition
I. Fill in the puppy's health record for the owner

Second Office Visit for Health Program—Usually at 9 Weeks of Age

A. Conduct a general physical examination and record body weight
B. Check for external parasites and dermatophytes, and initiate appropriate therapy
   1. Fleas, ticks, ear mites *(O. cynotis)*
   2. Mange mites, especially *D. canis* and *S. scabiei*
   3. Dermatophytes, particularly *Microsporum* spp. and *T. mentagrophytes*
C. Conduct a fecal examination including both direct smear and flotation
D. Adjust the dosage of heartworm preventive according to body weight
E. Administer an anthelmintic for hookworms and roundworms and, if tapeworms are present, administer praziquantel or epsiprantel
F. Vaccinate with DA_2PLPC* and, possibly, with kennel cough vaccine,[†] canine Lyme borreliosis vaccine, and *Giardia* vaccine
G. Adjust nutrition according to health needs, and, if needed, change the grooming procedures
H. Provide the owner with client education pamphlets on topics such as the following:
   1. Identification, treatment, and control of fleas, ticks, and ear mites
   2. Benefits of preventive management for canine heartworm disease
   3. Dental, skin, nail, and ear care
   4. "How to" on grooming and nutrition
   5. Management of normal and abnormal puppy behaviors
   6. Exercise and its importance
I. Fill in the puppy's health record for the owner

Third Office Visit for Health Program—Usually at 12 Weeks of Age

A. Conduct a general physical examination and record body weight
B. Check for external parasites and dermatophytes, and initiate appropriate therapy
   1. Fleas, ticks, ear mites *(O. cynotis)*
   2. Mange mites, especially *D. canis* and *S. scabiei*
   3. Dermatophytes, particularly *Microsporum* spp. and *T. mentagrophytes*
C. Conduct a fecal examination including both direct smear and flotation
D. Adjust the dosage of heartworm preventive according to body weight
E. Administer an anthelmintic for hookworms and roundworms and, if tapeworms are present, administer praziquantel or epsiprantel
F. Vaccinate with DA_2PLPC* and, possibly, with kennel cough vaccine,[†] canine Lyme borreliosis vaccine, and *Giardia* vaccine
G. Adjust nutrition according to health needs and, if needed, change grooming procedures
H. Provide the owner with client education pamphlets on topics such as the following:
   1. Identification, treatment, and control of fleas, ticks, and ear mites
   2. Dental, skin, nail, and ear care

BOX 17-1 General Outline of a Preventive Health Program for Dogs—cont'd

3. "How to" on grooming and nutrition
4. Management of normal and abnormal puppy behaviors
5. Recommendations for spaying and castration
6. Exercise and its importance

I. Fill in the puppy's health record for the owner

Subsequent Visits for Health Program—Usually Annual Visits‡

A. Conduct a general physical examination and record body weight
B. Check for external parasites and dermatophytes, and initiate appropriate therapy
   1. Fleas, ticks, ear mites *(O. cynotis)*
   2. Mange mites, especially *D. canis* and *S. scabiei*
   3. Dermatophytes, particularly *Microsporum* spp. and *T. mentagrophytes*
C. Conduct a fecal flotation and occult heartworm examination, or all tests for intestinal and heartworm infection screening
D. Adjust the dosage of heartworm preventive according to body weight
E. Administer an anthelmintic according to fecal examination findings
F. Vaccinate with DA_2PLPC* and rabies and, possibly, with kennel cough vaccine,† canine Lyme borreliosis vaccine, and *Giardia* vaccine
G. Adjust nutrition according to health needs and, if needed, change grooming procedures
H. Provide the owner with client education pamphlets on topics such as the following:
   1. Identification, treatment, and control of fleas, ticks, and ear mites
   2. Dental, skin, nail, and ear care
   3. "How to" on grooming and nutrition
   4. Management of normal and abnormal behaviors
   5. Exercise and its importance
I. Fill in the dog's health record for the owner

*This refers to the use of a vaccine to protect against the following: D, canine distemper; A_2 (canine adenovirus type 2), infectious canine hepatitis; P, canine parainfluenza; L, leptospirosis; P, canine parvovirus type 2 disease; and C, canine coronavirus disease.
†This refers to the use of a vaccine to protect against canine *Bordetella bronchiseptica*–induced disease. Puppies may be vaccinated with either an intranasal vaccine or a parenteral vaccine.
‡A fourth office visit may be desirable at 15 weeks of age for an additional parvovirus-2 vaccine booster in some puppies, especially high-risk breeds, such as Doberman pinscher, Rottweiler, Labrador retriever, and other presumed high-risk breeds.
From McCurnin DM, Bassert JM: Clinical textbook for veterinary technicians, ed 5, Philadelphia, 2002, WB Saunders.

horses with no history of recent tetanus toxoid vaccination. It provides immediate immunity, which lasts for about 2 weeks. Tetanus toxoid may be given to a horse to boost its immunity and provide longer protection. Manufacturer recommendations should be followed regarding age, route of administration, and follow-up boosters needed for each individual vaccine. Box 17-2 provides an example of a general preventive health program for horses.

Equine Vaccines

Tetanus
Equine rhinopneumonitis
Equine influenza
Strangles
Equine viral arteritis
Potomac horse fever
Botulism
Anthrax
Sarcocystis neurona
West Nile virus

Feline

A common polyvalent vaccine for cats is given for the prevention of feline viral rhinotracheitis (FVR), feline calicivirus (C), and feline panleukopenia (P). This combination may be referred to as *FVRCP.* Other available vaccines include those for feline chlamydiosis, feline leukemia, feline infectious peritonitis, *Bordetella,* and rabies. Manufacturer recommendations should be followed regarding age, route of administration, and follow-up boosters needed for each vaccine. Box 17-3 provides an example of a vaccination program for cats.

BOX 17-2 General Outline of a Preventive Health Program for Horses

First Quarter: January–March

All Horses

Deworm at least every 8 weeks. Exercise care in choice of anthelmintics for mares in the third trimester. Begin deworming foals at 2 months of age.

Trim feet every 6 weeks; do so more frequently in foals requiring limb correction.

Dentistry: check twice yearly and float teeth as needed. Remove wolf teeth in 2-year-olds and retained caps in 2-, 3-, and 4-year-olds.

Immunize for respiratory disease: influenza, strangles, and rhinopneumonitis.

In southeastern United States, immunize for equine encephalitis.

Stallions

Perform complete breeding examination. Maintain stallions under lights if being used for early breeding.

Pregnant Mares

Immunize with tetanus toxoid, and open sutured mares 30 days prepartum. Develop a colostrum bank. Ninth-day breeding only for mares with normal foaling history and normal reproductive tract. Wash udders of foaling mares.

Open Mares

Maintain under lights if being used for early breeding. Perform daily teasing. Perform reproductive tract examination during estrus. Mares should not be too fat but in gaining condition during breeding season.

Newborn Foals

Dip navel in disinfectant.

Carefully give a cleansing enema at birth.

Administer tetanus prophylaxis if indicated by history.

Perform immunoglobulin test at 12 to 24 hours.

Second Quarter: April–June

All Horses

Deworm at least every 8 weeks.

Trim feet every 6 weeks. Do not forget the foals and yearlings.

Dentistry: check teeth and remove or float teeth as needed.

Immunize for equine encephalomyelitis. Administer appropriate vaccine boosters.

Stallions

Maintain an exercise program.

Monitor the semen quality.

Broodmares

Palpate at 21, 42, and 60 days after successful breeding.

Foals

Creep-feed the foals and provide free-choice minerals. Immunize at 3 months of age.

Group foals by gender and size when weaned.

Third Quarter: July–September

All Horses

Deworm at least every 8 weeks. Clip and sweep the pastures.

Trim feet every 6 weeks. Continue corrective trimming on foals.

Dentistry: check teeth and remove or float teeth as needed.

Stallions

Maintain an exercise program.

Broodmares

Administer rhinopneumonitis boosters to pregnant mares according to manufacturer's labeled directions. Administer appropriate vaccine boosters to foals and yearlings.

Check condition of mare's udder at weaning, and reduce amount of feed given until milk flow is reduced.

Foals

Administer all appropriate immunizations. Provide free-choice minerals. Maintain a protein supplement in creep feeders.

Fourth Quarter: October–December

All Horses

Deworm at least every 8 weeks. Select an anthelmintic appropriate for the season.

Trim feet every 6 weeks. Continue corrective trimming on foals.

Dentistry: check teeth and remove or float teeth as needed.

Stallions

Continue exercise program.

Check immunizations.

Perform breeding examination.

Broodmares

Confirm pregnancy.

Begin treating open mares.

Check immunizations.

From McCurnin DM, Bassert JM: Clinical textbook for veterinary technicians, ed 5, Philadelphia, 2002, WB Saunders.

Feline Vaccines

Feline panleukopenia
Feline viral rhinotracheitis
Feline calicivirus
Rabies vaccine
Feline chlamydophila
Feline leukemia virus
Feline immunodeficiency virus
Feline infectious peritonitis
Feline *Bordetella*
Feline fungal vaccine
Feline *Giardia*

BOX 17-3 General Outline of a Preventive Health Program for Cats

First Office Visit for Health Program—Usually at 8 to 10 Weeks of Age

A. Perform a general physical examination and record body weight
B. Check for external parasites and dermatophytes, and initiate appropriate therapy for the following:
 1. Fleas and ear mites *(Otodectes cynotis)*
 2. Mange mites, especially *Notoedres cati*, *Demodex* spp., and *Cheyletiella* spp.
 3. Dermatophytes, particularly *Microsporum* spp. and *Trichophyton mentagrophytes*
C. Perform a fecal examination, including both direct smear and flotation
D. Administer anthelmintics, such as pyrantel pamoate for roundworms and hookworms and praziquantel or epsiprantel for tapeworms (if present)
E. Vaccinate with FVRC-P,*† *Chlamydia*,‡ FeLV§ (possibly test for FeLV/FIV before initial FeLV vaccination), FIP,¶ *Bordetella*, and *Giardia* vaccines
F. Advise on nutrition and routine grooming
G. Provide the owner with client education pamphlets on topics such as the following:
 1. Identification, treatment, and control of fleas, ticks, and ear mites
 2. Benefits of vaccination for FeLV infection
 3. Management of normal and abnormal cat behaviors
 4. Grooming "how to" and nutrition
H. Fill in the kitten's health record for the owner

Second Office Visit for Health Program—Usually at 12 to 14 Weeks of Age

A. Perform a general physical examination and record body weight
B. Check for external parasites and dermatophytes, and initiate appropriate therapy for the following:
 1. Fleas and ear mites *(O. cynotis)*
 2. Mange mites, especially *N. cati*, *Demodex* spp., and *Cheyletiella* spp.
 3. Dermatophytes, particularly *Microsporum* spp. and *T. mentagrophytes*
C. Perform a fecal examination, including both direct smear and flotation
D. Administer anthelmintics, such as pyrantel pamoate for roundworms and hookworms and praziquantel or epsiprantel for tapeworms (if present)
E. Vaccinate with FVRCP,* *Chlamydia*,‡ FeLV,§ rabies, FIP,¶ *Bordetella*, and *Giardia* vaccines
F. Adjust nutrition and grooming procedures
G. Provide the owner with client education pamphlets on topics such as the following:
 1. Identification, treatment, and control of fleas, ticks, and ear mites
 2. Benefits of vaccination for FeLV infection
 3. Dental, skin, nail, and ear care
 4. Management of normal and abnormal cat behaviors
 5. Exercise and its importance
 6. Recommendations for spaying, castration, and declawing
H. Fill in the kitten's health record for the owner

Subsequent Visits for Health Program—Usually Annual Visits

A. Perform a general physical examination and record body weight
B. Check for external parasites and dermatophytes, and initiate appropriate therapy for the following:
 1. Fleas and ear mites *(O. cynotis)*
 2. Mange mites, especially *N. cati*, *Demodex* spp., and *Cheyletiella* spp.
 3. Dermatophytes, particularly *Microsporum* spp. and *T. mentagrophytes*
C. Perform a fecal examination (fecal flotation)
D. Administer an anthelmintic, according to fecal examination findings
E. Vaccinate with FVRCP,* *Chlamydia*,‡ FeLV,§ rabies, FIP,¶ *Bordetella*, and *Giardia* vaccines

Continued

BOX 17-3 General Outline of a Preventive Health Program for Cats—cont'd

F. Adjust nutrition and grooming procedures
G. Provide the owner with client education pamphlets on topics such as the following:
 1. Identification, treatment, and control of fleas, ticks, and ear mites
 2. Benefits of vaccination for FeLV infection
 3. Dental, skin, nails, and ear care
 4. Management of normal and abnormal cat behaviors
 5. Exercise and its importance
 6. Recommendations for spaying, castration, and declawing
H. Fill in the cat's health record for the owner

FeLV, Feline leukemia virus; *FIP*, feline infectious peritonitis; *FIV*, feline immunodeficiency virus.
*FVRCP refers to the use of a vaccine to protect against feline viral rhinotracheitis (FVR), feline calicivirus infection (C), and feline panleukopenia (P).
†Cats being prepared for shipment or entering a boarding kennel, veterinary hospital, or clinic should be vaccinated at least 1 to 2 weeks before admission or shipment.
‡The vaccine currently available apparently produces effective protection only against *Chlamydia psittaci* infections. As with other vaccines for respiratory ailments, complete protection is not afforded; however, clinical signs of conjunctivitis or upper respiratory tract disease, if they do occur, can be restricted to short courses and are mild.
§Refers to the use of a vaccine to protect against FeLV infection. FeLV and FIV vaccines are administered subcutaneously in healthy kittens or older cats as two doses; the second dose is given 3 or 4 weeks after the first. Annual revaccination with a single dose is recommended.
¶The Primucell-FIP Vaccine (Pfizer Animal Health) is administered intranasally to healthy cats. Primary vaccination with two doses should be given; the second dose should be administered 3 to 4 weeks after the first, and single-dose annual revaccination is recommended.
From McCurnin DM, Bassert JM: Clinical textbook for veterinary technicians, ed 5, Philadelphia, 2002, WB Saunders.

Bovine

Many vaccines are available for cattle in many different combinations. Vaccine schedules for cattle vary depending on the type of cattle-raising operation; a veterinarian can best decide what program an individual operation needs. Examples of commonly used vaccines include those for leptospirosis, vibriosis, clostridial diseases, respiratory tract disease, and enteric disease. As with all vaccines, manufacturer recommendations should be carefully followed for the best results. Boxes 17-4 and 17-5 provide examples of preventive health programs for beef and dairy cattle.

Bovine Vaccines

Bovine respiratory disease complex vaccines are as follows:

PI3
IBR
BVD
Bovine respiratory syncytial virus
Mannheimia haemolytica (formerly known as *Pasteurella multocida*)
H. somnus
Clostridial vaccines
Leptospirosis
Campylobacteriosis (vibriosis)
Brucellosis
Trichomoniasis
Anthrax
Anaplasmosis
Enteric diseases
Bovine rotavirus
Bovine coronavirus
E. coli
Moraxella bovis (pinkeye)

Others

Vaccines are also available for sheep, poultry, and swine (Box 17-6). These animals may be raised in large numbers on farms, and similar to cattle-raising operations, vaccination schedules may vary according to the type of conditions and location. Ferrets have become common household pets and should be vaccinated for canine distemper according to the schedule used for dogs. Some rabies vaccines are

BOX 17-4 General Outline of a Preventive Health Program for Beef Cattle

Cow–Calf Herd Recommendations*

At Birth

Ingestion of colostrum within the first few hours after birth is an important factor in baby calf survival. Immunize with oral bovine rotavirus and coronavirus enteric disease vaccine if a calf diarrhea problem exists in the herd.

1- to 3-Month-Old Calves

Immunize with a seven-way clostridial disease product. Deworm with a commercial product that is safe for calves.

Preweaning Calves

Deworm with a broad-spectrum commercial dewormer, and immunize as follows:

IMMUNIZING VACCINE	AGE FOR VACCINE ADMINISTRATION
Brucella abortus, strain RB-51 (calfhood vaccination–replacement heifers only)	4 to 12 months
Clostridial diseases: *Clostridium perfringens* types C and D, *Clostridium chauvoei, Clostridium novyi, Clostridium septicum, Clostridium sordellii*	5 to 6 months
IBR and PI3 respiratory diseases (inactivated vaccines only)	5 to 6 months; booster at 12 to 13 months
BVD (inactivated vaccines only)	5 to 6 months; booster at 12 to 13 months
BRSV	5 to 6 months; booster at 12 to 13 months

Weaning Calves

Deworm with a broad-spectrum commercial dewormer, and treat for lice and grubs. Castrate the bull calves. Immunize with *Pasteurella* and *Haemophilus* (optional) vaccines.

Prebreeding Replacement Heifers

Deworm with a broad-spectrum commercial dewormer and treat for lice. Immunize as follows:

IMMUNIZING VACCINE	TIME OF VACCINE ADMINISTRATION
IBR and PI3 respiratory diseases	10 to 12 months
Clostridial diseases: *C. perfringens* types C and D, *C. novyi, C. septicum, C. sordellii, C. chauvoei*	10 to 12 months
BVD	10 to 12 months
BRSV	10 to 12 months
Leptospirosis	10 to 12 months
Campylobacteriosis	10 to 12 months

Prebreeding Cows

Deworm with a broad-spectrum dewormer and treat for lice. Immunize for leptospirosis and campylobacteriosis.

Precalving Cows

Immunize as follows:

IMMUNIZING VACCINE	TIME OF VACCINE ADMINISTRATION
IBR and PI3 respiratory diseases (inactivated vaccines only)	Before calving
BVD (inactivated vaccine only)	Before calving
BRSV	Before calving
Bovine rotavirus and coronavirus enteric diseases	Before calving
Escherichia coli enteric diseases	Before calving
Clostridial diseases: *C. perfringens* types C and D, *C. chauvoei, C. novyi, C. septicum, C. sordellii*	Before calving

Bulls

Deworm annually with a broad-spectrum dewormer, and treat for lice and grubs. Immunize as recommended for prebreeding replacement heifers annually (see the above section).

Continued

BOX 17-4 General Outline of a Preventive Health Program for Beef Cattle—cont'd

Feedlot Recommendations[†]

On Arrival into the Feedlot

Deworm with a broad-spectrum dewormer and immunize for IBR, PI3, BVD, BRSV, and clostridial diseases (use seven-way vaccine). Inactivated IBR, PI3, and BVD vaccines are the safest.

3-4 Weeks After Arrival into the Feedlot

Implant a commercial implant product. Treat for lice and grubs. Administer booster immunizations if necessary. Abort the heifers if necessary. Castrate and dehorn if necessary.

BRSV, Bovine respiratory syncytial virus; *BVD,* bovine virus diarrhea; *IBR,* infectious bovine rhinotracheitis; *PI3,* parainfluenza-3.

*Other optional vaccines that may be incorporated into the immunization program, depending on individual herd needs and diseases endemic to the area, include anthrax and anaplasmosis.

[†]Other optional vaccines that may be incorporated into the immunization program, depending on individual herd needs and diseases endemic to the area, include *Haemophilus somnus, Pasteurella* spp., leptospirosis, and anthrax.

From McCurnin DM, Bassert JM: Clinical textbook for veterinary technicians, ed 5, Philadelphia, 2002, WB Saunders.

BOX 17-5 General Outline of a Preventive Health Program for Dairy Cattle*

Calves

At Birth

Immunize with bovine rotavirus and coronavirus enteric disease vaccine,[†] and administer *Escherichia coli* enteric disease vaccine orally.

Weaning Age (about 2 months) to Breeding Age (about 15 months)

IMMUNIZING VACCINE	AGE FOR VACCINE ADMINISTRATION
Brucella abortus, strain RB-51 (calfhood vaccination—replacement heifers only)	4 to 12 months
Clostridial diseases: *Clostridium perfringens* types C and D, *Clostridium chauvoei, Clostridium novyi, Clostridium septicum, Clostridium sordellii*	2 to 4 months; booster in 2 weeks
IBR and PI3 respiratory diseases	4 to 6 months; booster at 12 to 13 months
BVD	6 to 8 months; booster at 12 to 13 months
BRSV	6 to 8 months; booster at 12 to 13 months
Leptospirosis	4 to 6 months; booster in 2 weeks
Campylobacteriosis	4 to 6 months; booster at 12 to 13 months

Fresh Cows and Heifers

IMMUNIZING VACCINE	TIME OF VACCINE ADMINISTRATION
IBR and PI3 respiratory diseases (inactivated vaccines only)	30 days postpartum
BVD (inactivated vaccines only)	30 days postpartum
BRSV	30 days postpartum
Leptospirosis	30 days postpartum
Campylobacteriosis	30 days postpartum

Dry Cows and Bred Heifers

The goal of dry cow immunization is to provide optimal protection for the newborn calf.

IMMUNIZING VACCINE	TIME OF VACCINE ADMINISTRATION
Leptospirosis	At time of dry-off
Bovine rotavirus and coronavirus enteric diseases[†]	At time of dry-off; booster in 2 to 3 weeks
Escherichia coli enteric disease[†]	At time of dry-off; booster in 2 to 3 weeks
Clostridial diseases: *C. perfringens* types C and D, *C. chauvoei, C. novyi, C. septicum, C. sordellii*	At time of dry-off; booster in 2 to 3 weeks

BRSV, Bovine respiratory syncytial virus; *BVD,* bovine virus diarrhea; *IBR,* infectious bovine rhinotracheitis; *PI3,* parainfluenza-3.

*Other vaccines that may be incorporated into the vaccination program, depending on individual herd needs and diseases endemic to the area, include *Haemophilus somnus, Pasteurella* spp., *Salmonella* spp., *Clostridium haemolyticum,* anthrax, and anaplasmosis.

[†]Use if problem of neonatal calf diarrhea exists on the farm.

From McCurnin DM, Bassert JM: Clinical textbook for veterinary technicians, ed 5, Philadelphia, 2002, WB Saunders.

BOX 17-6 General Outline of a Preventive Health Program for Swine

Prebreeding Recommendations for Boars
Purchase boars 60 days before intended use. Quarantine new boars for 30 days, then allow fence line contact with gilts and sows for 30 days before breeding. Immunize boars for leptospirosis and erysipelas. Treat for external and internal parasites before breeding.

Prebreeding Recommendations for Sows and Gilts
Immunize for leptospirosis, porcine parvovirus infection,* and pseudorabies* 2 to 4 weeks before breeding. Flush gilts by increasing ovulations. Treat for external and internal parasites before breeding.

Prefarrowing Recommendations for Sows and Gilts
Limit feed intake to about 4 lb per head per day or feed according to condition to avoid overweight sows or gilts at farrowing. Immunize for colibacillosis,* atrophic rhinitis, erysipelas, transmissible gastroenteritis (TGE), porcine rotavirus infection,* and *Clostridium perfringens* type C* according to manufacturer's labeled instructions. Treat for external and internal parasites before farrowing with approved products.

Farrowing Recommendations
Gradually increase feed intake so lactating swine are receiving full feed at peak milk production. (Rule of thumb: feed daily 1 lb of feed for every pig being nursed [e.g., a lactating sow with a litter of 12 pigs should receive at least 12 lb of feed daily].)

General Recommendations for Pigs
At Birth
Perform newborn pig procedures (e.g., clip needle teeth, dock tails, castrate, ear-notch, and inject iron dextran).

1 Week of Age
Immunize for TGE,* rotavirus,* and atrophic rhinitis.

4 to 5 Weeks of Age
Weaning occurs at this time. Immunize for atrophic rhinitis, erysipelas, and *Actinobacillus* infection.*

6 to 8 Weeks of Age
Treat for external and internal parasites with approved products.

Older Than 8 Weeks of Age
Repeated treatments for external and internal parasites with approved products may need to be done during the growing-finishing period.

*Dependent on problems in the individual swine herd.
From McCurnin DM, Bassert JM: Clinical textbook for veterinary technicians, ed 5, Philadelphia, 2002 WB Saunders.

approved for use in ferrets. Public health authorities can require a rabies-vaccinated ferret that bites a human to be euthanized and tested for rabies virus.

Swine Vaccines
Erysipelas
Leptospirosis
Transmissible gastroenteritis (TGE)
Porcine rotavirus
C. perfringens (type C)
Neonatal porcine colibacillosis
Porcine proliferative enteritis vaccine
Bordetella
Pasteurella
Actinobacillus
Mycoplasma
Porcine reproductive and respiratory syndrome (PRRS) vaccine
Porcine parvovirus
Pseudorabies
Streptococcus

Small Ruminant Vaccines
Enterotoxemia
Tetanus
Campylobacteriosis (vibriosis)
Chlamydia
Contagious ecthyma
Foot rot
Bluetongue

IMMUNOTHERAPEUTIC DRUGS

It may often be desirable to use drugs to stimulate the body's immunologic response. Immunotherapy involves using drugs to stimulate or suppress the body's immunologic response to diseases or conditions caused by agents such as bacteria, viruses, or cancer cells. Immunostimulants are agents that stimulate the immune response. Immunomodulators are agents used to adjust the immune response to a desired level. Table 17-1 lists some of the drugs commonly used in immunotherapy.

Immunostimulants act by stimulating macrophage activity, producing lymphokines, increasing natural killer cell activity, and enhancing cell-mediated immunity. These drugs may be used in the treatment of chronic pyoderma in dogs, equine sarcoids, and bovine ocular squamous cell carcinoma. They also may be used as adjunctive therapy for some other types of cancers, such as canine malignant lymphoma, fibrosarcoma, and feline retrovirus infection. Some immunostimulants may be used to help reduce the clinical signs and mortality associated with some infections such as *E. coli* diarrhea in calves. Many other immunostimulants, such as interferons, interleukin-1, and interleukin-2, are being investigated for potential use in veterinary medicine.

Immunosuppressive drugs are used to suppress the body's immunologic response. They are used in veterinary medicine to treat various immune-mediated disorders. Further information on immunosuppressive drugs may be found in Chapter 16.

IMMUNOSTIMULANTS

Complex Carbohydrates

Acemannan

This is a complex carbohydrate derived from aloe vera.

Clinical Uses

Acemannan is used as an aid in the treatment of fibrosarcoma in cats and dogs. It has also been used for stimulating wound healing and in the treatment of FeLV-infected and FIV-infected cats.

Dosage Form

- Acemannan Immunostimulant

Adverse Side Effects

There are no known side effects.

Immunomodulatory Bacterins

Staphylococcal Phage Lysate

Staphylococcal phage lysate (SPL) is prepared by lysing *Staphylococcus aureus* with a polyvalent bacteriophage.

TABLE 17-1 Immunotherapeutic Drugs and Indications for Their Use

PRODUCT NAME AND MANUFACTURER	PRODUCT TYPE	PRODUCT INDICATIONS
Acemannan Immunostimulant (Carrington)	A complex carbohydrate derived from aloe vera; stimulates macrophage activity	An aid in the treatment of fibrosarcoma in cats and dogs, and feline leukemia; also for stimulating wound healing
Staphage Lysate (SPL) (Delmont)	*Staphylococcus aureus* phage lysate	Treatment for canine pyoderma and related skin infections with a staphylococcal component
Rubeola Virus Immunomodulator (Eudaemonic)	Inactivated rubeola virus with histamine phosphate	Treatment of equine chronic myofascial inflammation
Nomagen (Fort Dodge)	A mycobacterial cell-wall fraction immunostimulant	Treatment of equine sarcoids and bovine ocular squamous cell carcinoma
ImmunoRegulin (Immuno Vet)	*Propionibacterium acnes* immunostimulant	Chronic recurrent pyoderma in dogs
CL/Mab 231 (Synbiotics)	Canine lymphoma monoclonal antibody	Adjunctive therapy for dogs with lymphoma

Clinical Uses

SPL is used in the treatment of canine pyoderma and related skin infections with a staphylococcal component.

Dosage Form

- Staphage Lysate (SPL)

Adverse Side Effects

These include malaise, fever, chills, and injection site irritation.

Propionibacterium acnes *Bacterin*

This is prepared from killed *Propionibacterium acnes.*

Clinical Uses

P. acnes is used in the treatment of chronic recurrent pyoderma and as an adjunctive therapy in the treatment of equine respiratory disease complex. It also has been used as an adjunctive therapy in the treatment of feline retrovirus infection.

Dosage Forms

- ImmunoRegulin
- EqStim

Adverse Side Effects

These include malaise, fever, and chills.

Mycobacterial Cell Wall Fraction

This is an emulsion of cell wall fractions that are modified to reduce their toxicity and allergic effects.

Clinical Uses

These include the treatment of equine sarcoids and bovine ocular squamous cell carcinoma. It is also used in the treatment of mixed mammary tumors and mammary adenocarcinoma in dogs.

Dosage Forms

- Regressin-V
- Nomagen

Adverse Side Effects

These include malaise, fever, and decreased appetite.

> *TECHNICIAN NOTES* The effects of immunotherapy may be decreased with the administration of immunosuppressive drugs.

REVIEW QUESTIONS

1. Immunizations should never take the place of regularly scheduled ____________.
2. What six factors may determine an animal's response to immunization? ____________
3. What is an inactivated vaccine? ____________
4. What is a live vaccine? ____________
5. What is a modified live vaccine? ____________
6. What is a toxoid? ____________
7. What is an antitoxin? ____________
8. When a shipment of vaccine arrives at a veterinary facility, what should occur immediately? ____________
9. What is immunotherapy? ____________
10. ____________ is a complex carbohydrate derived from aloe vera.
11. Vaccines are all that is needed to implement a comprehensive health care plan for animals.
    a. True
    b. False
12. All the following are important factors in a patient's response to vaccine, except ______.
    a. the health and age of the patient
    b. the type of vaccine given
    c. the route of administration
    d. administering a medicated bath before vaccination to clean the skin's surface

13. In the manufacture of _____ vaccines, organisms are treated most commonly by chemicals that kill the organisms, but very little change occurs in the antigens that stimulate protective immunity.
    a. live
    b. modified live
    c. inactivated (dead)
    d. recombinant
14. A ______ vaccine is prepared from live microorganisms or viruses. These organisms may be fully virulent or avirulent. Few vaccines of this origin are in use.
    a. live
    b. modified live
    c. inactivated (dead)
    d. recombinant
15. In _________ vaccines, organisms undergo a process (attenuation) to lose their virulence so that, when introduced to the body via inoculation, they cause an immune response instead of disease.
    a. live
    b. modified live
    c. inactivated (dead)
    d. recombinant
16. A(an) _______ vaccine is a specific antiserum aimed at a toxin that contains a concentration of antibodies extracted from the blood serum or plasma of a hyperimmunized animal (usually a horse).
    a. toxoid
    b. antitoxin
    c. recombinant
    d. autogenous
17. Most vaccines for small animals are most commonly administered by what route?
    a. intramuscular
    b. subcutaneous
    c. intravenous
    d. intranasal
18. All the following may be signs of anaphylaxis, except _____.
    a. vomiting
    b. blepharospasm
    c. salivation
    d. dyspnea
19. *Bordetella bronchiseptica* is a vaccine administered to _____.
    a. equines
    b. dogs
    c. cats
    d. both a and b
    e. both b and c
20. *Borrelia burgdorferi* is an example of a _________ vaccine.
    a. modified live
    b. autogenous
    c. recombinant
    d. toxoid

REFERENCES

Ford RB: Vaccines and vaccinations: issues for the 21st century, Suppl Compend Contin Educ Pract Vet 20(8C):19–24, 1998.

McCurnin DM, Bassert J, editors: Clinical textbook for veterinary technicians, ed 6, Philadelphia, 2006, WB Saunders.

Van Kampen KR: Recombinant technology, Suppl Compend Contin Educ Pract Vet 20(8):28–32, 1998.

CHAPTER 18

Miscellaneous Therapeutic Agents

KEY TERMS

Autologous
Chelating agent
Interleukins
Matrix
Methemoglobinemia
Nutraceutical
Stem cell

OUTLINE

LEARNING OBJECTIVES

After studying this chapter, you should be able to

1. Exhibit knowledge of polysulfated glycosaminoglycans and describe how they act as chondroprotectives.
2. List and describe three treatment methods used in regenerative medicine.
3. Generally describe the uses and adverse side effects of common antidotes.
4. Describe the use of naloxone and yohimbine HCl as reversal agents.
5. List the names of common lubricants.
6. Define *nutraceutical* and discuss the uses of nutraceuticals in veterinary medicine.
7. Discuss the advantages and disadvantages of herbal therapeutics and the evaluation of individual herbal products.

ALTERNATIVE MEDICINES

CHONDROPROTECTIVES

Chondroprotectives are substances that are able to decrease the progression of osteoarthritis by providing support to cartilage and promoting its repair.

Polysulfated Glycosaminoglycans

Polysulfated glycosaminoglycan (PSGAG) consists of a repeating chain of hexosamine and hexuronic acid (Boothe, 2012). The complex nature of the molecule allows water to be trapped in hyaline cartilage to provide resistance to compression and resiliency to the proteoglycan and collagen matrix. PSGAGs are extracted for commercial use from the tracheal tissue of the bovine. After intramuscular injection, PSGAG is deposited in articular cartilage and is preferentially taken up by osteoarthritic cartilage (Plumb, 2011). When used to treat degenerative joint conditions, these PSGAGs increase synovial fluid viscosity and inhibit enzymes that damage cartilage matrix within joints. PSGAGs also reduce inflammation by inhibiting prostaglandin released in joint injury.

Clinical Uses

PSGAG is used in the treatment of noninfectious degenerative or traumatic joint dysfunction and associated lameness of the carpal joints in horses. It also has been used to treat degenerative joint disorders in dogs and lameness in swine.

Dosage Forms

- Adequan I.A., for intraarticular injection
- Adequan I.M., for intramuscular injection
- Adequan Canine
- Chondroprotec

Adverse Side Effects

Adverse side effects are minimal with use of this product.

TECHNICIAN NOTES

- Amikacin may be used concurrently via the intraarticular route to prevent infection resulting from possible contamination.
- PSGAG should not be used in horses intended for food.
- Safety in breeding animals is undetermined.

REGENERATIVE MEDICINE

Regenerative medicine refers to the use of cells, cytokines, scaffolds, and growth factors to improve the repair of damaged or poorly functioning tissues or organs (Fitzwater, 2013). This therapy involves collecting tissue (generally fat, bone marrow, or blood) from the patient, isolating the desired cells or products, and administering the products back to the patient. These **autologous** products function to replace damaged tissue or stimulate the body's own repair mechanisms to bring about healing. Much of the focus of regenerative medicine is on the use of stem cells but also includes the use of **interleukin** antagonists, platelet-rich plasma (PRP), and other products. Regenerative medicine is used most often in the treatment of orthopedic disorders in horses and dogs. Other potential uses include chronic kidney disease and asthma in cats as well as immune-mediated disorders like inflammatory bowel disease and autoimmune hemolytic anemia in companion animals. The efficacy of regenerative medicine is somewhat controversial at this time because of questions related to the lack of extensive data from controlled studies. Some uncertainty remains whether positive results are due to tissue repair, an antiinflammatory effect, or postprocedure rest and restrictions.

Stem Cell Therapy

Stem cells are cells that reside in most native tissues of both the adult and the embryo and are essential for the maintenance of homeostasis. All organisms continuously renew various tissues and organs. This renewal process can occur because of a source of cells that are able to differentiate into the appropriate tissue or organ. These reserve cells are called **stem cells.**

The two types of stem cells are embryonic and adult. Embryonic stem cells are derived from the early embryo and are called totipotent or pluripotent because they can give rise to multiple tissue types and complete organs needed for the entire organism. These embryonic stem cells can be grown in vitro and form immortal cell lines. They are very useful in research but have two characteristics that limit their clinical use: (1) they form tumors called teratomas when implanted into a patient, and (2) they are foreign tissue that may be rejected by the host. Adult stem cells have a reduced capability for differentiation when compared with embryonic stem cells and are thus called *multipotent*. They are the cells that are used to make the daily renewals to tissues and organs. When used clinically, they do not form teratomas and because they are autologous they are not rejected as foreign. The use of adult stem cells also avoids the controversy of collecting from embryonic tissue. Stem cells derived from bone marrow or fat are called mesenchymal cells or stromal cells. Mesenchymal stem cells can differentiate into fat, cartilage, or bone and are the stem cells used clinically in veterinary medicine. The beneficial effect of stem cell therapy is a result of several mechanisms that include (1) production of growth factors and cytokines that foster growth and regeneration of tissue, (2) production and secretion of antiinflammatory mediators and other immune modulators, (3), differentiation into target tissues like cartilage and/or bone, and (4) the ability to "home" to an inflamed site through the vascular system. Stem cells are harvested from either bone marrow or fat. Fat yields a significantly larger number of cells than bone marrow but a definitive number of cells for therapy has not been established. In dogs and cats, fat tissue is usually harvested from the falciform ligament, the caudal scapular space, or the inguinal fold. The harvest site in the horse is usually the tail head area. Dogs and cats require general anesthesia for collection while collection can usually be performed with the use of sedation in the horse. After harvest, stem cells are sent to a commercial laboratory for isolation and culture or prepared in-hospital with the use of a bench-top technique. After preparation, the mesenchymal stem cells are injected with the use of aseptic technique either into the injury site or intravenously.

Companies providing stem cell products or services include the following:

- Vet Stem
- MediVet
- Animal Cell Therapies

Platelet-Rich Plasma

PRP is the platelet-concentrated plasma obtained from anticoagulated whole blood by a centrifugation process. The platelets are concentrated around the buffy coat near the top of the red cells at the distal end of the plasma. PRP provides several growth factors that signal local mesenchymal, epithelial, and endothelial cells to migrate, divide, and increase collagen and **matrix** formation. PRP therapy is used primarily by equine veterinarians for tendon and ligament injuries and to promote granulation of tissue defects. Blood is collected from the injured patient and centrifuged with a specialized tube. Plasma containing the autologous platelets is then separated from the red blood cells and injected into the injured tissue.

Companies supplying PRP products include:

- Vet Stem
- Vet Cell
- Vantus Laboratories

Interleukin-1 Antagonist Protein

Interleukin-1 (IL-1) is a proinflammatory cytokine that acts as a major mediator of joint disease. It is produced by synoviocytes, chondrocytes, and white blood cells and stimulates neutral proteinase production. Neutral proteinases promote synovial membrane thickening, cartilage breakdown, and general tissue destruction. The healthy joint has a balance of IL-1 and IL-1 antagonist (IL-1Ra). The theory of IL-1a therapy says that the injured or diseased joint has increased IL-1 that can be offset with IL-1Ra treatment. In this therapy blood is drawn from the equine patient with the use of a special syringe. This syringe contains glass beads that stimulate the production of IL-1Ra from white blood cells. The syringe containing the patient's blood and the glass beads is incubated and spun in a centrifuge to separate the plasma containing the IL-1Ra. The specially prepared plasma is then injected into the injured or diseased joint. This modality is mainly used to treat synovitis, capsulitis, arthritis, and, potentially, bursitis and tenosynovitis. Treatment with IL-1Ra is often called IRAP therapy.

Companies providing IRAP products include the following:
- Arthrex Vet Systems
- Dechra

NUTRACEUTICALS

The American Veterinary Medical Association (AVMA) defines **nutraceutical** medicine as "the use of micronutrients, macronutrients, and other nutritional supplements as therapeutic agents." In veterinary medicine, the term is generally used to refer to endogenous substances (not botanicals) that have been prepared or synthesized to support bodily functions. The popularity of these products, which may have characteristics of nutrients and pharmaceuticals, has seen tremendous growth in use by people in recent years. The medical community has acknowledged that some of them may have treatment or preventive effects (Boothe, 1997).

As people have become more aware of alternative medical options for themselves, they have come to expect similar options for their pets. Veterinarians and their clients can be expected to use nutraceuticals as treatment options to complement traditional medicine or when traditional treatment options have been exhausted.

The former North American Veterinary Nutraceutical Council proposed that a veterinary nutraceutical be defined as "a nondrug substance that is produced in a purified or extracted form and administered orally to provide agents required for normal body structure and function with the intent of improving the health and well-being of animals." Even though the definitions listed for nutraceutical and veterinary nutraceutical seem straightforward, a great deal of confusion exists over what is actually a nutraceutical. It has been stated that the term *nutraceutical* was developed to refer to a product marketed under the premise of being a dietary supplement but with the real intent of preventing or treating a disease (Warren, 2007).

The question often asked about these products is "Is it a food (nutrient) or a drug?" If it is a food, then it is not subject to U.S. Food and Drug Administration (FDA) approval; if it is a drug, it must go through the FDA approval process at a great deal of expense to the manufacturer. A product is usually determined to be a drug if its label has a claim that indicates a therapeutic or preventive intent. If the product has a label claim of a medical use and does not carry a new animal drug application (NADA) (indicating FDA approval), the product then becomes an unapproved drug and is subject to FDA regulation. Because the FDA has limited resources and higher priority issues, regulatory action may not be taken against these unapproved products. If a product is determined to be a food, it is usually determined to be "generally regarded as safe (GRAS)" by the FDA. Any product that is given by injection is considered a drug.

The Dietary Supplement Health and Education Act (DSHEA) of 1994 listed dietary supplements as vitamins, minerals, amino acids, herbal products, and substances that supplement the diet by increasing total dietary intake. This action made these products "food" and excluded them from FDA regulation. The Act does require, however, that the manufacturer show a disclaimer on the label after the product claim that says, "This statement has not been evaluated by the Food and Drug Administration. This product is not intended to diagnose, treat, cure, or prevent any disease." Because of concerns about potential residues and the potential differences in response across species, the Center for Veterinary Medicine (CVM) of the FDA has stated that the DSHEA does not apply to animals or animal feeds.

Because nutraceuticals have not been through an extensive evaluation process to validate their purity, safety, and efficacy, it is up to the veterinarian to evaluate the suitability of particular products for use in companion animals and to promote their use in the context of a valid veterinarian–client–patient relationship. Veterinary technicians should consult with their veterinarians to formulate sound advice to give to clients regarding use of these products. Some questions that should be answered when a nutraceutical product is evaluated include the following:
- What controlled studies have been done to determine whether the product does what it claims to do, and who performed the studies? Are these studies published in reputable veterinary journals?

- Does the product contain what it says it does, and is that product bioavailable? Bioavailability may be influenced by the source and form of the product (e.g., glucosamine HCl vs. glucosamine sulfate).
- Is the label easily understandable and are all ingredients listed in the same units? Ingredients should be listed by the order of magnitude by weight.
- Is the dosage listed on the label, along with clear instructions for use?
- Is the product free of contaminants? Were good manufacturing practices (GPAs) followed?
- Does the label carry a United States Pharmacopeia (USP)–verified label for the product or ingredient/s?

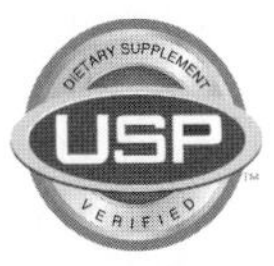

- Is the manufacturer a member of the National Animal Supplement Council (NASC)?

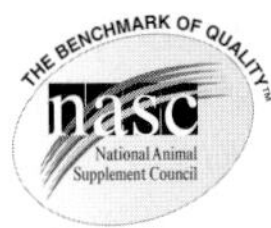

- Does the product have a lot number and expiration date on the label?
- Does the product rely on testimonials rather than scientific evidence for validation?

Clients should be urged to make use of information regarding nutraceutical quality by making use of the ConsumerLab (www.consumerlab.com) and USP (www.usp.org) websites.

The following is a partial list of the substances marketed as nutraceuticals. Some of these products may not be "endogenous substances" as defined earlier.

Glucosamine and Chondroitin Sulfate

Glucosamine is an amino sugar manufactured by animal cells from glucose and used by the body in the synthesis of glycoproteins and PSGAGs. Chondroitin sulfate is a glycosaminoglycan that combines with hyaluronic acid, proteins, and other glycosaminoglycans to form the basic cartilage matrix. Glucosamine and chondroitin sulfate are believed to act synergistically (Davidson, 2000) to exert a positive effect on cartilage metabolism and inhibition of cartilage breakdown. They have been used extensively in the treatment of osteoarthritis in dogs and horses. Four to six weeks of administration may be necessary for a therapeutic effect to be seen. A common veterinary product that contains these substances is called Cosequin; it is composed of glycosaminoglycan derived from the chitin of crab shell and chondroitin sulfate from bovine trachea. Dasuquin and Dasuquin for Cats are products that contain glucosamine and chondroitin sulfate with avocado/soybean unsaponifiables and decaffeinated tea with claims of enhanced chondroprotection. Glyco-Flex and SynoFlex derive their glycosaminoglycan from the *Perna canaliculus* mussel.

Fatty Acids

The omega-6 and omega-3 fatty acids are the ones most often found in commercial veterinary fatty acid supplements. Omega-6 fatty acids have a double bond six carbons from the methyl end, whereas omega-3 fatty acids have a double bond three carbons from the methyl end. Fatty acid supplementation has been shown to be useful in treating certain dermatologic conditions in dogs and cats because of their antiinflammatory effects. Omega-3 fatty acids are normally found in low concentrations in the cellular plasma membrane compared with omega-6 fatty acids, but the omega-3 level can be increased by a food or supplement that is enriched in this substance (Roudebush and Freeman, 2000). The breakdown products of the omega-3 acids are apparently less powerful mediators of the inflammatory response than those derived from the omega-6 fatty acids. The omega-3 and omega-6 fatty acids also may be helpful in treating heart disease, cancer, autoimmune disease, and rheumatoid arthritis. The proper ratio of omega-6 to omega-3 fatty acids in a product has apparently not been determined and is often debated. Fish oil and plant oils are common sources of these fatty acids. Side effects may include increased bleeding times and possible decreased immune function.

S-Adenosylmethionine

S-adenosylmethionine (SAMe) SD4 is a molecule produced in the body from methionine and adenosine triphosphate (ATP) by the enzyme SAMe synthetase (Davidson, 2002). It is recommended for veterinary use as a dietary supplement to support normal structure and function of the liver. Some studies have shown that this substance increases levels of glutathione in the liver. Glutathione is an antioxidant that may protect liver cells from injury. Denosyl is a SAMe product manufactured by Nutramax Laboratories.

Superoxide Dismutase

Superoxide dismutase from protein sources is an oxygen radical scavenger that has been used as an antiinflammatory agent for musculoskeletal problems.

Coenzyme Q

This substance is an enzyme cofactor of mitochondrial membranes that is important in electron transport and ATP formation. It is used in the treatment of cardiovascular problems.

HERBAL MEDICINES

The use of plants to treat veterinary patients is classified by the AVMA as a modality in the category of complementary and alternative veterinary medicine (CAVM). The AVMA in its policy guidelines states that "the theoretical bases and techniques for CAVM may diverge from veterinary medicine routinely taught in North American veterinary schools or may differ from current scientific knowledge or both." Even though it can be a controversial topic, the demand for herbal medicine by veterinary clients appears to have grown as an extension of the trend toward the increased use of "natural" dietary supplements and the "holistic" approach to good health in people. People may conclude that if herbal supplements make them feel better, the supplements will also make their pets feel better. The two main branches of herbal medicine are traditional and modern.

Traditional use of plant materials to treat ailments in people and animals can be traced to many ancient cultures, including highly refined traditions in China and India. The basis of Traditional Chinese Medicine (TCM), still practiced by some CAVM advocates, is the alteration of energetic systems in the body such as yin, yang, heat, cold, warm, dry, and moist through botanical interventions.

Modern herbal medicine makes use of the fact that plants or plant material contains chemicals (drugs) that may be used in a manner similar to drugs supplied by the pharmaceutical industry. Proponents of herbal medicine argue that whole plants (as opposed to a purified product) provide the advantages of synergy and safety. Synergy, they state, occurs when the primary therapeutic chemical in a plant/plants interacts with other chemicals in the plant/plants to provide a magnified or more efficacious effect. Safety, they believe, occurs because multiple chemicals in a plant may dilute any singly toxic ingredient. Some herbal practitioners report that plants "may contain antimicrobial, anticancer, and immune modulating factors" (Wynn, 2002) not presently known in currently used drugs. Herbal medicine, when used in conjunction with conventional medicine, can provide another dimension of service to the veterinary client and patient.

Very few controlled studies have been performed to document the safety and efficacy of herbal products. Veterinarians must rely on empiric data, anecdotal information, and personal experience to guide their use of botanicals. The Cochrane Collaboration provides a library of papers from studies conducted with the use of botanical medicine. Botanicals are classified as supplements by the FDA according to the DSHEA and fall into a regulatory gray zone where few monitoring programs are in place to ensure the potency and purity of these products. Plants may vary in their makeup according to climate conditions, soil type, fertilizer used, and other factors. Manufacturing practices, packaging procedures, and storage conditions also may influence the quality of the product. Quality control practices regarding the actual content of the product as well as its strength and purity may vary widely from manufacturer to manufacturer and from country to country. A coalition of animal supplement manufacturers formed the NASC, a voluntary membership group, to address issues of quality control in the industry in the United States. Some veterinarians have advised against using herbal products manufactured in China because of

TABLE 18-1 Potential Herb–Drug Interactions

HERB	INTERACTING DRUGS	RESULT
St. John's wort	Cyclosporine Fexofenadine Midazolam Digoxin Tacrolimus Amitriptyline Warfarin Theophylline	Decreased plasma drug concentrations
	Sertraline Buspirone	Serotonin syndrome
Gingko	Warfarin Heparin NSAIDs	Bleeding
	Omeprazole	Decreased plasma concentrations
Ginseng	Warfarin	Bleeding
	Heparin	Falsely elevated serum digoxin levels (laboratory test interaction with ginseng)
	NSAIDs	
	Opioids	Decreased analgesic effect
		Falsely elevated serum digoxin levels (laboratory test interaction with ginseng)
Garlic	Warfarin	Bleeding
Chamomile	Heparin	
Ginger	NSAIDs	

NSAIDs, Nonsteroidal antiinflammatory drugs.

reported contamination with heavy metals, herbs found in the product not listed on the label, or the presence of "spiked" (added) substances like anabolic steroids, glucocorticoids, thyroxine, and other substances (Rishniw, 2006). A useful resource for checking the quality of herbal products is the ConsumerLab website.

When choosing a product, veterinarians also must consider potential interactions of botanicals with conventional drugs that are being simultaneously administered and possible breed or species differences in drug responses. Certain herbs like ginkgo biloba, red clover, and feverfew may decrease platelet aggregation and should not be given before surgery or with conventional drugs that inhibit clotting. St. John's Wort should not be given with some drugs that modify behavior (monoamine oxidase inhibitors [MAOIs]). Potential herb–drug interactions are listed in Table 18-1. Other potential interactions can be found at the PubMed and ConsumerLab websites.

Botanicals are usually available from suppliers in three primary forms. These forms include the following:

Dried bulk herb: The plant has been harvested, dried, and often powdered. If powdered, it may be sold in loose powder form or placed in capsules.

Dried extracts: The plant is simmered in water, strained of residue, and sprayed into a vacuum chamber, which produces a powder or granules. A common extract is a 5:1 ratio that allows the use of less product because of the concentrated form. Water extracts may exclude plant substances that are alcohol soluble.

Liquid extracts: The ingredients are extracted in alcohol and the residue discarded. Advantages of alcohol extraction are thought to include concentration of the ingredient and improved absorption from the intestinal tract. Alcohol extractions usually taste bad to pets and must be added to another ingredient to improve palatability.

Most of the current dosing of botanicals for animals is extrapolated from human dosage information because few herbal products are produced specifically for animals. Dosage recommendations vary between forms and between extract dilutions (e.g., a 1:1 extract will be dosed differently than a 5:1 extract).

Summary of Herbal Medicines

Herbal medicine has added another dimension outside of conventional therapy to the treatment of veterinary patients. Its practice provides a holistic approach to veterinary health care for those veterinarians and clients who wish to use it as an ancillary method or when conventional methods have been exhausted. Until strict regulation of the botanical industry is achieved, however, veterinary technicians should counsel clients with judicious information about their use. The following factors may be helpful when one is advising clients about herbal use:

- The use of herbal medicine should not be started without discussion of the process with the attending veterinarian.
- Clients should purchase products from reputable manufacturers approved by the NASC.
- Clients can find product evaluation information at the ConsumerLab website.
- The recommended dosage should be followed closely.
- Herbs may cause harmful interactions with conventional drugs.
- Herb use may cause bleeding tendencies during surgical procedures.
- Adverse side effects of herbs should be reported to the Veterinary Botanical Medicine Association and to the manufacturer.

Box 18-1 includes a list of useful herbal references.

TECHNICIAN NOTES

The American Society of Anesthesiology recommends that patients should discontinue all herbal medicines 2 to 3 weeks before elective surgical procedures are performed.

BOX 18-1 Useful Herbal References

National Animal Supplement Council	www.nasc.cc
Veterinary Botanical Medicine Association	www.vbma.org
Drug Digest	www.drugdigest.org
PubMed	www.pubmed.gov
ConsumerLab	www.consumerlab.com
Cochrane Collaboration	www.cochrane.org
HerbMed	www.herbmed.org
American Association of Feed Control Officials	www.aafco.org
American Herbal Products Association	www.ahpa.org

Aloe

Aloe vera is a plant native to Africa that was used as early as 1500 BC for the treatment of various conditions and as a cathartic (Wynn and Fougere, 2007). Today, it is used primarily for the treatment of burns and skin inflammation. Some herbalists believe that aloe stimulates wound healing.

Bloodroot

The rhizome of *Sanguinaria canadensis* has traditionally been used as an expectorant and to treat respiratory conditions like bronchitis, asthma, and laryngitis. It is also reported to have antiinflammatory and antimicrobial effects.

Echinacea

Echinacea purpurea is a commonly used remedy for colds and flu in people in the United States and Europe, where research has been done to show that it is an immunostimulant. It is derived primarily from the American coneflower. No major side effects have been reported other than the occasional allergic reaction.

Garlic

Garlic is a perennial bulb in the lily family *(Allium sativum)* that is related to the onion. This plant has been used for centuries for its reported medicinal value. People have claimed that it produces disinfectant, diuretic, and/or expectorant effects. Evidence suggests that it does lower cholesterol values in people. No evidence, however, shows that garlic has any value in the treatment of parasites in animals. Garlic can produce Heinz body anemia in cats and possibly in dogs at high dosages.

Ginseng

Ginseng is made from the dried roots of several species of plants from the Panax family. Several varieties of ginseng, including American, Asian, Korean, and Siberian, have been identified. The Chinese believe that ginseng increases vitality and overall strength, possibly by improving aerobic metabolism. Side effects may include hypertension, nervousness, and excitement.

Ginkgo

Ginkgo biloba is thought to increase circulation to the brain and extremities and has been reported to improve memory and symptoms of senile dementia in people.

Goldenseal

The goldenseal plant *(Hydrastis canadensis)* produces an alkaloid ingredient called *berberine* that may have antimicrobial and vasoactive properties. Its potential veterinary indications include stomatitis, gastritis, enteritis, giardiasis, and focal bacterial skin infections (Wynn and Fougere, 2007). Goldenseal should not be used in pregnant animals because of its potential to cause uterine contractions (Romich, 2005). Goldenseal is becoming very scarce in the wild.

Milk Thistle

The milk thistle plant *(Silybum marianum)* contains an ingredient called *silymarin* that comprises biologically active flavonoids. This plant has been used as a hepatoprotectant and to enhance liver regeneration (Goodman and Trepanier, 2005). Milk thistle is thought to provide antioxidants that improve hepatocyte regeneration.

St. John's Wort

St. John's Wort is a plant that has reported (anecdotal) antianxiety and antidepression effects in people.

Saw Palmetto

Saw palmetto plant extract may be of value in treating benign prostatic hyperplasia because of its possible ability to reduce testosterone formation.

MISCELLANEOUS ANTIDOTES

Activated Charcoal

Activated charcoal is a fine, black, odorless, tasteless powder that is used to adsorb certain drugs or toxins to prevent or reduce their systemic absorption from the upper gastrointestinal tract.

Clinical Uses

These include oral administration to prevent or reduce the systemic absorption of certain drugs or toxins.

Dosage Forms

- Toxiban Suspension
- Toxiban Granules
- Activated charcoal powder (generic) (for reconstitution with water)

Adverse Side Effects

These include vomiting after very rapid administration of activated charcoal. Activated charcoal can also cause constipation or diarrhea, and the stool is black.

TECHNICIAN NOTES

- Activated charcoal is not considered effective against heavy metals (e.g., lead, mercury, or inorganic arsenic), mineral acids, caustic alkalis, nitrates, sodium, chloride/chlorate, ferrous sulfate, or petroleum distillates.
- Other oral therapeutic agents should not be administered within 3 hours after administration of activated charcoal therapy.
- Dairy products and mineral oil reduce the adsorptive properties of activated charcoal.

Calcium Ethylenediaminetetraacetic Acid

Calcium ethylenediaminetetraacetic acid (Ca-EDTA) is a heavy metal **chelating agent** that is available commercially (human label) as an injection. It also may be referred to as edetate calcium disodium, calcium disodium edetate, calcium edetate, calcium disodium ethylenediaminetetraacetate, and sodium calcium edetate.

Clinical Uses

In veterinary medicine, calcium EDTA is used for the treatment of lead poisoning.

Dosage Forms

- Calcium Disodium Versenate injection (human label)
- Meta-Dote

Adverse Side Effects

These include renal toxicity, depression (dogs), and vomiting/diarrhea (dogs). Zinc deficiency may occur from long-term therapy.

> **TECHNICIAN NOTES**
> - Calcium EDTA should not be used in anuric patients, and caution should be exercised when it is used in patients with renal insufficiency.
> - Calcium EDTA should not be administered orally.
> - Do not confuse with edetate disodium, which may cause severe hypocalcemia.
> - Magnesium sulfate (Epsom salt) or sodium sulfate may be used orally to prevent further intestinal absorption of lead.

Methylene Blue

Methylene blue is a thiazine dye that appears as dark green crystals or crystalline powder with a bronzelike luster. It is an oxidating agent that helps to convert methemoglobin (a compound formed from hemoglobin by oxidation of the iron atom) from the ferrous (Fe^{2+}) to the ferric (Fe^{3+}) state. It does not function as an oxygen carrier to hemoglobin.

Clinical Uses

Methylene blue is used for the treatment of **methemoglobinemia** caused by oxidative agents (e.g., nitrites, nitrates, and chlorates) in ruminants. It may be used for cyanide toxicity in ruminants. It can be used in dogs to intraoperatively stain pancreatic islet cell tumors preferentially and for treatment of acetaminophen poisoning.

Dosage Forms

- Methylene blue injection (generic) (human label)
- Methylene blue tablets (generic)
- Methylene blue powder (generic)

Adverse Side Effects

These include the development of Heinz body anemia or morphologic changes in red blood cells and decreased red blood cell life span. Methemoglobinemia may occur but is usually dose and species dependent. Tissue necrosis may occur with subcutaneous administration or extravasation during intravenous injection.

> **TECHNICIAN NOTES**
> - Methylene blue usually is contraindicated in cats.
> - Dogs and horses may show a greater occurrence of side effects than ruminants.
> - Methylene blue should not be used in patients with renal insufficiency.
> - Safety during pregnancy is unknown.

Acetylcysteine

Acetylcysteine is a white crystalline powder that is soluble in water or alcohol. It also may be referred to as *N*-acetylcysteine or *N*-acetyl-L-cysteine.

Clinical Uses

These include oral therapy for acetaminophen poisoning in dogs and cats. It also may be used as a mucolytic agent for pulmonary (via nebulization) or ophthalmic (via topical application) conditions.

Dosage Forms

- Mucomyst (human label)
- Mucosil (human label)
- Acetylcysteine (human label)

Adverse Side Effects

These include nausea, vomiting, and, occasionally, urticaria (hives) when administered orally. Chest tightness, bronchoconstriction, bronchial or tracheal irritation, and acetylcysteine hypersensitivity are rare but possible side effects when administered into the pulmonary tract. Acetylcysteine may cause bronchospasm in some patients receiving treatment via the pulmonary tract.

TECHNICIAN NOTES

- Acetylcysteine is incompatible with amphotericin B, chlortetracycline hydrochloride, erythromycin lactobionate, oxytetracycline hydrochloride, ampicillin sodium, tetracycline hydrochloride, iodized oil, hydrogen peroxide, chymotrypsin, and trypsin.
- Activated charcoal may adsorb acetylcysteine, reducing its effectiveness in treating acetaminophen toxicity.
- Carefully monitor patients that have bronchospastic diseases and that receive pulmonary treatment.
- The oral solution has a bad taste, and a masking agent (e.g., colas or juices) may be used.
- Open vials should be refrigerated and discarded after 96 hours.

Dimercaprol

Dimercaprol is a dithiol chelating agent that occurs as a colorless or nearly colorless viscous liquid with a disagreeable odor. The commercial solution may be cloudy or may contain small amounts of flaky material or sediment. This is normal and does not indicate deterioration of the product. It also may be referred to as BAL, British anti-Lewisite, dimercaptopropanol, or thioglycerol.

Clinical Uses

Dimercaprol is used primarily for the treatment of toxicity resulting from arsenic compounds but may be used for lead, mercury, or gold toxicity.

Dosage Forms

- Dimercaprol injection 100 mg/mL (human label)
- BAL in oil (human label)

Adverse Side Effects

Intramuscular injections are painful. Vomiting and seizures may occur with high doses. It is potentially nephrotoxic. Most side effects subside quickly because of rapid elimination of the drug.

Pralidoxime Chloride

Pralidoxime chloride is a quaternary ammonium oxime cholinesterase reactivator. It reverses the action of cholinesterase inhibitors such as certain organophosphates. It also may be referred to as a 2-PAM chloride or 2-pyridine aldoxime methyl chloride.

Clinical Uses

Pralidoxime chloride is used for oral treatment of organophosphate poisoning. It may be used in conjunction with atropine and supportive therapy.

Dosage Form

- Protopam injection (human label)

Adverse Side Effects

These are uncommon, but rapid intravenous injection may cause tachycardia, muscle rigidity, transient neuromuscular blockade, and laryngospasm.

TECHNICIAN NOTES

- Pralidoxime, similar to other anticholinesterases, may potentiate the action of barbiturates.
- Patients with impaired renal function require a lower dose and careful monitoring.

Penicillamine

Penicillamine is a chelating agent of metals such as copper, lead, iron, and mercury. It is a degradation product of penicillins but does not have antimicrobial activity. It also may be referred to as D-penicillamine, β,β-dimethylcysteine, or D,3-mercaptovaline.

Clinical Uses

Penicillamine is used for copper-associated hepatopathy and for long-term oral treatment of lead poisoning and cystine urolithiasis.

Dosage Forms

- Depen Titratabs, tablets (human label)
- Cuprimine capsules (human label)

Adverse Side Effects

These include nausea and vomiting. Other rare side effects include fever, lymphadenopathy, skin hypersensitivity reactions, and immune complex glomerulonephropathy.

TECHNICIAN NOTES Absorption of penicillamine may be reduced by concurrent administration of food, antacids, or iron salts.

Sodium Thiosulfate

Sodium thiosulfate uses the enzyme rhodanese to convert cyanide to a nontoxic thiocyanate ion, which is excreted in urine.

Clinical Uses

Sodium thiosulfate is used in the treatment of cyanide poisoning in horses and ruminants. It may be used in combination with sodium molybdate for the treatment of copper poisoning in ruminants. It also has been used for the treatment of arsenic poisoning. When applied topically, sodium thiosulfate has antifungal properties.

Dosage Forms

- Cyadote Injection
- Sodium Thiosulfate for Injection 25% (human label)

Adverse Side Effects

These are uncommon.

TECHNICIAN NOTES When sodium thiosulfate is administered intravenously, it should be given slowly.

Ethanol

Ethanol is an alcohol that is a competitive inhibitor of ethylene glycol metabolism. It also may be referred to as pure grain alcohol, grain alcohol, or ethyl alcohol.

Clinical Uses

Ethanol is used to treat ethylene glycol (antifreeze) poisoning.

Dosage Form

- Ethanol

Adverse Side Effects

Ethanol reduces body temperature and an overdose can be fatal.

TECHNICIAN NOTES

- A 20% to 50% solution of pure ethanol is administered intravenously until the animal is comatose and does not respond to a toe pinch. Administration is repeated as needed to maintain a comatose state for 3 days.
- Sodium bicarbonate is usually administered to control metabolic acidosis.

Fomepizole

Fomepizole is a competitive inhibitor of alcohol dehydrogenase. Its action prevents the conversion of ethylene glycol into glycoaldehyde and other toxic metabolites. This allows ethylene glycol to be excreted primarily unchanged. It also may be referred to as 4-methylpyrazole (4-MP).

Clinical Uses

Fomepizole is used to treat ethylene glycol (antifreeze) poisoning in dogs.

Dosage Form

- Antizol-Vet

Adverse Side Effects

Clinical signs of possible anaphylaxis include tachypnea, gagging, excessive salivation, and trembling.

TECHNICIAN NOTES

- Fomepizole must be diluted with 0.9% NaCl before intravenous injection.
- Dogs treated within 8 hours of ingestion have a better prognosis than those treated 10 to 12 hours after ingestion (Plumb, 2011).

Antivenin Polyvalent (Crotalidae)/ Antivenin *(Micrurus fulvius)* Coral Snake

These products are concentrated serum globulins collected from horses or other species vaccinated with different types of snake venoms. When the antivenin contains antibodies against only one species it is called monovalent and if it has antibodies against several species it is called polyvalent. Venom from the pit vipers like copperheads, rattlesnakes, and water moccasins has a different molecular structure from coral snake venom. This distinction requires treatment with the appropriate antivenin. Antivenin antibody combines with and inactivates venom at the time of administration but does not reverse damage done before administration. Treatment of snake bite often requires intensive supportive care of the patient with fluids, antibiotics, steroids, and pain medications in addition to antivenin.

Clinical Uses

These products are used in the treatment of snakebite in domestic animals from many of the poisonous snakes of North America. Because of the high price of antivenin, treatment with these products is potentially cost prohibitive.

Dosage Forms

- Antivenin (Crotalidae); polyvalent equine origin, labeled for dogs—Fort Dodge acquired by Boehringer.
- Antivenin (Crotalidae); polyvalent equine origin (human label)—Wyeth
- Antivenin (Crotalidae); CroFab Polyvalent Ovine Origin (human label)—Altana
- Antivenin *(Micrurus fulvius)*—Ayerst (no longer manufactured; supplies may exist)
- Antivenin (Crotalidae and *Micrurus*) veterinary labels in development—BioVeteria
- Antivenin (Crotalidae); polyvalent (labeled for horses)—Lake Immunogenics

Adverse Side Effects

Anaphylaxis may occur secondary to administration of equine- or ovine-origin products.

Vitamin K_1 (Phytonadione)

Vitamin K_1 is necessary for the synthesis of blood coagulation factors II, VII, IX, and X by the liver.

Clinical Uses

The main use of this product is for the treatment of anticoagulant rodenticide poisoning.

Dosage Forms

- Phytonadione; numerous veterinary-approved products are available, including oral capsules and an aqueous colloidal solution for injection.
- Phytonadione; Mephyton oral capsules and Aqua-Mephyton injectable (human label).

Adverse Side Effects

Anaphylaxis may occur with intravenous injection. The intramuscular route is usually recommended.

Thiamine HCl

Thiamine HCl is a water-soluble B vitamin used for the treatment or prevention of thiamine deficiency.

Clinical Uses

Thiamine HCl is used for thiamine deficiency in several species. It is used to treat polioencephalomalacia in cattle, sheep, and goats, as well as thiamine deficiencies associated with dietary lack or thiamine-destroying compounds in the diet.

Dosage Form

- Thiamine HCl; numerous veterinary and human label products are available.

Adverse Side Effects

Hypersensitivity or muscle soreness may be seen.

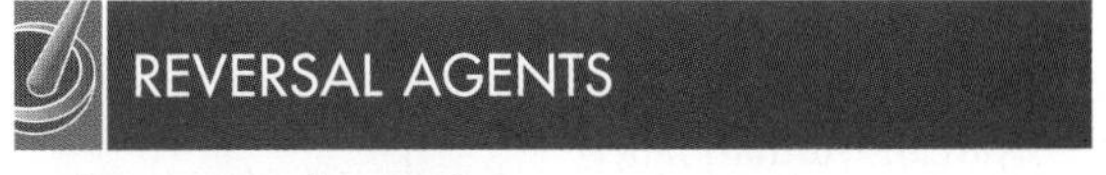

REVERSAL AGENTS

Atipamezole HCl

Atipamezole acts as a reversal agent for alpha-2–adrenergic agonists by competitively inhibiting alpha-2–adrenergic receptors.

Clinical Uses

Atipamezole HCl is used for the reversal of dexmedetomidine (Dexdomitor). It also has been used in the treatment of amitraz toxicity.

Dosage Form

- Antisedan

Adverse Side Effects

These include vomiting, diarrhea, hypersalivation, tremors, and apprehension.

> TECHNICIAN NOTES Pain perception returns after administration of atipamezole.

Flumazenil

Flumazenil acts as a benzodiazepine antagonist by competitively blocking benzodiazepines at benzodiazepine receptors.

Clinical Uses

Flumazenil is used for the reversal of benzodiazepine action.

Dosage Form

- Romazicon (human label)

Adverse Side Effects

Seizures may occur.

Naloxone HCl

Naloxone is a narcotic antagonist. It is structurally related to oxymorphone and may be referred to as *N*-allylnoroxymorphone HCl.

Clinical Uses

Naloxone is used for the treatment, prevention, or control of narcotic depression.

Dosage Forms

- P/M Naloxone HCl injection
- Narcan (human label)

Adverse Side Effects

These are uncommon.

> TECHNICIAN NOTES
> - Intravenous injection yields the quickest response.
> - A repeated dose may be necessary if the action of the narcotic outlasts the action of naloxone.
> - Naloxone also reverses the effects of butorphanol (Torbugesic), pentazocine (Talwin-V), and nalbuphine (Nubain).

Neostigmine

Neostigmine is a parasympathomimetic agent that competes with acetylcholine for acetylcholinesterase.

Clinical Uses

Neostigmine may be used to treat nondepolarizing neuromuscular blocking agent (curare-type) overdosages. It has also been used to treat ivermectin overdosages in cats.

Dosage Form

- Prostigmin ICN (human label)

Adverse Side Effects

Side effects are dose related and include nausea, vomiting, diarrhea, drooling, lacrimation, and others. Neostigmine may interact with atropine, corticosteroids, magnesium, dexpanthenol, and muscle relaxants.

Tolazoline HCl

Tolazoline is a competitive alpha-1–adrenergic and alpha-2–adrenergic receptor blocking agent that reverses the effects of alpha-2–adrenergic agonists.

Clinical Uses

Tolazoline HCl is used in horses for the reversal of xylazine (Rompun).

Dosage Form

- Tolazine

Adverse Side Effects

These include transient tachycardia, peripheral vasodilation, licking of lips, piloerection, clear lacrimal and nasal discharge, muscle fasciculations, and apprehension.

> TECHNICIAN NOTES
> - Tolazoline is not approved for use in food-producing animals.
> - Tolazoline has a short duration and may require repeated doses.

Yohimbine HCl

Yohimbine is an alpha-2–adrenergic receptor antagonist that reverses the effects of alpha-2–adrenergic agonists.

Clinical Uses

Yohimbine is used to reverse the effects of xylazine (Rompun). This action usually occurs within 1 to 3 minutes. It is approved for use in dogs and deer, but is also effective in other species.

Dosage Forms

- Yobine
- Antagonil (approved for deer)

TECHNICIAN NOTES

- Normal pain perception remains after administration of yohimbine.
- Caution should be exercised when used in epileptic or seizure-prone patients.
- Yohimbine should not be used in food-producing animals.
- Safety in pregnant or breeding animals is unknown.

LUBRICANTS

Lubricants are used to lubricate hands, arms, or instruments before gynecologic and rectal examinations are performed.

Dosage Forms

- K-Y Jelly
- Lube Jelly
- Lubri-Nert
- Lubrivet

Adverse Side Effects

Adverse side effects are uncommon.

TECHNICIAN NOTES Petroleum jelly (Vaseline) is not recommended for use as a lubricant because it is not water soluble and is not easily rinsed from instruments.

REVIEW QUESTIONS

1. A 2-year-old beagle has clinical signs of lead toxicity and a history to support the diagnosis. Which agent would be the drug of choice for treating this condition?
   a. Yohimbine HCl
   b. 2-PAM
   c. Calcium EDTA
   d. Methylene blue
2. A client calls and says that she has been giving her cat Tylenol for a limp. Now the cat is breathing fast, its face is swollen, and it is not active. You should tell the client to _____.
   a. give the cat hydrogen peroxide orally
   b. see whether she can get the cat to eat
   c. bring the cat to the hospital to start treatment with hydrogen peroxide
   d. bring the cat to the hospital to start treatment with acetylcysteine
3. Yohimbine HCl is a reversal agent for _____.
   a. Rompun
   b. acepromazine
   c. pentothal
   d. oxymorphone
4. Penicillamine should be administered _____.
   a. with food
   b. on an empty stomach
   c. with antacids
   d. with copper
5. Name four drugs that naloxone effectively reverses. ______________________
   ____
   ____
   ____
6. BAL has been administered to a 4-year-old mixed-breed dog for arsenic poisoning. Results of which of the following laboratory tests should be monitored closely?
   a. Packed cell volume (PCV)
   b. Blood urea nitrogen (BUN)
   c. White blood cell count (WBC)
   d. Alanine aminotransferase (ALT)
7. Glycosaminoglycans occur naturally in what part(s) of the body? ______________________.
8. What role do glycosaminoglycans (GAGs) provide in the treatment of degenerative joint conditions? ______________________

9. Define *nutraceutical.* Give an example.

____

10. A product usually is determined to be a drug if its label has a claim that indicates a therapeutic or preventive intent.
    a. True
    b. False
11. What Act defined dietary supplements, such as vitamins, minerals, amino acids, herbal products, and substances that supplement the diet by increasing total dietary intake, as "food" and excluded them from FDA regulation?
12. _______________ supplementation has been shown to be useful in treating certain dermatology conditions in dogs and cats.
13. What are two possible side effects of using fatty acids as a dietary supplement?

____

14. What is activated charcoal used for?

____

15. In veterinary medicine, calcium EDTA is used primarily for the treatment of

_______________.

16. Petroleum jelly is not recommended as a lubricant because it is not

_______________.

17. _______________ is a narcotic antagonist used for the treatment, prevention, or control of narcotic depression.
18. Flumazenil is used to reverse the effects of

_______________.

19. A dietary supplement for support of normal structure and function of the liver is

_______________.

20. Grain alcohol may be used to treat what poisoning? _______________
21. Echinacea may be used concurrently via the intraarticular route to prevent infections resulting from possible contamination.
    a. True
    b. False
22. Activated charcoal is effective in removing lead from the body.
    a. True
    b. False
23. After activated charcoal is administered, no other oral therapeutic agents should be administered within 3 hours.
    a. True
    b. False
24. It is permissible to use calcium EDTA in anuric patients.
    a. True
    b. False
25. Calcium EDTA can be administered orally.
    a. True
    b. False
26. Methylene blue should not be used in cats.
    a. True
    b. False
27. Ethanol is an alcohol that is a competitive inhibitor of ethylene glycol metabolism.
    a. True
    b. False
28. Sodium bicarbonate is contraindicated in the treatment of metabolic acidosis.
    a. True
    b. False
29. Naloxone reverses the effects of butorphanol, pentazocine, and nalbuphine.
    a. True
    b. False
30. Petroleum jelly (Vaseline) is an excellent choice for use in veterinary medicine because it is not easily rinsed from instruments and thereby prolongs the life of those instruments.
    a. True
    b. False
31. A 48-lb dog needs treatment for postanesthetic respiratory depression with naloxone (0.4 mg/mL). The dosage ordered is 0.02 mg/kg. What quantity (in milliliters) would you give?

____

32. An 8-lb cat requires treatment (at 0.2 mg/kg) with atipamezole (5 mg/mL) for the reversal of Dexdomitor administration. What quantity (milliliters) would you give?

____

33. A 455-kg horse requires reversal of xylazine sedation with yohimbine (2 mg/mL). The reversal dosage for yohimbine in horses is

0.075 mg/kg. How many milliliters would you draw up?

____

34. Prepare an injection of phytonadione (vitamin K_1) for an 80-lb dog that has ingested rodenticide. The dosage ordered is 2 mg/kg and the concentration of the K_1 solution is 10 mg/mL. What quantity will you draw up?

____

35. The order for a 65-lb arthritic dog is 5 mg/kg of Adequan (100 mg/mL). What quantity would you draw up for IM injection?

____

REFERENCES

Boothe DM: Antiinflammatory drugs. In Boothe DM, editor: Small animal clinical pharmacology and therapeutics, Philadelphia, 2012, WB Saunders.

Boothe DM: Nutraceuticals in veterinary medicine: part I definitions and regulations, Compend Contin Educ Pract Vet 19(11):1248–1255, 1997.

Davidson G: Glucosamine and chondroitin sulfate, Compend Contin Educ Pract Vet 22(5):454–458, 2000.

Davidson G: S-adenosylmethionine, Compend Contin Educ Pract Vet 24(8):600–603, 2002.

Fitzwater K: Regenerative stem cell, module 1: principles of stem cells—what is regenerative medicine? Veterinary Information Network (website). http://www.vin.com/members/proceedings/proceedings.plx?CID=ABVP2012&PID=83732. Accessed March 5, 2013.

Goodman L, Trepanier L: Potential drug interactions with dietary supplements, Compend Contin Educ Pract Vet 27(10):780–790, 2005.

Plumb DC: Veterinary drug handbook, ed 7, Ames, Iowa, 2011, Wiley-Blackwell.

Rishniw M: Evaluating herbal medicines, Davis, Calif, 2006, Veterinary Information Network.

Romich JA: Fundamentals of pharmacology for veterinary technicians, Clifton Park, NY, 2005, Thompson Delmar Learning.

Roudebush P, Freeman LM: Nutritional management of heart disease. In Bonagura JD, editor: Kirk's current veterinary therapy small animal practice, XIII, Philadelphia, 2000, WB Saunders.

Warren E: Nutraceuticals. Veterinary Information Network (website). http://www.vin.com/doc/?id=2994084. Accessed September 28, 2013.

Wynn SG: An introduction to herbal medicine, in Proceedings. West Vet Conf, Las Vegas, Nev, 2002.

Wynn SG, Fourgere BJ: Veterinary herbal medicine, St. Louis, 2007, Mosby Elsevier.

CHAPTER

Inventory: The Veterinary Technician's Role

KEY TERMS

Average cost of inventory on hand
DEA form
Delayed billing
FIFO
FOB
FOB destination
FOB shipping point
Full-service company
Inventory
Inventory control manager (ICM)
Invoice
Mail order discount house
Markup
Packing slip
Statement
Turnover
Veterinary supply distributor

OUTLINE

Introduction
Inventory
THE TIME EQUATION
TURNOVER
  Calculating Turnover Rate
Controlling Inventory
PROACTIVE INVENTORY CONTROL SYSTEM
KEEPING ACCURATE RECORDS
INVENTORY RECORDS
  Reorder Quantity
  Rabies Vaccine
ORGANIZING INVENTORY
  Pharmacy and Inventory Control Manager Office
  Organizing Inventory in the Veterinary Hospital
  Staff Memos
  Special Conditions
PHYSICAL INVENTORY
  Monthly Inventory Versus Rotating Inventory
PURCHASING INFORMATION
  Incoming Freight
  FOB Rules and Shipment Contracts
  Receiving Freight
  Stocking Shelves
  Vendors
  Communicating With Sales Representatives
  Drug Enforcement Administration Forms
  Special Orders
  Human Pharmacy
COMPUTERS AND INVENTORY
THE JOB OF INVENTORY CONTROL MANAGER

LEARNING OBJECTIVES

After studying this chapter, you should be able to

1. Explain why having an inventory control system is important.
2. Describe ways in which inventory control benefits a business.
3. Explain why inventory turnover is important.
4. Discuss ways of becoming an efficient inventory control manager.
5. Describe various inventory record-keeping systems.
6. Describe the differences in vendor types.
7. Describe good communication techniques that can be used with sales representatives.
8. Discuss ways that veterinary management computer software aids in tracking pharmaceutical inventory.

INTRODUCTION

Control of **inventory** is an important concern for companies both large and small, and veterinary businesses are no exception. Proactively maintaining pharmaceutical inventory is an ongoing endeavor for veterinary hospitals (Figure 19-1). Deciding how much trade or generic name product to buy, keeping expired items off the shelves, and performing a physical inventory are all integral parts of keeping a veterinary facility functioning as a healthy business. When a product is depleted before the next order arrives, it is frustrating for both veterinary staff and the clientele. When a product is not available, it cannot be sold and no profit can be made. Deciding which employee to entrust with this responsibility is an important decision for veterinary practice owners that should be made with careful consideration. Therefore, the employee chosen for this job should treat the position with respect and make every effort to be frugal with the employer's money.

The veterinary technician often is the employee chosen to perform this job. Therefore, knowledge of pharmaceutics and the ability to observe quantities of product used within a month are important talents that the veterinary technician must possess.

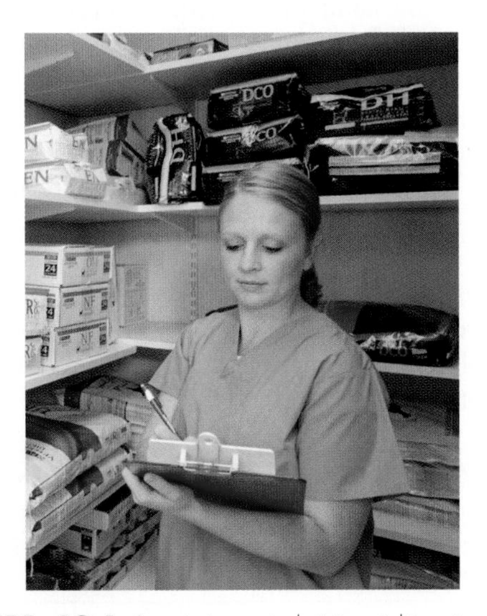

FIGURE 19-1 A veterinary technician taking inventory. (From Prendergast H: Front office management for the veterinary team, St. Louis, 2011, Saunders, Elseiver.)

> *TECHNICIAN NOTES* Along with knowledge of nursing skills, accepting the role of **inventory control manager (ICM)** boosts the veterinary technician's value as an employee.

In our technologically advanced society, pharmaceutics change rapidly because new products are constantly being developed. The veterinary technician who is charged with being the ICM must be willing to learn about new products and to pass this information on to the entire veterinary staff. Communication and good people skills are useful when one is dealing with pharmaceutical sales representatives. Sales representatives are invaluable to veterinary practices because they are armed with all available information about drugs, both old and new.

The ICM has many responsibilities. These responsibilities include keeping the staff informed regarding discontinued items, knowing the dates on which backordered items will be released from the vendor, packing up goods awaiting return to the vendor (e.g., expired items), rotating stock correctly, maintaining current prices on all products, organizing inventory for ease of location and counting, receiving and inspecting orders on arrival at the veterinary facility, and learning about new products. These are only a few of the responsibilities the ICM will meet daily. Inventory should be handled as an ongoing process. Each day, inventory must be visually counted, and physical inventory must be done at least once a month for good results.

INVENTORY

> *TECHNICIAN NOTES* The value of all assets owned by the veterinary facility has important tax and insurance implications.

Accounting of inventory items is very important when one is filing income taxes or in the event of a fire or natural disaster. Veterinary practices providing an accurate inventory of their business assets are assured that their insurance companies will reimburse the business accurately should a disaster occur.

The primary goal of inventory is to have sufficient quantities of inventory available to serve clients' needs, while at the same time minimizing the cost of carrying that inventory. Purchasing too many units of a slow-selling item can cost the practice money, and not purchasing enough of a high-selling item can result in the item being out of stock, which can cause frustration (Libby, Libby, and Short, 2004) for the veterinary team.

An accounting system plays three roles in the inventory management process:

1. The system must provide accurate information for preparation of periodic financial statements and tax returns.
2. It must provide up-to-date information on inventory quantities and costs, to facilitate ordering decisions.
3. Because inventories are subject to theft and other forms of misuse, the system also must provide the information needed to protect assets.

Thus, what exactly is the definition of inventory? It is tangible property that is sold in the normal course of a business day. In veterinary medicine, this would include such items as antibiotics, anthelmintics, shampoos, topical medications, prescription feeds, and even the dispensing bottles used to dispense liquid medication, as well as the syringes sold to clients that they must use to orally medicate their pets at home. Dispensing bottles, syringes, needles, ointment tins, and so forth could be classified as raw materials because they are carriers for the actual medicine that is being prescribed and dispensed. However, raw materials cost the practice money, just as pharmaceutics do. It is just as frustrating to run out of these items as it is to run out of a broad-spectrum antibiotic.

Most veterinary practices use the first in, first out (**FIFO**) method of inventory. This is not necessarily done by choice but rather because of the expiration dates on merchandise that the practice sells. Generally speaking, the expiration date that is the earliest should be sold first. A perpetual inventory control system, which is a detailed record for each type of merchandise stocked, shows the following:

- Units and costs of the beginning inventory
- Units and costs of each purchase
- Units and costs of the goods for each sale
- Units and costs of the goods on hand at any point in time

Luckily, most veterinary computer management software programs do the above listed items automatically. In today's business world, inventory is much easier to keep up with than it was in the days of periodic inventory, when businesses did not have computers (Libby, Libby, and Short, 2004). However, it is better to use a balance between a perpetual inventory control system and a periodic inventory because sometimes the amount of each item listed within the computer system may not be a true reflection of what is actually on hand. Nothing can ever take the place of a periodic inventory and physically counting the amount of each item on hand. The primary disadvantage of a periodic inventory system is the lack of inventory information that is available to the practice owner; that is, veterinary management software makes inventory easier because it shows up-to-date amounts of each item sold, along with trends during the summer or winter months that can help staff in deciding how much inventory needs to be purchased in the coming years.

Inventory is an ongoing process, and trends within the practice must be observed daily. The ICM must be able to recognize the products that each veterinarian in the practice uses and dispenses, to ensure that items are on hand when needed. Nothing is more frustrating than needing a drug or other inventory item to treat a patient with, only to find it is not in stock. Computer software designed for the veterinary business can help tremendously with tracking trends within the practice. Most software has the ability to provide printouts of day-by-day, week-by-week, month-by-month, and yearly sales trends (Figure 19-2).

Through establishment of a workable inventory control system within a realistic budget, expenses can be kept at a minimum.

> *TECHNICIAN NOTES* For many veterinary practices, inventory represents the second-highest expense. Payroll is usually the highest overhead item.

After determination and implementation of a realistic budget that might be based on the mission

Date: 05-21-13

Inventory report

Page: 4
Anthelmintics

Code	Description		U/M	Price	On hand	Avg cost	Stock value	Unit cost	Pkg. cost cost	Codes Cls	Last sold	Document
May	Jun	Jul	Aug	Sep	Oct	Nov	Dec	Jan	Feb	Mar	Apr	May
			Anthelmintics				**0.00**					
Canine vaccines												
1008	Bordetalla (Injection)		Ds	0.00	14	0.000	0.00	0.000	0.000	1		
Qty sold, last 12 months												
May	Jun	Jul	Aug	Sep	Oct	Nov	Dec	Jan	Feb	Mar	Apr	May
1009	Bordetalla (Intra-nasal)		Ds	0.00	1	0.000	0.00	0.000	0.000	0		
Qty sold, last 12 months												
May	Jun	Jul	Aug	Sep	Oct	Nov	Dec	Jan	Feb	Mar	Apr	May
9010	DA2PP/CV		Ds	0.00	15	0.000	0.00	0.000	0.000	0		
Qty sold, last 12 months												
May	Jun	Jul	Aug	Sep	Oct	Nov	Dec	Jan	Feb	Mar	Apr	May
9052	Rabies vaccine		Ds	0.00	21	0.000	0.00	0.000	0.000	1		
Qty sold, last 12 months												
May	Jun	Jul	Aug	Sep	Oct	Nov	Dec	Jan	Feb	Mar	Apr	May
			Canine vaccines				**0.00**					
Miscellaneous items												
1007	Large garbage sacks		Box	0.00	0	0.000	0.00	0.000	0.000	1		May
Qty sold, last 12 months												
May	Jun	Jul	Aug	Sep	Oct	Nov	Dec	Jan	Feb	Mar	Apr	
7022	Small garbage sacks		Box	0.00	0	0.000	0.00	0.000	0.000	1		May
Qty sold, last 12 months												
May	Jun	Jul	Aug	Sep	Oct	Nov	Dec	Jan	Feb	Mar	Apr	
7023	Computer printer paper		Pack	0.00	0	0.000	0.00	0.000	0.000	1		May
Qty sold, last 12 months												
May	Jun	Jul	Aug	Sep	Oct	Nov	Dec	Jan	Feb	Mar	Apr	

FIGURE 19-2 AVI-Mark Veterinary Software Management System (McAllister Software Systems, Piedmont, Mo.)

statement of the facility and practice needs, followed by implementation of that budget, there should be no danger of running out of inventory items because there always should be sufficient quantities of product on hand. An annual inventory evaluation is beneficial when a vision for the practice and its potential growth has been developed.

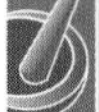

THE TIME EQUATION

When one is dealing with inventory, no equation is more important than the following:

$$\text{Time} = \text{Money}$$

Although it is important to have merchandise on hand for retail sale, a fine balance is needed to keep products from sitting too long on pharmacy shelves. Products that stay on the shelf for too long will not make money for the veterinary practice. Instead, this is similar to placing money in a jar and burying it in the backyard; the money is there, but it is not earning interest and it is not working for you. It is the same with inventory products. A fine inventory balance is crucial to the financial health of a business. In addition, clients do not like to buy products that have been sitting on pharmacy shelves for a long time because the labels begin to show signs of age or the products are dusty.

A periodic evaluation of inventory is crucial for keeping the balance in fine adjustment. Items that are not selling well or are used infrequently within the practice should be deleted from the inventory master list and should not be ordered in the future. Turnover, then, becomes an important issue.

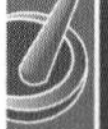

TURNOVER

TECHNICIAN NOTES

- **Turnover** is the number of times a product is sold or used in-house on an annual basis.
- Because there are 12 months in a year, the ideal situation is to use all inventory each month and reorder in time to begin the next month. However, in the real world, this simply does not happen.
- Four turnovers is a workable goal, and 12 turnovers may be set as the ideal goal. A mean turnover rate of eight turns per year is acceptable for most veterinary practices.

Calculating Turnover Rate

The following equation is used to determine turnover rate:

$$TurnoverRate = \frac{\text{Yearly inventory expense}}{\text{Average cost of inventory on hand}}$$

Example:

$$\frac{\$100{,}000}{\$20{,}000} = 5$$

The following equation determines the **average cost of inventory on hand:**

$$\text{Average cost of inventory on hand} = \frac{\text{Year's beginning inventory} + \text{Year's ending inventory}}{2}$$

Example:

$$\frac{\$150{,}000 + \$35{,}000}{2} = \$92{,}500$$

CONTROLLING INVENTORY

Establishing effective inventory control in a veterinary practice necessitates placing a person in charge of ordering and stocking supplies. An additional person trained as a backup is a must because when the ICM goes on vacation or is sick, someone else must be knowledgeable about the system. These two people can work effectively as a team to keep product supplies on hand.

The duties of the ICM are intense. This person is responsible for keeping an adequate supply of all products used, dispensed, and sold; organizing inventory items for easy location; identifying when products should be reordered; keeping accurate inventory records; ordering, receiving, and inspecting shipments; and maintaining price and price updates for all items. The ICM also is responsible for rotating stock, keeping expired items off the shelves, learning about new products, and keeping the practice owner apprised of the specials that suppliers may offer. This responsibility must be acted on every day. The veterinary technician who accepts the role of ICM must be able to perform clinical and nursing duties as well as manage inventory levels.

TECHNICIAN NOTES

The objectives of an inventory control system are twofold:

1. To make certain that items are on hand when needed
2. To be able to purchase needed items while staying within a budget

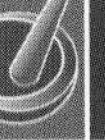

PROACTIVE INVENTORY CONTROL SYSTEM

For an inventory control system to be workable, it must be easy to use and have a turnover rate of at least four turns per year. It is the ICM's job to make sure that all supplies are on hand when needed. Expenses can be reduced when inventory amounts are ordered properly.

Proper handling of Drug Enforcement Administration (DEA) substances is an important concern.

TECHNICIAN NOTES Controlled substances (e.g., Sleepaway, diazepam) must be kept in a locked cabinet that has been bolted to the floor, and all amounts used must be correctly recorded in the controlled substance log.

Each pharmaceutical company has their own policy as concerns ordering controlled substances. Therefore, it is best to check with the company prior to placing an order so that proper policy can be followed.

Each **invoice** (Figure 19-3) that arrives at the veterinary hospital should be checked to verify amounts ordered and prices the practice is charged. A packing slip (Figure 19-4), an invoice, and a statement (Figure 19-5) are three different forms. Mistakes can be made on these forms unintentionally by the product vendor, but it may fall to the ICM to audit these mistakes and notify the vendor so the account can be adjusted to receive proper credit.

Backordered items can present problems. Backordered items are those items not on hand at the vendor for any number of reasons. Sometimes, the product may be on backorder for manufacturing reasons; another reason may be that the manufacturer is redesigning the product's label. Buyouts of large pharmaceutical corporations also can cause product to be on backorder until all minor details are worked out concerning the merger.

Identification of expired items may be one of the most frustrating experiences an ICM may face.

TECHNICIAN NOTES Most products have an expiration date on the label, and these must be checked frequently so they can be removed from the pharmacy when they are out-of-date.

Veterinary practice management systems software can be an invaluable aid in tracking expired items. When products are received, the *earliest* expiration date should be the one that is recorded in the computer system. Therefore, at the beginning of each month, the computer will reflect those products that expire first, and the ICM can print a list of the old drugs and quickly remove them from the pharmacy. As soon as the old products have been removed from the pharmacy shelves, the next earliest expiration date is recorded in the computer. Some pharmaceutical companies have policies that entitle the practice to free replacement of expired items. However, other vendors do not concur with this arrangement; therefore the ICM must be able to distinguish which expired product will produce a free product refund and which will not. Some pharmaceutical companies prefer to credit the facility's account instead of sending replacement merchandise; others offer no reimbursement whatsoever for expired items.

It is hoped that pilferage will not occur in the veterinary facility. However, an effective inventory control system will deter employees who may elect to steal because they know that inventory is counted on a regular basis. Likewise, merchandise displayed (e.g., leashes, collars, shampoo, grooming brushes) in the reception area of a veterinary facility can be enticing to some clients who may decide to "pick up" an item instead of paying for it. This is another reason why proper inventory control plays an important role.

The Pharmaceutical Warehouse
1546 Warehouse Road
Plains, Georgia 36945

INVOICE

Ship to:
All Pets Veterinary Hospital
1785 Lawrenceville Road
Lawrenceville, Georgia 37965

Bill to:
All Pets Veterinary Hospital
1785 Lawrenceville Road
Lawrenceville, Georgia 37965

Bill to	Invoice total
A7796	$335.10
Invoice number	**Invoice date**
953146-000	06-03-13
Customer account number	**Ship to**
198531	Lawrenceville, Georgia

Item code	Unit/Size	Description/ Strength	Quantity Ordered	Quantity Shipped	Item Status	Unit price	Extension	Box No.	REM
15637	18/box	Vetrap	3	3	Sent	$54.95	$164.85	1	
15937	9/pack	Gauze bandage rolls	5	5	Sent	$25.65	$128.25	1	
13465	Each	Roll cotton	12	12	Sent	$3.50	$42.00	1	

• *Please note that late payments are subject to a 1.5% monthly finance charge*

Merchandise total
$335.10

Invoice total
$335.10

*** Please pay within thirty days of receipt of this invoice.**

FIGURE 19-3 A sample invoice.

KEEPING ACCURATE RECORDS

An orderly way of keeping track of data regarding inventory should be employed. Most veterinary facilities in this age of computer technology use software designed especially for the veterinary business. Remember, when dealing with computers, the old adage—"garbage in, garbage out" ("GIGO")—can detract from the quality of information that a computer contains.

INVENTORY RECORDS

Many types of inventory records may be used in a veterinary facility. At least some of the following should be used, although some practices may elect to use them all.

A reorder log, sometimes called a "want book" (Figure 19-6), is an effective way to track products to be ordered. Each member of the veterinary staff can use this log to record items that should be ordered.

The Pharmaceutical Warehouse

PACKING LIST

Ship to:
All Pets Veterinary Hospital
1785 Lawrenceville Road
Lawrenceville, Georgia 37965

Bill to:
All Pets Veterinary Hospital
1785 Lawrenceville Road
Lawrenceville, Georgia 37965

Customer account number	Ship to
198531	Lawrenceville, Georgia

Item code	Unit/Size	Description/ Strength	Quantity Ordered	Quantity Shipped	Item Status	Unit price	Extension	Box No.	REM
15637	18/box	Vetrap	3	3	Sent	$54.95	$164.85	1	
15937	9/pack	Gauze bandage rolls	5	5	Sent	$25.65	$128.25	1	
13465	Each	Roll cotton	12	12	Sent	$3.50	$42.00	1	

FIGURE 19-4 A sample packing slip. (Some vendors do not record prices on their packing slips.)

TECHNICIAN NOTES All veterinary personnel should know the importance of maintaining inventory and should make every effort to record in the reorder log any product that has been depleted.

In a busy practice, this habit is of utmost importance because once supplies have been exhausted, obtaining interim product from the neighboring veterinary facility becomes an "emergency." Afterward, the amounts borrowed must be replaced or paid for.

TECHNICIAN NOTES The reorder point is the level reached that necessitates a product reorder.

It is the responsibility of the ICM to set the reorder point. If orders are placed each week, then a minimum of a 3-week supply should be kept in stock. Larger veterinary hospitals, emergency clinics, and colleges of veterinary medicine may require that inventory be ordered via a purchase order. A purchase order is a written form accompanied by a purchase order number. Generally, the form is mailed, although it may be faxed to the vendor, who then will send the merchandise.

TECHNICIAN NOTES In keeping basic order records, it is imperative to keep a copy of each order.

Regardless of whether a purchase order form is mailed to the vendor or an order is given over the phone, all of the following items should be recorded: order date, order amount, order size, name of the product, vendor(s), product catalog number, unit cost, total cost, receive date, amount received, and discount or special cost (if applicable). When these items are kept in a written form, an inaccurate order can be corrected easily by contacting the company involved.

An inventory master list provides endless quantities of information. Each veterinary practice should

The Pharmaceutical Warehouse
1546 Warehouse Road
Plains, Georgia 36945

STATEMENT

01000000345697862213213132132132456654

Statement Date	Account Number	Due Date
06-03-13	198531	07-03-13
New Balance	**Indicate Amount Enclosed**	
$335.10		

The Pharmaceutical Warehouse
1546 Warehouse Road
Plains, Georgia 36945

Please detach here and return the above portion with yhour payment

Questions? Call 1-800-897-3679

Account Name	Account Number	Statement Date	Statement Number	Page
All Pets Veterinary Hospital	198531	06-03-13	3596342	1 of 1

BALANCE SUMMARY

Previous Balance	Add Purchases	Payments	Credits	Late Charge	Adjustments	Balance Due
$120.00	$335.10	$120.00	0.00	0.00	0.00	$335.10

ACCOUNT AGING

1-30 Days Past Due	31-60 Days Past Due	61-90 Days Past Due	91-120 Days Past Due	>120 Days Past Due	Current Balance
0.00	0.00	0.00	0.00	0.00	**$335.10**

FIGURE 19-5 A sample statement.

strive to keep a current list of all products in stock. An inventory master list provides information such as name of the product, item number code, usage, order status, and price. Some veterinary management software includes information regarding the seasonal use of products. One category in which this may be important is the area of flea and tick products. Today's computer software designed for veterinary businesses has the ability to reflect the months during which the greatest amount of product was sold. For instance, it may be that flea and tick shampoo is purchased more frequently during the months of March through September as compared with other times of the year. By using this information, the ICM can better predict how much merchandise should be ordered. The master list also reflects

Reorder Log

Date of Order	Amount	Item Description	Catalog Number	Cost		Extended Cost	
3-14-13	6	Sharps' containers	796029	$ 3	79	$ 22	74
3-15-13	3 boxes	Tuberculin slyringes	194356	$ 9	59	$ 28	77
3-15-13	6 boxes	Needles 22ga. x 3/4"	355796	$ 7	50	$ 45	00

FIGURE 19-6 An example of a reorder log.

trade names, generic names, unit size, strength, name of the product's manufacturer, phone numbers, addresses, practice account numbers, order information, unit price, and a formula for calculating markup. (Some of these items are optional.)

> TECHNICIAN NOTES **Markup** is the amount of money (usually a percentage) over cost that an item is sold for.

There is a difference between cost and retail value. Cost is what the practice pays for an item. *Total cost* is the amount the item costs plus tax. The retail price is the amount the practice charges a client for an item. Retail price usually includes a profit margin (i.e., markup). Each practice has a way of figuring markup, and the percentages used may vary. A common way to figure total cost is to multiply the product's cost by the appropriate tax. When the total cost of an item is obtained and is multiplied by 2, a 100% markup (i.e., retail price) is the result. This is illustrated below.

The following is an equation to figure total cost:

$$\text{Cost} + \text{Tax} = \text{Total cost}$$

Example:

$$\text{Amoxicillin (100 mg, 100-count bottle) cost} = \$26.75$$

$$\text{Tax (@ 10\%)} = 0.100$$

$$\$26.75 \times 0.100 = \$2.675$$

$$\$26.75 + \$2.675 = \$29.425$$

The following shows how to find retail price @ 100% markup:

$$\text{Total cost of the item} \times 2 = \text{Retail Price @ 100\% markup}$$

$$\$29.43 \times 2 = \$58.86$$

Then: \$58.86 divided by 100 tablets in the bottle = 0.5886 or \$0.59 each

Thus, each tablet can be retailed for \$0.59 (or \$0.60 to make accounting easier).

Reorder Quantity

When the reorder quantity is determined, a good idea is to set the amount equal to a 1-month supply. By ordering a 1-month supply of product, the ICM will not have to micromanage inventory. The reorder quantity can be posted on the computer's master inventory list.

Rabies Vaccine

Records regarding rabies vaccine are very important. Each rabies certificate reflects the vaccine's expiration date and serial number (Figure 19-7). Therefore, the ICM must ensure that the certificates reflect those numbers by checking that the serial number and expiration date are posted correctly in the computer. This is not optional; it *must* be done.

ORGANIZING INVENTORY

Pharmacy and Inventory Control Manager Office

> TECHNICIAN NOTES A room in the veterinary facility that is set up to serve as the pharmacy office and the ICM office provides a place to organize catalogs, journals, magazines, and sales lists.

Other items, such as DEA order records, Occupational Safety and Health Administration (OSHA) manuals, material safety data sheets (MSDSs), and suppliers' catalogs, also can be stored in the pharmacy office.

Organizing Inventory in the Veterinary Hospital

The ideal situation for organizing inventory in the veterinary hospital is to establish a centrally located pharmacy area. In this manner, all pharmaceutics can be counted easily.

> TECHNICIAN NOTES Inventory within the pharmacy area can be arranged in a variety of ways. The most common ways to arrange products are alphabetically, by therapeutic use, or by classification of the drug.

An easy way to organize inventory is to print the master inventory list and then stock products on the

CERTIFICATE OF VACCINATION

Date of rabies vaccination	29 APR 12
Next rabies vaccination on	29 APR 13
Certificate number	N/A
Previous rabies vaccination	N/A
Best Veterinary Hospital	
Taylor Lane, DVM	
621 Banner Street	
Camden, Arkansas 71701	
501-536-8390	
Owner's name	**Best Veterinary Client**
Owner's address	**1313 Schnauzer Lane** **Camden, Arkansas 71701**
County of owner's residence	Ouachita

This is to certify...
That I have vaccinated against rabies the animal described below:

Patient Information and Signalment	
Patient's name	Tangent
Species	Canine
Breed	Mix
Gender	Male/Neutered
Color and markings	Brindle/White on chest
Tag number	N/A
Weight	101.4 lbs.
Age	2 years

Signed: Taylor Lane, DVM

Vaccinations administered:

Vaccines administered
RV/DA2PP/CV/Bordetella

Rabies Vaccine Information	
Manufactured by	Zoetis Animal Health
Serial number	A232705A
Lot expiration date	26 AUG 13
Administration of vaccine	SC on right side

FIGURE 19-7 A sample rabies certificate.

shelf in the same way that they are listed on the master list. In this way, when it is time to perform inventory, products are arranged on the pharmacy shelves in the same order they appear on the master inventory list, thereby enabling inventory to be performed in a timely fashion.

Staff Memos

> TECHNICIAN NOTES The ICM should designate a bulletin board for memos to the veterinary staff.

Memos attached to a bulletin board can alert all hospital staff of company buyouts, discontinued items, and backordered items. The use of a bulletin board provides the ICM with freedom from frustrating interruptions by office staff concerning inventory questions. Additionally, this bulletin board is a good location for the reorder log (i.e., "want book").

Special Conditions

Some special conditions must be recognized when one is arranging inventory. Products that require refrigeration have only a limited amount of storage space in the refrigerator. Care should be taken to avoid ordering too large a quantity of these items because the available amount of refrigeration may not be able to contain the order amount. DEA substances should be kept in a locked cabinet that has been bolted to the floor. The space within the cabinet should be considered before increased amounts of merchandise are ordered.

PHYSICAL INVENTORY

Monthly Inventory Versus Rotating Inventory

When and how often to perform this necessary function needs to be decided. One effective method is to perform a rotating inventory. A rotating inventory necessitates the division of like products into categories. These categories are given a number of one through four. For example, each category designated as one is counted during the month of January. Each category designated as two is counted during the month of February; three is counted in March, and four in April. During the month of May, the inventory begins again, starting with those categories designated with number one. Thus, each category is counted three times a year (Figure 19-8). Although this may not be acceptable to all veterinary practice owners, it certainly can be an efficient way to perform a physical inventory. Often, only one person is responsible for inventory control within the veterinary facility, and counting every item stocked in a practice may take a single person 1 to 2 days to complete. If inventory is done on a monthly basis (i.e., all items counted each month), the ICM cannot perform other nursing or technical duties on the day inventory is taken. When a rotating method is used, a smaller amount of inventory is counted each month, thus enabling the ICM to have time available to perform other job duties.

> TECHNICIAN NOTES Nothing is as effective as performing a physical inventory.

Some practice owners may require a monthly inventory count. However, performing inventory on a rotational 3- to 4-month cycle makes the ICM's job easier. A veterinary technician may perform many functions in a veterinary practice; use of a rotating inventory ensures an accurate count and good use of the veterinary technician's nursing skills.

PURCHASING INFORMATION

In a busy veterinary facility, an ideal situation is to deal with as few suppliers as possible. The ICM will constantly be involved in an appointment with sales representatives if various vendors are used. Dealing with as few suppliers as possible releases the ICM to perform regular nursing and technical duties required by the facility. If sales representatives are asked to make an appointment, the ICM will know when to expect a visit and can better prepare the normal work schedule around this visit. The ICM should ensure that sales representatives are aware of lunch breaks and quitting time; otherwise, they may just "pop in" to make a sale without considering the ICM's schedule.

Anthelmintics (1) Dry Goods (1) In-house Products (1) Anesthetics (1) Bovine Vaccines (1) Equine Vaccines (1) Equine Products (1)	Large Animal Sprays (2) Flea Products and Shampoo (2) Large Animal Powders (2) Otic Products (2) Ophthalmics (2)
Lab Test Kits (3) Small Animal Pharmacy (3) Dietary Items (3) Heartworm Preventive (3) Porcine Vaccines (3)	Large Animal Injectables (4) Large Animal Gallons (4) Large Animal Products (4) Small Animal Vaccines (4) Vitamins (4)

Start rotating inventory in January by counting all items with a #1 beside them. In February, count all items with a #2 beside them. Proceed in the same manner for the rest of the year and thus, all inventory will be counted three times a year.

FIGURE 19-8 An example of how to divide inventory.

In dealing with pharmaceutical and supplier sales representatives, it is advantageous to be aware of several things. (Knowledge of the following information will make the ICM more effective in the responsibility of inventory maintenance.) Quantity and assortment discounts are ways that pharmaceutical companies can offer increased quantities of goods. Usually, the company will offer a discount for buying larger amounts, but several conditions must be considered by the ICM. First, how fast can amounts of the product sold in the practice be increased? Remember, time is money, and product left sitting in the pharmacy for extended periods will end up costing the practice money, even though the merchandise may have been bought at a discounted rate. Also, where will the overstock be stored? Does the practice have sufficient room to store increased quantities of product? Sometimes, quantity discounts are not what they appear to be.

Delayed billing is another feature that some pharmaceutical and supplier companies may offer. When discounts for quantity buying are offered to the veterinary practice, the statement often will reflect a delayed billing option (i.e., the statement does not have to be paid within the usual 30-day span). Instead, the option of paying within a 60- to 90-day period will extend the discount. Usually, no interest is charged to the buyer, and the practice owner may be able to purchase increased amounts of stock at a reduced rate without the trial of coming up with funds to pay for it all within a 30-day limit. Consideration must still be given to whether sufficient room exists for storage of overstock and how soon the product can be sold.

When an order is placed, many companies waive the shipping fee if the veterinary practice orders a minimum amount of product. For example, if the minimum order amount is $250 per order, the ICM can save the practice shipping fees by ordering the minimum amount. Keep in mind that a shipping fee of $10 when multiplied over 10 orders adds up to $100. Shipping costs multiplied by 12 months could be used to buy other products instead of being spent on shipping fees.

Some pharmaceutical and supplier companies offer discounts for early payment. Veterinary practices can save money by paying the **statement** early. This too is a way to save the practice money. On the other hand, penalties may be imposed for statements paid after the 30-day time limit. The amount paid in penalties can also buy product instead of being spent on late fees. Every practice should endeavor to pay within 30 days.

The ICM should be familiar with each vendor's return policy. Items that are expired may have to be returned, along with any item that is not selling well. Some vendors will allow product to be returned and will credit the practice's account accordingly. Items that have expired may be picked up by a sales representative and replaced. It should be noted that expired controlled substances cannot be picked up by the sales representative for return to the pharmaceutical company.

Incoming Freight

The inventory control manager must be alert to possible damage incurred to freight during shipping.

> *TECHNICIAN NOTES* At the time freight is being unloaded at the veterinary facility, the ICM should visually check for damage by noting any boxes that are not intact. Wetness to the cardboard container may indicate breakage of the contents, and boxes should be counted and the number should be compared with the number of containers listed on the **packing slip.**

As soon as freight arrives, it should be opened and any damage should be noted. Evidence of damage should be reported to the vendor as soon as possible so that credit can be received and/or damaged items replaced. Some companies have a 24-hour reporting period (i.e., all damaged items must be reported within 24 hours of arrival time). Damaged goods should be returned to the vendor from which they were ordered, in the original shipping carton with the damaged goods inside. In this way, the vendor can assess the damage and correctly apply credit to the veterinary facility's account.

FOB Rules and Shipment Contracts

A vendor delivers freight to the purchaser. The veterinary facility may make an order with a telephone representative, send or fax a purchase order, or make an order with the sales representative during his or her appointment at the veterinary facility. A shipment contract is one in which the seller turns the goods over to a carrier for delivery to the buyer. The seller has no responsibility for seeing that the goods reach their destination. In a shipment contract, both title and risk of loss pass to the buyer when the goods are given to the carrier. Shipment contracts are often designated by the term *FOB Place of Shipment* (such as FOB Camden, Arkansas). When goods are sent **FOB** (free on board) followed by place of shipment, they will be delivered free to the place of shipment. The buyer must pay all shipping charges from there to the place of destination. The terms indicate that title to the goods and risk of loss pass at the point of origin. Delivery to the carrier by the seller and acceptance by the carrier completes the transfer of both title and risk of loss. Therefore, the buyer accepts full responsibility during the transit of goods (Brown and Sukys, 2006).

A vendor uses a form of transportation to send required items to the veterinary hospital (e.g., UPS [United Parcel Service], Averitt Express, Federal Express, or U.S. Postal Service). Once the vendor releases freight to the carrier, the freight becomes subject to two FOB rules: FOB destination and FOB shipping point.

> *TECHNICIAN NOTES* Vendors place different terms of delivery on freight that is leaving a pharmaceutical facility. Basically, FOB rules state which business (vendor or buyer) has the title to freight and who will be responsible in cases of loss of freight when the vendor uses outside transportation companies to deliver goods. **FOB destination** means that the title of ownership (freight) is being passed from the vendor to the purchaser, and said freight becomes the property of the purchaser when the shipment is delivered to the veterinary hospital. **FOB shipping point** means that the title of ownership (freight) passes from the vendor to the purchaser when the vendor places the goods in possession of a carrier. FOB shipping point requires the purchaser to determine what responsibility the carrier will take if damage or loss occurs to freight. The ICM should realize that

shipments can be refused (not signed for) on delivery. In such cases, if the ICM deems that damage has or may have occurred because of the condition of the shipping container, the shipment may be refused, in which case the carrier will send the goods back to the vendor.

Receiving Freight

TECHNICIAN NOTES It is best to allow the person who placed the order to unpack the freight once the order has been received.

If the order is incorrect, the person who placed the order will know it immediately, whereas a person unpacking freight who did not place the order will not know what is correct. Several important questions should be asked when one is unpacking an order, such as "Did I get exactly what I ordered?"; "Did I get the right drug form (i.e., capsules, tablets, or powder)?"; "Did I receive the correct size and/or strength?"; "Is the product's expiration date far enough into the future?"; "Does the invoice list the price I was quoted by the phone representative or sales representative?"; "Does this order cost more than the last order of the same items?"; "Is anything backordered, and if so, when will that item be shipped?"; "Is any freight damaged or missing?"; and "Is the order correct, and if so, can the bill be paid?" (Lukens and Landon, 1993). By asking all these questions, the ICM is assured that the veterinary facility will be treated fairly by the vendor.

Stocking Shelves

TECHNICIAN NOTES It should be remembered when shelves are stocked that newly received items should be placed behind older items, so that the old is used and/or sold first.

When stock is rotated in this manner, the facility is assured that the product is sold or used by the hospital before the expiration date. When stocking shelves, the ICM should record expiration dates. The earliest date should be the one recorded in the computer, so the software will present an accurate list of expired items when the command is given to print an expired items list. Stocking shelves also presents a convenient time to dust and wipe off labels and lids on products that have been sitting on the shelf for extended periods. It should be noted that after cleaning, products should be replaced in specific locations to facilitate accurate inventory.

Vendors

Several different types of vendors may be used. The ICM must have adequate knowledge of these types to correctly place an order. Some vendors allow ordering by phone; others require that the order be given to a sales representative. Still others require a faxed order or an order sent through the mail.

Full-service companies are those that send a sales representative to visit the veterinary facility and offer full service. A technical staff, usually made up of veterinarians, is employed. Full-service companies usually carry a limited product line. Some products may be newly developed products that still retain a patent with the federal government and cannot be ordered through a distributorship. A full-service company has sales representatives who call on the veterinary hospital and take orders. Most full-service companies will replace outdated product with new or will credit the hospital's account accordingly.

TECHNICIAN NOTES The sales representative may not pick up expired controlled substances; these must be mailed back to the company.

A full-service company may have several "deals" that the ICM must decide to accept or decline. Examples of full-service companies include Pfizer Animal Health, Pharmacia-Upjohn, Schering-Plough Animal Health, and Fort Dodge Animal Health. These companies employ veterinarians as technical support staff, and their product lines are often limited as compared with distributorships. However, full-service companies are forerunners in the development of new drugs protected under U.S. patent laws, in which case they may not be sold under a generic name until the patent expires.

Mail order discount houses provide a good source for ordering items such as gauze, syringes, needles, paper towels, paper drapes, and even isopropyl alcohol. Ordering from this type of vendor occurs over the telephone because most do not employ sales representatives to visit the hospital, although catalogs may be supplied and mailed to the buyer.

Veterinary supply distributors provide the most common way of acquiring supplies for the veterinary facility. A distributor is an intermediate between a full-service company and the mail order discount house. If a full-service company gives its approval and a contract is signed between two companies, some products normally sold only through a full-service company may be obtained from a distributor. Many times, products sold by the full-service company to the distributor are those with a patent about to expire or those with an already expired patent. The distributor may elect to sell under a generic name instead of the full-service company's trade name. A distributorship usually maintains a huge inventory and employs sales representatives who call on veterinary facilities. Products ordered from a distributorship should be documented carefully. Should expired product need to be returned, the ICM may have to provide invoice numbers to prove which distributorship the product was purchased from before credit is applied to the facility's account.

Communicating With Sales Representatives

It is important for the ICM to be certain that sales representatives that visit the facility are aware of certain things. Sales representatives should know the ICM's scheduled lunch and quitting times. Additionally, the ICM should make sure that the sales representative is aware that all emergencies take priority over scheduled sales appointments. It is usually best to schedule an appointment with a visiting sales representative because this is much easier than having to drop other responsibilities in order to talk to the representative.

Drug Enforcement Administration Forms

Dealing with U.S. Drug Enforcement Administration (DEA) forms can be a frustrating experience if they are not handled correctly. However, if certain rules are kept in mind, ordering controlled substances need not be stressful.

> *TECHNICIAN NOTES* All veterinarians have a DEA number assigned to them and their veterinary license. This number is private and should never be given out for any reason.

Forms must be ordered from the DEA and kept in a secure location once mailed to the veterinarian. **DEA forms** are multicopy forms (i.e., carbon copies are made). The veterinarian keeps a copy of the order for his or her records. All information contained on these forms must be correct. Important considerations to keep in mind when one is filling out these forms include no markouts, no use of correction fluid or tape, no misspellings or incorrect drug strength, and inclusion of the veterinarian's signature on the form. These forms must be filled out with an ink pen or typewriter.

Special Orders

Often, clients may require "special orders." Clients must be made aware that once a "special order" is made, it must be purchased. If this is not understood, the veterinary facility may have to hold on to a slow-moving item or one that is never sold at all. Once this "special order" has been received by the hospital, the ICM should let the client know that the item has arrived. It is best to place these "special orders" near the receptionist's desk because the ICM may be busy with other duties when the client arrives to pick up the order.

Human Pharmacy

At various times, the veterinary practitioner may have to use a human pharmacy to supply drugs for clients' pets. A veterinarian may call the order into the pharmacy or provide the order on a written prescription. Keeping a good working relationship between pharmacist and veterinarian is important because a pharmacist may have additional knowledge about pharmaceutical products.

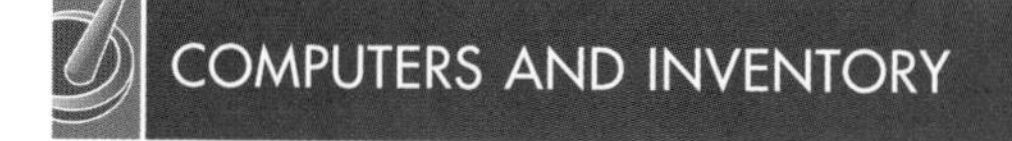

COMPUTERS AND INVENTORY

The advent of computer software technology has made inventory easier for all businesses. Many types of veterinary management software programs are available. Most programs offer features such as provisions for entering client information, inventory control, printout of common forms (e.g., rabies certificates), medical history, and accounting information. It is important to enter all inventory products used for each patient because the software has the ability to automatically subtract inventory amounts used. This is where "GIGO" is very important. Although each employee has good intentions, the ICM may find discrepancies in the total amount of product on hand. Staff meetings represent a good time to remind employees how important "GIGO" is. All newly received inventory items must be added to amounts already posted in the computer. Bar coding is available on most pharmaceutical products. Using a device capable of reading bar codes greatly enhances the counting and maintaining of inventory.

Additionally, most software can be used to produce automatic expiration lists from computer files each month. The total amount of money spent on inventory in a day, week, month, or year can be obtained when computer software systems are used.

THE JOB OF INVENTORY CONTROL MANAGER

It cannot be overemphasized how important inventory control is to the veterinary facility. Veterinary technician who are willing to take on this added responsibility will find themselves to be invaluable members of the staff. Keeping in mind that inventory is the second highest expense for the veterinary hospital will enable the ICM to use care when considering sales offers. Understanding the practice's mission is crucial in inventory control. Remember, time is money, and product left sitting on the shelf for extended periods does not benefit the facility. Keeping a turnover of at least four turns per year is a minimum goal. Training a backup person to monitor inventory during times of vacation or sickness experienced by the ICM is crucial. Reminding employees during staff meetings of the importance of "GIGO" and documenting items in low supply on the reorder log will allow the facility to keep a continuous supply of needed product on hand. DEA products must be controlled by effective documentation of their use in a log book kept solely for this purpose (e.g., controlled substance log book).

Many other factors are also important. Establishing a formula for markup is critical. The way inventory is arranged within the pharmacy has a great deal to do with the ease of counting it. No better method of counting inventory can replace doing a physical inventory. Keep sales representatives abreast of lunch breaks and leaving times. Carefully observe all freight for damage, and report claims as soon as possible after receiving the product. Always rotate product on shelves so that the oldest product is sold first. Be knowledgeable about the different types of vendors. Decide which method of inventory counting is most advantageous to your particular situation by deciding whether to count all inventory monthly or on a rotating basis. Keep a good relationship with a local pharmacy because these businesses serve as a valuable source of knowledge and enable the veterinarian to order human products not normally sold through veterinary vendors. Decide whether a manual or a computerized system is best for your facility. However, keep in mind that, in this age of technology, a computer system facilitates efficient work flow.

REVIEW QUESTIONS

1. What is inventory? ____________________
2. Name the five principles used to control expenses:
   a. ____________________
   b. ____________________
   c. ____________________
   d. ____________________
   e. ____________________
3. When dealing with inventory, it is crucial to remember that time is ____________________.
4. What is turnover? ____________________
5. Calculate the turnover rate by using the following information: Yearly inventory expense = $125,000; average cost of inventory on hand = $31,250. ____________________

6. Calculate the average cost of inventory on hand by using the following information: Year's beginning inventory = $75,000; year's ending inventory = $130,000. ______________________
7. Name two objectives of an inventory control system. ______________________
8. What is a packing slip?

____
9. What is an invoice? ______________________
10. What is a statement? ______________________
11. What is the reorder point?

____
12. Why is recording the expiration date and serial number for rabies vaccine so important?

____
13. Once the reorder point is reached, a basic rule of thumb is to order a ______________________-month supply.
14. List some rules for filling out a DEA form.

____
15. Time = Money.
    a. True
    b. False
16. A mean turnover rate of ______ is acceptable for most veterinary practices.
    a. 12
    b. 4
    c. 2
    d. 8
17. Inventory should be placed on pharmacy shelves in such a way so as to ensure ______.
    a. LILO
    b. FIFO
    c. FOB
    d. ICM
18. DEA forms are issued by ______.
    a. state governments
    b. county governments
    c. city governments
    d. the federal government
19. An item may be placed on backorder just because the pharmaceutical company is changing the color of the drug's label.
    a. True
    b. False
20. The price a veterinary hospital pays for an item is known as ______, and the amount the hospital sells the item to a client for is known as ______ price.
    a. retail; cost
    b. cost; retail
21. The expiration date and the serial number of rabies vaccine administered must be recorded on each pet's rabies certificate.
    a. True
    b. False
22. Delayed billing has no perks for a veterinary practice owner.
    a. True
    b. False
23. When a shipment arrives at a veterinary hospital, if the delivery carton appears to be damaged, the ICM does not have to accept the shipment from the carrier.
    a. True
    b. False
24. When a DEA form is used to order a controlled substance, it is acceptable to draw a line through a misspelled word and then write it correctly beside the mistake.
    a. True
    b. False

REFERENCES

Brown GW, Sukys PA: Business law with UCC applications, ed 11, New York, 2006, McGraw-Hill Irwin.

Libby R, Libby P, Short DG: Financial accounting, ed 4, New York, 2004, McGraw-Hill Irwin.

Lukens RL, Landon RM: A guide to inventory management for veterinary practices: effective inventory control, Westchester, Pa, 1993, SmithKline Beecham Animal Health.

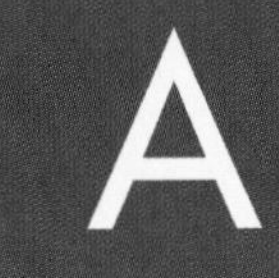

Common Abbreviations Used in Veterinary Medicine

AD	right ear (auris dextra)
ad lib	freely, as wanted (ad libitum)
AL	left ear (auris laeva)
A.M.	morning
AMA	against medical advice
ASAP	as soon as possible
A.U.	each ear (aures unitas)
b.i.d.	twice daily (bis in die)
bol.	large pill, bolus
Bute	Phenylbutazone
c– (cum)	with
caps	capsule
cc	cubic centimeters
cwt.	Hundredweight
DDx	differential diagnosis
DES	diethylstilbestrol
DMSO	dimethyl sulfoxide
DS	dose or days not acceptable
D/S or D-S	dextrose in saline
D_5W or D5W	5% dextrose with water
Dx	Diagnosis
e.o.d	every other day
g or gm	gram
gal	gallon
GI	gastrointestinal
gtt	drops (guttae)
GU	genitourinary
h or hr	hour
IM	intramuscular
IP	intraperitoneal
IV	intravenous
IVP	intravenous pyelogram
K	potassium
l or L	liter
lt	left
LA	long-acting
lb	pound
LRS	lactated Ringer's solution
mcg or μg	microgram
mEq	milliequivalent
mg	milligram
mm	millimeters
Na	sodium
non repetat.	do not repeat (non repetatur)
NPO	nothing by mouth (nil per os)
O	pint
O.D.	right eye (oculus dexter)
O.S.	left eye (oculus sinister)
O.U.	both eyes (oculi unitas)
oz	ounce
p.c.	after meals (post cibum)
per os or PO	by mouth, orally
Phos	phosphorus
p.r.n.	as needed (pro re nata)
PTA	prior to administration
pwd	powder
q2h	every 2 hours (quaque secunda hora)
q4h	every 4 hours (quaque quarta hora)
q.d.	every day (quaque die)
q.h. or o.h.	every hour (quaque hora)
q.i.d.	four times a day (quater in die)
q.o.d.	every other day
r or rt	right
Rx	take thou of (prescription)
s–	(sine) without
SC or SQ	subcutaneous
s.i.d.	once a day (semel in die)
sig.	directions, instructions
SOB	shortness of breath
SR	sustained release
STAT	immediately (statim)
Sx	surgery
T, Tbs, Tbsp	tablespoon
t, tsp	teaspoon

Tab tablet
t.i.d. three times a day (ter in die)
TLC tender loving care
TR trace
Tx treatment
U unit
UG urogenital
μL microliter
ung. ointment
Ut dict. as directed (ut dictum)
V-D vomiting/diarrhea
× times, multiply

APPENDIX B

Weights and Measures

Metrologic and Pharmaceutic Weights and Measures

The Metric System of Weight
1 microgram (mcg) = 0.000001 gram (g) (μg)
1 milligram (mg) = 0.001 g = 1000 mcg (μg)
1 gram (g) = 1.0 g = 1000 mg
1 kilogram (kg) = 1000.0 g

The Metric System of Liquid Measure
1 milliliter (mL) = 0.001 L
1 liter (L) = 1000 mL

The Avoirdupois System of Weights
437.5 grains (gr) = 1 ounce (oz)
16 oz = 1 pound (lb) = 7000 gr

Apothecaries' System of Weights
20 gr = 1 scruple
3 scruples (ε) = 1 dram = 60 gr
8 drams = 1 oz = 480 gr
12 oz = 1 lb = 5760 gr

Apothecaries' System of Liquid Measures (U.S. Wine Measure)
60 minims = 1 fluid dram
8 fluid drams = 1 fluid ounce (fl oz)
16 fl oz = 1 pint
8 pints = 1 gallon (cong.)

From Boothe DM: Small animal clinical pharmacology & therapeutics, ed 2, St. Louis, 2012, Elsevier.

Equivalents (Approximate)

1 grain (gr)	64.8 milligram (mg)	60 mg
1 ounce (oz)	28.35 gram (g)	30 g
1 pound (lb)	453.6 g	454 g
1 dram (60 gr)	3.9 g	4 g
1 apothecary ounce (480 gr)	31.1 g	30 g
1 minim	0.06 (mL) milliliter	0.06 mL
1 fluid dram	3.7 mL	4 mL
1 fluid ounce	29.573 mL	30 mL
1 pint	473.1 mL	480 or 500 mL
1 gallon	3785.4 mL	4000 mL
1 mg	$\frac{1}{64.8}$ gr	$\frac{1}{65}$ or $\frac{1}{60}$ gr
1 g	15,432 gr	15 gr
1 kilogram (kg)		2.2 pounds (lb)
1 gallon (water)	8.337 lb (8 lb approx.)	3.8 kg (approx.)
1 gallon occupies 231 cubic inches		
1 mL	1.000027 cubic centimeters	
1 pint	473 mL	500 mL
1 quart	946 mL	1000 mL
1 drop	0.06 mL	1 minim
1 dessert spoonful		8 mL
1 teaspoonful (tsp)		5 mL
1 tablespoonful (Tb)		15 mL

From Boothe DM: Small animal clinical pharmacology & therapeutics, ed 2, St. Louis, 2012, Elsevier.

Conversions for Calculating Dosage

w/v%*	μg/mL	μg/mL (mcg/mL)	Dilution g to mL
10%	100	100,000	1:10
5%	50	50,000	1:20
2%	20	20,000	1:50
1%	10	10,000	1:100
0.1%	1	1000	1:1000
0.2%	0.2	200	1:5000
0.01%	0.1	100	1:25,000
0.004%	0.04	40	1:25,000
0.002%	0.02	20	1:50,000
0.001%	0.01	10	1:100,000
0.0001%	0.001	1	1:1,000,000

*The definition of w/v is grams/dL

From Boothe DM: Small animal clinical pharmacology & therapeutics, ed 2, St. Louis, 2012, Elsevier.

Dry Weight and Volume Conversions

DRY WEIGHT	VOLUME CONVERSIONS
1 pound (lb)	453.6 grams (g)
1 gram (g)	0.0022 pound (lb)
1 gram (g)	1000 milligrams (mg)
1 gram (g)	1,000,000 micrograms (μg)
1 kilogram (kg)	1000 grams
1 kilogram (kg)	2.205 pounds (lb)
1 milligram (mg)	0.001 gram (g)
1 microgram (μg)	0.001 milligrams (mg)
1 microgram per gram (μg.g)	1 part per million (ppm)
1 part per million (ppm)	0.454 milligram/pound (mg/lb)
1 part per million (ppm)	0.907 gram per ton (g/T)
1 liter (L)	1000 milliliter (mL)
1 milliliter (mL)	1000 microliter (μL or lambda)

From Boothe DM: Small animal clinical pharmacology & therapeutics, ed 2, St. Louis, 2012, Elsevier.

Common Units and Conversion Factors

UNIT	ABBREVIATION
CONCENTRATION OF SOLUTIONS	
grams per deciliter	g/dL
grams per liter	g/L
international units per liter	IU/L
micrograms per deciliter	μg/dL
micromoles per liter	μmol/L
microunits per milliliter	μU/mL
milliequivalents per liter	mEq/L
milligrams per deciliter	mg/dL
millimoles per kilogram	mmol/kg
millimoles per liter	mmol/L
milliosmoles per kilogram	mOsm/kg
parts per million	ppm
percent	g/dL
units per liter	U/L
DISTANCE	
centimeter	cm
meter squared	m^2
millimeter	mm
FLUIDS	
deciliter (10^2 mL)	dL
liter (10^3 mL)	L
microliter (10^{-6})	μL
milliliter (1 mL or 10^{-3} L)	mL
PRESSURE	
centimeters of water	cm H_2O
millimeters of mercury	mm Hg
TIME	
every	q
hour	h
minute	min
month	mo
second	sec
week	wk
year	yr

UNIT	ABBREVIATION
WEIGHTS	
grain (1 gr = 65 mg)	gr
gram (1 g or 10^{-3} kg)	g
kilogram (10^3 g)	kg
microgram (10^{-6} g)	μg
milligram (10^{-3} g)	mg
nanogram (10^{-9} g)	ng
pictogram (10^{-12} g)	pg

COMMON CONVERSIONS

VOLUME OR WEIGHT	EQUIVALENT
1 dram	3.9 grams
1 drop (gt)	0.06 milliliter
15 drops	1 milliliter (1 cc)
1 fluid dram	3.7 milliliters
1 glass	240 milliliters (8 ounces)
1 grain	0.065 gram or 65 milligrams
1 gram	15.43 grains
1 kilogram	2.20 pounds (avoirdupois)
1 kilogram	2.65 pounds (Troy)
1 liter	1.06 quarts
1 liter	33.80 fluid ounces
1 measuring cup	240 milliliters ($\frac{1}{2}$ pint)
2 measuring cups	500 milliliters (1 pint)
1 milligram	1/65 grain
1 milliliter	16.23 minims
1 minim	0.062 milliliter
1 ounce	31.1 grams
1 ounce	30 milliliters or 28.35 grams
1 pint	473.2 milliliters
1 quart	15 milliliters
1 tablespoon	15 milliliters
2 tablespoons	30 milliliters
1 teacup	180 milliliters (6 ounces)
1 teaspoon	5 milliliters
1 unit (e.g., penicillin)	0.000625 mg

Temperature Equivalents

FAHRENHEIT (°F)	CELSIUS (°C)
TEMPERATURE CONVERSIONS	
°Fahrenheit to °Celsius: (°F − 32°)(5/9)	°Celsius to °Fahrenheit: (°C)(9/5) + 32°
98.6	37.0
99.0	37.2
100.0	37.7
101.0	38.3
102.0	38.8
103.0	39.4
104.0	40.0
105.0	40.5
106.0	41.1

Table of Weight Equivalents

POUND (LB)	KILOGRAM (KG)
lb = kg × 2.2	kg = lb ÷ 2.2
5	2.27
10	4.5
15	6.8
20	9.0
25	11.4
30	13.6
35	15.9
40	18.2
45	20.5
50	22.7
55	25.0
60	27.3
65	29.5
70	31.8
75	34.1
80	36.4
85	38.6
90	40.9
95	43.2
100	45.5

APPENDIX C

Antidotes

TOXIC AGENT	SYSTEMIC ANTIDOTE	DOSAGE AND METHOD FOR TREATMENT
Acetaminophen	N-acetylcysteine (Mucomyst)	150 mg/kg loading dose, PO or IV, then 50 mg/kg every 4 hours for 17 to 20 additional doses
	Cimetidine	5 mg/kg, orally, every 6 to 8 hours for 2 to 3 days; prevents biotransformation of acetaminophen
Amphetamines	Chlorpromazine	1 mg/kg IM, IP, IV; administer only half dose if barbiturates have been given: blocks excitation. Higher doses (10 to 18 mg/kg IV) may be beneficial if large volumes are consumed. Treatment of increased intracranial pressure may be indicated (mannitol, furosemide)
	Urinary alkalinization: Ammonium chloride	100 to 200 mg/kg per day divided every 8 to 12 hours (contraindicated with myoglobinuria, renal failure, or acidosis)
Amitraz	Atipamezole	50 g/kg IM. Signs should reverse in 10 minutes. Repeat every 3 to 4 hours as needed. Can follow with 0.1 mg/kg yohimbine IM every 6 hours
	Yohimbine	Dogs: 0.11 mg/kg IV slowly Cats: 0.5 mg/kg IV slowly
Antitussives	Naloxone	If narcotic (e.g., hydrocodone, codeine)
Arsenic, mercury and other heavy metals except cadmium, lead, silver, selenium, and thallium	Dimercaprol (BAL)	10% solution in oil; give small animals 2.5 to 5 mg/kg IM every 4 hours for 2 days, bid for the next 10 days or until recovery. Note: In severe acute poisoning, 5-mg/kg dosage should be given only for the first day.
	D-Penicillamine (Cuprimine)	Developed for chronic mercury poisoning; now seems most promising drug; no reports on dosage in animals. Dosage for humans is 250 mg orally, every 6 hours for 10 days (3 to 4 mg/kg)
Aspirin	No specific antidote (see also, nonsteroidal antiinflammatory drugs)	Acute toxicosis: urinary alkalinization, other supportive therapy; doses of 50 mg/kg per day (dog) and 25 mg/kg/day (cat); 7 mL/kg per day of bismuth subsalicylate (dogs and cats) may be toxic.
Atropine, belladonna alkaloids	Physostigmine salicylate	0.1 to 0.6 mg/kg (do not use neostigmine)
Barbiturates	Doxapram (Dopram)	2% solution: give small animals 3 to 5 mg/kg IV only (0.14 to 0.25 mL/kg); repeat as necessary

TOXIC AGENT	SYSTEMIC ANTIDOTE	DOSAGE AND METHOD FOR TREATMENT
Barium, bismuth salts	Sodium sulfate/ magnesium sulfate	20% solution given orally, 2 to 25 g
Bleach	Treat as alkali	Use of emetics is controversial; treat as an alkali poisoning. Therapies have included milk or water (large volumes), milk of magnesia (2 to 3 mg/kg), egg whites, or powdered milk slurry. Sodium bicarbonate is *not* recommended.
Borates (roach killers, fleas products, fertilizers, herbicides, antiseptics, disinfectants, contact lens solutions)	No specific antidote	Supportive therapy includes emetics and gastric lavage, fluid therapy and diuresis; treatment of seizures and hyperthermia as indicated.
Botulism	Antitoxin	Use is controversial. Supportive care may be sufficient. Supportive therapy may include penicillin, physostigmine or neostigmine, and atropine.
Bromethalin	No specific antidote	Supportive care may include treatment of cerebral edema.
Bromides	Chlorides (sodium or ammonium salts)	0.5 to 1 g daily for several days; hasten excretion.
Caffeine/chocolate	No specific antidote	General treatment, diazepam (2 to 5 mg/kg) for tremors; treat arrhythmias as indicated.
Carbon monoxide	Oxygen	Pure oxygen at normal or high pressure; artificial respiration; blood transfusion
Cholinergic agents	Atropine sulfate	0.02 to 0.04 mg/kg, as needed
Cholinesterase inhibitors	Atropine sulfate	Dosage is 0.2 to 0.4 mg/kg, repeated as needed for atropinization. Treat cyanosis (if present) first. Blocks only muscarinic effects. Atropine in oil may be injected for prolonged effect during the night. *Avoid atropine intoxication!*
	Pralidoxime chloride (2-PAM) (organophosphates, some carbamates; but not carbaryl, dimethan, or carbam piloxime)	5% solution; five 20- to 50-mg/kg IM or by slow IV (0.2 to 1.0 mg/kg) injection (maximum dose is 500 mg/min), repeat as needed. 2-PAM alleviates nicotinic effect and regenerates cholinesterase. Morphine, succinylcholine, and phenothiazine tranquilizers are contraindicated.
	Diphenhydramine	1-4 mg/kg IM, PO every 8 hours to block nicotinic effects.
Cocaine	No specific antidote	Chlorpromazine (up to 15 mg/kg; may lower seizure threshold, use cautiously); butylcholinesterase may convert cocaine to inactive metabolites (currently under investigation); fluids, metoprolol, or isopropanol to treat cardiac arrhythmias; phentolamine or sodium nitroprusside if beta blockers cause hypertension; lidocaine (instead of beta blockers) to control cardiac arrhythmias.

TOXIC AGENT	SYSTEMIC ANTIDOTE	DOSAGE AND METHOD FOR TREATMENT
Crayons (aniline dyes)	Ascorbic acid	20-30 mg/kg PO or 20 mg/kg IV slowly
	Methylene blue (if ascorbic acid fails)	Dogs: 3 to 4 mg/kg IV Cats: 1.5 mg/kg. (Methylene blue may cause Heinz body formation in the absence of methemoglobinemia, and sometimes in the presence of methemoglobinemia.)
Copper	D-Penicillamine (Cuprimine)	52 mg/kg for 6 days (also see arsenic)
	Ammonium molybdate	50 to 500 mg, PO, once a day
	Sodium thiosulfate	300 to 1000 mg, PO, once a day
	Ammonium tetrathiomolybdate	100 to 500 mg, PO on alternate days for 3 treatments
Coumarin-derivative anticoagulants	Vitamin K_1 (Aqua-mephyton, 5-mg caps) (Vita K_1, Eschar, 25-mg caps) Whole blood or plasma	Give 3 to 5 mg/kg/day with canned food. Treat 7 days for warfarin-type, treat 21 to 30 days for second-generation anticoagulant rodenticides. Oral therapy is more efficacious than IV. Blood transfusion, 25 mL/kg
Curare	Neostigmine methylsulfate	Solution: 1 : 5000 for 1 : 2000. (1 mL = 0.2 or 0.5 mg/mL). Dose is 0.005 mg/5 kg, SC. Follow with IV injection of atropine (0.04 mg/kg).
	Edrophonium chloride (Tensilon) Artificial respiration	1% solution; give 0.05 to 1.0 mg/kg IV.
Cyanide	Methemoglobin (sodium nitrite is used to form methemoglobin) Sodium thiosulfate	1% solution of sodium nitrite, dosage is 16 mg/kg IV (1.6 mL/kg). Follow with sodium thiosulfate 20% solution at dosage of 30 to 40 mg/kg (0.15 to 0.2 mL/kg) IV. If treatment is repeated, use only sodium thiosulfate. Note: These may be given simultaneously as follows: 0.5 mL/kg of combination consisting of 10 g sodium nitrite, 15 g sodium thiosulfate, distilled water quantity sufficient 250 mL. Dosage may be repeated once. If further treatment is required, give only 20% solution of sodium thiosulfate at level of 0.2 mL/kg.
Decongestants	No specific antidote	Treat symptomatically.
Detergents: anionic (Na, K, NH_4^+)		Milk or water followed by demulcent (e.g., oils, acacia, gelatin, starch, egg white)
Detergents: cationic (chlorides, iodides)		Castile soap dissolved in four times bulk of hot water. Albumin.
Diatomaceous earth		No treatment indicated unless pulmonary, then supportive.

TOXIC AGENT	SYSTEMIC ANTIDOTE	DOSAGE AND METHOD FOR TREATMENT
Digitalis glycosides, oleander, and *Bufo* toads	Potassium chloride	Dog: 0.5 to 2.0 g, orally in divided doses or, in serious cases, as diluted solution given IV by slow drip (ECG control is essential).
	Diphenylhydantoin Propranolol (β -blocker)	25 mg/minute IV control is established. 0.5 to 1.0 mg/kg IV or IM as needed to control cardiac arrhythmias (ECG control is essential).
	Atropine sulfate	0.02 to 0.04 mg/kg as needed for cholinergic control; 2 to 5 mg/kg, control convulsions
	Diazepam (Valium)	2 to 5 mg/kg; in the case of *Bufo* toads, must treat convulsions first
Ethylene glycol	Ethanol	See methanol and ethylene glycol. Minimal lethal dose of ethylene glycol is 4.2 to 6.6 mL/kg (4.5 ounces in 20-lb dog) and 1.5 mL for cats. Give IV, 1.1 g/kg (4.4 mL/kg) of 25% solution. Give 0.5 g/kg (2.0 mL/kg) every 4 hours for 4 days. To prevent or correct acidosis, use sodium bicarbonate IV, 0.4 g/kg. Activated charcoal: 5 g/kg orally if within 4 hours of ingestion.
	4-Methylpyrazole	20 mg/kg, 15 mg/kg at 12 and 24 hours, 5 mg/kg at 36 hours
	Sodium bicarbonate 5%	8 mL/kg (dog) or 6 mg/kg (cat) IP every 4 hours for five treatments, then every 6 hours for four more treatments.
Fertilizer	No specific antidote	Supportive therapy may include treatment for electrolyte disorders, vomiting, H_2 receptor blockers for gastritis, (sucralfate and analgesics as needed)
Fluoride	Calcium borogluconate	3 to 10 mL of 5% to 10% solution
Fluoroacetate (Compound 1080)	Glyceryl monoacetin	0.1 to 0.5 mg/kg IM hourly for several hours (total 2 to 4 mg/kg), or diluted (0.5 to 1%) IV (danger of hemolysis). Monoacetin is available only from chemical supply houses.
	Acetamide	Animal may be protected if acetamide is given before or simultaneously with Compound 1080 (experimental).
	Pentobarbital Note: All treatments are generally unrewarding.	May protect against lethal dose (experimental).
Formaldehyde		Ammonia water (0.2% orally) or ammonium acetate (1% for lavage). Starch: 1 part to 15 parts hot water, added gradually. Gelatin soaked in water for 30 minutes. Albumin (4-6 egg whites to 1 quart warm water); sodium thiosulfate (10% solution given orally). 0.5 to 3 g for small animals, followed by lavage or emesis
Garbage	No specific therapy	Supportive therapy may include antiemetics (metoclopramide or phenothiazines) and treatment of endotoxemia.
Hallucinogens (LSD, PCP)	Diazepam (Valium)	As needed; avoid respiratory depression (2 to 5 mg/kg)

TOXIC AGENT	SYSTEMIC ANTIDOTE	DOSAGE AND METHOD FOR TREATMENT
Heparin	Protamine sulfate	1% solution; give 1 to 1.5 mg to antagonize each 1 mg of heparin; slow IV injection. Reduce dose as time increases between heparin injection and start of treatment (after 30 minutes give only 0.5 mg).
Iron salts	Deferoxamine (Desferal)	Dose for animals not yet established. Dose for humans is 5 g of 5% solution given orally, then 20 mg/kg IM every 4 to 6 hours. In case of shock, dose is 40 mg/kg by IV drip over 4-hour period; may be repeated in 6 hours, then 15 mg/kg by drip every 8 hours.
Ivermectin	Physostigmine	0.06 mg/kg IV very slowly; actions should last 30 to 90 minutes.
	Picrotoxin (GABA antagonist)	Use is controversial. May cause severe seizures. Other treatment may include epinephrine and, if the product causing toxicosis is Eqvalan, an antihistamine to counteract polysorbate 80 (releases histamine in dogs) and atropine.
Lead	Calcium disodium edetate ($CaNa_2EDTA$)	Dosage: maximum safe dose is 75 mg/kg per 24 hours (only for severe case). EDTA is available in 20% solution; for IV drip, dilute in 5% glucose to 0.5%; for IM, add procaine to 20% solution to give 0.5% concentration of procaine.
	EDTA and BAL	BAL is given as 10% solution in oil. Treatment: (1) In severe case (CNS involvement with >100 μg Pb/100 g whole blood) give 4 mg/kg. BAL only as initial dose; follow after 4 hours, and every 4 hours for 3 to 4 days, with BAL and EDTA (12.5 mg/kg) at separate IM sites; skip 2 or 3 days, and then treat again for 3 to 4 days. (2) In subacute case with <100 μg Pb/100 g whole blood, give only 50 mg EDTA/kg per 24 hours for 3 to 5 days.
	Penicillamine (Cuprimine)	(3) May use after treatments either *1* or *2*; 100 mg/kg/day orally for 1 to 4 weeks.
	Thiamine HCl	Experimental for nervous signs; 5 mg/kg, IV, bid, for 1 to 2 weeks; give slowly and watch for untoward reactions
	Succimer (Chemet)	Oral human dose: 10 mg/kg every 8 hours for 5 days, then 10 mg/kg bid for 2 weeks (total of 19 days of therapy). Animal dosages have not been established. (Used if blood lead levels >45 ppm.)
Local anesthetics	See treatment for methemoglobinemia	Particularly cats
Marijuana	No effective antidotes	Protein: milk, egg whites (4-6 egg whites to 1 quart warm water). Magnesium oxide (1:25 dilution with warm water). Sodium formaldehyde sulfoxylate: 5% solution for lavage. Starch (1 part to 15 parts hot water, added gradually) Activated charcoal: 5 to 50 g.

TOXIC AGENT	SYSTEMIC ANTIDOTE	DOSAGE AND METHOD FOR TREATMENT
Metaldehyde	Diazepam (Valium)	2 to 5 mg/kg IV to control tremors.
	Triflupromazine	0.2 to 2 mg/kg IV
	Pentobarbital	To effect; Note: should monitor liver function and treat accordingly
Methanol and ethylene glycol	Ethanol	Give IV, 1.1 g/kg (4.4 mL/kg) of 25% solution. Give 0.5 g/kg (2 mL/kg) every 4 hours for 4 days. To prevent or correct acidosis, use sodium bicarbonate IV, 0.4 g/kg. Activated charcoal: 5 g/kg orally if within 4 hours of ingestion.
	4-Methylpyrazole	20 mg/kg, 15 mg/kg at 12 and 24 hours, 5 mg/kg at 36 hours
Methemoglobinemia-producing agents (nitrites, chlorates)	Methylene blue	1% solution (maximum concentration), give by *slow* IV injection, 8.8 mg/kg (0.9 mL/kg); repeat if needed. To prevent fall in blood pressure in case of nitrite poisoning, use a sympathomimetic drug (ephedrine or epinephrine). (Not recommended for cats.)
	Ascorbic acid	20 to 30 mg/kg PO or 20 mg/kg IV slowly; methylene blue; dogs: 3 to 4 mg/kg IV slowly if ascorbic acid not effective; cats: 1.5 mg/kg
Morphine and related drugs	Naloxone chloride (Narcan)	0.1 mg/kg IV Do not repeat if respiration is not satisfactory. See Note.
	Levallorphan tartrate (Lorfan)	Give IV, 0.1 to 0.5 mL of solution containing 1 mg/mL. Note: Use either of these antidotes only in acute poisoning. Artificial respiration may be indicated. Activated charcoal is also indicated.
Mothballs (naphthalene, paradichlorobenzene)	No specific antidote	Supportive care includes fluid therapy and maintenance of renal and hepatic function.
Narcotics	Naloxone	Emesis: indicated only if patient is sufficiently alert. Dog: 0.02 to 0.04 mg/kg IV; repeat as needed. Cat: 0.05 to 0.1 mg/kg IV; repeat as needed. Supportive therapy may include anticonvulsants (especially for meperidine), fluid therapy.
Nicotine	No specific antidote	Emesis: indicated only within 60 minutes and in absence of clinical signs. Atropine indicated to control parasympathetic signs.
Nonsteroidal antiinflammatory drugs	Sucralfate	500 to 100 mg PO every 8 hours
	Misoprostol	3 to 5 μg/kg every 8 to 12 hours
	Omeprazole	0.7 mg/kg every 24 hours (dog); alternative, ranitidine or famotidine (dog and cat)
Oxalates	Calcium	Treatment: 23% solution of calcium gluconate IV. Give 3 to 20 mL (to control hypocalcemia). Or calcium hydroxide as 0.15% solution or chalk or other calcium salts. Magnesium sulfate as cathartic. Other alkalines are contraindicated because their salts are more soluble. Maintain diuresis to prevent calcium oxalate deposition in kidney.

TOXIC AGENT	SYSTEMIC ANTIDOTE	DOSAGE AND METHOD FOR TREATMENT
Onion/garlic	No specific antidote	Supportive therapy should address methemoglobinemia and hemoglobinuria. Avoid acidic urine.
Organic solvents: acetone, benzene, benzol, methanol, methylene chloride, naphtha, trichloroethane, acetonitrile, chloroform, trichloroethylene, toluene, xylene, xylol	No specific antidote	Emesis contraindicated. Supportive therapy includes treatment of cardiac arrhythmias, methemoglobinemia, renal failure, chemical pneumonia.
Petroleum distillates (aliphatic hydrocarbons)		Olive oil, other vegetable oils, or mineral oil given orally. After 30 minutes, sodium sulfate as cathartic. Emesis and lavage are contraindicated for ingested volatile solvents, but petroleum distillates are used as carrier agents for more toxic agents.
Phenols and cresols		Soap and water or alcohol lavage of skin. Sodium bicarbonate (0.5%) dressings. Activated charcoal and/or mineral oil given orally.
Phenothiazine	Methylamphetamine (Desoxyn)	0.1 to 0.2 mg/kg IV; also transfusion. Only available in tablet form.
	Diphenhydramine HCl	For CNS depression, 2 to 5 mg/kg IV for extrapyramidal signs.
Phytotoxins and botulin	Antitoxins not available commercially, except for botulism.	As indicated for specific antitoxins; examples of phytotoxins: ricin, abrin, robin, crotin
Plants		Treat signs as necessary.
Red squill	Atropine sulfate, propranolol, potassium chloride	See Digitalis and oleander
Scorpion sting	Antivenin (may not be recommended)	Supportive therapy includes analgesia to control pain (morphine and meperidine, but not butorphanol, are contraindicated because of potential synergy with scorpion venom); methocarbamol (if muscle spasms evident) and fluid therapy.
Smoke inhalation	Supportive therapy	Supportive therapy should target the respiratory system and treatment of carbon monoxide intoxication. Oxygen therapy; intermittent positive pressure ventilation with positive end-expiratory pressure with positive inotropic support, bronchodilators, treatment for cyanide poisoning if indicated, and treatment for cerebral edema.
Snake bite Rattlesnake Copperhead Water moccasin	Antivenin; Trivalent Crotalidae	Caution: equine origin. Administer 1 to 2 vials, IV, slowly, diluted in 250 to 500 mL of saline or lactated Ringer's. Also administer antihistamines. *Corticosteroids are contraindicated.*
Coral snake	Antivenin	Caution: equine origin. May be used as with pit viper antivenin.

TOXIC AGENT	SYSTEMIC ANTIDOTE	DOSAGE AND METHOD FOR TREATMENT
Spider bite Black widow	Antivenin	Caution: equine origin. Administer IV undiluted. Supportive therapy should include muscle relaxants (dantrolene or methocarbamol) analgesics, calcium gluconate for severe muscle cramping.
	Dantrolene sodium (Dantrium)	1 mg/kg IV, followed by 1 mg/kg PO every 4 hours
Brown recluse	Dapsone	1 mg/kg, bid for 10 days
Strontium	Calcium salts	Usual dose of calcium borogluconate
	Ammonium chloride	0.2 to 0.5 g orally three to four times daily
	Potassium chloride	Give simultaneously with thiocarbazone or Prussian blue, 2 to 6 g orally daily in divided doses.
Strychnine and brucine	Pentobarbital	Give IV to effect; higher dose is usually required than that required for anesthesia. Place animal in warm, quiet room.
	Amobarbital	Give by slow IV infusion; inject to effect. Duration of sedation is usually 4 to 6 hours.
	Methocarbamol (Robaxin)	10% solution; average first dose is 149 mg/kg IV (range: 40 to 300 mg). Repeat half dose as needed.
	Glyceryl guaiacolate (Guaifenison)	110 mg/kg IV, 5% solution. Repeat as necessary.
	Diazepam (Valium)	2 to 5 mg/kg, control convulsions, induce emesis, then use other agents.
Thallium	Prussian blue	0.2 gm/kg orally in three divided doses daily.
	Potassium chloride	Give simultaneously with Prussian blue, 2 to 6 g orally, daily in divided doses.
Theobromine	See Caffeine/chocolate	
Toad poisoning (*Bufo alvarius, Bufo marinus*)	Propranolol (*Bufo* poisoning only)	1.5 to 5 mg/kg IV; repeat in 20 minutes if ECG does not normalize; supportive therapy includes fluid therapy
	Atropine	0.04 mg/kg IV to control hypersalivation or asystole
	Lidocaine	Dogs: 1 to 2 mg/kg IV followed by continuous infusion of 25 to 75 μg/kg/min; cats: 0.25 to 1 mg/kg IV bolus followed by 5 to 40 μg/kg/min continuous IV infusion
	Diazepam (Valium)	2 to 5 mg/kg in the case of *Bufo* toads; must treat convulsions first
Tricyclic antidepressants	No specific antidote	Supportive therapy should target seizures (diazepam, phenobarbital, or general anesthesia with pentobarbital or short-acting thiobarbiturates; or, if unsuccessful, neuromuscular blockade with pancuronium (0.03 to 0.06 mg/kg IV) or vecuronium (10 to 20 μg/kg IV in dogs or 20 to 40 μg/kg in cats); cardiotoxicity (see Toad poisoning): propranolol, lidocaine (quinidine, procainamide, disopyramide are contraindicated); sodium bicarbonate (1 to 3 mEq/kg)
Unknown (e.g., toxic plants or other materials)	No specific antidote	Activated charcoal 2 to 5 g/kg (replaces universal antidote). For small animals: through stomach tube, as a slurry in water. Follow with emetic or cathartic, and repeat procedure.

TOXIC AGENT	SYSTEMIC ANTIDOTE	DOSAGE AND METHOD FOR TREATMENT
Vitamin D_3 rodenticides	Treatment of hypercalcemia	Supportive therapy should target treatment of hypercalcemia (0.9% saline solution); control of seizures and treatment of hyperthermia. Calciuria can be promoted with furosemide (1 to 5 mg/kg every 6 to 12 hours for 2 to 4 weeks); prednisolone; calcitonin (4 to 6 IU/kg every 6 to 12 hours if calcium > 18 mg/dL); sodium bicarbonate if severe metabolic acidosis.
	Amphojel, Basagel	As phosphate binders (aluminum hydroxide 30 to 90 mg/kg PO every 8 to 24 hours for 2 weeks)
Xylitol		Hypoglycemia: 1 to 2 mL of 25% dextrose followed by 2.5% to 5% dextrose infusion as needed to maintain normoglycemia. Add potassium to fluids to maintain serum potassium (treat for 12 to 24 hours). Hepatic necrosis: 140 to 280 mg/kg *N*-acetylcysteine IV followed by 70 mg/kg qid IV or PO; S-adenosylmethionine 17 to 20 mg/kg/day PO, silymarin 20 to 50 mg/kg/day PO
Zinc	Chelation therapy (see Lead)	CaEDTA, Succimer. Other supportive therapy includes fluid therapy and antisecretory drugs such as ranitidine, famotidine, or omeprazole to decrease oral absorption of zinc.

BAL, British anti-Lewisite; *bid,* twice a day; *CNS,* central nervous system; *ECG,* electrocardiogram; *EDTA,* ethylenediaminetetraacetic acid; *GABA,* gamma-aminobutyric acid; *IM,* intramuscular; *IP,* intraperitoneal; *IV,* intravenous; *LSD,* lysergic acid diethylamide; *PCP,* phencyclidine; *PO,* by mouth; *qid,* four times a day; *SC,* subcutaneous.
From Boothe DM: Small animal clinical pharmacology and therapeutics, St. Louis, 2010, Elsevier.

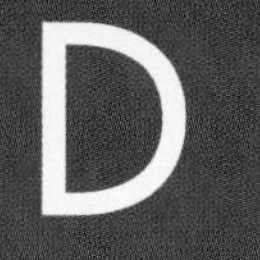

Appendix D Common Drugs: Approximate Dosages

DRUG NAME	OTHER NAMES	FORMULATIONS AVAILABLE	DOSAGE
Acetaminophen	Tylenol and many generic brands	120-, 160-, 325-, and 500-mg tablets	Dog: 15 mg/kg PO q8h Cat: Not recommended
Acetaminophen with codeine	Tylenol with codeine and many generic brands	Oral solution and tablets. Many forms (e.g., 300 mg acetaminophen plus either 15-, 30-, or 60-mg codeine)	Follow dosing recommendations for codeine
Acetazolamide	Diamox	125- and 250-mg tablets	5–10 mg/kg PO q8–12h (glaucoma) 4 to 8 mg/kg PO q8–12h (other diuretic uses)
Acetylcysteine	Mucomyst	20% solution	Antidote: 140 mg/kg (loading dose) then 70 mg/kg IV or PO q4h for five doses. Eye: 2% solution topically q2h
Acetylsalicylic acid	*See* Aspirin		
ACTH	*See* Corticotropin		
Activated charcoal	*See* Charcoal, activated		
Adequan	*See* Polysulfated glycosaminoglycan (PSGAG)		
Albendazole	Valbazen	113.6-mg/mL suspension and 300-mg/mL paste	25–50 mg/kg PO q12h for 3 days. For *Giardia* use 25 mg/kg q12h for 2 days
Albuterol	Proventil or Ventolin	2-, 4-, and 5-mg tablets; 2 mg/5 mL syrup	20–50 mcg/kg q6–8h; up to maximum of 100 mcg/kg q6–8h PO
Allopurinol	Lopurin, Zyloprim	100- and 300-mg tablets	10 mg/kg q8h, then reduce to 10 mg/kg q24h
Aluminum carbonate gel	Basaljel	Capsule (equivalent to 500 mg aluminum hydroxide)	10–30 mg/kg PO q8h (with meals)
Aluminum hydroxide gel	Amphojel	64-mg/mL oral suspension; 600-mg tablet	10–30 mg/kg PO q8h (with meals)

DRUG NAME	OTHER NAMES	FORMULATIONS AVAILABLE	DOSAGE
Amikacin	Amiglyde-V (veterinary) and Amikin (human)	50- and 250-mg/mL injection	Dog: 15–30 mg/kg IV, SC, IM q24h Cat: 10–14 mg/kg IV, SC, IM q24h
Amiodarone	Cordarone	200-mg tablets; 50-mg/mL injection	Dog: Start with 15-mg/kg loading dose, then 10 mg/kg/day thereafter
Aminopentamide	Centrine	0.2-mg tablet; 0.5-mg/mL injection	Dog: 0.01–0.03 mg/kg IM, SC, PO q8–12h Cat: 0.1 mg/cat IM, SC, PO q8–12h
Aminophylline	Many (generic) (Theophylline is preferred for oral therapy)	100- and 200-mg tablets; 25-mg/mL injection	Dog: 10 mg/kg PO, IM, IV q8h Cat: 6.6 mg/kg PO q12h
6-Aminosalicylic acid	*See* Mesalamine, Olsalazine		
Amitraz	Mitaban	10.6-mL concentrated dip (19.9%). 10.6 mL per 7.5 L water (0.025% solution)	Apply three to six topical treatments q2wk. For refractory cases, this dose has been exceeded to produce increased efficacy. Doses that have been used include 0.025%, 0.05%, and 0.1% concentration applied twice per week and 0.125% solution applied to one-half body every day for 4 weeks to 5 months.
Amitriptyline	Elavil	10-, 25-, 50-, 75-, 100-, and 150-mg tablets; 10-mg/mL injection	Dog: 1–2 mg/kg PO q12–24h (range: 0.25–4 mg/kg q12–24h) Cat: 2–4 mg/cat/day PO; for cystitis: 2 mg/kg/day (2.5–7.5 mg/cat/day)
Amlodipine besylate	Norvasc	2.5-, 5-, and 10-mg tablets	Dog: 2.5 mg/dog or 0.1 mg/kg PO once daily Cat: 0.625 mg/cat/day PO initially and increase if needed to 1.25 mg/cat/day (average is 0.18 mg/kg)
Ammonium chloride	Generic	Available as crystals	Dog: 100 mg/kg PO q12h Cat: 800 mg/cat (approx. ⅓ to ¼ tsp) mixed with food daily
Amoxicillin trihydrate	Amoxi-Tabs, Amoxi-drops, Amoxil, and others	50-, 100-, 200-, and 400-mg tablets; 50-mg/mL oral suspension	6.6–20 mg/kg PO q8–12h

DRUG NAME	OTHER NAMES	FORMULATIONS AVAILABLE	DOSAGE
Amoxicillin/ clavulanic acid	Clavamox	62.5-, 125-, 250-, and 375-mg tablets; 62.5-mg/mL suspension	Dog: 12.5–25 mg/kg PO q12h Cat: 62.5 mg/cat PO q12h; consider administering these doses q8h for gram-negative infections
Amphotericin B	Fungizone	50-mg injectable vial	0.5 mg/kg IV (slow infusion) q48h, to a cumulative dose of 4 to 8 mg/kg
Amphotericin B (liposomal)	Amphotec, Abelcet, AmBisome		Dog: 2–3 mg/kg IV 3 times/wk for 9–12 treatments for a cumulative dose of 24–27 mg/kg Cat: 1 mg/kg IV 3 times/wk for 12 treatments
Ampicillin	Omnipen, Principen, others	250-, and 500-mg capsules; 125-, 250-, and 500-mg vials of ampicillin sodium	10–20 mg/kg IV, IM, SC q6–8h (ampicillin sodium); 20–40 mg/kg PO q8h
Ampicillin + sulbactam	Unasyn	1.5- and 3- g vials in 2 : 1 combination for injection	110–120 mg/kg IV, IM q8h
Ampicillin trihydrate	Polyflex	10- and 25-mg vials for injection	Dog: 10–50 mg/kg SC, IM q24h Cat: 10–20 mg/kg SC, IM q24h
Amprolium	Amprol, Corid	9.6% (9.6 g/dL) oral solution; soluble powder	1.25 g of 20% amprolium powder to daily feed, or 30 mL of 9.6% amprolium solution to 3.8 L of drinking water for 7 days
Antacid drugs	*See* Aluminum hydroxide gel, Magnesium hydroxide, and Calcium carbonate		
Apomorphine hydrochloride	Generic	6-mg tablet	0.44 mg/kg IM; 0.05 mg/kg IV; 0.1 mg/kg SC, or instill 0.25 mg in conjunctiva of eye (dissolve 6-mg tablet in 1–2 mL of saline)
Ascorbic acid	Vitamin C	Various forms	100–500 mg/animal/day (diet supplement) or 100 mg/animal q8h (urine acidification)
L-Asparaginase	Elspar	10,000 U per vial for injection	400 U/kg IV, IP, IM weekly; or 10,000 U/m^2 weekly for 3 wk
Aspirin	Many generic and brand names (Bufferin, Ascriptin)	81-mg and 325-mg tablets	Dog: Mild analgesia: 10 mg/kg q12h Antiinflammatory: 20–25 mg/kg q12h Antiplatelet: 5–10 mg/kg q24–48h Cat: 81 mg q48h PO

DRUG NAME	OTHER NAMES	FORMULATIONS AVAILABLE	DOSAGE
Atenolol	Tenormin	25-, 50-, and 100-mg tablets; 25-mg/mL oral suspension; and 0.5-mg/mL ampule for injection	Dog: 6.25–12.5 mg/dog q12h (or 0.25–1.0 mg/kg q12–24h) PO Cat: 6.25–12.5 mg/cat q12h (approx. 3 mg/kg) PO
Atipamezole	Antisedan	5-mg/mL injection	Inject same volume as used for medetomidine
Atracurium	Tracrium	10-mg/mL injection	0.2 mg/kg IV initially, then 0.15 mg/kg q30min (or IV infusion at 4–9 mcg/kg/min)
Atropine	Many generic brands	400-, 500-, and 540- mcg/mL injection; 15-mg/mL injection	0.02–0.04 mg/kg IV, IM, SC q6–8h;0.2–0.5 mg/kg (as needed) for organophosphate and carbamate toxicosis
Auranofin (triethylphosphine gold)	Ridaura	3-mg capsule	0.1–0.2 mg/kg PO q12h
Aurothioglucose	Solganal	50-mg/mL injection	Dog <10 kg: 1 mg IM first wk, 2 mg IM second wk, 1 mg/kg/wk maintenance Dog >10 kg: 5 mg IM first wk, 10 mg IM second wk, 1 mg/kg/wk maintenance Cat: 0.5–1 mg/cat IM q7 days
Azathioprine	Imuran	50-mg tablet; 10-mg/mL for injection	Dog: 2 mg/kg PO q24h initially then 0.5–1 mg/kg q48h Cat (use cautiously): 0.3 mg/kg PO q48h
Azithromycin	Zithromax	250-mg capsule; and 250- and 600-mg tablets; 20-mg/mL oral suspension	Dog: 10 mg/kg PO q48h or 3.3 mg/kg once daily Cat: 5–10 mg/kg PO every other day
AZT (azidothymidine)	*See* Zidovudine		
Bactrim (sulfamethoxazole + trimethoprim)	*See* Trimethoprim-sulfonamide combinations		
BAL	*See* Dimercaprol		
Benazepril	Lotensin	5-, 10-, 20-, and 40-mg tablets	Dog: 0.25–0.5 mg/kg PO q24h Cat: 0.5–1 mg/kg q24h PO or 2.5 mg/cat/day up to a maximum of 5 mg/cat/day
Betamethasone	Celestone	600-mcg (0.6-mg) tablet; 3-mg/mL sodium phosphate injection	0.1–0.2 mg/kg PO q12–24h
Bethanechol	Urecholine	5-, 10-, 25-, and 50-mg tablets; 5-mg/mL injection	Dog: 5–15 mg/dog PO q8h Cat: 1.25–5 mg/cat PO q8h

DRUG NAME	OTHER NAMES	FORMULATIONS AVAILABLE	DOSAGE
Bisacodyl	Dulcolax	5-mg tablet	5 mg/animal PO q8–24h
Bismuth subsalicylate	Pepto-Bismol	Oral suspension: 262 mg/15 mL or 525 mg/mL in extra-strength formulation; 262-mg tablet	1–3 mL/kg/day (in divided doses) PO
Bleomycin	Blenoxane	15-U vials for injection	10 U/m^2 IV or SC for 3 days, then 10 U/m^2 weekly (maximum cumulative dose 200 U/m^2)
Bromide	*See* Potassium bromide		
BSP (Bromsulphalein)	*See* Sulfobromophthalein (BSP)		
Budesonide	Entocort	3-mg capsule	Dog, cat: 0.125 mg/kg q6–8h PO; dose interval may be increased to q12h when condition improves
Bunamidine hydrochloride	Scolaban	400-mg tablet	20–50 mg/kg PO
Bupivacaine	Marcaine and generic	2.5- and 5-mg/mL solution injection	1 mL of 0.5% solution per 1–1.5 mg/kg for an epidural
Buprenorphine	Temgesic (Vetergesic in the UK)	0.3-mg/mL solution	Dog: 0.006–0.02 mg/kg IV, IM, SC q4–8h Cat: 0.005–0.01 mg/kg IV, IM q4–8h Buccal administration in cats: 0.01–0.02 mg/kg q12h
Buspirone	BuSpar	5- and 10-mg tablets	Dog: 2.5–10 mg/dog PO q12–24h; or 1 mg/kg q12h PO Cat: 2.5–5 mg/cat PO q24h (may be increased to 5–7.5 mg/cat twice daily for some cats)
Busulfan	Myleran	2-mg tablet	3–4 mg/m^2 PO q24h
Butorphanol	Torbutrol, Torbugesic	1-, 5-, and 10-mg tablets; 0.5- or 10-mg/mL injection	Dog: Antitussive: 0.055 mg/kg SC q6–12h or 0.55 mg/kg PO Preanesthetic: 0.2–0.4 mg/kg IV, IM, SC (with acepromazine) Analgesic: 0.2–0.4 mg/kg IV, IM, SC q2–4h or 0.55–1.1 mg/kg PO q6–12h Cat: Analgesic: 0.2–0.8 mg/kg IV, SC q2–6h, or 1.5 mg/kg PO q4–8h

DRUG NAME	OTHER NAMES	FORMULATIONS AVAILABLE	DOSAGE
Calcitriol	Rocaltrol, Calcijex	Available as injection (Calcijex) and capsules (Rocaltrol): 0.25- and 0.5-mcg capsules; 1- or 2-mcg/mL injection	Dog: 0.25–0.5 mcg/dog/day or approx. 0.12 mg/kg Cat: 0.25 mcg/cat every other day; or 0.01–0.04 mcg/kg/day
Calcium carbonate	Many brands available: Titralac, Tums, generic	Many tablets or oral suspension (e.g., 650-mg tablet contains 260 mg calcium ion)	For phosphate binder: 60–100 mg/kg/day in divided doses PO For calcium supplementation: 70–180 mg/kg/day added to food
Calcium chloride	Generic	10% (100 mg/mL) solution	0.1–0.3 mL/kg IV (slowly)
Calcium citrate	Citracal (OTC)	950-mg tablet (contains 200 mg calcium ion)	Dog: 20 mg/kg/day added to food Cat: 10–30 mg/kg PO q8h (with meals)
Calcium disodium	*See* Edetate calcium disodium		
EDTA			
Calcium gluconate	Kalcinate and generic	10% (100 mg/mL) injection	0.5–1.5 mL/kg IV (slowly)
Calcium lactate	Generic	OTC tablet	Dog: 0.5–2.0 g/dog/day PO (in divided doses) Cat: 0.2–0.5 g/cat/day PO (in divided doses)
Captopril	Capoten	25-mg tablet	Dog: 0.5–2 mg/kg PO q8–12h Cat: 3.12–6.25 mg/cat PO q8h
Carbenicillin	Geopen, Pyopen	1-, 2-, 5-, 10-, and 30-g vials for injection	40–50 mg/kg and up to 100 mg/kg IV, IM, SC q6–8h
Carbenicillin indanyl sodium	Geocillin	500-mg tablet	10 mg/kg PO q8h
Carbimazole	Neomercazole	Available in Europe	Cat: 5 mg/cat PO q8h (induction), followed by 5 mg/cat PO q12h
Carboplatin	Paraplatin	50- and 150-mg vial for injection	Dog: 300 mg/m^2 IV q3–4wk Cat: 200 mg/m^2 IV q4wk
Carprofen	Rimadyl (Zenecarp in the UK), Novox, generic	25-, 75-, and 100-mg tablets; 50 mg/mL solution	Dog: 2.2 mg/kg PO q12h; or 4.4 mg/kg once daily PO; 2.2 mg/kg q12h or 4.4 mg/kg once daily SC Cat: doses not available
Carvedilol	Coreg	3.125-, 6.25-, 12.5-, and 25-mg tablets	Dog: 0.2 to 0.4 mg/kg q12h PO; titrate dose up to 1.5 mg/kg q12h PO if needed
Cascara sagrada	Many brands (e.g., Nature's Remedy)	100- and 325-mg tablets	Dog: 1–5 mg/kg day PO Cat: 1–2 mg/cat/day

DRUG NAME	OTHER NAMES	FORMULATIONS AVAILABLE	DOSAGE
Castor oil	Generic	Oral liquid (100%)	Dog: 8–30 mL/day PO Cat: 4–10 mL/day PO
Cefadroxil	Cefa-Tabs, Cefa-Drops	50-mg/mL oral suspension; 50-, 100-, 200-, and 1000-mg tablets	Dog: 22–30 mg/kg PO q12h Cat: 22 mg/kg PO q24h
Cefazolin sodium	Ancef, Kefzol, and generic	50 and 100 mg/50 mL for injection	20–35 mg/kg IV, IM q8h For perisurgical use: 22 mg/kg q2h during surgery
Cefdinir	Omnicef	300-mg capsules; 25-mg/mL oral suspension	Dose not established (human dose is 7 mg/kg PO q12h)
Cefixime	Suprax	20-mg/mL oral suspension and 200- and 400-mg tablets	10 mg/kg PO q12h For cystitis: 5 mg/kg PO q12–24h
Cefotaxime	Claforan	500-mg and 1-, 2-, and 10-g vials for injection	Dog: 50 mg/kg IV, IM, SC q12h Cat: 20–80 mg/kg IV, IM q6h
Cefotetan	Cefotan	1-, 2-, and 10-g vials for injection	30 mg/kg IV, SC q8h
Cefovecin	Convenia	80 mg/mL injection	Dog, cat: 8 mg/kg SC once every 14 days
Cefoxitin sodium	Mefoxin	1-, 2-, and 10-g vials for injection	30 mg/kg IV q6–8h
Cefpodoxime proxetil	Simplicef	100- and 200-mg tablets; 10- or 20-mg/mL human label suspension	Dog: 5–10 mg/kg PO once daily Cat: Dose not established
Ceftazidime	Fortaz, Ceptaz, Tazicef	0.5-, 1-, 2- and 6-g vials reconstituted to 280 mg/mL	30 mg/kg IV, IM q6h
Ceftiofur	Naxcel (ceftiofur sodium); Excenel (ceftiofur HCl)	50-mg/mL injection	2.2–4.4 mg/kg SC q24h (for urinary tract infections)
Cephalexin	Keflex and generic forms	250- and 500-mg capsules; 250- and 500-mg tablets; 100-mg/mL or 125- and 250-mg/5-mL oral suspension	10–30 mg/kg PO q6–12h; for pyoderma, 22–35 mg/kg PO q12h
Cetirizine	Zyrtec	1-mg/mL oral syrup; 5- and 10-mg tablets	Dog: 5–10 mg/dog q12h, PO, up to a dose of 2 mg/kg q12h, PO Cat: 5 mg/cat, PO, q24h
Charcoal, activated	Acta-Char, Charcodote, Toxiban, generic	Oral suspension	1–4 g/kg PO (granules); 6–12 mL/kg (suspension)

DRUG NAME	OTHER NAMES	FORMULATIONS AVAILABLE	DOSAGE
Chlorambucil	Leukeran	2-mg tablet	Dog: 2–6 mg/m^2 or 0.1–0.2 mg/kg PO q24h initially, then q48h Cat: 0.1–0.2 mg/kg q24h initially, then q48h PO
Chloramphenicol and chloramphenicol palmitate	Chloromycetin, generic forms	30-mg/mL oral suspension (palmitate); 250-mg capsule; and 100-, 250-, and 500-mg tablets	Dog: 40–50 mg/kg PO q8h Cat: 12.5–20 mg/kg PO q12h
Chlorothiazide	Diuril	250- and 500-mg tablets; 50-mg/mL oral suspension and injection	20–40 mg/kg PO q12h or IV
Chlorpheniramine maleate	Chlor-Trimeton, Phenetron, and others	4- and 8-mg tablets	Dog: 4–8 mg/dog PO q12h (up to a maximum of 0.5 mg/kg q12h) Cat: 2 mg/cat PO q12h
Chlorpromazine	Thorazine	25-mg/mL injection solution	Dog: 0.5 mg/kg IM, SC q6–8h (before cancer chemotherapy administer 2 mg/kg SC q3h) Cat: 0.2–0.4 mg/kg q6–8h IM, SC
Chorionic gonadotropin	*See* Gonadotropin		
Cimetidine	Tagamet (OTC and prescription)	100-, 150-, 200-, and 300-mg tablets and 60-mg/mL injection	10 mg/kg IV, IM, PO q6–8h (in renal failure administer 2.5–5 mg/kg IV, PO q12h)
Ciprofloxacin	Cipro and generic	250-, 500-, and 750-mg tablets; 2-mg/mL injection	Dog: 10–20 mg/kg PO, IV q24h Cat: Not recommended
Cisapride		Must be compounded	Dog: 0.1–0.5 mg/kg PO q8–12h (doses as high as 0.5–1.0 mg/kg have been used in some dogs) Cat: 2.5–5 mg/cat PO q8–12h (as high as 1 mg/kg q8h has been administered to cats)
Cisplatin	Platinol	1-mg/mL injection; 50-mg vials	Dog: 60–70 mg/m^2 q3–4wk (administer fluid for diuresis with therapy) Cat: Not recommended
Clavamox	*See* Amoxicillin-clavulanic acid combination		
Clavulanic acid	*See* Amoxicillin–clavulanic acid combination		

DRUG NAME	OTHER NAMES	FORMULATIONS AVAILABLE	DOSAGE
Clemastine	Tavist, Contac 12-hour allergy, and generic	1.34-mg tablet (OTC); 2.64-mg tablet (Rx); 0.134-mg/mL syrup	Dog: 0.05–0.1 mg/kg PO q12h
Clindamycin	Antirobe, Cleocin, and generic	Oral liquid 25-mg/mL; 25-, 75-, 150-, and 300-mg capsule; and 150-mg/mL injection (Cleocin)	Dog: 11–33 mg/kg q12h PO; for oral and soft tissue infection: 5.5–33 mg/kg q12h PO Cat: 11–33 mg/kg q24h PO for skin and anaerobic infections Toxoplasmosis: 12.5–25 mg/kg PO q12h for 4 wks
Clofazimine	Lamprene	50- and 100-mg capsules	Cat: 1 mg/kg PO up to a maximum of 4 mg/kg/day
Clomipramine	Anafranil (human label); Clomicalm (veterinary label)	10-, 25-, and 50-mg tablets (human); 5-, 20-, and 80-mg tablets (veterinary)	Dog: 1–2 mg/kg PO q12h up to a maximum of 3 mg/kg PO q12h Cat: 1–5 mg/cat PO q12–24h
Clonazepam	Klonopin	0.5-, 1-, and 2-mg tablets	Dog: 0.5 mg/kg PO q8–12h Cat: 0.1–0.2 mg/kg q12–24h PO
Clopidogrel	Plavix	75-mg tablets	Dog: 2–4 mg/kg q24h PO; give oral loading dose of 10 mg/kg Cat: 19 mg per cat (¼ tablet) q24h PO
Clorazepate	Tranxene	3.75-, 7.5-, 11.25-, 15-, and 22.5-mg tablets	Dog: 2 mg/kg PO q12h Cat: 0.2–0.4 mg/kg q12–24h PO (up to 0.5–2 mg/kg)
Cloxacillin	Cloxapen, Orbenin, Tegopen	250- and 500-mg capsules; 25-mg/mL oral solution	20–40 mg/kg PO q8h
Codeine	Generic	15-, 30-, and 60-mg tablets; 5-mg/mL syrup; 3-mg/mL oral solution	Analgesia: 0.5–1 mg/kg PO q4–6h Antitussive: 0.1–0.3 mg/kg PO q4–6h
Colchicine	Generic	500- and 600-mcg tablets; 500-mcg/mL ampule injection	0.01–0.03 mg/kg PO q24h
Colony-stimulating factor	Sargramostim (Leukine) and filgrastim (Neupogen)	300 mcg/mL (Neupogen) and 250 or 500 mcg/mL (Leukine)	Leukine: 0.25 mg/m^2 q12h SC or IV infusion. Neupogen: 0.005 mg/kg (5 mcg/kg) q24h SC for 2 wk
Corticotropin (ACTH)	ActharGel 80 U/mL	Response test: collect pre-ACTH sample and inject	2.2 IU/kg IM; collect post-ACTH sample in 2 hours in dogs and at 1 and 2 hours in cats
Cosequin	*See* Glucosamine chondroitin sulfate		

DRUG NAME	OTHER NAMES	FORMULATIONS AVAILABLE	DOSAGE
Cosyntropin	Cortrosyn	250 mcg per vial (can be stored in freezer for 6 months)	Response test: Dog: Collect pre-ACTH sample and inject 5 mcg/kg IV or IM and collect sample at 30 and 60 min Cat: 0.125 mg IV or IM and collect sample at 30 min and 60 min after IV administration and 30 and 60 min after IM administration
Cyanocobalamin (vitamin B_{12})	Many	100-mcg/mL injection	Dog: 200–500 mcg/day IM, SC Cat: 250 mcg/day IM, SC
Cyclophosphamide	Cytoxan, Neosar	25-mg/mL injection; 25- and 50-mg tablets	Dog: Anticancer: 50 mg/m^2 PO once daily 4 days/wk or 150–300 mg/m^2 IV and repeat in 21 days Immunosuppressive therapy: 50 mg/m^2 (approx. 2.2 mg/kg) PO q48h or 2.2 mg/kg once daily for 4 days/wk Cat: 6.25–12.5 mg/cat once daily 4 days/wk
Cyclosporine (cyclosporin A)	Atopica, Neoral, Optimmune (ophthalmic)	Atopica: 10-, 25-, 50-, and 100-mg capsule, 100 mg/mL oral solution. Neoral: 25-mg and 100-mg microemulsion capsules; 100-mg/mL oral solution (for microemulsion). Optimmune: 0.2% ointment	Dog: 3–7 mg/kg/day; for atopic dermatitis some dogs are controlled with q48h dosing Cat: 5 mg/kg PO q24h
Cyproheptadine	Periactin	4-mg tablet; 2-mg/5-mL syrup	Antihistamine: 1.1 mg/kg PO q8–12h Appetite stimulant: 2 mg/cat PO
Cytarabine (cytosine arabinoside)	Cytosar-U	100-mg vial	Dog (lymphoma): 100 mg/m^2 IV, SC once daily or 50 mg/m^2 twice daily for 4 days Cat: 100 mg/m^2 once daily for 2 days
Dacarbazine	DTIC	200-mg vial for injection	200 mg/m^2 IV for 5 days q3wk; or 800–1000 mg/m^2 IV q3wk
Dalteparin	Fragmin	2500 units/0.2mL or 5000 units/0.2ml prefilled syringes, or 10,000 unit/mL multidose vials for injection	Dog: 100–150 units/kg q8hr SC Cat: 180 units/kg q6h SC

DRUG NAME	OTHER NAMES	FORMULATIONS AVAILABLE	DOSAGE
Danazol	Danocrine	50-, 100-, and 200-mg capsules	5–10 mg/kg PO q12h
Dantrolene	Dantrium	100-mg capsule and 0.33-mg/mL injection	For prevention of malignant hyperthermia: 2–3 mg/kg IV For muscle relaxation: Dog: 1–5 mg/kg PO q8h Cat: 0.5–2 mg/kg PO q12h
Dapsone	Generic	25- and 100-mg tablets	Dog: 1.1 mg/kg PO q8–12h Cat: Do not use
Deferoxamine	Desferal	500-mg vial for injection	10 mg/kg IV, IM q2h for two doses; then 10 mg/kg q8h for 24 hours
Deprenyl (l-deprenyl)	*See* Selegiline (Anipryl)		
Deracoxib	Deramaxx	25-, 100-mg tablets	Dog: 3–4 mg/kg q24h PO for 7 days; or 1–2 mg/kg q24h PO for long-term use Cat: Dose not established
Desmopressin acetate	DDAVP	100-mcg/mL injection and desmopressin acetate nasal solution (0.01% metered spray); 0.1- and 0.2-mg tablets	Diabetes insipidus: 2–4 drops (2 mcg) q12–24h intranasally or in eye Animal oral dose: 0.05–0.1 mg/dog q12h PO initially, then increase to 0.1–0.2 mg/dog q12h as needed von Willebrand's disease treatment: 1 mcg/kg (0.01 mL/kg) SC, IV, diluted in 20 mL saline administered over 10 min
Desoxycorticosterone pivalate	Percorten-V, DOCP, or DOCA pivalate	25 mg/mL injection	1.5–2.2 mg/kg IM q25days
Dexamethasone (dexamethasone solution and dexamethasone sodium phosphate)	Azium solution in polyethylene glycol. Sodium phosphate forms include DexaJect SP, Dexavet, and Dexasone. Tablets include Decadron and generic	Azium solution, 2 mg/mL; sodium phosphate forms are 3.33 mg/mL; 0.25-, 0.5-, 0.75-, 1-, 1.5-, 2-, 4-, and 6-mg tablets	Antiinflammatory: 0.07–0.15 mg/kg IV, IM, PO q12–24h Dexamethasone suppression test: Dog: 0.01 mg/kg IV Cat: 0.1 mg/kg IV Collect sample at 0, 4, and 8 hours
Dexmedetomidine	Dexdomitor	0.5-mg/mL injectable solution	Dog: Sedative and analgesic: 375 mg/m^2 IV or 500 mg/m^2 IM Dog: Preanesthetic: 125 mg/m^2 IM Cat: Sedative and analgesic: 40 mcg/kg IM

DRUG NAME	OTHER NAMES	FORMULATIONS AVAILABLE	DOSAGE
Dextran	Dextran 70, Gentran-70	Injectable solution: 250, 500, and 1000 mL	10–20 mL/kg IV to effect
Dextromethorphan	Benylin and others	Available in syrup, capsule, and tablet; many OTC products	0.5–2 mg/kg PO q6–8h has been reported, but effective dose not established
Dextrose solution 5%	D5W	Fluid solution for IV administration	40–50 mL/kg IV q24h
Diazepam	Valium and generic	2- and 5-mg tablets; 5-mg/mL solution for injection	Preanesthetic: 0.5 mg/kg IV Status epilepticus: 0.5 mg/kg IV, 1.0 mg/kg rectal; repeat if necessary Appetite stimulant (cat): 0.2 mg/kg IV
Dichlorophen	Vermiplex (*See* Toluene)		
Dichlorphenamide	Daranide	50-mg tablet	3–5 mg/kg PO q8–12h
Dichlorvos	Task	10- and 25-mg tablets	Dog: 26.4–33 mg/kg PO Cat: 11 mg/kg PO
Dicloxacillin	Dynapen	125-, 250-, and 500-mg capsules; 12.5-mg/mL oral suspension	25 mg/kg IM q6h Oral doses not absorbed
Diethylcarbamazine (DEC)	Caricide, Filaribits	Chewable tablets; 50-, 60-, 180-, 200-, and 400-mg tablets	Heartworm prophylaxis: 6.6 mg/kg PO q24h
Diethylstilbestrol (DES)	DES, generic (no longer manufactured in the United States)	1- and 5-mg tablet; 50-mg/mL injection	Dog: 0.1–1.0 mg/dog PO q24h Cat: 0.05–0.1 mg/cat PO q24h
Difloxacin	Dicural	11.4-, 45.4-, and 136-mg tablets	Dog: 5–10 mg/kg/day PO Cat: Safe dose not established
Digoxin	Lanoxin, Cardoxin	0.0625-, 0.125-, 0.25-mg tablets; 0.05- and 0.15-mg/mL elixir.	Dog: (rapid digitalization): 0.0055-0.011 mg/kg IV q1h to effect Cat: 0.0080.01 mg/kg PO q48h (approx. ¼ of a 0.125-mg tablet/cat) Dog: <20 kg body weight: 0.01 mg/kg q12h; >20 kg use 0.22 mg/m^2 PO q12h (subtract 10% for elixir)
Dihydrotachysterol (vitamin D)	Hytakerol, DHT	0.125-mg tablet; 0.5- mg/mL oral liquid	0.01 mg/kg/day PO; for acute treatment administer 0.02 mg/kg initially, then 0.01–0.02 mg/kg PO q24–48h thereafter

DRUG NAME	OTHER NAMES	FORMULATIONS AVAILABLE	DOSAGE
Diltiazem	Cardizem, Dilacor	30-, 60-, 90-, and 120-mg tablets; 50-mg/mL injection	Dog: 0.5–1.5 mg/kg PO q8h, 0.25 mg/kg over 2 min IV (repeat if necessary) Cat: 1.75–2.4 mg/kg PO q8h For Dilacor XR or Cardizem CD: dose is 10 mg/kg PO once daily
Dimenhydrinate	Dramamine (Gravol in Canada)	50-mg tablets; 50-mg/mL injection	Dog: 4–8 mg/kg PO, IM, IV q8h Cat: 12.5 mg/cat IV, IM, PO q8h
Dimercaprol (BAL)	BAL in oil	Injection	4 mg/kg IM q4h
Dinoprost tromethamine	*See* Prostaglandin $F_{2\alpha}$ 5-mg/mL injection		
Dioctyl calcium sulfosuccinate	*See* Docusate calcium		
Dioctyl sodium sulfosuccinate	*See* Docusate sodium		
Diphenhydramine	Diphenhydramine	Available OTC: 2.5-mg/mL elixir; 25- and 50-mg capsules and tablets; 50-mg/mL injection	Dog: 25–50 mg/dog IV, IM, PO q8h Cat: 2–4 mg/kg q6–8h PO or 1 mg/kg IM, IV q6–8h
Diphenoxylate	Lomotil	2.5 mg	Dog: 0.1–0.2 mg/kg PO q8–12h Cat: 0.05–0.1 mg/kg PO q12h
Diphenylhydantoin	*See* Phenytoin		
Diphosphonate disodium etidronate	*See* Etidronate disodium		
Dipyridamole	Persantine	25-, 50-, 75-mg tablets; 5-mg/mL injection	4–10 mg/kg PO q24h
Dirlotapide	Slentrol	5-mg/mL oral oil-based solution	Dog: Start with 0.01 mL/kg/day PO Adjust by doubling the dose in 2 weeks Monthly adjustments to dose should be done on the basis of animal's weight loss. Do not exceed 0.2 mL/kg/day Cat: Do not administer to cats
Disopyramide	Norpace (Rythmodan in Canada)	100- and 150-mg capsules (10-mg/mL injection in Canada only)	6–15 mg/kg PO q8h
Dithiazanine iodide	Dizan	10-, 50-, 100-, and 200-mg tablets	Heartworm: 6.6–11 mg/kg PO q24h for 7–10 days; for other parasites: 22 mg/kg PO

DRUG NAME	OTHER NAMES	FORMULATIONS AVAILABLE	DOSAGE
Divalproex sodium	*See* Valproic acid		
Dobutamine	Dobutrex	250-mg/20 mL vial for injection (12.5 mg/mL)	Dog: 5–20 mcg/kg/min IV infusion Cat: 2 mcg/kg/min IV infusion
Docusate calcium	Surfak, Doxidan	60-mg tablet (and many others)	Dog: 50–100 mg/dog PO q12–24h Cat: 50 mg/cat PO q12–24h
Docusate sodium	Colace, Doxan, Doss, many OTC brands	50-, and 100-mg capsules; 10-mg/mL liquid	Dog: 50–200 mg/dog PO q8–12h Cat: 50 mg/cat PO q12–24h
Dolasetron mesylate	Anzemet	50-, 100-mg tablets; 20-mg/mL injection	Dog, cat: Prevention of nausea and vomiting: 0.6 mg/kg IV or PO q24h Treating vomiting and nausea: 1.0 mg/kg PO or IV once daily
Domperidone	Motilium	Not available in the United States	2 to 5 mg/animal PO
Dopamine	Intropin	40-, 80-, or 160-mg/mL	Dog, cat: 2–10 mcg/kg/min IV infusion
Doxapram	Dopram, Respiram	20-mg/mL injection	5–10 mg/kg IV Neonate: 1–5 mg SC, sublingual, or via umbilical vein
Doxorubicin	Adriamycin	2-mg/mL injection	30 mg/m^2 IV q21 days, or >20 kg use 30 mg/m^2 and <20 kg use 1 mg/kg Cat: 20 mg/m^2 or approx. 1–1.25 mg/kg IV q3wk
Doxycycline	Vibramycin and generic forms	10-mg/mL oral suspension; 100-mg injection vial; 50- or 100-mg tablets or capsules	3–5 mg/kg PO, IV q12h or 10 mg/kg PO q24h For *Rickettsia* in dogs: 5 mg/kg q12h
Edetate calcium disodium ($CaNa_2EDTA$)	Calcium disodium versenate	20-mg/mL injection	25 mg/kg SC, IM, IV q6h for 2–5 days
Edrophonium	Tensilon and others	10-mg/mL injection	Dog: 0.11–0.22 mg/kg IV Cat: 0.25–0.5 mg/cat (total dose) IV
Enalapril	Enacard, Vasotec	2.5-, 5-, 10-, and 20-mg tablets	Dog: 0.5 mg/kg PO q12–24h Cat: 0.25–0.5 mg/kg PO q12–24h
Enflurane	Ethrane	Available as solution for inhalation	Induction: 2%-3% Maintenance: 1.5%-3%

DRUG NAME	OTHER NAMES	FORMULATIONS AVAILABLE	DOSAGE
Enilconazole	Imaverol, Clinafarm-EC	10% or 13.8% emulsion	Nasal aspergillosis: 10 mg/kg q12h instilled into nasal sinus for 14 days (10% solution diluted 50/50 with water) Dermatophytes: Dilute 10% solution to 0.2% and wash lesion with solution four times at 3- to 4-day intervals
Enoxaparin	Lovenox	30 mg/0.3 mL, 40 mg/0.4 mL, 60 mg/0.6 mL, 80 mg/0.8 mL, and 100 mg/1 mL in prefilled syringes for injection	Dog: 0.8 mg/kg SC q6h Cat: 1.25 mg/kg SC q6h
Enrofloxacin	Baytril	68-, 22.7-, and 5.7-mg tablets. Taste Tabs are 22.7 and 68 mg; 22.7-mg/mL injection	Dog: 5–20 mg/kg/day PO, IM Cat: 5 mg/kg/day PO (do not exceed dose)
Ephedrine	Many, generic	25- and 50-mg/mL injection	Vasopressor: 0.75 mg/kg, IM, SC; repeat as needed
Epinephrine	Adrenaline and generic forms	1-mg/mL (1 : 1000) injection solution	Cardiac arrest: 10–20 mcg/kg IV or 200 mcg/kg intratracheal (may be diluted in saline before administration) Anaphylactic shock: 2.5–5 mcg/kg IV or 50 mcg/kg intratracheal (may be diluted in saline)
Epoetin alpha (Erythropoietin) (r-HuEPO)	Epogen, epoetin alfa (r-HuEPO)	2000-U/mL injection	Doses range from 35 or 50 U/kg three times/wk to 400 U/kg/wk IV, SC (adjust dose to hematocrit of 0.30–0.34) Cat: Start with 100 units/kg three times/wk and adjust dose based on hematocrit
Epsiprantel	Cestex	Coated tablet	Dog: 5.5 mg/kg PO Cat: 2.75 mg/kg PO
Ergocalciferol (vitamin D_2)	Calciferol, Drisdol	400-U tablet (OTC); 50,000-U tablet (1.25 mg); 500,000-U/mL (12.5 mg/mL) injection	500–2000 U/kg/day PO
Erythromycin	Many brands and generic	250- or 500-mg capsule or tablet	Antibacterial dose: 10–20 mg/kg PO q8–12h Prokinetic dose: 0.5–1.0 mg/kg PO q8h

DRUG NAME	OTHER NAMES	FORMULATIONS AVAILABLE	DOSAGE
Esmolol	Brevibloc	10-mg/mL injection	500 mcg/kg IV, which may be given as 0.05–0.1 mg/kg slowly every 5 min or 50–200 mcg/kg/min infusion
Estradiol cypionate (ECP)	ECP, Depo-Estradiol, generic	2-mg/mL injection	Dog: 22–44 mcg/kg IM (total dose not to exceed 1.0 mg Cat: 250 mcg/cat IM between 40 hours and 5 days of mating
Etidronate disodium	Didronel	200- and 400-mg tablets; 50-mg/mL injection	Dog: 5 mg/kg/day PO Cat: 10 mg/kg/day PO
Etodolac	EtoGesic, veterinary; Lodine, human	150- and 300-mg tablets	Dog: 10–15 mg/kg PO once daily Cat: Dose not established
Etretinate	Tegison	10- and 25-mg capsules	Dog: 1 mg/kg PO, with food/day, or for <15 kg 10 mg/dog PO q24h; >15 kg 10 mg/dog PO q12h Cat: 2 mg/kg/day
Famotidine	Pepcid	10-mg tablet; 10-mg/mL injection	Dog: 0.1–0.2 mg/kg IM, SC, PO, IV q12h; or 0.5 mg/kg PO q24h, or 0.5 mg/kg IM, SC, PO, IV q24h Cat: 0.2–0.25 mg/kg IM, IV, SC, PO q12–24h
Felbamate	Felbatol	400- and 600-mg tablets; 120-mg/mL oral flavored suspension	Dog: Start with 15 mg/kg PO q8h and increase gradually to maximum of 65 mg/kg q8h
Fenbendazole	Panacur, Safe-Guard	Panacur granules 22.2% (222 mg/g); 100-mg/mL liquid	50 mg/kg/day PO for 3 days
Fentanyl	Sublimaze, generic	50-mcg/ mL injection	0.02–0.04 mg/kg IV, IM, SC q2h or 0.01 mg/kg IV, IM, SC (with acetylpromazine or diazepam) For analgesia: 0.01 mg/kg IV, IM, SC q2h
Fentanyl transdermal	Duragesic	25-, 50-, 75-, and 100-mcg/h patch	Dog: 10–20 kg, 50- mcg/h patch q72h Cat: 25-mcg patch every 120h
Ferrous sulfate	Many OTC brands	Many	Dog: 100–300 mg/dog PO q24h Cat: 50–100 mg/cat PO q24h
Finasteride	Proscar	5-mg tablets	Dog (BPH): 5-mg tablet/dog PO q24h
Firocoxib	Previcox	57- or 227-mg tablets	Dog: 5 mg/kg PO, once daily Cat: 1.5 mg/kg, once; long-term safety in cats has not been determined

DRUG NAME	OTHER NAMES	FORMULATIONS AVAILABLE	DOSAGE
Florfenicol	Nuflor	300 mg/mL (cattle)	Dog: 20 mg/kg q6h PO, IM Cat: 22 mg/kg q12h IM, PO
Fluconazole	Diflucan	50-, 100-, 150-, and 200-mg tablets; 10- or 40-mg/mL oral suspension; 2-mg/mL IV injection	Dog: 10–12 mg/kg day PO For *Malassezia*, 5 mg/kg q12h PO Cat: 50 mg/cat PO q12h or 50 mg/cat/day PO
Flucytosine	Ancobon	250-mg capsule; 75-mg/mL oral suspension	25–50 mg/kg PO q6–8h (up to a maximal dose of 100 mg/kg PO q12h)
Fludrocortisone	Florinef	100-mcg (0.1 mg) tablet	Dog: 0.2–0.8 mg/dog or 0.02 mg/kg PO q24h (13–23 mcg/kg) Cat: 0.1–0.2 mg/cat PO q24h
Flumazenil	Romazicon	100-mcg/mL (0.1 mg/mL) injection	0.2 mg (total dose) IV as needed
Flumethasone	Flucort	0.5-mg/mL injection	Dog, cat: Antiinflammatory: 0.15–0.3 mg/kg IV, IM, SC q12–24h
Flunixin meglumine	Banamine	10- and 50-mg/mL injection	1.1 mg/kg IV, IM, SC once or 1.1 mg/kg/day PO 3 days/wk Ophthalmic: 0.5 mg/kg IV once
5-Fluorouracil	Fluorouracil	50-mg/mL vial	Dog: 150 mg/m^2 IV once/week Cat: Do not use
Fluoxetine	Prozac, Reconcile	8-, 16-, 32-, and 64-mg chewable tablets for dogs. Human formulation is 10- and 20-mg capsules and 4-mg/mL oral solution	Dog: 1–2 mg/kg/day PO q24h Cat: 0.5–4 mg/cat PO q24h
Follicle-stimulating hormone (FSH)	*See* Urofollitropin		
Fomepizole	4-Methylpyrazole, Antizole, and Antizol-vet	5% solution	Dog: 20 mg/kg initially IV, then 15 mg/kg at 12- and 24-hour intervals, then 5 mg/kg at 36hours; repeat q12h if necessary
Furazolidone	Furoxone	100-mg tablet	4 mg/kg PO q12h for 7–10 days
Furosemide	Lasix, generic	12.5-, 20-, and 50-mg tablets; 10-mg/mL oral solution; 50-mg/mL injection	Dog: 2–6 mg/kg IV, IM, SC, PO q8–12h (or as needed) Cat: 1–4 mg/kg IV, IM, SC, PO q8–24h
Gabapentin	Neurontin	100-, 300-, 400-mg capsules; 100-, 300-, 400-, 600-, 800-mg scored tablets; 50-mg/mL oral solution (contains xylitol)	Dog, cat: Anticonvulsant dose: 2.5–10 mg/kg q8–12h PO For analgesia: 10–15 mg/kg q8h PO

DRUG NAME	OTHER NAMES	FORMULATIONS AVAILABLE	DOSAGE
Gemfibrozil	Lopid	300-mg capsules; 600-mg tablets	7.5 mg/kg PO q12h
Gentamicin	Gentocin	50- and 100-mg/mL solution for injection	Dog: 9–14 mg/kg IV, IM, SC q24h Cat: 5–8 mg/kg IV, IM, SC q24h
Glipizide	Glucotrol	5- and 10-mg tablets	Dog: Not recommended Cat: 2.5–7.5 mg/cat PO q12h. Usual dose is 2.5 mg/cat initially, then increase to 5 mg/cat q12h
Glucosamine chondroitin sulfate	Cosequin and others	Regular (RS) and double-strength (DS) capsules	Dog: 1–2 RS capsules/day (2–4 capsules of DS for large dogs) Cat: 1 RS capsule/day
Glyburide	Diabeta, Micronase, Glynase	1.25-, 2.5-, and 5-mg tablets	0.2 mg/kg/day PO or 0.625 mg/cat
Glycerin	Generic	Oral solution	1–2 mL/kg, up to PO q8h
Glycopyrrolate	Robinul-V	0.2-mg/mL injection	0.005 to 0.01 mg/kg IV, IM, SC
Gold sodium thiomalate	Myochrysine	10-, 25- and 50-mg/mL injection	1–5 mg IM on first wk, then 2–10 mg IM on second wk, then 1 mg/kg once/wk IM maintenance
Gold therapy	*See* Aurothioglucose, Gold sodium thiomalate, or Auranofin		
GoLYTELY	*See* Polyethylene glycol electrolyte solution		
Gonadorelin (GnRH, LHRH)	Factrel	50-mcg/mL injection	Dog: 50–100 mcg/dog/day IM q24–48h Cat: 25 mcg/cat IM once
Gonadotropin, chorionic (hCG)	Profasi, Pregnyl, generic, A.P.L.	Injection sizes of 5000, 10,000 and 20,000 U	Dog: 22 U/kg IM q24–48h or 44 U IM once Cat: 250 U/cat IM once
Gonadotropin-releasing hormone	*See* Gonadorelin		
Granisetron	Kytril	1-mg/mL injection; 1-mg tablet	0.01 mg/kg (10 mcg/kg) IV
Griseofulvin (microsize)	Fulvicin U/F	125-, 250-, and 500-mg tablets; 25-mg/mL oral suspension; 125-mg/mL oral syrup	50 mg/kg PO q24h (up to a maximum dose of 110–132 mg/kg/day in divided treatments)
Griseofulvin (ultramicrosize)	Fulvicin P/G, Gris-PEG	100-, 125-, 165-, 250-, and 330-mg tablets	30 mg/kg/day in divided treatments PO
Growth hormone (hGH, somatrem, somatropin)	Protropin, Humatrope, Nutropin	5- and 10-mg/vial	0.1 U/kg SC, IM three times/wk for 4–6 weeks (Usual human pediatric dose is 0.18–0.3 mg/kg/wk)

DRUG NAME	OTHER NAMES	FORMULATIONS AVAILABLE	DOSAGE
Guaifenesin	Glyceryl guaiacolate, Guaiphenesin, Mucinex	Tablets: 100-, 200-mg; 600-mg extended-release tablets Oral solution: 20 mg/mL or 40 mg/mL	Dog, cat: Expectorant: 3–5 mg/kg q8h PO Dog: Anesthetic adjunct: 2.2 mL/kg/h of a 5% solution IV
Halothane	Fluothane	250-mL bottle	Induction: 3% Maintenance: 0.5%-1.5%
Hemoglobin glutamer	Oxyglobin	13-g/dL in 125-mL single-dose bags	Dog: One-time dose of 1030 mL/kg IV at a rate not to exceed 10 mL/kg/h Cat: One-time dose of 3–5 mL/kg slowly IV
Heparin sodium	Liquaemin (United States); Hepalean (Canada)	1000- and 10,000-U/mL injection	100–200 U/kg IV loading dose; then 100–300 U/kg SC q6–8h Low-dose prophylaxis (dog and cat): 70 U/kg SC q8–12h
Hetastarch	Hydroxyethyl starch (HES)	Injectable solution	Dog: 10–20 mL/kg/day IV Cat: 5–10 mL/kg/day IV
Hycodan	*See* Hydrocodone bitartrate		
Hydralazine	Apresoline	10-mg tablet; 20-mg/mL injection	Dog: 0.5 mg/kg (initial dose); titrate to 0.5–2 mg/kg PO q12h Cat: 2.5 mg/cat PO q12–24h
Hydrochlorothiazide	HydroDIURIL and generic	10- and 100-mg/mL oral solution and 25-, 50-, and 100-mg tablets	24 mg/kg PO q12h
Hydrocodone bitartrate	Hycodan	5-mg tablet; 1-mg/mL syrup	Dog: 0.22 mg/kg PO q4–8h Cat: No dose available
Hydrocortisone	Cortef, and generic	5-, 10-, 20-mg tablets	Replacement therapy: 1–2 mg/kg PO q12h Antiinflammatory: 2.5–5 mg/kg PO q12h
Hydrocortisone sodium succinate	Solu-Cortef	Various size vials for injection	Shock: 50–150 mg/kg IV Antiinflammatory: 5 mg/kg IV q12h
Hydromorphone	Dilaudid, Hydrostat, and generic	1-, 2-, 4-, 10-mg/mL injection	Oral forms are available, but there is no assurance of oral absorption in dogs; 0.22 mg/kg IM or SC Repeat every 4–6 hours, or as needed for pain treatment
Hydroxyethyl starch (HES)	*See* Hetastarch		
Hydroxyurea	Hydrea	500-mg capsule	Dog: 50 mg/kg PO once daily, 3 days/wk Cat: 25 mg/kg PO once daily, 3 days/wk

DRUG NAME	OTHER NAMES	FORMULATIONS AVAILABLE	DOSAGE
Hydroxyzine	Atarax	10-, 25-, and 50-mg tablets; 2-mg/mL oral solution	Dog: 2 mg/kg q12h PO, IV, IM Cat: Safe dose not established
Ibuprofen	Motrin, Advil, Nuprin	200-, 400-, 600-, and 800-mg tablets	Safe dose not established
Imipenem	Primaxin	250- or 500-mg vials for injection	3–10 mg/kg q6–8h IV, SC, or IM; usually 5 mg/kg q6–8h IM, IV, or SC q6–8h
Imipramine	Tofranil	10-, 25-, and 50-mg tablets	Dog: 2–4 mg/kg PO q12–24h Cat: 0.5 to 1.0 mg/kg q12–24h PO
Indomethacin	Indocin		Safe dose not established
Insulin, regular crystalline		100-U/mL injection	Ketoacidosis: animals <3 kg, 1 U/animal initially, then 1 U/animal q1h; animals 3–10 kg, 2 U/animal initially, then 1 U/animal q1h; animals >10 kg, 0.25 U/kg initially, then 0.1 U/kg IM q1h
Insulin	NPH isophane, Ultralente, or PZI	100-U/mL injection	Dog <15 kg: 1 U/kg SC q24h (to effect) Dog >25 kg: 0.5 U/kg SC q24h (to effect) Cat: PZI or Ultralente initial dose 0.5–1.0 U/kg SC, usually twice/day
Interferon (interferon alpha, HuIFN-alpha)	Roferon	5- and 10-million U/vial	Dog: 2.5 million U/kg IV once daily for 3 days Cat: 1 million U/kg IV once daily for 5 consecutive days at 0, 14, and 60 days
Iodide	*See* Potassium iodide		
Ipecac syrup	Ipecac	Oral solution: 30-mL bottle	Dog: 3–6 mL/dog PO Cat: 2–6 mL/cat PO
Ipodate	Cholecystographic agent	50-mg capsules	Cat: 15 mg/kg q12h PO (usually 50 mg/cat q12h)
Iron	*See* Ferrous sulfate		
Isoflurane	AErrane	100-mL bottle	Induction: 5% Maintenance: 1.5%-2.5%
Isoproterenol	Isuprel	0.2-mg/mL ampules for injection	10 mcg/kg IM, SC q6h; or dilute 1 mg in 500 mL of 5% dextrose or Ringer's solution and infuse IV 0.5–1 mL/min (1–2 mcg/min) or to effect
Isosorbide dinitrate	Isordil, Isorbid, Sorbitrate	2.5-, 5-, 10-, 20-, 30-, and 40-mg tablets; 40-mg capsules	2.5–5 mg/animal PO q12h (or 0.22–1.1 mg/kg PO q12h)

DRUG NAME	OTHER NAMES	FORMULATIONS AVAILABLE	DOSAGE
Isosorbide mononitrate	Monoket	10- and 20-mg tablets	5 mg/dog PO two dose/day 7 hours apart
Isotretinoin	Accutane	10-, 20-, and 40-mg capsules	Dog: 1–3 mg/kg/day (up to a maximum recommended dose of 3–4 mg/kg/day PO) Cat: Dose not established
Itraconazole	Sporanox	100-mg capsules; 10-mg/mL oral solution	Dog: 2.5 mg/kg PO q12h or 5 mg/kg PO q24h For dermatophytes: 3 mg/kg/day PO for 15 days For *Malassezia:* 5 mg/kg q24h PO for 2 days, repeated each week for 3 weeks Cat: 1.5–3.0 mg/kg, up to 5 mg/kg PO for 15 days
Ivermectin	Heartguard, Ivomec, Eqvalan liquid	1% (10 mg/mL) injectable solution; 10-mg/mL oral solution; 18.7-mg/mL oral paste; 68-, 136-, and 272-mcg tablets	Heartworm preventative: Dog: 6 mcg/kg PO q30 days Cat: 24 mcg/kg PO q30 days Microfilaricide: 50 mcg/kg PO 2 weeks after adulticide therapy Ectoparasite therapy (dog and cat): 200–300 mcg/kg IM, SC, PO Endoparasites (dog and cat): 200–400 mcg/kg SC, PO weekly Demodex therapy: Start with 100 mcg/kg, then increase to 600 mcg/kg/day PO for 60–120 days
Kanamycin	Kantrim	200- and 500-mg/mL injection	10 mg/kg IV, IM, SC q6–8h; or 20 mg/kg q24h IV, IM, SC
Kaopectate (kaolin + pectin)	Kaopectate	Oral suspension	12 oz (1–2 mL/kg) PO q2–6h
Ketamine	Ketalar, Ketavet, Vetalar	100-mg/mL injection solution	Dog: 5.5–22 mg/kg IV, IM (recommend adjunctive sedative or tranquilizer treatment) Cat: 2–25 mg/kg IV, IM (recommend adjunctive sedative or tranquilizer treatment)
Ketoconazole	Nizoral	200-mg tablet; 100-mg/mL oral suspension (only available in Canada)	Dog: 10–15 mg/kg PO q8–12h For *Malassezia canis* infection use 5 mg/kg PO q24h Hyperadrenocorticism: 15 mg/kg PO q12h Cat: 5–10 mg/kg PO q8–12h
Ketoprofen	Orudis-KT (human OTC tablet); Ketofen (veterinary injection)	12.5-mg tablet (OTC); 100-mg/mL injection	Dog, cat: 1 mg/kg PO q24h for up to 5 days or 2.0 mg/kg IV, IM, SC for one dose

DRUG NAME	OTHER NAMES	FORMULATIONS AVAILABLE	DOSAGE
Ketorolac tromethamine	Toradol	10-mg tablet; 15- and 30-mg/mL injection in 10% alcohol	Dog: 0.5 mg/kg PO, IM, IV q12h for not more than two doses
L-Dopa	*See* Levodopa		
Lactated Ringer's solution	Generic	250-, 500-, and 1000-mL bags	Maintenance: 55–65 mL/kg/day IV For severe dehydration: 50 mL/kg/h IV or for shock 90 mL/kg IV (dogs) and 60–70 mL/kg IV (cats)
Lactulose	Chronulac, generic	10 g/15 mL	Constipation: 1 mL/4.5 kg PO q8h (to effect) Hepatic encephalopathy: Dog: 0.5 mL/kg PO q8h Cat: 2.5–5 mL/cat PO q8h
Leucovorin (folinic acid)	Wellcovorin, generic	5-, 10-, 15-, and 25-mg tablets; 3- and 5- mg/mL injection	With methotrexate administration: 3 mg/m^2 IV, IM, PO Antidote for pyrimethamine toxicosis: 1 mg/kg PO q24h
Levamisole	Levasole, Tamisol, Ergamisol	0.184-g bolus; 11.7 g/13-g packet; 50-mg tablet (Ergamisol)	Dog (hookworms): 5–8 mg/kg PO once (up to 10 mg/kg PO for 2 days) Microfilaricide: 10 mg/kg PO q24h for 6–10 days Immunostimulant: 0.5–2 mg/kg PO three times/wk Cat: 4.4 mg/kg once PO For lungworms: 20–40 mg/kg PO q48h for five treatments
Levetiracetam	Keppra	250-, 500-, 750-mg tablets	Dog: Start with 20 mg/kg q8h PO; increase gradually as necessary Cat: 30 mg/kg q12h PO
Levodopa (L-dopa)	Larodopa, l-dopa	100-, 250-, and 500-mg tablets or capsules	Hepatic encephalopathy: 6.8 mg/kg initially then 1.4 mg/kg q6h
Levothyroxine sodium (T_4)	Soloxine, Thyro-Tabs, Synthroid	0.1- to 0.8-mg tablets (in 0.1-mg increments)	Dog: 18–22 mcg/kg PO q12h (adjust dose via monitoring) Cat: 10–20 mcg/kg/day PO (adjust dose via monitoring)
Lidocaine	Xylocaine, generic	5-, 10-, 15-, and 20-mg/mL injection	Antiarrhythmic: Dog: 2–4 mg/kg IV (to a maximum dose of 8 mg/kg over 10-minute period); 25–75 mcg/kg/min IV infusion; 6 mg/kg IM q1.5h Cat: 0.25–0.75 mg/kg IV slowly; or 10–40 mcg/kg/min infusion For epidural (dog and cat): 4.4 mg/kg of 2% solution

DRUG NAME	OTHER NAMES	FORMULATIONS AVAILABLE	DOSAGE
Lincomycin	Lincocin	100-, 200-, and 500-mg tablets	15–25 mg/kg PO q12h For pyoderma: Doses as low as 10 mg/kg q12h have been used
Linezolid	Zyvox	400- and 600-mg tablets; 20-mg/mL oral suspension; 2-mg/mL injection	Dog, cat: 10 mg/kg q8–12h PO, IV
Liothyronine (T_3)	Cytomel	60-mcg tablet	4.4 mcg/kg PO q8h For T_3 suppression test (cats): Collect presample for T_4 and T_3; administer 25 mcg q8h for seven doses, then collect post samples for T_3 and T_4 after last dose
Lisinopril	Prinivil, Zestril	2.5-, 5-, 10-, 20-, and 40-mg tablets	Dog: 0.5 mg/kg PO q24h Cat: No dose established
Lithium carbonate	Lithotabs	150-, 300-, and 600-mg capsules; 300-mg tablet; 300-mg/5 mL syrup	Dog: 10 mg/kg PO q12h Cat: Not recommended
Lomotil	*See* Diphenoxylate		
Lomustine	CCNU, CeeNU	10-, 40-, 100-mg capsules	Dog: 70–90 mg/m^2, every 4 weeks PO For brain tumors: Use 60–90 mg/m^2 q6–8wk PO Cat: 50–60 mg/m^2 PO q3–6 wk or 10 mg/cat PO every 3 weeks
Loperamide	Imodium, generic	2-mg tablet; 0.2-mg/mL oral liquid	Dog: 0.1 mg/kg PO q8–12h Cat: 0.08–0.16 mg/kg PO q12h
Lufenuron	Program	45-, 90-, 135-, 204.9-, and 409.8-mg tablets; 135- and 270-mg suspension per unit pack	Dog: 10 mg/kg PO q30 days Cat: 30 mg/kg PO q30 days, 10 mg/kg SC q6mo
Lufenuron + milbemycin oxime	Sentinel tablets and Flavor Tabs	Milbemycin/lufenuron ratio is as follows: 2.3/46-mg tablets; 5.75/115–11.5/230-, and 23/460-mg Flavor Tabs	Administer 1 tablet q30 days; each tablet formulated for size of dog
Luteinizing hormone	*See* Gonadorelin		
L-Lysine	Enisyl-F	250-mg/mL paste	Paste formulation: 1–2 mL/cat, PO, to adult cats (approx. 400 mg/cat) and 1 mL/cat, PO, for kittens
Magnesium citrate	Citroma, Citro-Nesia (Citro-Mag in Canada)	Oral solution	2 to 4 mL/kg PO

DRUG NAME	OTHER NAMES	FORMULATIONS AVAILABLE	DOSAGE
Magnesium hydroxide	Milk of Magnesia	Oral liquid	Antacid: 5–10 mL/kg PO q4–6h Cathartic: Dog: 15–50 PO mL/kg Cat: 2–6 mL/cat PO q24h
Magnesium sulfate	Epsom salts	Crystals, many generic preparations	Dog: 8–25 g/dog PO q24h; for treating arrhythmias: 0.15–0.3 mEq/kg slowly IV over 5–15 min followed by 0.75–1.0 mEq/kg/day; fluid supplementation: 0.75–1.0 mEq/kg/day Cat: 2–5 g/cat PO q24h
Mannitol	Osmitrol	5%–25% solution for injection	Diuretic: 1 g/kg of 5%-25% solution IV to maintain urine flow. Glaucoma or central nervous system edema: 0.25–2 g/kg of 15%-25% solution IV over 30–60 min (repeat in 6 hours if necessary)
Marbofloxacin	Marbocyl, Zeniquin	25-, 50-, 100-, and 200-mg tablets	Dog, cat: 2.75–5.55 mg/kg PO q24h
Maropitant	Cerenia	10-mg/mL injection; 16-, 24-, 60-, 160-mg tablets	Dog: 1 mg/kg SC once daily for up to 5 days; 2 mg/kg PO once daily for up to 5 days For motion sickness: 8 mg/kg PO once daily for up to 2 days Cat: Dose not established
MCT oil	MCT oil (many sources)	Oral liquid	1–2 mL/kg/day in food
Mebendazole	Telmintic	Each gram of powder contains 40 mg	22 mg/kg (with food) q24h for 3 days
Meclizine	Antivert, generic	12.5-, 25-, and 50-mg tablets	Dog: 25 mg PO q24h (for motion sickness, administer 1 hour before traveling) Cat: 12.5 mg PO q24h
Meclofenamic acid (meclofenamate sodium)	Arquel, Meclomen	50- and 100-mg capsules	Dog: 1 mg/kg/day PO for up to 5 days Cat: Not recommended
Medium-chain triglycerides	*See* MCT oil		
Medroxyprogesterone acetate	Depo-Provera (injection); Provera (tablets)	150- and 400-mg/mL suspension injection; 2.5-, 5-, and 10-mg tablets	1.1–2.2 mg/kg IM q7 days; for behavioral use, 10–20 mg/kg SC; for prostate, 3–5 mg/kg SC, IM

DRUG NAME	OTHER NAMES	FORMULATIONS AVAILABLE	DOSAGE
Megestrol acetate	Ovaban	5-mg tablet	Dog: Proestrus: 2 mg/kg PO q24h for 8 days Anestrus: 0.5 mg/kg PO q24h for 30 days Behavior: 2–4 mg/kg q24h for 8 days (reduce dose for maintenance) Cat: Dermatologic therapy or urine spraying: 2.5–5 mg/cat PO q24h for 1 week, then reduce to 5 mg once or twice/wk Suppress estrus: 5 mg/cat/day for 3 days, then 2.5–5 mg once/wk for 10 weeks
Melarsomine	Immiticide	25-mg/mL injection; after reconstitution retains potency for 24 hours	Administer via deep IM injection. Class 1–2 dogs: 2.5 mg/kg/day for 2 consecutive days Class 3 dogs: 2.5 mg/kg once, then in 1 month two additional doses 24 hours apart
Meloxicam	Metacam (veterinary); Mobic (human)	Veterinary: 1.5-mg/mL oral suspension and 5-mg/mL injection Human: 7.5-mg tablets	Dog: 0.2 mg/kg initially PO, then 0.1 mg/kg q24h PO thereafter; injection 0.1 mg/kg IV or SC Cat: 0.3 mg/kg SC one-time injection; 0.05 mg/kg q24–48h PO for chronic use
Melphalan	Alkeran	2-mg tablet	1.5 mg/m^2 (or 0.1–0.2 mg/kg) PO q24h for 7–10 days (repeat every 3 weeks)
Meperidine	Demerol	50- and 100-mg tablets; 10-mg/mL syrup; 25-, 50-, 75-, and 100-mg/mL injection	Dog: 5–10 mg/kg IV, IM as often as q2–3h (or as needed) Cat: 3–5 mg/kg IV, IM q2–4h (or as needed)
Mepivacaine	Carbocaine-V	2% (20 mg/mL) injection	Variable dose for local infiltration. For epidural: 0.5 mL of 2% solution q30sec until reflexes are absent
6-Mercaptopurine	Purinethol	50-mg tablet	Dog: 50 mg/m^2 PO q24h Cat: Do not use
Meropenem	Merrem	500 mg in 20-ml vial, or 1-gm vial in 30-ml vial for injection	Dogs, cats: 8.5 mg/kg SC q12hr up to 12 mg/kg SC q12hr or 24 mg/kg IV q12hr
Mesalamine	Asacol, Mesasal, Pentasa	400-mg tablet; 250-mg capsule	Veterinary dose has not been established, the usual human oral dose is 400–500 mg q6–8h (*also see* Sulfasalazine, Olsalazine)
Metaproterenol	Alupent, Metaprel	10- and 20-mg tablets; 5-mg/mL syrup; inhalers	0.325–0.65 mg/kg PO q4–6h

DRUG NAME	OTHER NAMES	FORMULATIONS AVAILABLE	DOSAGE
Methadone	Methadose, generic	2-mg/mL oral solution; 10- and 20-mg/mL solution for injection; 5-, 10-, 40-mg tablets	Dog: 0.5–2.2 mg/kg IV, SC, IM, or 0.5–1.0 mg/kg IV q3–4 h for analgesia Cat: 0.2–0.5 mg/kg SC or IM, or 0.05–0.1 mg/kg up to 0.2 mg/kg IV q3–4h for analgesia
Methazolamide	Neptazane	25- and 50-mg tablets	2–3 mg/kg PO q8–12h
Methenamine hippurate	Hiprex, Urex	1-g tablet	Dog: 500 mg/dog PO q12h Cat: 250 mg/cat PO q12h
Methenamine mandelate	Mandelamine, generic	1-g tablet; granules for oral solution; 50- and 100-mg/mL oral suspension	10–20 mg/kg PO q8–12h
Methimazole	Tapazole	5- and 10-mg tablets	Cat: 2.5 mg/cat q12h PO for 7–14 days then 5–10 mg/cat PO q12h and adjust by monitoring T_4
DL-Methionine	*See* Racemethionine		
Methocarbamol	Robaxin-V	500- and 750-mg tablets; 100-mg/mL injection	44 mg/kg PO q8h on the first day then 22–44 mg/kg PO q8h
Methohexital	Brevital	0.5-, 2.5-, and 5-g vials for injection	3 to 6 mg/kg IV (give slowly to effect)
Methotrexate	MTX, Mexate, Folex, Rheumatrex, generic	2.5-mg tablet; 2.5- or 25-mg/mL injection	2.5–5 mg/m_2 PO q48h (dose depends on specific protocol) Dog: 0.3–0.5 mg/kg IV once/wk Cat: 0.8 mg/kg IV q2–3wk
Methoxamine	Vasoxyl	20-mg/mL injection	200–250 mcg/kg IM or 40–80 mcg/kg IV
Methoxyflurane	Metofane	4-oz bottle for inhalation	Induction: 3% Maintenance: 0.5%-1.5%
Methylene Blue	0.1% Generic, also called New Methylene Blue	1% solution (10 mg/mL)	1.5 mg/kg IV, slowly
Methylprednisolone	Medrol	1-, 2-, 4-, 8-, 18-, and 32-mg tablets	0.22–0.44 mg/kg PO q12–24h
Methylprednisolone acetate	Depo-Medrol	20- or 40-mg/mL suspension for injection	Dog: 1 mg/kg (or 20–40 mg/dog) IM q1–3wk Cat: 10–20 mg/cat IM q1–3wk
Methylprednisolone sodium succinate	Solu-Medrol	1- and 2-g and 125- and 500-mg vials for injection	For emergency use: 30 mg/kg IV and repeat at 15 mg/kg IV in 2–6 hours
4-Methylpyrazole (fomepizole)	Antizole, Antizol-Vet (Fomepizole)	5% solution	*See* Fomepizol for dose
Methyltestosterone	Android, generic	10- and 25-mg tablets	Dog: 5–25 mg/dog PO q24–48h Cat: 2.5–5 mg/cat PO q24–48h
Metoclopramide	Reglan, Clopra, and others	5- and 10-mg tablets; 1-mg/mL oral solution; 5- mg/mL injection	0.2–0.5 mg/kg IV, IM, PO q6–8h or IV loading dose at 0.4 mg/kg followed by 0.3 mg/kg/h IV

DRUG NAME	OTHER NAMES	FORMULATIONS AVAILABLE	DOSAGE
Metoprolol tartrate	Lopressor	50- and 100-mg tablets; 1-mg/mL injection	Dog: 5–50 mg/dog (0.5–1.0 mg/kg) PO q8h Cat: 2–15 mg/cat PO q8h
Metronidazole and metronidazole benzoate	Flagyl, generic	250- and 500-mg tablets; 50-mg/mL suspension; 5-mg/mL injection; the benzoate form is not available commercially and must be obtained from a compounding pharmacist	For anaerobes: Dog: 15 mg/kg PO q12h or 12 mg/kg q8h Cat: 10–25 mg/kg PO q24h For *Giardia:* Dog: 12–15 mg/kg PO q12h for 8 days Cat: 17 mg/kg ⅓ tablet/cat) q24h for 8 days
Mexiletine	Mexitil	150-, 200-, and 250-mg capsules	Dog: 5–8 mg/kg PO q8–12h (use cautiously) Cat: Do not use
Mibolerone	Cheque drops	55-mcg/mL oral solution	Dog: 0.45–11.3 kg, 30 mcg; 11.8–22.7 kg, 60 mcg; 23–45.3 kg, 120 mcg; >45.8 kg, 180 mcg; or approx. 2.6–5 mcg/kg/day PO Cat: Safe dose not established
Midazolam	Versed	5-mg/mL injection	Dog: 0.1–0.25 mg/kg IV, IM (or 0.1–0.3 mg/kg/h IV infusion) Cat: 0.05 mg/kg IV; or 0.3–0.6 mg/ kg IV (combine with 3 mg/kg ketamine)
Milbemycin oxime	Interceptor Flavor Tabs	11.5-, 5.75-, and 2.3-mg tablets	Dog: Microfilaricide; 0.5 mg/kg; Demodex: 2 mg/kg PO q24h for 60–120 days Heartworm prevention: 0.5 mg/kg PO q30 days Cat: 2 mg/kg q30 days PO
Milk of Magnesia	*See* Magnesium hydroxide		
Mineral oil	Generic	Oral liquid	Dog: 10–50 mL/dog PO q12h Cat: 10–25 mL/cat PO q12h
Minocycline	Minocin	50-, 75-, and 100-mg tablets or capsules; 10-mg/mL oral suspension	5–12.5 mg/kg PO q12h
Misoprostol	Cytotec	0.1-mg (100 mcg), 0.2-mg (200 mcg) tablets	Dog: 2–5 mcg/kg PO q6–8h; for atopic dermatitis: 5 mcg/kg q8h PO Cat: Dose not established
Mithramycin	*See* Plicamycin (Mithracin)		

DRUG NAME	OTHER NAMES	FORMULATIONS AVAILABLE	DOSAGE
Mitotane (o,p′-DDD)	Lysodren	500-mg tablet	Dog: For pituitary-dependent hypercorticism: 50 mg/kg/day (in divided doses) PO for 5–10 days, then 50–70 mg/kg/wk PO For adrenal tumor: 50–75 mg/kg day for 10 days, then 75–100 mg/kg/wk PO
Mitoxantrone	Novantrone	2-mg/mL injection	Dog: 6 mg/m^2 IV q21 days Cat: 6.5 mg/m^2 IV q21 days
Morphine	Generic	1- and 15-mg/mL injection; 30- and 60-mg delayed-release tablets	Dog: 0.1–1 mg/kg IV, IM, SC (dose is escalated as needed for pain relief) q4–6h Dog: 0.5 mg/kg q2h IV, IM, or CRI 0.2 mg/kg followed by 0.1 mg/kg/h IV Epidural: 0.1 mg/kg Cat: 0.1 mg/kg q3–6h IM, SC (or as needed)
Moxidectin	Cydectin	Injection	Dog: Heartworm prevention: 3 mcg/kg Endoparasites: 25–300 mcg/kg *Demodex:* 400 mcg/kg/day up to 500 mcg/kg/day for 21–22 weeks
Moxifloxacin	Avelox	400-mg tablet	10 mg/kg q24h PO
Mycochrysine	*See* Gold sodium thiomalate		
Mycophenolate	Cell Cept	250-mg capsule	Dog: 10 mg/kg q8h PO Cat: No dose established
Naloxone	Narcan	20- or 400-mcg/mL injection	0.01–0.04 mg/kg IV, IM, SC as needed to reverse opiate
Naltrexone	Trexan	50-mg tablet	For behavior problems: 2.2 mg/kg PO q12h
Nandrolone decanoate	Deca-Durabolin	Nandrolone decanoate injection: 50-, 100-, and 200-mg/mL	Dog: 1–1.5 mg/kg/wk IM Cat: 1 mg/cat/wk IM
Naproxen	Naprosyn, Naxen, Aleve (naproxen sodium)	220-mg tablet (OTC); 25-mg/mL suspension liquid; 250-, 375-, and 500-mg tablets (Rx)	Dog: 5 mg initially, then 2 mg/kg q48h Cat: Not recommended
Neomycin	Biosal	500-mg bolus; 200-mg/mL oral liquid	10–20 mg/kg PO q6–12h

DRUG NAME	OTHER NAMES	FORMULATIONS AVAILABLE	DOSAGE
Neostigmine bromide and neostigmine methylsulfate	Prostigmin; Stiglyn	15-mg tablet	Neostigmine bromide: 0.25- and 0.5-mg/mL injection; neostigmine methylsulfate: 2 mg/kg/day PO (in divided doses, to effect) Injection: Antimyasthenic: 10 mcg/kg IM, SC, as needed Antidote for nondepolarizing neuromuscular block: 40 mcg/kg IM, SC Diagnostic aid for myasthenia gravis: 40 mcg/kg IM or 20 mcg/kg IV
Nifedipine	Adalat, Procardia	10- and 20-mg capsules	Dose not established; in humans, the dose is 10 mg/human three times/day and increased in 10-mg increments to effect
Nitenpyram	Capstar	11.4- or 57-mg tablet	1 mg/kg PO daily as needed to kill fleas
Nitrates	*See* Nitroglycerin, Isosorbide dinitrate, or Nitroprusside		
Nitrofurantoin	Macrodantin, Furalan, Furantoin, Furadantin, or generic	Macrodantin and generic 25-, 50-, and 100-mg capsules; Furalan, Furantoin, and generic 50- and 100-mg tablets; Furadantin 5-mg/mL oral suspension	10 mg/kg/day divided into four daily treatments, then 1 mg/kg PO at night
Nitroglycerin ointment	Nitrol, Nitro-Bid, Nitrostat	0.5-, 0.8-, 1-, 5-, and 10-mg/mL injection; 2% ointment; transdermal systems (0.2 mg/h patch)	Dog: 4–12 mg (up to 15 mg) topically q12 Cat: 2–4 mg topically q12h (or ¼ inch of ointment per cat)
Nitroprusside	Nitropress	50-mg vial for injection	1–5, up to a maximum of 10 mcg/kg/min IV infusion
Nizatidine	Axid	150- and 300-mg capsules	Dog: 5 mg/kg PO q24h
Norfloxacin	Noroxin	400-mg tablet	22 mg/kg PO q12h
o,p'-DDD	*See* Mitotane (Lysodren)		
Olsalazine	Dipentum	500-mg tablet	Dose not established (usual human dose is 500 mg or 5–10 mg/kg PO twice daily)
Omeprazole	Prilosec (formerly Losec), Gastrogard (equine paste)	20-mg capsule	Dog: 20 mg/dog PO once daily (or 0.7 mg/kg q24h) Cat: 0.5–0.7 mg/kg q24h PO

DRUG NAME	OTHER NAMES	FORMULATIONS AVAILABLE	DOSAGE
Ondansetron	Zofran	4- and 8-mg tablets; 2-mg/mL injection	0.5–1.0 mg/kg IV, PO 30 minutes before administration of cancer drugs
Orbifloxacin	Orbax	5.7-, 22.7-, and 68-mg tablets	2.5–7.5 mg/kg PO once daily
Ormetoprim	*See* Primor (ormetoprim-sulfadimethoxine)		
Oxacillin	Prostaphlin, generic	250- and 500-mg capsules; 50-mg/mL oral solution	22–40 mg/kg PO q8h
Oxazepam	Serax	15-mg tablet	Cat: Appetite stimulant: 2.5 mg/cat PO
Oxtriphylline	Choledyl-SA	400- and 600-mg tablet (oral solutions and syrup available in Canada but not the United States)	Dog: 47 mg/kg (equivalent to 30 mg/kg theophylline) PO q12h
Oxybutynin chloride	Ditropan	5-mg tablet	Dog: 5 mg/dog PO q6–8h
Oxymetholone	Anadrol	50-mg tablet	1–5 mg/kg/day PO
Oxymorphone	Numorphan	1.5- and 1-mg/mL injection	Dog, cat: Analgesia: 0.1–0.2 mg/kg IV, SC, IM (as needed), redose with 0.05–0.1 mg/kg q1–2h Preanesthetic: 0.025–0.05 mg/kg IM, SC
Oxytetracycline	Terramycin	250-mg tablets; 100- and 200-mg/mL injection	7.5–10 mg/kg IV q12h; 20 mg/kg PO q12h
Oxytocin	Pitocin and Syntocinon (nasal solution) and generic	10- and 20- U/mL injection; 40-U/mL nasal solution	Dog: 5–20 U/dog SC, IM (repeat every 30 min for primary inertia) Cat: 2.5–3 U/cat SC, IM (repeat every 30 min)
2-PAM	*See* Pralidoxime chloride		
Pamidronate	Aredia	30-, 60-, 90-mg vials for injection	Dog: 2 mg/kg IV, SC For treatment of cholecalciferol toxicosis: 1.3–2 mg/kg for two treatments
Pancreatic enzyme	*See* Pancrelipase		
Pancrelipase	Viokase	16,800 U of lipase, 70,000 U of protease, and 70,000 U of amylase per 0.7 g; also capsules and tablets	Mix 2 tsp powder with food per 20 kg body weight or 1–3 tsp/0.45 kg of food 20 min before feeding
Pancuronium bromide	Pavulon	1- and 2-mg/mL injection	0.1 mg/kg IV or start with 0.01 mg/kg and additional 0.01-mg/kg doses every 30 min

DRUG NAME	OTHER NAMES	FORMULATIONS AVAILABLE	DOSAGE
Pantoprazole	Protonix	40-mg tablets, 0.4-mg/mL vials for injection	Dog, cat: 0.5 mg/kg q24h IV or 0.5–1 mg/kg IV infusion over 24 hours
Paregoric	Corrective mixture	2 mg morphine per 5 mL of paregoric	0.05–0.06 mg/kg PO q12h
Paroxetine	Paxil	10-, 20-, 30-, and 40-mg tablets	Cat: ⅛ to ¼ of a 10-mg tablet daily PO
D-Penicillamine	Cuprimine, Depen	125- and 250-mg capsules and 250-mg tablets	10–15 mg/kg PO q12h
Penicillin G benzathine	Benzapen and other names	150,000 U/mL, combined with 150,000 U/mL of procaine penicillin G	24,000 U/kg IM q48h
Penicillin G potassium; penicillin G sodium	Many brands	5- to 20-million U vials	20,000–40,000 U/kg IV, IM q6–8h
Penicillin G procaine	Generic	300,000 U/mL suspension	20,000–40,000 U/kg IM q12–24h
Penicillin V	Pen-Vee	250- and 500-mg tablets	10 mg/kg PO q8h
Pentobarbital	Nembutal and generic	50 mg/mL	25–30 mg/kg IV to effect; or 2–15 mg/kg IV to effect, followed by 0.2–1.0 mg/kg/h IV
Pentoxifylline	Trental	400-mg tablet	Dog: For use in canine dermatology and for vasculitis, 10 mg/kg PO q12h and up to 15 mg/kg q8h Cat: ¼ of 400-mg tab PO, q8–12h
Pepto Bismol	*See* Bismuth subsalicylate		
Phenobarbital	Luminal, generic	15-, 30-, 60-, and 100-mg tablets; 30-, 60-, 65-, and 130-mg/mL injection; 4-mg/mL oral elixir solution	Dog: 2–8 mg/kg PO q12h Cat: 2–4 mg/kg PO q12h Dog and cat: Adjust dose by monitoring plasma concentration Status epilepticus: Administer in increments of 10–20 mg/kg IV (to effect)
Phenoxybenzamine	Dibenzyline	10-mg capsule	Dog: 0.25 mg/kg PO q8–12h or 0.5 mg/kg q24h Cat: 2.5 mg/cat q8–12h or 0.5 mg/cat PO q12h (in cats, doses as high as 0.5 mg/kg IV have been used to relax urethral smooth muscle)

DRUG NAME	OTHER NAMES	FORMULATIONS AVAILABLE	DOSAGE
Phentolamine	Regitine (Rogitine in Canada)	5-mg vial for injection	0.02–0.1 mg/kg IV
Phenylbutazone	Butazolidin, generic	100-, 200-, 400-mg and 1-g tablets; 200-mg/mL injection	Dog: 15–22 mg/kg PO, IV q8–12h (44 mg/kg/day) (800 mg/dog maximum) Cat: 6–8 mg/kg IV, PO q12h
Phenylephrine	Neo-Synephrine	10-mg/mL injection; 1% nasal solution	0.01 mg/kg IV q15min; 0.1 mg/kg IM, SC q15min
Phenylpropanolamine	PPA, Propalin, Proin PPA	25-, 50-, and 75-mg tablets and 25-mg/mL liquid	Dog: 1 mg/kg q12h PO and increase to 1.5–2.0 mg/kg as needed q8h PO
Phenytoin	Dilantin	30- and 125-mg/mL oral suspension; 30- and 100-mg capsules; 50-mg/mL injection	Antiepileptic dog: 20–35 mg/kg q8h Antiarrhythmic: 30 mg/kg PO q8h or 10 mg/kg IV over 5 min
Physostigmine	Antilirium	1-mg/mL injection	0.02 mg/kg IV q12h
Phytomenadione	*See* Vitamin K_1		
Phytonadione	*See* Vitamin K_1		
Pimobendan	Vetmedin	2.5- and 5-mg capsules (Europe and Canada); 1.25-, 2.5-, 5-mg chewable tablets (United States)	Dog: 0.05 mg/kg/day in divided treatments q12h Cat: Dose not established
Piperacillin	Pipracil	2-, 3-, 4-, and 40-g vials for injection	40 mg/kg IV or IM q6h
Piperazine	Many	860-mg powder; 140-mg capsule, 170-, 340-, and 800-mg/mL oral solution	44–66 mg/kg PO administered once
Piroxicam	Feldene, generic	10-mg capsule	Dog: 0.3 mg/kg PO q48h Cat: 0.3 mg/kg q24h PO
Pitressin (ADH)	*See* Vasopressin, Desmopressin acetate		
Plicamycin (old name is mithramycin)	Mithracin	2.5-mg injection	Dog: Antineoplastic: 25–30 mcg/kg day IV (slow infusion) for 8–10 days Antihypercalcemic: 25 mcg/kg/day IV (slow infusion) over 4 h Cat: Not recommended
Polyethylene glycol electrolyte solution	GoLYTELY	Oral solution	25 mL/kg PO; repeat in 2–4 hours PO
Polysulfated glycosaminoglycan (PSGAG)	Adequan Canine	100-mg/mL injection in 5-mL vial (for horses vials are 250 mg/mL)	4.4 mg/kg IM twice weekly for up to 4 weeks

DRUG NAME	OTHER NAMES	FORMULATIONS AVAILABLE	DOSAGE
Potassium bromide (KBr)	No commercial formulation	Usually prepared as oral solution; must be compounded	Dog and cat: 30–40 mg/kg PO q24h; if administered without phenobarbital, higher doses of up to 40–50 mg/kg may be needed. Adjust doses by monitoring plasma concentrations. Loading doses of 600–800 mg/kg divided over 3–4 days have been administered.
Potassium chloride (KCl)	Generic	Various concentrations for injection (usually 2 mEq/mL); oral suspension and oral solution	0.5 mEq potassium/kg/day; or supplement 10–40 mEq/500 mL of fluids, depending on serum potassium
Potassium citrate	Generic, Urocit-K	5-mEq tablet; some forms are in combination with potassium chloride	0.5 mEq/kg/day PO
Potassium gluconate	Kaon, Tumil-K, generic	2-mEq tablet; 500-mg tablet; Kaon elixir is 20-mg/15- mL elixir	Dog: 0.5 mEq/kg PO q12–24h Cat: 2–8 mEq/day PO divided twice daily
Potassium iodide			30–100 mg/cat daily (in single or divided doses) for 10–14 days
Pralidoxime chloride (2-PAM)	2-PAM, Protopam Chloride	50-mg/mL injection	20 mg/kg q8–12h (initial dose) IV slow or IM
Praziquantel	Droncit	23- and 34-mg tablets; 56.8-mg/mL injection	Dog (PO): <6.8 kg, 7.5 mg/kg, once; >6.8 kg, 5 mg/kg, once (IM, SC): <2.3 kg, 7.5 mg/kg, once; 2.7–4.5 kg, 6.3 mg/kg, once; >5 kg, 5 mg/kg, once Cat (PO): <1.8 kg, 6.3 mg/kg, once; >1.8 kg, 5 mg/kg, once (for *Paragonimus* use 25 mg/kg q8h for 2–3 days) (IM, SC): 5 mg/kg
Prazosin	Minipress	1-, 2-, and 5-mg capsules	0.5- and 2-mg/animal (1 mg/15 kg) PO q8–12h
Prednisolone	Delta-Cortef and many others	5- and 20-mg tablets	Dog (cat often requires two times dog dose) Antiinflammatory: 0.5–1 mg/kg IV, IM, PO q12–24h initially, then taper to q48h Immunosuppressive: 2.2–6.6 mg/kg/day IV, IM, PO initially, then taper to 2–4 mg/kg q48h Replacement therapy: 0.2–0.3 mg/kg/day PO

DRUG NAME	OTHER NAMES	FORMULATIONS AVAILABLE	DOSAGE
Prednisolone sodium succinate	Solu-Delta-Cortef	100- and 200-mg vials for injection (10 and 50 mg/mL)	Shock: 15–30 mg/kg IV (repeat in 4–6 hours) Central nervous system trauma: 15–30 mg/kg IV, taper to 1–2 mg/kg q12h
Prednisone	Deltasone and generic; Meticorten for injection	1-, 2.5-, 5-, 10-, 20-, 25-, and 50-mg tablets; 1 mg/mL syrup (LiquidPred in 5% alcohol) and 1-mg/mL oral solution (in 5% alcohol); 10- and 40-mg/mL prednisone suspension for injection	Same as prednisolone, except that prednisone is not recommended for cats
Primidone	Mylepsin, Neurosyn (Mysoline in Canada)	50- and 250-mg tablets	8–10 mg/kg PO q8–12h as initial dose, then is adjusted via monitoring to 10–15 mg/kg q8h
Primor (ormetoprim + sulfadimethoxine)	Primor	Combination tablet (ormetoprim + sulfadimethoxine)	27 mg/kg on first day, followed by 13.5 mg/kg PO q24h
Procainamide	Pronestyl, generic	250-, 375-, 500-mg tablets or capsules; 100- and 500-mg/mL injection	Dog: 10–30 mg/kg PO q6h (to a maximum dose of 40 mg/kg), 8–20 mg/kg IV IM; 25–50 mcg/ kg/ min IV infusion Cat: 3–8 mg/kg IM, PO q6–8h
Prochlorperazine	Compazine	5-, 10-, and 25-mg tablets (prochlorperazine maleate); 5-mg/mL injection (prochlorperazine edisylate)	0.1–0.5 mg/kg IM, SC q6–8h
Progesterone, repositol	*See* Medroxyprogesterone acetate		
Promethazine	Phenergan	6.25- and 25-mg/5-mL syrup; 12.5-,25-, 50-mg tablets; 25- and 50-mg/mL injection	0.2–0.4 mg/kg IV, IM PO q6–8h (up to a maximum dose of 1 mg/ kg)
Propantheline bromide	Pro-Banthine	7.5- and 15-mg tablet	0.25–0.5 mg/kg PO q8–12h
Propionylpromazine	Tranvet	5-, 10-mg/mL injection or 20-mg tablet	1.1–4.4 mg/kg q12–24h PO or 0.1–1.1 mg/kg IM, IV (range of dose depends on degree of sedation needed)

DRUG NAME	OTHER NAMES	FORMULATIONS AVAILABLE	DOSAGE
Propofol	Rapinovet and PropoFlo (veterinary); Diprivan (human)	1% (10 mg/mL) injection in 20-mL ampules	6.6 mg/kg IV slowly over 60 seconds; constant-rate infusions have been used at 5 mg/kg slowly IV, followed by 100–400 mcg/kg/min IV
Propranolol	Inderal	10-, 20-, 40-, 60-, 80-, and 90-mg tablets; 1-mg/mL injection; 4- and 8-mg/mL oral solution	Dog: 20–60 mcg/kg over 5–10 min IV; 0.2–1 mg/kg PO q8h (titrate dose to effect) Cat: 0.4–1.2 mg/kg (2.5–5 mg/cat) PO q8h
Propylthiouracil (PTU)	Generic, Propyl-Thyracil	50- and 100-mg tablets	11 mg/kg PO q12h
Prostaglandin F_2 alpha (dinoprost)	Lutalyse	5-mg/mL solution for injection	Pyometra: Dog: 0.1–0.2 mg/kg SC once daily for 5 days Cat: 0.1–0.25 mg/kg SC once daily for 5 days Abortion: Dog: 0.025–0.05 mg (25–50 mcg)/kg IM q12h Cat: 0.5–1 mg/kg IM for two injections
Pseudoephedrine	Sudafed and many others (some formulations have been discontinued)	30- and 60-mg tablets; 120-mg capsule; 6-mg/mL syrup	0.2–0.4 mg/kg (or 15–60 mg/dog) PO q8–12h
Psyllium	Metamucil and others	Available as powder	1 tsp/5–10 kg (added to each meal)
Pyrantel pamoate	Nemex, Strongid	180-mg/mL paste and 50-mg/mL suspension	Dog: 5 mg/kg PO once and repeat in 7–10 days Cat: 20 mg/kg PO once
Pyridostigmine bromide	Mestinon, Regonol	12-mg/mL oral syrup; 60-mg tablet; 5-mg/mL injection	Antimyasthenic: 0.02–0.04 mg/kg IV q2h or 0.5–3 mg/kg PO q8–12h Antidote (nondepolarizing muscle relaxant): 0.15–0.3 mg/kg IM, IV
Pyrimethamine	Daraprim, ReBalance (Equine)	25-mg tablet equine formulation (ReBalance) contains 250 mg sulfadiazine and 12.5 mg pyrimethamine per milliliter	Dog: 1 mg/kg PO q24h for 14–21 days (5 days for *Neospora caninum*) Cat: 0.5–1 mg/kg PO q24h for 14–28 days
Quinidine gluconate	Quinaglute, Duraquin	324-mg tablets; 80-mg/mL injection	Dog: 6–20 mg/kg IM q6h; 6–20 mg/kg PO q6–8h (of base)
Quinidine sulfate	Cin-Quin, Quinora	100-, 200-, and 300-mg tablets; 200- and 300-mg capsules; 20-mg/mL injection	Dog: 6–20 mg/kg PO q6–8h (of base); 5–10 mg/kg IV

DRUG NAME	OTHER NAMES	FORMULATIONS AVAILABLE	DOSAGE
Quinidine polygalacturonate	Cardioquin	275-mg tablet	Dog: 6–20 mg/kg PO q6h (of base) (275 mg quinidine polygalacturonate = 167 mg quinidine base)
Racemethionine (DL-methionine)	Uroeze, MethioForm, generic; Human forms include Pedameth, Uracid, and generic	500-mg tablets and powders added to animal's food; 75-mg/5 mL pediatric oral solution; 200-mg capsule	Dog: 150–300 mg/kg/day PO Cat: 1–1.5 g/cat PO (added to food each day)
Ranitidine	Zantac	75-, 150-, and 300-mg tablets; 150- and 300-mg capsules; 25-mg/mL injection	Dog: 2 mg/kg IV, PO q8h Cat: 2.5 mg/kg IV q12h, 3.5 mg/kg PO q12h
Retinoids	*See* Isotretinoin (Accutane), Retinol (Aquasol A), or Etretinate (Tegison)		
Retinol	*See* Vitamin A (Aquasol A)		
Riboflavin (vitamin B_2)	*See* Vitamin B_2		
Rifampin	Rifadin	150- and 300-mg capsules	5–15 mg/kg PO q24h
Ringer's solution	Generic	250-, 500-, and 1000-mL bags for infusion	55–65 mL/kg/day IV, SC, or IP; 50 ml/kg/h IV for severe dehydration
Ronidazole		No commercial formulations are available. However, compounding pharmacies have prepared formulations for cats.	Dog: Dose not established Cat: 30–60 mg/kg/day PO for 2 weeks
Salicylate	*See* Aspirin, acetylsalicylic acid		
Selegiline (deprenyl)	Anipryl (also known as deprenyl, and *l*-deprenyl); human dose form is Eldepryl	2-, 5-, 10-, 15-, and 30-mg tablets	Dog: Begin with 1 mg/kg PO q24h; if no response within 2 months, increase dose to maximum of 2 mg/kg PO q24h Cat: 0.25–0.5 mg/kg q12–24h PO
Senna	Senokot	Granules in concentrate or syrup	Dog: Syrup; 5–10 mL/dog q24h; Granules: 1/2 to 1 tsp/dog q24h PO with food Cat: Syrup: 5 mL/cat q24h; granules: ½ teaspoon/cat q24h (with food)

DRUG NAME	OTHER NAMES	FORMULATIONS AVAILABLE	DOSAGE
Septra (sulfamethoxazole + trimethoprim)	*See* Trimethoprim + sulfonamides		
Sildenafil	Viagra	25-, 50-, 100-mg tablets	Dog: 0.5–1 mg/kg q12h PO; higher dose of 2–3 mg/kg q8h may be needed in some cases
Silymarin	Silybin, Marin, "milk thistle"	Silymarin tablets are widely available OTC. Commercial veterinary formulations (Marin) also contain zinc and vitamin E in a phosphatidylcholine complex in tablets for dogs and cats.	30 mg/kg/day PO
Sodium bicarbonate ($NaHCO_3$)	Generic, Baking Soda, Soda Mint	325-, 520-, and 650-mg tablets; injection of various strengths (4.2% to 8.4%), and 1 mEq/mL	Acidosis: 0.5–1 mEq/kg IV Renal failure: 10 mg/kg PO q8–12h Alkalization of urine: 50 mg/kg PO q8–12h (1 tsp is approx. 2 g)
Sodium bromide	No commercial form	Must be compounded	Same as potassium bromide, except dose is 15% lower (30 mg/kg potassium bromide is equivalent to 25 mg/kg sodium bromide)
Sodium chloride	0.9%, Generic	500- and 1000-mL infusion	15–30 mL/kg/h IV
Sodium chloride	7.5%, Generic	Infusion	2–8 mL/kg IV
Sodium thiomalate	*See* Gold sodium thiomalate		
Somatrem, Somatropin	*See* Growth hormone		
Sotalol	Betapace	80-, 160-, 240-mg tablets	Dog: 1–2 mg/kg PO q12h (one can start with 40 mg/dog q12h, then increase to 80 mg if no response) Cat: 1–2 mg/kg PO q12h
Spironolactone	Aldactone	25-, 50-, and 100-mg tablets	2–4 mg/kg/day (or 1–2 mg/kg PO q12h)
Stanozolol	Winstrol-V	50-mg/mL injection; 2-mg tablet	Dog: 2 mg/dog (or range of 1–4 mg/dog) PO q12h; 25–50 mg/dog/wk IM Cat: 1 mg/cat PO q12h; 25 mg/cat/wk IM
Succimer	Chemet	100-mg capsule	Dog: 10 mg/kg PO q8h for 5 days, then 10 mg/kg PO q12h for 2 more weeks Cat: 10 mg/kg q8h for 2 weeks

DRUG NAME	OTHER NAMES	FORMULATIONS AVAILABLE	DOSAGE
Sucralfate	Carafate (Sulcrate in Canada)	1-g tablet; 200-mg/mL oral suspension	Dog: 0.5–1 g/dog PO q8–12h Cat: 0.25 g/cat PO q8–12h
Sufentanil citrate	Sufenta	50-mcg/mL injection	2 mcg/kg IV, up to a maximum dose of 5 mcg/kg
Sulfadiazine	Generic, combined with trimethoprim in Tribrissen	500-mg tablet; trimethoprim-sulfadiazine 30-, 120-, 240-, 480-, and 960-mg tablets	100 mg/kg IV, PO (loading dose), followed by 50 mg/kg IV, PO q12h (*see also* Trimethoprim)
Sulfadimethoxine	Albon, Bactrovet, generic	125-, 250-, and 500-mg tablets; 400-mg/mL injection; 50-mg/mL suspension	55 mg/kg PO (loading dose), followed by 27.5 mg/kg PO q12h (*see also* Primor)
Sulfamethoxazole	Gantanol	50-mg tablet	100 mg/kg PO (loading dose), followed by 50 mg/kg PO q12h (*see also* Bactrim, Septra)
Sulfasalazine (sulfapyridine + mesalamine)	Azulfidine (Salazopyrin in Canada)	500-mg tablet	Dog: 10–30 mg/kg PO q8–12h (*see also* Mesalamine, Olsalazine) Cat: 20 mg/kg q12h PO
Sulfisoxazole	Gantrisin	500-mg tablet; 500-mg/5 mL syrup	50 mg/kg PO q8h (urinary tract infections)
Tamoxifen	Nolvadex	10- and 20-mg tablets (tamoxifen citrate)	Veterinary dose not established; 10 mg PO q12h is human dose
Taurine	Generic	Available in powder	Dog: 500 mg PO q12h Cat: 250 mg/cat PO q12h
Telazol	*See* Tiletamine + zolazepam		
Terbinafine	Lamisil	125-, 250-mg tablets	Dog: *Malassezia* dermatitis: 30 mg/kg/day PO Cat: Dermatophytosis: 30–40 mg/kg PO q24h
Terbutaline	Brethine, Bricanyl	2.5- and 5-mg tablets; 1-mg/mL injection (equivalent to 0.82 mg/mL)	Dog: 1.25–5 mg/dog PO q8h Cat: 0.1–0.2 mg/kg PO q12h (or 0.625 mg/cat, ¼ of 2.5-mg tablet) For acute treatment in cats: 5–10 mcg/kg q4h SC or IM
Testosterone cypionate ester	Andro-Cyp, Andronate, Depo-Testosterone	100- and 200-mg/mL injection	1–2 mg/kg IM q2–4wk (*see also* Methyltestosterone)
Testosterone propionate ester	Testex (Malogen in Canada)	100-mg/mL injection	0.5–1 mg/kg 2–3 times/wk IM
Tetracycline	Panmycin	250- and 500-mg capsules; 100-mg/mL suspension	15–20 mg/kg PO q8h; or 4.4–11 mg/kg IV, IM q8h

DRUG NAME	OTHER NAMES	FORMULATIONS AVAILABLE	DOSAGE
Thenium closylate	Canopar	500-mg tablet	Dog: >4.5 kg: 500 mg PO once, repeat in 2–3 weeks; 2.5–4.5 kg: 250 mg q12h for 1 day, repeat in 2–3 weeks
Theophylline	Many brands and generic	100-, 125-, 200-, 250-, and 300-mg tablets; 27-mg/5 mL oral solution or elixir; injection in 5% dextrose	Dog: 9 mg/kg PO q6–8h Cat: 4 mg/kg PO q8–12h
Theophylline extended-release	Inwood Labs Extended Release	100-, 200-, 300-, and 400-mg tablets or 125-, 200-, 300-mg capsules	Dog: 10 mg/kg q12h PO of extended-release tablet or capsule Cat: 20 mg/kg q24–48h PO extended-release tablet or 25 mg/kg q24–48h PO extended-release capsule
Thiamine (vitamin B_1)	Bewon and others	250-mcg/5 mL elixir; tablets of various size from 5 mg to 500 mg; 100- and 500-mg/mL injection	Dog: 10–100 mg/dog/day PO or 12.5–50 mg/dog IM or SC/day Cat: 5–30 mg/cat/day PO (up to a maximum dose of 50 mg/cat/day) or 12.5–25 mg/cat IM or SC/day
Thiamylal sodium		No longer available	
Thioguanine (6-TG)	Generic	40-mg tablet	40 mg/m^2 PO q24h Cat: 25 mg/m^2 PO q24h for 1–5 days, then repeat every 30 days
Thiomalate sodium	*See* Gold sodium thiomalate		
Thiotepa	Generic	15-mg injection (usually in solution of 10 mg/mL)	0.2–0.5 mg/m^2 weekly, or daily for 5–10 days IM, intracavitary, or intratumor
Thyroid hormone	*See* Levothyroxine sodium (T_4), or Liothyronine		
Thyrotropin, thyroid-stimulating hormone (TSH)	Thytropar, Thyrogen	10-U vial; old forms difficult to obtain; Thyrogen is 1000 mcg/vial	Dog: Collect baseline sample, followed by 0.1 U/kg IV (maximum dose is 5 U); collect post-TSH sample at 6 hours Cat: Collect baseline sample, followed by 2.5 U/cat IM and collect a post-TSH sample at 8–12 hours
Ticarcillin	Ticar, Ticillin	Vials containing 1, 3, 6, 20, and 30 g	33–50 mg/kg IV, IM q4–6h

DRUG NAME	OTHER NAMES	FORMULATIONS AVAILABLE	DOSAGE
Ticarcillin + clavulanate	Timentin	3-g/vial for injection	Dose according to rate for ticarcillin
Tiletamine + zolazepam	Telazol, Zoletil	50 mg of each component per milliliter	Dog: 6.6–10 mg/kg IM (short term) or 10–13 mg/kg IM (longer procedure) Cat: 10–12 mg/kg IM (minor procedure) or 14–16 mg/kg IM (for surgery)
Tobramycin	Nebcin	40-mg/mL injection	Dog: 9–14 mg/kg IM, IV, SC q24h Cat: 5–8 mg/kg IM, SC, IV q24h
Tocainide	Tonocard	400- and 600-mg tablets	Dog: 15–20 mg/kg PO q8h Cat: No dose established
Toluene	Vermiplex		267 mg/kg PO (of toluene), repeat in 2–4 weeks
Tramadol hydrochloride	Ultram, generic	Tramadol immediate-release tablets are available in 50-mg tablets	Dog: 5 mg/kg PO q6–8h Cat: Safe dose not established
Trandolapril	Mavik	1-, 2-, and 4-mg tablets	Not established for dogs; human dose is 1 mg/person/day to start, then increase to 2–4 mg/day
Triamcinolone	Vetalog, Trimtabs, Aristocort, generic	Veterinary (Vetalog) 0.5- and 1.5-mg tablets. Human form: 1-, 2-, 4-, 8-, and 16-mg tablets; 10-mg/mL injection	Antiinflammatory: 0.5–1 mg/kg PO q12–24h, then taper dose to 0.5–1 PO mg/kg q48h; however, manufacturer recommends doses of 0.11 to 0.22 mg/kg/day
Triamcinolone acetonide	Vetalog	2- or 6-mg/mL suspension injection	0.1–0.2 mg/kg IM, SC, repeat in 7–10 days Intralesional: 1.2–1.8 mg, or 1 mg for every centimeter diameter of tumor
Triamterene	Dyrenium	50- and 100-mg capsules	1–2 mg/kg PO q12h
Tribrissen	*See* Trimethoprim-sulfadimethoxine combination		
Trientine hydrochloride	Syprine	250-mg capsule	10–15 mg/kg PO q12h
Trifluoperazine	Stelazine	10-mg/mL oral solution; 1-, 2-, 5-, and 10-mg tablets; 2-mg/mL injection	0.03 mg/kg IM q12h
Triflupromazine	Vesprin	10- and 20-mg/mL injection	0.1–0.3 mg/kg IM, PO q8–12h

DRUG NAME	OTHER NAMES	FORMULATIONS AVAILABLE	DOSAGE
Tri-iodothyronine	*See* Liothyronine		
Trilostane	Vetoryl	10-, 30-, 60-, and 120-mg capsules; no formulations approved in the United States; must be imported	Dog: 3.9–9.2 mg/kg/day PO (most common dose is 6.1 mg/kg/day); adjust dose based on cortisol measurements
Trimeprazine tartrate	Temaril (Panectyl in Canada)	2.5-mg/5 mL syrup; 2.5-mg tablet	0.5 mg/kg PO q12h
Trimethobenzamide	Tigan and others	100-mg/mL injection; 100- and 250-mg capsules	Dog: 3 mg/kg IM, PO q8h Cat: Not recommended
Trimethoprim + sulfonamides (sulfadiazine or sulfamethoxazole)	Tribrissen and others	30-, 120-, 240-, 480-, and 960-mg tablets with trimethoprim to sulfa ratio 1 : 5	15 mg/kg PO q12h, or 30 mg/kg PO q12–24h For *Toxoplasma:* 30 mg/kg PO q12h
Tripelennamine	Pelamine, PBZ	25- and 50-mg tablets; 20-mg/mL injection	1 mg/kg PO q12h
TSH (thyroid-stimulating hormone)	*See* Thyrotropin		
Tylosin	Tylocine, Tylan, Tylosin tartrate	Available as soluble powder 2.2 g tylosin per tsp (tablets for dogs in Canada)	Dog, cat: 7–15 mg/kg PO q12–24h Dog: For colitis: 10–20 mg/kg q8h with food initially, then increase interval to q12–24h
Urofollitropin (FSH)	Metrodin	75 U/vial for injection	75 U/day IM for 7 days
Ursodiol (ursodeoxycholate)	Actigall	300-mg capsule, 250-mg tablets	10–15 mg/kg PO q24h
Valproic acid, divalproex	Depakene (valproic acid); Depakote (divalproex)	125-, 250-, and 500-mg tablets (Depakote); 250-mg capsule; 50-mg/mL syrup (Depakene)	Dog: 60–200 mg/kg PO q8h; or 25–105 mg/kg/day PO when administered with phenobarbital
Vancomycin	Vancocin, Vancoled	Vials for injection (0.5 to 10 g)	Dog: 15 mg/kg q6–8h IV infusion Cat: 12–15 mg/kg q8h IV infusion
Vasopressin (ADH)	Pitressin	20 U/mL (aqueous)	10 U IV, IM
Verapamil	Calan, Isoptin	40-, 80-, and 120-mg tablet; 2.5-mg/mL injection	Dog: 0.05 mg/kg IV q10–30 min (maximum cumulative dose is 0.15 mg/kg)
Vinblastine	Velban	1-mg/mL injection	2 mg/m^2 IV (slow infusion) once/week
Vincristine	Oncovin, Vincasar, generic	1-mg/mL injection	Antitumor: 0.5–0.7 mg/m^2 IV (or 0.025–0.05 mg/kg) once/week For thrombocytopenia: 0.02 mg/kg IV once/week
Viokase	*See* Pancrelipase		

DRUG NAME	OTHER NAMES	FORMULATIONS AVAILABLE	DOSAGE
Vitamin A (retinoids)	Aquasol A	Oral solution: 5000 U (1500 RE) per 0.1 mL; 10,000-, 25,000-, and 50,000-U tablets	625–800 U/kg PO q24h
Vitamin B_1	*See* Thiamine		
Vitamin B_2 (riboflavin)	Riboflavin	Various size tablets in increments from 10 to 250 mg	Dog: 10–20 mg/day PO Cat: 5–10 mg/day PO
Vitamin B_{12} (cyanocobalamin)	Cyanocobalamin	Various size tablets in increments from 25 to 100 mcg and injections	Dog: 100–200 mcg/day PO Cat: 50–100 mcg/day PO
Vitamin C (ascorbic acid)	*See* Ascorbic acid	Tablets of various sizes and injection	100–500 mg/day
Vitamin D	*See* Dihydrotachysterol or Ergocalciferol		
Vitamin E (alpha-tocopherol)	Aquasol E, generic	Wide variety of capsules, tablets, oral solution available (e.g., 1000 units per capsule)	100–400 U PO q12h (or 400–600 U PO q12h for immune-mediated skin disease)
Vitamin K_1 (phytonadione, phytomenadione)	Aquamephyton (injection), Mephyton (tablets); Veta-K1 (capsules)	2- or 10-mg/mL injection; 5-mg tablet (Mephyton); 25-mg capsule (Veta-K1)	Short-acting rodenticides: 1 mg/kg/day IM, SC, PO for 10–14 days Long-acting rodenticides: 2.5–5 mg/kg/day and up to 6 weeks IM, SC, PO for 3–4 weeks Birds: 2.5–5 mg/kg q24h
Warfarin	Coumadin, generic	1-, 2-, 2.5-, 4-, 5-, 7.5-, and 10-mg tablets	Dog: 0.1–0.2 mg/kg PO q24h Cat: Thromboembolism: Start with 0.5 mg/cat/day and adjust dose based on clotting time assessment
Xylazine	Rompun and generic	20- and 100-mg/mL injection	Dog: 1.1 mg/kg IV, 2.2 mg/kg IM Cat: 1.1 mg/kg IM (emetic dose is 0.4–0.5 mg/kg IV)
Yohimbine	Yobine	2-mg/mL injection	0.11 mg/kg IV or 0.25–0.5 mg/kg SC, IM
Zidovudine (AZT)	Retrovir	10-mg/mL syrup; 10-mg/mL injection	Cat: 15 mg/kg PO q12h to 20 mg/kg q8h (doses as high as 30 mg/kg/day also have been used)
Zolazepam	*See* Tiletamine + zolazepam combination		

DRUG NAME	OTHER NAMES	FORMULATIONS AVAILABLE	DOSAGE
Zonisamide	Zonegran	100-mg capsule	Dog: 3 mg/kg q8h PO; it has also been administered to dogs at 10 mg/kg q12h PO Cat: Dose not established

Note: Doses listed are for dogs *and* cats, unless otherwise listed. Many of the doses listed are extralabel or are human drugs used in an off-label or extralabel manner. Doses listed are based on the best available evidence at the time of table preparation; however, the author cannot ensure the efficacy of drugs used according to recommendations in this table. Adverse effects may be possible from drugs listed in this table of which the author was not aware at the time of table preparation. Veterinarians using these tables are encouraged to check current literature, product labels, and the manufacturer's disclosures for information regarding efficacy and any known adverse effects or contraindications not identified at the time of table preparation.
ACTH, Adrenocorticotropic hormone; *ADH,* antidiuretic hormone; *BPH,* benign prostatic hyperplasia; *CRI,* continuous rate infusion; *GnRH,* gonadotropin-releasing hormone; *hCG,* human chorionic gonadotropin; *IM,* intramuscular; *IP,* intraperitoneal; *IV,* intravenous; *LHRH,* luteinizing hormone-releasing hormone; *MCT,* medium-chain triglycerides; *OTC,* over-the-counter (without prescription); *PO,* per os (oral); *PSGAG,* polysulfated glycosaminoglycan; *Rx,* prescription only; *SC,* subcutaneous; *U,* units.
From Papich MG: Kirk's current veterinary therapy, St. Louis, 2008, Saunders Elsevier.

APPENDIX E

Listing of Drugs According to Functional and Therapeutic Classification

DRUG CLASSIFICATION	DRUG NAME
Acidifying agent	Ammonium chloride
	Racemethionine
Adrenal suppressant	Trilostane
Adrenergic agonist	Ephedrine hydrochloride
	Epinephrine
	Fenoldopam mesylate
	Phenylpropanolamine hydrochloride
	Pseudoephedrine hydrochloride
Adrenolytic agent	Mitotane
Alkalinizing agent	Potassium citrate
	Sodium bicarbonate
Alpha-2 antagonist	Atipamezole hydrochloride
	Yohimbine
Analgesic	Acetaminophen
	Amantadine
	Gabapentin
	Pregabalin
	Tramadol
Analgesic, nonsteroidal antiinflammatory drug	Aspirin
	Carprofen
	Deracoxib
	Etodolac
	Firocoxib
	Flunixin meglumine
	Ibuprofen
	Indomethacin
	Ketoprofen
	Ketorolac tromethamine
	Meclofenamate sodium; Meclofenamic acid
	Meloxicam
	Naproxen
	Phenylbutazone
	Piroxicam
	Tepoxalin
Analgesic, opioid	Acetaminophen–codeine
	Buprenorphine hydrochloride
	Butorphanol tartrate
	Fentanyl citrate
	Fentanyl transdermal
	Hydrocodone
	Hydromorphone
	Loperamide hydrochloride
	Meperidine
	Methadone hydrochloride
	Morphine sulfate
	Oxymorphone hydrochloride
	Pentazocine
	Remifentanil
	Sufentanil citrate
Analgesic, opioid, antitussive	Butorphanol
	Codeine
	Hydrocodone
Anesthetic	Alfaxalone
	Ketamine hydrochloride
	Propofol
	Tiletamine–zolazepam
Anesthetic, alpha-2 agonist	Detomidine hydrochloride
	Dexmedetomidine
	Medetomidine hydrochloride
	Romifidine hydrochloride
	Xylazine hydrochloride

DRUG CLASSIFICATION	DRUG NAME
Anesthetic, barbiturate	Methohexital sodium
	Pentobarbital sodium
	Thiopental sodium
Anesthetic, inhalant	Enflurane
	Halothane
	Isoflurane
	Methoxyflurane
	Sevoflurane
Antacid	Aluminum hydroxide and aluminum carbonate
Antiarrhythmic	Amiodarone
	Carvedilol
	Disopyramide
	Lidocaine
	Mexiletine
	Procainamide hydrochloride
	Quinidine
	Quinidine gluconate
	Quinidine polygalacturonate
	Quinidine sulfate
	Tocainide hydrochloride
Antiarrhythmic, calcium channel blocker	Diltiazem hydrochloride
	Verapamil hydrochloride
Antiarthritic agent	Chondroitin sulfate
	Glucosamine–chondroitin sulfate
	Polysulfated glycosaminoglycan
Antibacterial	Chloramphenicol
	Clofazimine
	Dapsone
	Florfenicol
	Fosfomycin
	Isoniazid
	Linezolid
	Methenamine
	Nitrofurantoin
	Polymyxin B
	Pyrimethamine
	Rifampin
Antibacterial, aminoglycoside	Amikacin
	Gentamicin sulfate
	Kanamycin sulfate
	Neomycin
	Tobramycin sulfate
Antibacterial, antidiarrheal	Sulfasalazine
Antibacterial, antiparasitic	Metronidazole
	Ronidazole
Antibacterial, beta-lactam	Amoxicillin
	Amoxicillin–clavulanate potassium
	Ampicillin
	Ampicillin–sulbactam
	Carbenicillin
	Cefaclor
	Cefadroxil
	Cefazolin sodium
	Cefdinir
	Cefepime
	Cefixime
	Cefotaxime sodium
	Cefotetan disodium
	Cefovecin
	Cefoxitin sodium
	Cefpodoxime proxetil
	Cefquinome
	Ceftazidime
	Ceftiofur crystalline free acid
	Ceftiofur hydrochloride
	Ceftiofur sodium
	Cephalexin
	Cloxacillin sodium
	Dicloxacillin sodium
	Doripenem
	Ertapenem
	Imipenem–cilastatin
	Meropenem
	Oxacillin sodium
	Penicillin G
	Piperacillin sodium

DRUG CLASSIFICATION	DRUG NAME
	Ticarcillin–clavulanate potassium
	Ticarcillin disodium
Antibacterial, fluoroquinolone	Ciprofloxacin hydrochloride
	Danofloxacin mesylate
	Difloxacin hydrochloride
	Enrofloxacin
	Marbofloxacin
	Moxifloxacin
	Norfloxacin
	Orbifloxacin
	Pradofloxacin
Antibacterial, glycopeptide	Vancomycin
Antibacterial, lincosamide	Clindamycin hydrochloride
	Clindamycin palmitate
	Clindamycin phosphate
	Lincomycin hydrochloride
	Lincomysin hydrochloride monohydrate
Antibacterial, macrolide	Azithromycin
	Clarithromycin
	Erythromycin
	Tilmicosin phosphate
	Tulathromycin
	Tylosin
Antibacterial, potentiated sulfonamide	Ormetoprim–sulfadimethoxine
	Trimethoprim–sulfadiazine
	Trimethoprim–sulfamethoxazole
Antibacterial, sulfonamide	Sulfachlorpyridazine
	Sulfadiazine
	Sulfadimethoxine
	Sulfamethazine
	Sulfamethoxazole
	Sulfaquinoxaline
Antibacterial, tetracycline	Chlortetracycline
	Doxycycline

DRUG CLASSIFICATION	DRUG NAME
	Minocycline hydrochloride
	Oxytetracycline
	Tetracycline
Antibiotic, aminocyclitol	Spectinomycin
Anticancer agent	Asparaginase (L-asparaginase)
	Bleomycin sulfate
	Busulfan
	Carboplatin
	Chlorambucil
	Cisplatin
	Cyclophosphamide
	Cytarabine
	Dacarbazine
	Doxorubicin hydrochloride
	Fluorouracil
	Hydroxyurea
	Lomustine
	Melphalan
	Mercaptopurine
	Methotrexate
	Mitoxantrone hydrochloride
	Plicamycin
	Streptozocin
	Thioguanine
	Thiotepa
	Toceranib
	Vinblastine sulfate
	Vincristine sulfate
Anticholinergic	Aminopentamide
	Atropine sulfate
	Glycopyrrolate
	Hyoscyamine
	Oxybutynin chloride
Anticholinesterase agent	Neostigmine
	Physostigmine
	Pyridostigmine bromide
Anticoagulant	Dalteparin
	Dipyridamole
	Enoxaparin
	Heparin sodium
	Warfarin sodium

DRUG CLASSIFICATION	DRUG NAME
Anticonvulsant	Bromide
	Clonazepam
	Clorazepate dipotassium
	Felbamate
	Levetiracetam
	Lorazepam
	Midazolam hydrochloride
	Oxazepam
	Phenobarbital
	Phenobarbital sodium
	Phenytoin
	Phenytoin sodium
	Primidone
	Valproate sodium
	Valproic acid
	Zonisamide
Anticonvulsant, analgesic	Gabapentin
	Pregabalin
Anticonvulsant, tranquilizer	Diazepam
Antidiarrheal	Bismuth subsalicylate
	Diphenoxylate
	Kaolin–pectin
	Mesalamine
	Olsalazine sodium
	Paregoric
	Propantheline bromide
Antidote	Charcoal, activated
	Deferoxamine mesylate
	Dimercaprol
	Edetate calcium disodium
	Flumazenil
	Fomepizole
	Leucovorin calcium
	Methylene blue 0.1%
	Penicillamine
	Pralidoxime chloride
	Succimer
	Trientine hydrochloride
Antiemetic	Aprepitant
	Dolasetron mesylate
	Dronabinol
	Granisetron hydrochloride
	Maropitant
	Meclizine
	Mirtazapine
	Ondansetron hydrochloride
	Trimethobenzamide
Antiemetic, antidiarrheal	Prochlorperazine edisylate
	Prochlorperazine maleate (with isopropamide iodide)
Antiemetic, phenothiazine	Chlorpromazine
	Prochlorperazine edisylate
	Prochlorperazine maleate
	Trifluoperazine hydrochloride
	Triflupromazine hydrochloride
	Trimeprazine tartrate
Antiemetic, phenothiazine, antihistamine	Promethazine hydrochloride
	Propiopromazine hydrochloride
Antiemetic, prokinetic agent	Metoclopramide hydrochloride
Antiestrogen	Tamoxifen citrate
Antifungal	Amphotericin B
	Enilconazole
	Fluconazole
	Flucytosine
	Griseofulvin
	Itraconazole
	Ketoconazole
	Posaconazole
	Terbinafine hydrochloride
	Voriconazole
Antifungal, expectorant	Potassium iodide
Antihistamine	Cetirizine hydrochloride
	Chlorpheniramine maleate

DRUG CLASSIFICATION	DRUG NAME
	Clemastine fumarate
	Cyproheptadine hydrochloride
	Dimenhydrinate
	Diphenhydramine hydrochloride
	Hydroxyzine
	Tiludronate disodium
	Tripelennamine citrate
Antihypercalcemic agent	Alendronate
	Etidronate disodium
	Pamidronate disodium
	Zoledronate
Antihyperglycemic agent	Gemfibrozil
	Glipizide
	Glyburide
	Metformin
Antiinflammatory	Allopurinol
	Colchicine
	Dimethyl sulfoxide (DMSO)
	Niacinamide
	Pentoxifylline
Antiinflammatory, corticosteroid	Betamethasone
	Budesonide
	Desoxycorticosterone pivalate
	Dexamethasone
	Dexamethasone sodium phosphate
	Flumethasone
	Hydrocortisone
	Isoflupredone acetate
	Methylprednisolone
	Prednisolone
	Prednisolone acetate
	Prednisolone sodium succinate
	Prednisone
	Triamcinolone acetonide
	Triamcinolone diacetate
	Triamcinolone hexacetonide
Antimyasthenic	Edrophonium chloride
Antiobesity	Dirlotapide
	Mitratapide
Antiparasitic	Albendazole
	Amitraz
	Amprolium
	Bunamidine hydrochloride
	Dichlorvos
	Diethylcarbamazine citrate
	Dithiazanine iodide
	Doramectin
	Epsiprantel
	Febantel
	Fenbendazole
	Furazolidone
	Ivermectin
	Ivermectin–praziquantel
	Levamisole hydrochloride
	Lufenuron
	Lufenuron–milbemycin oxime
	Mebendazole
	Melarsomine
	Metaflumizone
	Milbemycin oxime
	Moxidectin
	Nitenpyram
	Oxfendazole
	Oxibendazole
	Paromomycin sulfate
	Piperazine
	Praziquantel
	Pyrantel pamoate
	Pyrantel tartrate
	Quinacrine hydrochloride
	Selamectin
	Spinosad
	Thenium closylate
	Thiabendazole
	Thiacetarsamide sodium
Antiplatelet agent	Clopidogrel

DRUG CLASSIFICATION	DRUG NAME
Antiprotozoal	Atovaquone
	Diclazuril
	Imidocarb hydrochloride
	Metronidazole
	Nitazoxanide
	Ponazuril
	Pyrimethamine–sulfadiazine
	Ronidazole
	Tinidazole
	Toltrazuril
Antispasmodic	N-butylscopolammonium bromide
	(Butylscopolamine bromide)
Antithyroid agent	Carbimazole
	Iopanoic acid
	Ipodate
	Methimazole
	Propylthiouracil
Antitussive, analgesic	Butorphanol
	Dextromethorphan
	Hydrocodone bitartrate
Antiulcer agent	Misoprostol
	Sucralfate
Antiulcer agent, H_2-blocker	Cimetidine hydrochloride
	Famotidine
	Nizatidine
	Ranitidine hydrochloride
Antiulcer agent, proton-pump inhibitor	Omeprazole
	Pantoprazole
Antiviral	Acyclovir
	Famciclovir
	Lysine (L-Lysine)
	Zidovudine
Antiviral analgesic	Amantadine
Behavior-modifying drug	Buspirone hydrochloride
	Trazodone
Behavior-modifying drug, SSRI	Fluoxetine hydrochloride
	Paroxetine
Behavior-modifying drug, Tricyclic	Amitriptyline hydrochloride
	Clomipramine hydrochloride
	Doxepin
	Imipramine hydrochloride
Beta-agonist	Isoproterenol hydrochloride
Beta-blocker	Atenolol
	Bisoprolol
	Esmolol hydrochloride
	Metoprolol tartrate
	Propranolol hydrochloride
	Sotalol hydrochloride
Bronchodilator	Aminophylline
	Oxtriphylline
	Theophylline
Bronchodilator, beta-agonist	Albuterol sulfate
	Clenbuterol
	Metaproterenol sulfate
	Terbutaline sulfate
	Zilpaterol
Calcium supplement	Calcitriol
	Calcium carbonate
	Calcium chloride
	Calcium citrate
	Calcium gluconate and calcium borogluconate
	Calcium lactate
Cardiac inotropic agent	Digitoxin
	Digoxin
	Dobutamine hydrochloride
	Pimobendan
Cholinergic	Bethanechol chloride
Corticosteroid, hormone	Fludrocortisone acetate
Dermatologic agent	Isotretinoin
Diuretic	Acetazolamide
	Chlorothiazide
	Dichlorphenamide
	Furosemide

DRUG CLASSIFICATION	DRUG NAME
	Hydrochlorothiazide
	Mannitol
	Methazolamide
	Spironolactone
	Triamterene
Diuretic, laxative	Glycerin
Dopamine agonist	Bromocriptine mesylate
	Levodopa
	Pergolide
	Pergolide mesylate
	Selegiline hydrochloride
Emetic	Apomorphine hydrochloride
	Ipecac
Expectorant; muscle relaxant	Guaifenesin
Fluid replacement	Dextran
	Dextrose solution
	Hetastarch
	Lactated Ringer's solution
	Pentastarch
	Ringer's solution
	Sodium chloride 0.9%
	Sodium chloride 7.2%
Hepatic protectant	S-adenosylmethionine (SAMe)
	Silymarin
Hormone	Altrenogest
	Colony-stimulating factors
	Corticotropin
	Cosyntropin
	Danazol
	Desmopressin acetate
	Diethylstilbestrol
	Epoetin alpha (erythropoietin)
	Estradiol cypionate
	Estriol
	Gonadorelin hydrochloride, gonadorelin diacetate tetrahydrate
	Gonadotropin, chorionic
	Growth hormone
	Insulin
	Levothyroxine sodium
	Liothyronine sodium
	Medroxyprogesterone acetate
	Megestrol acetate
	Mibolerone
	Testosterone
	Urofollitropin
	Vasopressin
Hormone, anabolic agent	Boldenone undecylenate
	Methyltestosterone
	Nandrolone decanoate
	Oxymetholone
	Stanozolol
Hormone, antagonist	Finasteride
Hormone, labor induction	Oxytocin
Hormone, thyroid	Thyroid-releasing hormone
	Thyrotropin
Immunostimulant	Interferon
	Lithium carbonate
Immunosuppressive agent	Auranofin
	Aurothioglucose
	Azathioprine
	Cyclophosphamide
	Cyclosporine
	Gold sodium thiomalate
	Mycophenolate
	Tacrolimus
Iodine supplement	Iodide
	Potassium iodide
	Sodium iodide (20%)
Laxative	Bisacodyl
	Cascara sagrada
	Castor oil
	Docusate
	Lactulose
	Magnesium citrate
	Magnesium hydroxide
	Mineral oil
	Polyethylene glycol electrolyte solution

DRUG CLASSIFICATION	DRUG NAME
	Psyllium
	Senna
	Ursodeoxycholic acid
	Ursodiol
Laxative, antiarrhythmic	Magnesium sulfate
Local anesthetic	Bupivacaine hydrochloride
	Mepivacaine
Local anesthetic, antiarrhythmic	Lidocaine hydrochloride
Mucolytic, antidote	Acetylcysteine
Muscle relaxant	Atracurium besylate
	Dantrolene sodium
	Methocarbamol
	Pancuronium bromide
Nutritional supplement	Ferrous sulfate
	Iron dextran
	MCT oil
	Taurine
	Zinc
Opioid antagonist	Naloxone hydrochloride
	Naltrexone
Pancreatic enzyme	Pancrelipase
Phosphate supplement, urine acidifier	Potassium phosphate
Potassium supplement	Potassium chloride
	Potassium gluconate
Prokinetic agent	Cisapride
	Domperidone
	Methylnaltrexone
	Metronidazole
	Tegaserod
Prostaglandin	Cloprostenol
	Dinoprost tromethamine
	Prostaglandin F_2 alpha
Respiratory stimulant	Doxapram hydrochloride
Tranquilizer, benzodiazepine	Alprazolam
Tranquilizer, phenothiazine	Acepromazine maleate
Vasodilator	Hydralazine hydrochloride
	Irbesartan
	Isosorbide dinitrate
	Isosorbide mononitrate
	Isoxsuprine
	Nitroglycerin
	Nitroprusside (sodium nitroprusside)
	Phenoxybenzamine hydrochloride
	Phentolamine mesylate
	Prazosin
	Sildenafil
Vasodilator, ACE inhibitor	Benazepril hydrochloride
	Captopril
	Enalapril maleate
	Lisinopril
	Ramipril
	Trandolapril
Vasodilator, calcium channel blocker	Amlodipine besylate
	Losartan
	Nifedipine
Vasopressor	Arginine vasopressin
	Methoxamine
	Phenylephrine hydrochloride
Vitamin	Ascorbic acid
	Cyanocobalamin
	Dihydrotachysterol
	Ergocalciferol
	Phytonadione
	Riboflavin
	Thiamine hydrochloride
	Vitamin A
	Vitamin E
	Vitamin K

From Papich MG: Handbook of veterinary drugs, St. Louis, 2010, Saunders.

Controlled Substances Information Summary

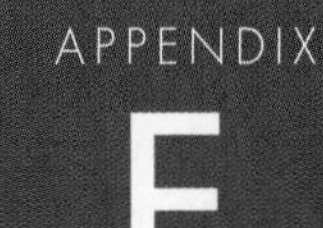

APPENDIX F

Drugs that have been determined to have potential for abuse by people are classified as controlled substances. Controlled substances are regulated through the efforts of the U.S. Drug Enforcement Administration (DEA), which enforces the regulations of the Controlled Substances Act (CSA) and the DEA regulations of Title 21, Code of Federal Regulations (CFR), Parts 1300 to 1316. Much valuable information related to the CSA and the CFR is available online at www.deadiversion.usdoj.gov.

Information that may be found at the DEA Diversion website includes but is not limited to the following:

- Applications and online forms, including Form 106, Report of Theft and Loss of Controlled Substances
- A complete list of controlled substances and the schedule of each
- A list of Drugs and Chemicals of Concern that includes both controlled and noncontrolled drugs (e.g., Tramadol) whose abuse potential concerns the DEA
- Information about proposed or new regulations under the CFR
- Offices and directories, including a list of DEA offices and officials throughout the United States
- A *Practitioner's Manual* that summarizes much of the CSA and CFR

SCHEDULES OF CONTROLLED SUBSTANCES

Drugs that are under the control of the Controlled Substances Act are placed into five schedules, or classes, according to their potential for abuse. This schedule is designated by a *C* with a Roman numeral (I, II, III, IV, or V) inside the C.

Schedule I substances have no (or controversial) accepted medical use and a high potential for abuse. Lysergic acid diethylamide (LSD), heroin, crack cocaine, marijuana, and peyote are substances in this class. The use of medicinal marijuana in human medicine is controversial but may be permitted in some states.

Schedule II drugs have accepted medical uses but have a high potential for abuse. A partial list of schedule II drugs includes morphine, meperidine, codeine, cocaine, oxymorphone, amphetamines, and pentobarbital. Orders for schedule II drugs must be made using the DEA Form 222.

Schedule III substances have less potential for abuse than those in schedule II and include Hycodan, paregoric, barbiturates such as thiamylal or thiopental, and anabolic steroids.

Schedule IV drugs have lower abuse potential than those in schedule III. Included in this class are phenobarbital, diazepam, and pentazocine.

Schedule V drugs are the lowest on the scale of abuse potential and include mostly antidiarrheal and anticough medications. Lomotil and Robitussin with codeine are in this schedule.

REGISTRATION REQUIREMENTS

Every person or entity that handles controlled substances must be registered with the DEA or be exempt under the regulations. DEA registration gives practitioners the authority to handle controlled substances. The DEA-registered practitioner may engage only in those activities that are allowed under state law in the state in which the practice is located. In some cases, state law is more stringent than federal law. In all cases, the most stringent regulation takes precedence. To obtain DEA registration, a practitioner must apply using DEA Form 224, which can be submitted as a hard copy or online.

A practitioner must be registered with the DEA in each state in which controlled substances are prescribed, administered, or dispensed. Also, a separate registration is required for each place of business or practice where controlled substances are stored or dispensed. An exemption is made that allows affiliated (employee) veterinarians to act on behalf of registered veterinarians to administer or dispense controlled substances. The affiliated practitioner cannot write prescriptions under this exemption and may need state registration.

The person who holds the registration must keep the information on the registration certificate current. A letter of request must be made to alter the name or address or to approve a change in schedule on the certificate. A DEA modification must be issued before applications related to the request may be carried out by the registrant. Registrations must be renewed every 3 years.

SECURITY REQUIREMENTS

CFR regulations require that all registrants provide effective measures and procedures to guard against theft or diversion of controlled substances. The *DEA Practitioner's Manual* lists several factors that may be used to determine the adequacy of security measures. Those factors include the following:

- Location of the premises
- Type of building and its construction
- Type and quantity of controlled substances kept on the premises
- Type of storage container
- Control of public access to the facility
- Adequacy of premise monitoring systems
- Availability of police protection

Regulations require that schedule II through V controlled substances be stored in a "securely locked, substantially constructed cabinet." If the registrant stores carfentanil, etorphine, and/or diprenorphine, a safe or steel cabinet equivalent to a U.S. Government Class V security container (General Services Administration specifications) must be used.

Regulations state that a registrant should limit access to controlled substances according to the following guidelines. Access should be denied to the following:

- Any person convicted of a felony related to a controlled substance
- Any person denied a DEA registration
- Any person who has had a DEA registration revoked
- Any person who has surrendered a DEA license for cause

Registrants must notify the DEA of any theft or "significant loss" of controlled substances using DEA Form 106 as soon as the theft or loss is discovered.

RECORD-KEEPING REQUIREMENTS

Registrants under the CSA must maintain specific records. The *Practitioner's Manual* states that records, inventories, and records of substances in schedules I and II must be maintained separately from all other records. It further states that records of substances in schedules III, IV, and V must be maintained separately or on a form that is readily retrievable from ordinary business records of the practitioner. Thus, the registrant must have two separate sets of records for controlled substances. The records for schedules III, IV, and V can be kept with records for noncontrolled substances if they can be easily retrieved. Schedule II records are usually kept in a controlled substances log, and schedule III, IV, and V drugs are kept in a controlled substances log and/or in a computer inventory system. The American Animal Hospital Association publishes a controlled substances log for purchase that may avoid pitfalls of hospital/clinic-constructed logs. Entries in the log should be made in ink with great care, and mistakes should be marked through, corrected, and initialed.

Each registrant must maintain a "complete and accurate record of the controlled substances on hand and date the inventory was conducted." This record must be in written, typewritten, or printed form and maintained at the registration location for 2 years. After the first inventory is taken, a new inventory must be carried out every 2 years. Regulations state that each inventory must contain the following information:

- Whether the inventory was taken at the beginning or the end of the business day

- Names of the controlled substances
- Each form of the controlled substances (e.g., 50-mg tablet)
- Number of dosage units in each container (e.g., 100-tablet bottles)
- Number of commercial containers of each form (e.g., two 100-tablet bottles)
- Disposition of the controlled substances
- Name, address, and DEA registration number of the registrant
- Signature of the person performing the inventory

DISPOSAL OF CONTROLLED SUBSTANCES

A practitioner may dispose of out-of-date, damaged, or otherwise unusable or unwanted controlled substances by transferring them to a registrant who is authorized to receive them. These registrants are referred to as "reverse distributors." A list of authorized reverse distributors can be found in Appendix E of the *Practitioner's Manual.* Practitioners are advised to keep for 2 years copies of the records that document such transfer. Another method of disposal involves destruction of drugs in the presence of a DEA agent or other authorized person. This method is not generally encouraged by the DEA. The "pour-it-down-the-drain" method should be discouraged because it may contaminate the water supply.

VALID PRESCRIPTION REQUIREMENTS

Controlled substances are also prescription drugs. The dispensing or administering of a prescription drug requires a valid veterinarian–client–patient relationship (VCPR). The dispensing or administering of such a drug without a valid VCPR is illegal under federal law. A prescription for a controlled substance must be signed and dated on the date of issue. The prescription must include the patient's (owner's) full name and address, the practitioner's full name and address, and the practitioner's DEA number. It must be written in ink or indelible pencil or printed, and it must be manually signed by the practitioner on the date issued. A designated individual may be assigned to prepare prescriptions for the practitioner's signature. The prescription also must include the following:

- Drug name
- Drug strength
- Dosage form
- Quantity prescribed
- Directions for use
- Number of refills authorized

Bibliography

Ahrens AA: Pharmacology, the national veterinary medical series for independent study, Philadelphia, 1996, Lippincott Williams & Wilkins.

Anderson KN, Anderson L, editors: Mosby's pocket dictionary of medicine, nursing, and allied health, St. Louis, 1998, Mosby.

Anderson KN, Anderson L, editors: Mosby's pocket dictionary of medicine, nursing, and allied health, ed 4, St. Louis, 2002, Mosby.

Anonymous: *White paper: rogue Internet pharmacies* (website). http://www.avma.org/noah/members/scientific/prescribing/white_paper.asp. Accessed March 10, 2001.

Barragry TB: Cardiac disease: veterinary drug therapy, Philadelphia, 1994, Lea & Febiger.

Barton CL: Chemotherapy. In Boothe DM, editor: Small animal clinical pharmacology and therapeutics, Philadelphia, 2001, WB Saunders.

Bill R, editor: Pharmacology for veterinary technicians, Goleta, Calif, 1993, American Veterinary Publications.

Birchard S, Sherding R, editors: Saunders manual of small animal practice, Philadelphia, 1994, WB Saunders.

Blankenship J, Campbell JB, editors: Laboratory mathematics: medical and biological applications, St. Louis, 1976, Mosby.

Bonagura JD, editor: Kirk's current veterinary therapy XIII: small animal practice, Philadelphia, 2000, WB Saunders.

Boothe DM: Nutraceuticals in veterinary medicine: part I: definitions and regulations, Compend Contin Educ Pract Vet 19(11):1248–1255, 1997.

Boothe DM, editor: The veterinary clinics of North America, small animal practice, Philadelphia, 1998, WB Saunders.

Boothe DM: Small animal clinical pharmacology and therapeutics, Philadelphia, 2001, WB Saunders.

Brander GC, Pugh DM, Bywater RJ, et al, editors: Veterinary applied pharmacology and therapeutics, ed 5, London, 1991, Bailliere Tindall.

Carter GR, Chengappa MM, Roberts AW, editors: Essentials of veterinary microbiology, Baltimore, 1995, Williams & Wilkins.

Cowgill LD: Managing renal disease and hypertension, 1991, Harmon-Smith.

Crow SE, Walshaw SO, editors: Manual of clinical procedures in the dog and cat, Philadelphia, 1987, JB Lippincott.

Davidson G: Pharmacy update: new FDA policy gives clear guidance for compounding, Vet Tech 18(3):195–201, 1997.

Davidson G: Glucosamine and chondroitin sulfate, Compend Contin Educ Pract Vet 22(5):454–458, 2000.

Davidson G: S-adenosylmethionine, Compend Contin Educ Pract Vet 24(8):600–603, 2002.

DeLahunta A, editor: Veterinary neuroanatomy and clinical neurology, Philadelphia, 1983, WB Saunders.

DeNovo RC: Chronic vomiting in the cat and dog, in Proceedings. Am Vet Med Assoc, Nashville, Tenn, 2002.

DiBartola SP, editor: Fluid therapy in small animal practice, ed 2, Philadelphia, 2000, WB Saunders.

Dowling PM: Respiratory drugs, in Proceedings. Annu Meet Am Vet Med Assoc, Boston, 2001.

Ettinger SJ, editor: Textbook of veterinary internal medicine, ed 3, Philadelphia, 1989, WB Saunders.

Ettinger SJ, editor: Textbook of veterinary internal medicine, ed 5, vol I and II, Philadelphia, 1993, WB Saunders.

Fascetti AJ: *Nutraceuticals and food faddism* (website). http://www.avma.org/noah/-default.asp. Accessed January 8, 1998.

Ford RB: Vaccines and vaccinations: issues for the 21st century, Suppl Compend Contin Educ Pract Vet 20(8C):19–24, 1998.

Foushee LL: Omeprazole, Compend Contin Educ Pract Vet 22(8):746–749, 2000.

Ganong WF: Review of medical physiology, ed 21, New York, 2003, McGraw-Hill.

Gelatt KN: Textbook of veterinary ophthalmology, Philadelphia, 1981, Lea & Febiger.

Giovanoni R, Warren RC: Cardiovascular drugs. In Giovanoni R, Warren RC, editors: Principles of pharmacology, St. Louis, 1983, Mosby.

Hall JA, Washabau RJ: Gastrointestinal prokinetic therapy: dopaminergic antagonist drugs, Compend Contin Educ Pract Vet 19(2):214–219, 1997.

Hamlin RL: Cardiovascular system, introduction, in Proceedings. Music City Vet Conf, Nashville, Tenn, 2003.

Hand MS, Thatcher CD, Remillard RL, et al, editors: Small animal clinical nutrition, ed 4, Topeka, Kan, 2000, Mark Morris Institute.

Haskins SC: Fluid overload: how to identify and manage, in Proceedings. Int Vet Emerg Crit Care Symp, Orlando, Fla, 2000.

Hendrix CM, Robinson E, editors: Diagnostic veterinary parasitology, ed 2, St. Louis, 1998, Mosby.

Hoffman AM: What's new with aerosol medications in the horse, in Proceedings. Annu Meet Am Vet Med Assoc, Boston, 2001.

Jenkins WL: Chemotherapeutic agents affecting host cellular functions: antineoplastics and immunomodulators. In Brander GC, Pugh DM, Bywater RJ, et al, editors: Veterinary applied pharmacology and therapeutics, ed 5, London, 1991, Bailliere Tindall.

Kirk RW, editor: Current veterinary therapy VIII: small animal practice, Philadelphia, 1983, WB Saunders.

Kirk RW, Bonagura JD, editors: Current veterinary therapy X: small animal practice, Philadelphia, 1989, WB Saunders.

Kirk RW, Bonagura JD, editors: Current veterinary therapy XII: small animal practice, Philadelphia, 1995, WB Saunders.
Lane DR, Cooper BC, editors: Veterinary nursing, ed 2, Oxford, England, 1999, Butterworth-Heinemann.
Lane DR, Cooper VN, editors: Veterinary nursing, ed 3, Oxford, 2003, Butterworth-Heinemann.
Langston VC, Mercer HD: Nonsteroidal antiinflammatory drugs, in Proceedings. 17th Semin Vet Techs, West Vet Conf, Las Vegas, 1988.
Lavoie JP: Inhalation therapy for equine heaves, Comp Contin Educ Pract Vet 23(5):475–477, 2001.
Locklar CF Jr, Locklar MS: Personal interview, March 12, 2003.
Lukens RL, Landon RM: A guide to inventory management for veterinary practices: effective inventory control, West Chester, Pa, 1993, SmithKline Beecham Animal Health.
MacEwen EG, Rosenthal RC: Approach to treatment of cancer patients. In Ettinger SJ, editor: Textbook of veterinary internal medicine, ed 5, Philadelphia, 2000, WB Saunders.
McCurnin DM, Bassert JM, editors: Clinical textbook for veterinary technicians, ed 5, Philadelphia, 2002, WB Saunders.
McCurnin DM, Bassert JM, Thomas J, editors: Clinical textbook for veterinary technicians, ed 8, St. Louis, 2014. Elsevier.
McKiernan B: Respiratory therapeutics, in Proceedings. 17th Semin Vet Techs, West Vet Conf, Las Vegas, 1988.
Mealey KL: Clinically significant drug interactions, Compend Contin Educ Pract Vet 24(1):10–22, 2002.
Muir WW, DiBartola SP: Fluid therapy. In Kirk RW, editor: Current veterinary therapy VIII: small animal practice, Philadelphia, 1983, WB Saunders.
Muir WW, Hubbell JA: Handbook of veterinary anesthesia, ed 3, St. Louis, 2000, Mosby.
Muller GH, Kirk RW, Scott DW: Small animal dermatology, ed 4, Philadelphia, 1989, WB Saunders.
Norsworthy GD: Clinical aspects of feline blood transfusions, Comp Contin Educ Pract Vet 14:470, 1992.
Paddleford RR: Manual of small animal anesthesia, Philadelphia, 1999, WB Saunders.
Papich MG: Handbook of veterinary drugs, Philadelphia, 2002, WB Saunders.
Parker AR: Domperidone, Compend Contin Educ Pract Vet 23(10):906–908, 2001.
Plumb DC: Veterinary drug handbook, ed 4, Ames, Iowa, 2002, Iowa State University Press.
Plumb DC: Veterinary drug handbook, ed 7, Ames, Iowa, 2011, Wiley-Blackwell.
Quinn PJ, Donnelly ME, Carter BK, et al, editors: Microbial and parasitic diseases of the dog and cat, London, 1997, Saunders.
Scott DW, Miller WH, Griffin CE: Small animal dermatology, ed 6, Philadelphia, 2001, WB Saunders.
Shull EA: Psychopharmacology in veterinary behavioral medicine, in Proceedings. Annu Conf Vet Tech, UT-CVM, Knoxville, Tenn, 1998.
Simpson BS, Simpson DM: Behavioral pharmacotherapy: part I: antipsychotics and antidepressants, Compend Contin Educ Pract Vet 18(10):1067–1081, 1996.
Simpson BS, Simpson DM: Behavioral pharmacotherapy: part II: anxiolytics and mood stabilizers, Compend Contin Educ Pract Vet 18(11):1203–1210, 1996.
Smith P: New studies, products fuel heartworm debate. Vet Prod News 11(4):34–36, 1999.
Snyder S, editor: Drugs and the brain, New York, 1986, Scientific American Library.
Spinelli JS, Enos LR, editors: Drugs in veterinary practice, St. Louis, 1978, Mosby.
Tilley LP, Smith WK: The 5-minute veterinary consult canine and feline, ed 2, Baltimore, 2000, Lippincott Williams & Wilkins.
Tizard I: Veterinary immunology: an introduction, ed 4, Philadelphia, 1992, WB Saunders.
Tizard I: Veterinary immunology: an introduction, ed 6, Philadelphia, 2000, WB Saunders.
Upson DW: Handbook of clinical veterinary pharmacology, ed 4, Manhattan, Kan, 1988, Dan Upson Enterprises.
Ware WA: Problems in chronic heart failure management, in Proceedings. Am Vet Med Assoc Annu Conf, Nashville, Tenn, 2002.
Webb AI, Aeschbacher G: Animal drug container labels: a guide to the reader, J Am Vet Med Assoc 202:1591–1599, 1993.
Williams BR, Baer C, editors: Essentials of clinical pharmacology in nursing, Springhouse, Pa, 1990, Springhouse Corp.

Glossary

acetylcholine A neurotransmitter that allows a nerve impulse to cross the synaptic junction (gap) between two nerve fibers or between a nerve fiber and an organ (e.g., muscle, gland).

acetylcholinesterase An enzyme that brings about the breakdown of acetylcholine in the synaptic gap.

active immunity Immunity that occurs by an animal's own immune response after exposure to foreign antigen.

Addison's disease A disease or syndrome characterized by inadequate amounts of corticosteroid hormones.

adjuvant A substance given with an antigen to enhance the immune response to the antigen. Adjuvants may form a localized granuloma at the injection site or may produce systemic hypersensitivity. Adjuvants have received much attention as a result of a possible (but not proven) link with the increased incidence of fibrosarcomas in vaccinated cats. Examples of adjuvants are aluminum hydroxide, aluminum phosphate, aluminum potassium sulfate, water in oil, saponin, and diethylaminoethyl (DEAE) dextran.

adrenergic A term used to describe an action or a receptor that is activated by epinephrine or norepinephrine.

adsorbent A drug that inhibits gastrointestinal absorption of drugs, toxins, or chemicals by attracting and holding them to its surface.

adverse drug event Harm to a patient caused by a therapeutic or preventive intervention. It could be due to a medication error or adverse drug reaction.

adverse drug reaction An undesirable response to a drug by a patient. It may vary in severity from mild to fatal.

aerosolization The conversion of a liquid into a fine mist or colloidal suspension in air.

afterload The resistance (pressure) in arteries that must be overcome to empty blood from the ventricle.

agonist A drug that brings about a specific action by binding with the appropriate receptor.

alkylation Formation of a linkage between a substance and DNA that causes irreversible inhibition of the DNA molecule. Alkylating drugs are used in chemotherapy treatment of cancer.

anabolism The constructive phase of metabolism in which body cells repair and replace tissue.

analgesia The absence of the sensation of pain.

analogue A chemical compound having a structure similar to another but differing from it in some way.

anaphylaxis A systemic, severe allergic reaction.

anesthesia The loss of all sensation. May be described as local (affecting a small area), regional, or surgical (accompanied by unconsciousness).

angiogenesis The development of blood vessels.

antagonist A drug that inhibits a specific action by binding with a particular receptor.

anthelmintic Drug used to eliminate helminth parasites (e.g., roundworms) from a host.

antibacterial An agent that inhibits bacterial growth, impedes replication of bacteria, or kills bacteria.

antibiotic An agent produced by a microorganism or semi-synthetically that has the ability to inhibit the growth of or kill microorganisms.

antibody An immunoglobulin molecule that combines with the specific antigen that induced its formation.

anticholinergic Blocking nerve impulse transmission through the parasympathetic nervous system; also called *parasympatholytic.* Anticholinergic drugs may be used for the treatment of diarrhea or vomiting.

antigen Any substance that can induce a specific immune response, such as toxins, foreign proteins, bacteria, and viruses.

antimicrobial An agent that kills microorganisms or suppresses their multiplication or growth.

antiseptic A substance used on the skin to prevent the growth of bacteria or to provide preoperative cleansing of the skin.

antitussive A drug that inhibits or suppresses the cough reflex.

arrhythmia (dysrhythmia) A variation from the normal rhythm.

astringent An agent that causes contraction after application to tissue.

atony The absence or lack of normal tone or strength.

autologous Belonging to the same organism.

automaticity The ability of cardiac muscle to generate impulses.

autonomic nervous system That portion of the nervous system that controls involuntary activities.

average cost of inventory on hand Average cost of inventory on hand is determined by adding the year's beginning inventory to the year's ending inventory and dividing by 2.

avirulent The inability of an infectious agent to produce pathologic effects.

bacteria Single-celled microorganisms that usually have a rigid cell wall and a round, rod-like, or spiral shape.

bactericidal An agent with the capability to kill bacteria.

bacterin A killed bacterial vaccine.

bacteriostatic An agent that inhibits the growth or reproduction of bacteria.

beta-Lactamase Enzymes that reduce the effectiveness of certain antibiotics; beta-lactamase I is penicillinase; beta-lactamase II is cephalosporinase.

blepharospasm Squinting of the eye.

bots Larvae of several fly species (e.g., *Gasterophilus* [horse bot]).

bradyarrhythmia Bradycardia associated with an irregularity of heart rhythm.

bradycardia A slower-than-normal heart rate.

bronchoconstriction Narrowing of the bronchi and bronchioles, which results in increased airway resistance and decreased airflow.

bronchodilation Widening lumen of bronchi and bronchioles, which results from relaxation of smooth muscle in the walls of the bronchi and bronchioles. Airway resistance is decreased, and airflow is increased.

buffer A substance that decreases the change in pH when an acid or base is added.

callus Hypertrophy of the horny layer of the epidermis in a localized area as a result of pressure or friction.

cardiac remodeling Change in the size, shape, structure, and physiology of the heart due to damage to the myocardium.

catalepsy A state of involuntary muscle rigidity that is accompanied by immobility, amnesia, and variable amounts of analgesia. Some reflexes may be preserved.

catecholamine The class of neurotransmitters that includes dopamine, epinephrine, and norepinephrine. When given therapeutically, catecholamines mimic the effects of stimulating the sympathetic nervous system.

cell cycle–nonspecific Capable of acting in several or all cell cycle phases.

cell cycle–specific Capable of acting during a particular cell cycle phase only.

cerumen A waxy secretion of the glands of the external ear canal.

cestode A tapeworm.

chelating agent An agent used in chemotherapy for metal poisoning.

chemoreceptor trigger zone (CRTZ) An area in the brain that activates the vomiting center when stimulated by toxic substances in the blood.

cholinergic Activated by or transmitted through acetylcholine; also called parasympathomimetic. Cholinergic drugs increase activity in the gastrointestinal tract.

chronotropic Affecting the heart rate.

closed-angle glaucoma A type of primary glaucoma of the eye that is characterized by a shallow anterior chamber and a narrow angle that compromises filtration because the iris is blocking the angle and is causing an increase in intraocular pressure.

collagen A fibrous substance found in skin, tendon, bone, cartilage, and all other connective tissues.

colloid A chemical system composed of a continuous medium throughout which small particles are distributed and do not settle out under the influence of gravity.

colony forming unit (CFI) An estimate of viable bacterial or fungal numbers.

comedo (pl. comedones) A plug of keratin and sebum within a hair follicle of the skin.

compounding Any manipulation (e.g., diluting, combining) performed to produce a dosage-form drug, other than the manipulations described in the directions for use on the labeling of an approved drug product.

conjunctivitis Inflammation of the conjunctiva.

counterirritant An agent that produces superficial irritation that is intended to relieve some other irritation.

cream A semisolid preparation of oil, water, and a medicinal agent.

Cushing's disease or syndrome Hyperadrenocorticism; a disease or syndrome characterized by an overabundance of corticosteroid hormones.

cycloplegia Paralysis of the ciliary muscle.

cytotoxic Capable of destroying cells.

DEA form An official federal government carbon form from the Drug Enforcement Administration used for ordering controlled substances.

decongestant A substance that reduces the swelling of mucous membranes.

deep pain Pain arising from deep receptors in the periosteum, tendons, and joint structures.

delayed billing A benefit that some companies offer to the buyer who is purchasing increased amounts of merchandise. The date the statement must be paid is usually longer than 30 to 60 days away.

dentifrice A preparation for cleansing teeth that is available in a powder, paste, or liquid.

depolarization Neutralizing of the polarity of a cardiac cell by an inflow of sodium ions. Depolarization results in contraction of the cardiac cell and renders it incapable of further contraction until repolarization occurs.

dermatitis Inflammation of the skin.

dermatophyte Fungi parasitic on the skin.

dermatophytosis A fungal skin infection.

detergent An agent that cleanses.

detrusor The smooth muscle of the urinary bladder that is mainly responsible for emptying the bladder during urination.

detrusor areflexia The absence of detrusor contractions.

disinfect To make free of pathogens or make them inactive.

disseminated intravascular coagulation (DIC) Widespread formation of clots (thrombi) in the microscopic blood vessels of the circulatory system. DIC occurs as a complication of a wide variety of disorders and consumes clotting factors, with resultant bleeding.

dissociation The act of separating into ionic components (NaCl → Na and Cl).

distichia (distichiasis) Eyelashes emerge through the meibomian gland opening at the eyelid margin in a misdirected way, causing the eyelashes to touch and irritate the corneal surface.

dosage rate Determination of the amount of dose to be administered (e.g., 10 mg/kg).

dose The amount of drug to be administered to a patient (e.g., 100 mg).

downregulation A decrease in the number of cellular receptors to a molecule resulting in reduced sensitivity to the molecule.

drug A substance used to diagnose, prevent, or treat disease.

dystocia Difficult birth.

ectoparasite A parasite that lives on the outside body surface of its host.

ectropion A rolling outward (i.e., away from the eye) or sagging of the eyelid. Many times, the conjunctiva is plainly visible.

effector A gland, organ, or tissue that responds to nerve stimulation with a specific action.

efficacy The extent to which a drug causes the intended effects in a patient.

electrolyte A substance that dissociates into ions when placed in solution, becoming capable of conducting electricity.

elixir A hydroalcoholic liquid that contains sweeteners, flavoring, and a medicinal agent.

emesis The act of vomiting.

empirical Based on observation and personal experience.

emulsion A medicinal agent that consists of oily substances dispersed in an aqueous medium with an additive to stabilize the dispersion.

endometrium The mucous membrane lining of the uterus.

endoparasite A parasite that lives inside the body of its host.

endothelial layer The smooth layer of epithelial cells that line blood vessels.

entropion A rolling inward (i.e., toward the cornea) of the eyelid.

equivalent weight One gram molecular weight (from periodic chart) divided by the total positive valence of the material.

erythema Redness of the skin caused by congestion of the capillaries.

erythropoiesis The formation of erythrocytes.

erythropoietin A glycoprotein hormone secreted mainly by the kidney; it acts on stem cells of the bone marrow to stimulate red blood cell production.

euthyroid A normal thyroid gland.

expectorant A drug that enhances the expulsion of secretions from the respiratory tract.

extralabel use The use of a drug that is not specifically listed on the U.S. Food and Drug Administration (FDA)-approved label.

exudation Leakage of fluid, cells, or cellular debris from blood vessels and their deposition in or on the tissue.

fatty acid Organic compound of carbon, hydrogen, and oxygen that is esterified with glycerol to form fat.

feed efficiency The rate at which animals convert feed into tissue. It is expressed as the number of pounds or kilograms of feed needed to produce 1 lb or 1 kg of animal.

feedback The return of some of the output product of a process as input in a way that controls the process.

fibrinolysis Fibrin (clot) breakdown through the action of the enzyme plasmin.

FIFO Acronym for "first in, first out."

FOB Acronym for "free on board."

FOB destination Title of possession passes from the pharmaceutic company to the buyer (i.e., the purchaser) when the shipment is delivered to the buyer's business destination (i.e., the veterinary facility).

FOB shipping point Title passes from the pharmaceutic company to the purchaser when the vendor places the goods in the possession of the carrier (e.g., United Parcel Service, Federal Express, Averitt Express).

full-service company A pharmaceutic company that offers full service (e.g., the company employs sales representatives [reps] who visit veterinary facilities), usually with a limited number of products.

fungicidal An agent that kills fungi.

fungistatic An agent that inhibits the growth of fungi.

furuncle (furunculosis) A focal suppurative inflammation of the skin and subcutaneous tissue; also known as a *boil.*

ganglionic synapse The site of the synapse between neuron one and neuron two of the autonomic nervous system.

glaucoma A group of eye diseases characterized by increased intraocular pressure that results in damage to the retina and the optic nerve.

gonadotropin A hormone that stimulates the ovaries or testes.

granulation tissue New tissue formed in the healing of wounds of the soft tissue, consisting of connective tissue cells and ingrown young vessels; it ultimately forms a scar.

Green Book An on-line resource listing all FDA approved animal drugs.

half-life The amount of time (usually expressed in hours) that it takes for the quantity of a drug in the body to be reduced by 50%.

helminths Parasitic worms, including nematodes, cestodes, and trematodes.

hematemesis Vomiting of blood (the vomitus often resembles coffee grounds).

hematuria Blood in the urine.

histamine A chemical mediator of the inflammatory response released from mast cells. Histamine may cause dilation and increased permeability of small blood vessels, constriction of small airways, increased secretion of mucus in the airways, and pain.

Horner's syndrome Paralysis of the sympathetic nerve supply to the eye that may cause enophthalmos, ptosis of the upper eyelid, slight elevation of the lower eyelid, constriction of the pupil, and narrowing of the palpebral tissue.

humidification Addition of moisture to the air.

hybridoma A cell culture that consists of a clone of a hybrid cell formed by fusing cells of different types, such as stimulated mouse plasma cells and myeloma cells.

hyperalgesia A heightened sense of pain.

hyperkalemia An excess of potassium in the blood.

hypernatremia An excess of sodium in the blood.

hyphema A condition in which red blood cells are present in the anterior chamber of the eye(s).

hypertension Persistently high blood pressure.

hypertonus The state characterized by an increased tonicity or tension.

hypokalemia Abnormally low potassium concentration in the blood.

hyponatremia A deficiency of sodium in the blood.

hypophyseal portal system This is the portal system of the pituitary gland in which venules from the hypothalamus connect with capillaries of the anterior pituitary.

hypovolemia Decreased volume of circulating blood.

iatrogenic Caused by the physician (veterinarian).

Immunoglobulin A (IgA) Class of antibody produced on mucous membrane surfaces, such as those of the respiratory tract.

in vitro Within an artificial environment.

in vivo Within the living body.

inotropic Affecting the force of cardiac muscle contraction.

inspissated Thickened or dried out.

integumentary system Pertaining to, or composed of, skin.

interleukins A group of polypeptide cytokines that carry signals between cells in the immune system.

intracameral injection An injection into the anterior chamber of the eye.

inventory The quantity of goods or assets that a veterinary facility possesses, requiring proactive control to keep supplies stable and current.

inventory control manager (ICM) A person (many times a licensed veterinary medical technician [LVMT]) responsible for monitoring, ordering, and maintaining inventory in a veterinary facility.

invoice A form generated by a company that documents the quantity and price of each item ordered by the inventory control manager.

involution The return of a reproductive organ to normal size after delivery.

iodophor An iodine compound with a longer activity period that results from the combination of iodine and a carrier molecule that releases iodine over time.

keratitis Inflammation of the cornea.

keratolytic An agent that promotes loosening or separation of the horny layer of the epidermis.

keratoplastic An agent that promotes normalization of the development of keratin.

levo isomer Left-sided arrangement of a molecule that may exist in a left- or a right-sided configuration. Levo and dextro isomers have the same molecular formula.

liniment A medicine in an oily, soapy, or alcoholic vehicle to be rubbed on the skin to relieve pain or to act as a counterirritant.

lower motor neurons Peripheral neurons whose cell bodies lie in the central gray columns of the spinal cord and whose terminations lie in skeletal muscle. A sufficient number of lesions of lower motor neurons cause muscles supplied by the nerve to atrophy, resulting in weak reflexes and flaccid paralysis.

MRSA Methicillin-resistant *Staphylococcus aureus.*

mail order discount house A company that accepts orders from the buyer by telephone; a good source for ordering items such as gauze, cotton, isopropyl alcohol, or paper towels.

manufacturing The bulk production of drugs for resale outside of the veterinarian–client–patient relationship.

markup The amount of money over cost for which a product sells. Markup percentages vary from practice to practice, but all markups reflect a retail value over wholesale value.

matrix The intercellular substance of tissues like cartilage and bone.

melena Dark or black stools that result from blood staining. Bleeding has occurred in the anterior part of the gastrointestinal tract.

metabolic acidosis Decreased body pH caused by excess hydrogen ions in the extracellular fluid.

metabolic alkalosis Increased body pH caused by excess bicarbonate in the extracellular fluid.

metabolism (biotransformation) The biochemical process that alters a drug from an active form to a form that is inactive or that can be eliminated from the body.

metastasis Generally refers to the transfer of cancer cells from one site to another.

metered dose inhaler (MDI) A hand held device that uses a propellant to deliver a specific amount of medication that is inhaled into the lungs by the patient.

methemoglobinemia The presence of methemoglobin in the blood caused by injury or toxic agents that convert a larger-than-normal proportion of hemoglobin into methemoglobin, which does not function as an oxygen carrier.

microfilaria A prelarval stage of a filarial worm transmitted to the biting insect from the principal host (e.g., filarial stage of *Dirofilaria immitis*).

microorganism An organism that is microscopic (e.g., bacterium, protozoan, Rickettsia, virus, and fungus).

milliequivalent A term used to express the concentration of electrolytes in a solution; 1/1000 of an equivalent weight.

miosis Contraction of the pupil.

modulation The modification of nociceptive transmission.

monovalent A vaccine, antiserum, or antitoxin developed specifically for a single antigen or organism.

motilin A hormone secreted by cells in the duodenal mucosa that causes contraction of intestinal smooth muscle.

mucolytic Having the ability to break down mucus.

multimodal analgesia The use of different drugs with different actions to produce optimal analgesia and minimize individual drug quantities when possible.

muscarinic receptors Receptors activated by acetylcholine and muscarine that are found in glands, the heart, and smooth muscle. An acronym for remembering muscarinic effects is SLUD: S, salivation; L, lacrimation; U, urination; D, defecation.

mydriasis Dilation of the pupil.

myeloma A malignant neoplasm of plasma cells (B lymphocytes).

myelosuppression Inhibition of bone marrow activity that results in decreased production of blood cells and platelets.

myofibril A muscle fibril composed of numerous myofilaments.

nasogastric (intubation) Passing a flexible tube through the nasal passages into the stomach.

nebulization The process of converting liquid medications into a spray that can be carried into the respiratory system by inhaled air.

nematodes Parasitic worms, including intestinal roundworms, filarial worms, lungworms, kidney worms, heartworms, and others.

nephrology The study of the urinary (renal) system.

nephron The basic functional unit of the kidney.

nephrotoxic Toxic to the kidneys.

nerve block A loss of feeling or sensation produced by injecting an anesthetic agent around a nerve to interfere with its ability to conduct impulses.

neuropathic pain Pain that originates from injury or involvement of the peripheral or central nervous system.

nicotinic receptors Receptors activated by acetylcholine and nicotine found at the neuromuscular junction of the skeletal muscle and at the ganglionic synapses.

nitrogen balance The condition of the body as it relates to protein intake and use. Positive nitrogen balance implies a net gain in body protein.

nociception The reception, conduction, and central nervous system processing of nerve signals generated by nociceptors.

nonproductive cough A cough that does not result in coughing up of mucus, secretions, or debris (a dry cough).

nutraceutical Any nontoxic food component that has scientifically proven health benefits.

ointment A semisolid preparation that contains medicinal agents for application to the skin or eyes.

oncotic pressure The osmotic pressure generated by plasma proteins in the blood.

open-angle glaucoma A type of primary glaucoma of the eye in which the angle of the anterior chamber remains open, but filtration of the aqueous humor is gradually reduced, causing an increase in intraocular pressure.

organophosphate A substance that can interfere with the function of the nervous system by inhibiting the enzyme cholinesterase.

osmotic pressure The ability of solute molecules to attract water.

otoacariasis Infestation of ear mites.

ototoxic Toxic to the ears.

packing slip A document supplied by the vendor that accompanies a purchase. A packing slip generally reflects quantities ordered, not prices.

parasitiasis A condition in which an animal harbors an endoparasite or an ectoparasite but no clinical signs of infection or infestation are evident.

parasitosis A condition in which an animal harbors an endoparasite or an ectoparasite and clinical signs of infection or infestation are evident.

parasympathetic nervous system That portion of the autonomic nervous system that arises from the craniosacral portion of the spinal cord, is mediated by the neurotransmitter acetylcholine, and is concerned primarily with conserving and restoring a steady state in the body.

parasympathomimetic A drug that mimics the effects of stimulating the parasympathetic nervous system.

parenteral The route of administration of injectable drugs.

parenteral administration By a route other than the alimentary canal (e.g., intramuscular, subcutaneous, intravenous).

parietal cell A cell located in the gastric mucosa that secretes hydrochloric acid.

partition coefficient The ratio of the solubility of substances (e.g., gas anesthetics) between two states in which they may be found (e.g., blood and gas, gas and rubber goods).

passive immunity Immunity that occurs by administration of antibody produced in another individual.

pathologic pain Pain with an exaggerated response; it is often associated with tissue injury due to trauma or surgery.

percent concentration An expression of the strength of a substance based on the ratio of parts per hundred (e.g., 25%).

perception The processing and recognition of pain in the cerebral hemispheres.

peristalsis A wave of smooth muscle contraction that passes along a tubular structure (gastrointestinal or other) and moves the contents of that structure forward.

physiologic pain The protective sensation of pain that allows individuals to move away from potential tissue damage.

polydipsia Excessive thirst manifested by increased water consumption.

polyuria Excessive urination.

polyvalent A vaccine, antiserum, or antitoxin active against multiple antigens or organisms; mixed vaccine.

preemptive analgesia Analgesia administered before the painful stimulus to help prevent sensitization and windup.

preload The volume of blood in the ventricles at the end of diastole.

premature ventricular contraction (PVC) Contraction of the ventricles without a corresponding contraction of the atria. PVCs arise from an irritable focus or foci in the ventricles.

prescription (legend) drug A drug that is limited to use under the supervision of a veterinarian because of potential danger, difficulty of administration, or other considerations. The legend that designates a prescription drug states the following: "Caution: Federal law restricts this drug to use by or on the order of a licensed veterinarian."

preservative A substance, such as an antibiotic, antiinfective, or fungistat, that is added to a product to destroy or inhibit multiplication of microorganisms.

primary hypothyroidism Hypothyroidism resulting from a pathologic condition in the thyroid.

productive cough A cough that results in coughing up of mucus, secretions, or debris.

prostaglandin A substance synthesized by cells from arachidonic acid that serves as a mediator of inflammation and has other physiologic functions.

pruritus Itching.

pseudomembranous colitis A severe acute inflammation of the bowel mucosa.

pyoderma Any skin disease characterized by the presence or formation of pus.

ratio concentration An expression of the strength of a substance based on the ratio of its parts (e.g., 1:32).

recombinant DNA technology A process that removes a gene from one organism or pathogen and inserts it into the DNA of another. This also may be referred to as *gene splicing.*

regimen A program for administration of a drug that includes the route, the dose (how much), the frequency (how often), and the duration (for how long) of administration.

regional anesthesia Loss of feeling or sensation in a large area (region) of the body after injection of an anesthetic agent into the spinal canal or around peripheral nerves.

regurgitation Casting up of undigested or semidigested (ruminant) foodstuff from the esophagus or rumen.

releasing factor (releasing hormone) A hormone produced by the hypothalamus and transported to the anterior pituitary to stimulate the release of trophic hormones.

repolarization The return of the cell membrane to its resting polarity after depolarization.

residue An amount of a drug still present in animal tissue or products (e.g., meat, milk, eggs) at a particular point (slaughter or collection).

retroperitoneal Located behind the peritoneum.

reverse sneeze Aspiration reflex—short periods of noisy inspiratory effort in dogs.

seborrhea An increase in scaling of the skin; sebum production may or may not be increased.

seborrhea oleosa Condition characterized by scaling and excess lipid production that forms brownish yellow clumps, which adhere to the hair and skin.

seborrhea sicca Characterized by dry skin and white to gray scales that do not adhere to the hair or skin.

seborrheic dermatitis An inflammatory type of seborrhea characterized by scaling and greasiness.

segmentation Periodic constriction of segments of the intestine without movement backward or forward; a mixing rather than a propulsive movement.

solute A substance dissolved in a solvent to form a solution.

solution A mixture of two substances not chemically combined with each other.

somatic pain Pain arising from bones, joints, muscle or skin. Somatic pain is described in humans as localized, sharp, constant, aching, or throbbing.

speculum An instrument for dilating a body orifice or cavity to allow visual inspection.

sporicidal An agent capable of killing spores.

statement A document generated by the vendor that details the quantity and pricing of all goods purchased (usually in 1 month) by the buyer. The total balance is generally expected to be paid in full within 30 days.

stem cell Cells found in embryonic tissue and the adult animal that have the ability for self-renewal, a lack of cellular specialization, and can give rise to other more specialized cells.

stock solution A concentrated solution that will be diluted to a weaker solution for use.

stroke volume The amount of blood ejected by the left ventricle with each beat.

surfactant A mixture of phospholipids secreted by type II alveolar cells that reduce surface tension in pulmonary fluids.

suspension A preparation of solid particles dispersed in a liquid but not dissolved in it.

symbiosis Two living organisms of different species living together.

sympathetic nervous system That portion of the autonomic nervous system that arises from the thoracolumbar spinal cord, is mediated by catecholamines, and is concerned with the fight-or-flight response.

sympathomimetic A drug that mimics the effects of stimulating the sympathetic nervous system.

tachyarrhythmia Tachycardia associated with an irregularity in normal heart rhythm.

tachycardia A faster-than-normal heart rate.

tachypnea Rapid breathing.

teratogenic An agent that causes harm to the developing fetus.

thrombocytopenia A decreased number of platelets.

thromboembolism The condition that occurs when thrombus material becomes dislodged and is transported by the bloodstream to another site.

thrombophlebitis Inflammation of a vein associated with a thrombus formation.

thrombus A clot in the circulatory system.

total nutrient admixture A solution used for parenteral administration that contains amino acids, lipids, dextrose, vitamins, and minerals.

totipotent (stem cell) A cell existing in the zygote and fertilized oocyte that is capable of creating an entire animal including extra-embryonic membranes.

transcellular fluid Cerebrospinal fluid, aqueous humor of the eye, synovial fluid, gastrointestinal fluid, lymph, bile, and glandular and respiratory secretions.

transdermal application The use of a patch applied to the skin to deliver a drug through an intact cutaneous surface to the systemic circulation.

transduction The process that involves translation of noxious stimuli into electric activity at sensory nerve endings.

transmission Conduction of pain impulses from peripheral pain receptors to the spinal cord.

trophic hormone A hormone that results in production of a second hormone in a target gland.

turgor Degree of fullness or congestion; describes the degree of elasticity of the skin.

turnover The number of times a product is sold or used up in a veterinary facility. The minimum turnover rate should be established at four times a year.

upper motor neurons Neurons in the cerebral cortex that conduct impulses from the motor cortex to the motor nuclei of the cerebral nerves or to the ventral gray columns of the spinal column. A sufficient number of lesions of upper motor neurons interrupt the inhibitory effect that upper motor neurons have on lower motor neurons, resulting in exaggerated or hyperactive reflexes.

upregulation An increase in the number of cellular receptors to a molecule resulting in an increased sensitivity to the molecule.

uremia Abnormally high concentrations of urea, creatinine, and other nitrogenous end products of protein and amino acid metabolism in the blood.

urinary incontinence Lack of voluntary control over the normal excretion of urine.

urinary tract infection Infection of the urinary tract. Infection may be localized or may affect the entire urinary tract.

uvea The vascular layer of the eye that comprises the iris, ciliary body, and choroid.

uveitis Inflammation of the uvea.

vesicant A substance that causes blister formation.

veterinarian–client–patient relationship The set of circumstances that must exist between the veterinarian, the client, and the patient before the dispensing of prescription drugs is appropriate.

veterinary supply distributor An intermediate company (i.e., not full service, not mail order) that generally stocks a large inventory and employs sales representatives who visit veterinary facilities.

virulence The ability of an infectious agent to produce pathologic effects.

visceral pain Pain arising from stretching, distension, or inflammation of viscera, described in humans as deep, cramping, or aching and difficult to localize.

viscid Sticky.

vomiting center An area in the medulla that may be stimulated by the chemoreceptor trigger zone, the cerebrum, or peripheral receptors to induce vomiting.

withdrawal time The length of time it takes for a drug to be eliminated from animal tissue or products after it is no longer used.

Index

Note: Pages number followed by "b" indicate boxes; "f" figures; "t" tables.

C

F

G

H

I

O

P

S

T